Handbook of Skull Base Surgery

T0260069

Antonio Di Ieva, MD, PhD
Neurosurgeon and Associate Professor
Macquarie University Hospital
Honorary Research Fellow
Garvan Institute of Medical Research
Sydney, Australia
Privatdozent of Neuroanatomy
Medical University of Vienna
Vienna, Austria
Alumnus of the University of Toronto
Toronto, Ontario, Canada

John M. Lee, MD, FRCSC, MSc
Assistant Professor
Department of Otolaryngology–Head & Neck Surgery
St. Michael's Hospital
University of Toronto
Toronto, Ontario, Canada

Michael D. Cusimano, MD, MHPE, FRCSC, PhD, FACS, FAANS
Professor of Neurosurgery, Education and Public Health
Division of Neurosurgery
St. Michael's Hospital
University of Toronto
Toronto, Ontario, Canada

174 illustrations

Thieme
New York • Suttgart • Delhi • Rio de Janeiro

Executive Editor: Timothy Hiscock
Managing Editor: Elizabeth Palumbo
Director, Editorial Services: Mary Jo Casey
Editorial Assistant: Haley Paskalides
Production Editor: Barbara A. Chernow
International Production Director: Andreas Schabert
Vice President, Editorial and E-Product Development:
    Vera Spillner
International Marketing Director: Fiona Henderson
International Sales Director: Louisa Turrell
Director of Sales, North America: Mike Roseman
Senior Vice President and Chief Operating Officer:
    Sarah Vanderbilt
President: Brian D. Scanlan
Typesetting by Carol Pierson, Chernow Editorial
    Services, Inc.

Cover image: Leonardo da Vinci, Milan, Italy, 1489. Royal Collection Trust/©Her Majesty Queen Elizabeth II, 2014

Library of Congress Cataloging-in-Publication Data

Di Ieva, Antonio, author.
    Handbook of skull base surgery / Antonio Di Ieva,
John M. Lee, Michael D. Cusimano.
    p. ; cm.
    Includes bibliographical references and index.
    ISBN 978-1-62623-025-5 (alk. paper) — ISBN
978-1-62623-026-2 (eISBN)
    I. Lee, John M., author. II. Cusimano, Michael D.,
author. III. Title. [DNLM: 1. Skull Base Neoplasms—
surgery—Handbooks. 2. Skull Base—surgery—
Handbooks. WE 39]
    RD529
    617.5'14—dc23   2015031249

Important note: Medicine is an ever-changing science undergoing continual development. Research and clinical experience are continually expanding our knowledge, in particular our knowledge of proper treatment and drug therapy. Insofar as this book mentions any dosage or application, readers may rest assured that the authors, editors, and publishers have made every effort to ensure that such references are in accordance with **the state of knowledge at the time of production of the book.**

Nevertheless, this does not involve, imply, or express any guarantee or responsibility on the part of the publishers in respect to any dosage instructions and forms of applications stated in the book. **Every user is requested to examine carefully** the manufacturers' leaflets accompanying each drug and to check, if necessary in consultation with a physician or specialist, whether the dosage schedules mentioned therein or the contraindications stated by the manufacturers differ from the statements made in the present book. Such examination is particularly important with drugs that are either rarely used or have been newly released on the market. Every dosage schedule or every form of application used is entirely at the user's own risk and responsibility. The authors and publishers request every user to report to the publishers any discrepancies or inaccuracies noticed. If errors in this work are found after publication, errata will be posted at www.thieme.com on the product description page.

Some of the product names, patents, and registered designs referred to in this book are in fact registered trademarks or proprietary names even though specific reference to this fact is not always made in the text. Therefore, the appearance of a name without designation as proprietary is not to be construed as a representation by the publisher that it is in the public domain.

©2016 Thieme Medical Publishers, Inc.
Thieme Publishers New York
333 Seventh Avenue, New York, NY 10001 USA
+1 800 782 3488, customerservice@thieme.com

Thieme Publishers Stuttgart
Rüdigerstrasse 14, 70469 Stuttgart, Germany
+49 [0]711 8931 421, customerservice@thieme.de

Thieme Publishers Delhi
A-12, Second Floor, Sector-2, Noida-201301
Uttar Pradesh, India
+91 120 45 566 00, customerservice@thieme.in

Thieme Publishers Rio de Janeiro Thieme
Publicações Ltda.
Edifício Rodolpho de Paoli, 25º andar
Av. Nilo Peçanha, 50 – Sala 2508
Rio de Janeiro 20020-906, Brasil
+55 21 3172 2297

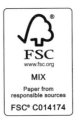

FSC
www.fsc.org
MIX
Paper from
responsible sources
FSC® C014174

Printed in the United States at Sheridan Books. 5 4 3 2 1

ISBN 978-1-62623-025-5

Also available as an e-book:
eISBN 978-1-62623-026-2

This book, including all parts thereof, is legally protected by copyright. Any use, exploitation, or commercialization outside the narrow limits set by copyright legislation without the publisher's consent is illegal and liable to prosecution. This applies in par- ticular to photostat reproduction, copying, mimeographing or duplication of any kind, translating, preparation of microfilms, and electronic data processing and storage.

The editors personally wish to acknowledge and dedicate the book:

To my beloved parents, Tina and Pino, my constant anchors in always supporting my peregrinations, forever, and to my sister Leonarda Vanessa. And to Jennilee, who has lovingly supported me and patiently attended to the entire gestation of this book. A special appreciation goes to Michael Cusimano, for having believed in me since the first moment and for all his teachings during my clinical fellowship in skull base surgery, and to all of the amazing people I've had the opportunity to know and to work with in Toronto . . . and around the world!

Antonio Di Ieva

To my wonderful wife Rania, who has truly taught me what is important in this world. Without your love, support, and sacrifice, I would not be where I am today. To my parents, King and Maggie, thank you for your unwavering dedication and guidance. To my teachers, mentors, residents, and students, thank you for always challenging and inspiring me to provide the best possible care to our patients. Last but not least, thank you to Antonio and Michael, for the opportunity and privilege to work with both of you as colleagues and friends in this most rewarding project.

John M. Lee

To my immediate and extended family for the endless hours they have put up with for the last 25 years of practicing this specialty. In the last year, they have put up with even more hours, as every available weekend, weeknight, and holiday went to making this book happen! To my formal teachers, colleagues, staff, and especially my patients for the lessons they give me every day. For my faith that provides inner strength. And finally, to my fellow editors, whom I have seen grow into wonderful and valued colleagues.

Michael D. Cusimano

Contents

Section III.   Postoperative and Surgery-Related Aspects

Preface

Skull base surgery is one of the most complex fields of medicine. The field spans several specialties and literally requires the mastery of the anatomy, pathology, and pathophysiology of at least four surgical specialties, to say nothing of the content knowledge of several others. Because of these facts, the education of the skull base surgeon can be long and arduous and one could argue that the learning is lifelong. While this is a challenge of the specialty, it is also one of its great gems. Successful application of the specialty also requires an open mind to bring together the efforts of multiple disciplines in a mutually collaborative way that enhances care of the patient. This ability to continually work with colleagues from different disciplines and be constantly learning is also a gem of the specialty. Few areas of medicine or of human endeavor provide the individual with such a unique blend of challenges, new learning, and continual stimulation. The intellectual and other challenges of the field are a constant source of motivation for those who are devoted to helping patients afflicted by lesions of the skull base.

Over the last century, skull base surgery has matured and had its advances and setbacks, but there is no doubt that patients have benefited most from the multidisciplinary collaboration of the field. Several radical changes have occurred over the last quarter century in parallel with improvements in technology. The developments of radiosurgery, advanced imaging, endoscopic techniques, and the multidisciplinary clinic have all enhanced the field. Most relevant to surgeons have been the renaissance of surgical anatomy and the development of new approaches to the skull base.

All this subspecialization has meant that skull base surgery has become increasingly concentrated in centers of excellence around the world. This has benefited the care of patients but also benefited the education of future generations. A holistic approach to the patient is time consuming and complicated but is also extremely rewarding. The future will expect more subspecialization and surgeons will increasingly become coordinators, conductors, and mentors.

We hope that this book will be a small contribution that helps to advance the field for years to come.

Antonio Di Ieva, MD, PhD
John M. Lee, MD, FRCSC, MSc
Michael D. Cusimano, MD, MHPE,
FRCSC, PhD, FACS, FAANS

Structure of the Handbook

This handbook focuses on the multidisciplinary management of the skull base, where neurosurgeons, otolaryngologists-head and neck surgeons, and craniomaxillofacial, plastic, and orbital surgeons, as well as neuroophthalmologists, interventional neuroradiologists, radiation oncologists, endocrinologists, and researchers bring together their respective expertise. Rather than creating a surgical atlas, the editors' goal was to present the sequence of steps needed to perform specific operations, while also describing variations that allow surgeons to perform procedures according to their interpretation.

The handbook is divided into three sections. Section I, "History, Principles, and Preoperative Assessment" (Chapters 1–13), deals with the "nuts and bolts" that form the foundation of the field. This includes anatomical, embryological, and radiological summaries relevant to the skull base. Principles of pathology, neurology, otorhinolaryngology, endocrinology, and neuroophthalmology are also summarized in the dedicated chapters. Chapter 1 introduces the historical background of several eponyms used in the daily practice of skull base surgery ("Who named what"), while Chapter 13 summarizes the high-tech instruments used in the field. Principles of anesthesia in skull base surgery (Chapter 11) and the endovascular interventions for skull base lesions (Chapter 12) are also treated in this first section.

Section II, "Skull Base Surgery" (Chapters 14 to 28), focuses on surgical approaches and specific pathologies affecting the skull base. Throughout the section, the symbol ◈ identifies the surgical step of an approach, while the ◈◈ indicates a possible variation. Chapters 14 to 17 summarize the surgical steps used in the approaches for skull base lesions. The transcranial approaches are covered in Chapter 14, while the transfacial approaches are reviewed in Chapter 15. Chapters 16 and 17 cover the endoscopic transsphenoidal approaches and endscopic transcranial keyhole approaches, respectively. Chapters 19 to 28 are oriented more toward a succinct but complete coverage of topics based on the skull base compartment affected by the most typical diseases. Each chapter contains sections relevant to the specific pathology. Specific chapters in this section are dedicated to the vascular neurosurgery in the skull base (25), management of the dural sinuses (26), skull base (27) and cranial nerve (28) reconstruction.

Section III, "Postoperative and Surgery-Related Aspects" (Chapters 29 to 41), deals with the postsurgical treatment of patients. Chapter 29 addresses postoperative care and complications management, while Chapters 30 and 31 cover the principles of radiation therapy and chemotherapy, respectively. Topics of specific relevance such as cerebrospinal fluid leakage, skull base infections, traumatology, and pediatrics are also covered in this section. Biology and genetics of skull base tumors are covered in Chapter 38, while quality of life issues, education, and skull base surgery nursing are covered in Chapters 39 to 41.

Antonio Di Ieva, MD, PhD

Acknowledgments

We would like to thank all of the contributors who have shared their expertise with us in writing this handbook, as well as the following persons for their help and careful proofreading of some chapters: Jennilee Davidson, Joseph Di Michele, Stefan St. George, Nadia Khan, Marzia Niamah, Shubham Sharma, Michael Solarski, and Adriana Workewych. Some junior residents in neurosurgery at the University of Toronto, including Ali Akbar, Kyle Juraschka, Farshad Nassiri, and Jetan Badhiwala, also gave useful feedback.

In addition, we would like to thank Professor Manfred Tschabitscher for his invaluable advice on the anatomy and history chapters; Professor Kalman Kovacs for his comments on the pathology chapter; Dr. Joseph Barfett for his contribution to the paragraph on nuclear medicine in the imaging chapter; Professor Marcus Stoodley for his suggestions on the Chiari malformation paragraph; and Drs. Angela Liching Ng, Stephen Santoreneos, and Amal Abou-Hamden for their contribution to the chapter on foramen magnum meningiomas.

We would also like to acknowledge the wonderful editorial staff at Thieme for their continuous support in this editorial project and Anthony Pazos for his superb illustrations and constant brainstorming by email. Angela Lee gave her time voluntarily to prepare many illustrations, as did Gian-Marco Busato, Madeline Di Michele, Angela Lee, Olivia So, and Adriana Workewych. A special acknowledgment goes to Stanley Zhang for his assistance in the coordination of several students who helped with the illustrations and reviews of chapters.

A special mention to the philanthropic support of many very grateful patients and their families, especially Mr. and Mrs. Dennis and Julia Bausch, Mrs. Wei Ren, Mr. and Mrs. Boesch, Mr. and Mrs. Sam and Sandra Sturino, and the Lucy Colavita Foundation.

Last but not least, we wish to thank our patients and the great secretary who superbly manages them, Cristina Lucarini.

Contributors

The following individuals contributed to the chapters listed below their names.

Alessandra Alfieri, MD
Neurosurgeon
Neurosurgery Department
S. Anna and S. Sebastiano Hospital
Caserta, Italy
Chapters 24 and 36

Jennifer Anderson, MD, MSc, FRCS(C)
Chief and Associate Professor
Department of Otolaryngology-Head & Neck Surgery
St. Michael's Hospital
University of Toronto
Toronto, Ontario, Canada
Chapter 8

Gian-Marco Busato, MD, MSc
Resident
Department of Otolaryngology-Head & Neck Surgery
University of Toronto
Toronto, Ontario, Canada
Chapters 2–4

Joseph M. Chen, MD, FRCSC
Professor and Chief
Department of Otolaryngology
Head & Neck Surgery
Sunnybrook Health Sciences Center
University of Toronto
Toronto, Ontario, Canada
Chapter 14.4

Michael D. Cusimano, MD, MHPE, FRCSC, PhD, FACS, FAANS
Professor
Professor of Neurosurgery, Education and Public Health
Departments of Neurosurgery, Education and Public Health
St. Michael's Hospital
University of Toronto
Toronto, Ontario, Canada
Chapters 14, 18, 19, 21, 22.1–22.5, 22.7, 22.8, 24, and 41

Iacopo Dallan, MD
First ENT Unit
Azienda Ospedaliero
Universitaria Pisana
Head and Neck Surgery and Forensic Dissection Research Center (HNS and FDRC)
DBSV, University of Insubria
Varese, Italy
Chapters 2.7 and 20

Roberto J. Diaz, BSc, MD, PhD, FRCSC
Surgical Neuro-Oncology Fellow
Department of Neurological Surgery
University of Miami School of Medicine
University of Miami Hospital & Jackson Memorial Hospital
Miami, Florida, USA
Chapters 31 and 38

Claudio De Tommasi, MD
Skull Base/Vascular Fellow
Walton Centre for Neurology and
    Neurosurgery
Liverpool, UK
Chapter 32

Antonio Di Ieva, MD, PhD
Neurosurgeon and Associate Professor
Macquarie University Hospital
Honorary Research Fellow
Garvan Institute of Medical Research
Sydney, Australia
Privatdozent of Neuroanatomy
Medical University of Vienna
Vienna, Austria
Alumnus of the University of Toronto
Toronto, Ontario, Canada
Chapters 1, 2, 3, 4, 6, 7, 9, 13, 14, 18,
    19, 21, 22.1–22.5, 22.7, 22.8, 23, 24,
    26, 28, 32, 34, 35, 40, and 41

Khaled Effendi, MD, FRCPC
Endovascular Neurosurgery Fellow
St. Michael's Hospital
Toronto, Ontario, Canada
Chapter 12

Hussein Fathalla, MD, PhD
Clinical and Research Fellow in Skull
    Base Surgery
St. Michael's Hospital
Toronto, Ontario, Canada
Chapter 33

Andrew Gao, MD
Neuropathology Resident
Department of Laboratory Medicine
    and Pathobiology
University of Toronto
Toronto, Ontario, Canada
Chapter 6

Marco Garavaglia, MD
Assistant Professor, Department of
    Anesthesia
St. Michael's Hospital
University of Toronto
Toronto, Ontario, Canada
Chapter 11

Menno Germans, MD
Neurosurgeon
Neurosurgical Center Nijmegen
Amsterdam, The Netherlands
Chapters 2.12 and 25

**Ralph W. Gilbert, MD, FRCSC, BSC
(HONS)**
Professor and Head
Division of Head and Neck
Department of Otolaryngoogy
University of Toronto
Toronto, Ontario, Canada
Chapter 27

Alberto Goffi, MD
Intensivist
Assistant Professor
Department of Medicine
    Interdepartmental
Division of Critical Care
Medicine University of Toronto
Toronto Western Hospital MSNICU
University Health Network
Toronto, Ontario, Canada
Chapter 29

**Jeannette Marie Goguen, MD, Med,
    FRCPC**
Associate Professor
Program Director, Endocrinology
University of Toronto
Toronto, Ontario, Canada
Chapter 9

Cristian Gragnaniello, MD, PhD, MSurg, MAdvSurg
Neurosurgery Fellow at the Royal Adelaide Hospital
Adelaide, Australia
Chapters 14.6 and 22.7

Edsel Ing, MD, FRCSC
Associate Professor, University of Toronto Ophthalmology and Vision Sciences
Toronto East General Hospital
Toronto, Ontario, Canada
Chapter 10

Fuminari Komatsu, MD, PhD
Neurosurgeon, Assistant Professor
Department of Neurosurgery
Tokai University Hachioji Hospital
Tokyo, Japan
Chapters 17 and 39

Mika Komatsu, MD
Ota Neurosurgical Clinic
Tokyo, Japan
Chapters 17 and 39

Jafri Kuthubutheen, MBBS (Hons), FRACS
Department of Otolaryngology Head and Neck Surgery
Fiona Stanley Hospital, Western Australia
University of Western Australia
Perth, Australia
Chapter 14.4

John M. Lee, MD, FRCSC, MSc
Assistant Professor
Department of Otolaryngology–Head & Neck Surgery
St. Michael's Hospital
University of Toronto
Toronto, Ontario, Canada
Chapters 6, 15, 16, 23, and 37

James K. Liu, MD, FAANS
Associate Professor of Neurological Surgery
Director, Center for Skull Base and Pituitary Surgery
Departments of Neurological Surgery and Otolaryngology-Head and Neck Surgery
Neurological Institute of New Jersey
Rutgers University-New Jersey Medical School
Newark, New Jersey, USA
Chapter 22.6

R. Loch Macdonald, MD, PhD, FRCS, FAANS, FACS
Chair, Division of Neurosurgery
St. Michael's Hospital
Professor of Surgery, University of Toronto
Toronto, Ontario, Canada
Chapter 25

Kimberly Mah-Poy, MD, FRCPC
Adjunct Lecturer, Department of Medicine, Division of Endocrinology University of Toronto
Staff Physician
St. Michael's Hospital
Toronto, Ontario, Canada
Chapter 9

Renuka K. Reddy, MD
Research Fellow
Department of Neurological Surgery
Rutgers University – New Jersey
    Medical School
Newark, New Jersey, USA
Chapter 22.6

Arjun Sahgal, MD
Associate Professor
Deputy Chief of Radiation Oncology
Sunnybrook Health Sciences Centre
University of Toronto
Toronto, Ontario, Canada
Chapter 30

Dipanka Sarma, MBBS, MD
Assistant Professor
Diagnostic and Therapeutic
    Neuroradiology
Medical Imaging
St. Michael's Hospital
University of Toronto
Toronto, Ontario, Canada
Chapter 5

Julian Spears, MD, SM, FRCS, FACS
Assistant Professor
Division of Neurosurgery &
    Department of Medical Imaging
St. Michael's Hospital
University of Toronto
Toronto, Ontario, Canada
Chapter 12

Irene Vanek, MD
Assistant Professor
Neuroophthalmologist Staff
St. Michael's Hospital
Toronto, Ontario, Canada
Chapter 10

Ian J. Witterick, MD, MSc, FRCSC
Professor and Chair
Department of Otolarngology – Head
    & Neck Surgery
Mount Sinai Hospital
University of Toronto
Toronto, Ontario, Canada
Chapter 15

Husein Zain, MD
Assistant Professor
Department of Therapeutic Radiology
Yale School of Medicine
New Haven, Connecticut, USA
Chapter 30

Figures

Illustrator: Anthony Pazos.

In additional, the editors thank the following persons for contributing the figures listed after their names.

Jennifer Anderson: Fig. 8.1

Gian-Marco Busato: Figs. 16.1B–16.8

Madeline Di Michele: Figs. 2.4, 14.14, 15.1, 20.1, 20.2

Angela Y. Lee: Figs. 2.4, 2.5, 2.17, 2.18, 14.2, 14.4, 14.5, 14.7, 14.9–14.14, 14.19, 14.22, 14.23, 14.25, 15.1, 17.2, 20.1, 20.2, 21.4, 21.5, 22.12, Table 34.1

Olivia So: Figs. 2.16, 14.24, 22.3, 22.4, 22.14, 26.2

Adriana Workewych: Figs. 2.8, 2.21, 3.3, 10.1, 10.2, 14.20, 22.1, 22.6, 22.17

Abbreviations

ABI	auditory brainstem implant	CRT	conformal radiation therapy
ABR	auditory brainstem-evoked response	CSB	central skull base
		CVR	cerebrovascular resistance
AC	anterior clinoidectomy	CS	cavernous sinus
ACA	anterior cerebral artery	CSF	cerebrospinal fluid
AcomA	anterior communicating artery	CT	computed tomography
		CTA	computer tomography angiography
ACP	anterior clinoid process		
ACTH	adenocorticotropic hormone	CTV	computed tomography venography
ADC	apparent diffusion coefficient	CVD	cortical venous drainage
		CVJ	craniovertebral junction
ADH	antidiuretic hormone	dAVF	dural arteriovenous fistula
AEA	anterior ethmoidal artery	DDAVP	Desmopressin
AFP	alpha-fetoprotein	DI	diabetes insipidus
AICA	anterior inferior cerebellar artery	DL	dentate ligament
		DSA	digital subtraction angiography
ALT	anterolateral thigh		
ASB	anterior skull base	DST	dexamethasone testing
AVM	arteriovenous malformation	DTI	diffusion tensor imaging
BA	basilar artery	DVT	deep venous thrombosis
BAEP	brainstem auditory evoked potential	DWI	diffusion weighted imaging
		EABR	evoked auditory brainstem responses
BCC	basal cell carcinoma		
BCM	brainstem cavernous malformation	EAC	external auditory canal
		ECA	external carotid artery
BPPV	benign paroxysmal positional vertigo	ECoG	electrocochleography
		EDNAC	extradural neural axis compartment
BSAER	brainstem auditory evoked responses	EEG	electroencephalography
		ELANA	excimer laser-assisted nonocclusive anastomosis
BTO	balloon test occlusion		
CBF	cerebral blood flow	EMA	epithelial membrane antigen
CBV	cerebral blood volume		
CCF	carotid-cavernous fistula	EMG	electromyography
CFR	craniofacial resection	ENB	esthesioneuroblastoma
CI	cochlear implant	ENG	electronystagmogram
CM	Chiari malformation	ENT	ears, nose, and throat (otorhinolaryngology)
CN	cranial nerve		
CNS	central nervous system	EVD	external ventricular drain
CPA	cerebellopontine angle	EWS	Ewing's sarcoma
CPP	cerebral perfusion pressure	FESS	functional endoscopic sinus surgery
CRH	corticotropin releasing hormone		

FLAIR	fluid attenuation inversion recovery	IMAX	internal maxillary artery
FM	foramen magnum	IMRT	intensity modulated radiation therapy
FMM	foramen magnum meningioma	INR	interventional neuroradiology
FO	foramen ovale	IOF	inferior orbital fissure
FR	foramen rotundum	IPSS	inferior petrosal sinus sampling
FS	foramen spinosum	ITF	infratemporal fossa
FSH	follicle-stimulating hormone	ITT	insulin tolerance test
FTOZ	frontotemporal-orbitozygomatic	JB	jugular bulb
		JNA	juvenile nasopharyngeal angiofibroma
GCS	Glasgow Coma Scale/Score	KPS	Karnofsky performance status
GFAP	glial fibrillary acidic protein		
GG	Gasser ganglion	LAE	long-acting release
Gg	geniculate ganglion	LD	lumbar drain
GH	growth hormone	LH	luteinizing hormone
GHRH	growth-hormone-releasing-hormone	LINAC	linear accelerator
		LMWH	low molecular weight heparin
GK	Gamma Knife	LSPN	lesser superficial petrosal nerve
GSPN	greater superficial petrosal nerve		
GSW	guns shot wound	LTBR	lateral temporal bone resection
GTR	gross total resection		
Gy	gray	MAP	mean arterial pressure
H–B	House-Brackmann	MCA	middle cerebral artery
Hb	haemoglobin	MCF	middle cranial fossa
HCG	human chorionic gonadotropin	MEN	multiple endocrine neoplasia
HFS	hemifacial spasm	MEP	motor evoked potentials
HPA	hypothalamic-pituitary-adrenal	MF	middle fossa
		MHT	meningohypophyseal trunk
HPC	hemangiopericytoma	MMA	middle meningeal artery
HPL	human placental lactogen	MMSE	mini-mental state examination
IAC	internal auditory canal		
ICA	internal carotid artery	MOCA	Montreal cognitive assessment
ICG	indocyanine green		
ICH	intracerebral hemorrhage	MRA	magnetic resonance angiography
ICP	intracranial pressure		
ICU	intensive care unit	MRI	magnetic resonance imaging
IGF	insulin-like growth factor		
IGRT	image guided radiation therapy		

MRV	magnetic resonance venography	RAPD	relative afferent pupillary defect
MSB	middle skull base	RBC	red blood cell
MVD	microvascular decompression	RFFF	radial forearm free flap
NAP	nerve direct potentials	RION	radiation-induced optic neuropathy
NF	neurofibromatosis	RMS	rhabdomyosarcoma
NPS	nasopharyngeal carcinoma	ROI	region of interest
OA	occipital artery	RS	radiosurgery
OAE	otoacoustic emissions	RSPC	retrosigmoid paracerebellar
OC	orbitocranial	RT	radiotherapy
OCT	optical coherence tomography	SAH	subarachnoid hemorrhage
		SBF	skull base fracture
OGF	insulin growth factor	SBM	skull base meningioma
OGTT	oral glucose tolerance test	sc	subcutaneous
OMC	ostiomeatal complex	SCA	superior cerebellar artery
OND	optic nerve decompression	SCC	semicircular canal / squamous cell carcinoma
OPG	optic pathway glioma		
OZ	orbitozygomatic	SDH	subdural hemorrhage
PA	pituitary adenoma	SDS	speech discrimination score
PCA	posterior cerebral artery	SFT	solitary fibrous tumor
PcomA	posterior communicating artery	SHa	superior hypophyseal artery
		SNL	superior nuchal line
PCP	posterior clinoid process	SNUC	sinonasal undifferentiated carcinoma
PET	positron emission tomography		
		SO	suboccipital
PICA	posteroinferior cerebellar artery	SOF	superior orbital fissure
		SPECT	single photon emission computed tomography
PLAP	placental alkaline phosphatase		
		SPV	superior petrosal vein
PO	per os	SRS	stereotactic radiosurgery
PONV	post-operative nausea and vomiting	SRT	stereotactic radiotherapy / speech reception threshold
PPF	pterygopalatine fossa	SSA	somatostatin analog
PPG	pterygopalatine ganglion	SSC	superior semicircular canal
PRL	prolactin	SSEP	somatosensory evoked potentials
PSR	primary spontaneous rhinorrhea		
		SSS	superior sagittal sinus
PTA	pure tone audiometry	STA	superior temporal artery
PTTG	pituitary tumor transforming gene	STIR	short tau inversion recovery
		STL	superior temporal line
PVA	polyvinyl alcohol	STR	subtotal resection
QOL	quality of life	TCR	trigeminocardiac reflex

TDAST	thoracodorsal artery scapular tip	UFH	unfractioned heparin
		VA	vertebral artery
TL	translabyrinthine	VACS	vacuum-assisted closure systems
TM	tympanic membrane		
TMJ	temporomandibular joint	VEGF	vascular endothelial growth factor
TN	trigeminal neuralgia		
TOF	time of flight	VEP	visual evoked potentials
TPFF	temporoparietal fascia flap	VHL	von Hippel-Lindau
		VOR	vestibular ocular reflex
TS	tuberculum sellae	VS	vestibular schwannoma
TSH	thyroid-stimulating hormone	VTE	venous thromboembolism
		VTO	venous test occlusion
TSS	transsphenoidal surgery	WHO	World Health Organization

History, Principles, and Preoperative Assessment

1 History of Skull Base Anatomy and Its Eponyms

The earliest records of anatomic dissections on human beings date to the third century BC and are from Alexandria, Egypt. The eponyms and descriptions of several anatomic structures are still associated with these early anatomists, who probably also performed vivisections. Despite their observations, Galenic theories, based on observations in animals, dominated the study of human anatomy for more than 1,500 years. It is known that Galen performed dissections on animals only, and the arbitrary application of his observations to humans led to erroneous descriptions of human anatomy.

In the Western world, the origin of modern human anatomy can be traced back to the University of Bologna, Italy, during the Middle Ages when Mondino de' Luzzi (1270–1326) and his pupil Guido da Vigevano (1280–1349) "restored" anatomy from Galen's dogmas.[1] Guido introduced the use of anatomic illustrations, creating a milestone in the development of anatomy as a scientific and artistic field. Cadaver dissections, as a scientific method for the description and understanding of the human body, gave rise to the recognition of anatomy as a specific field of medical science.

The development of modern anatomy occurred during the Renaissance, with the establishment of many anatomy theaters, such as the one in Padua, Italy.[2] During the Italian Renaissance, many multitalented men of genius contributed to the artistic and scientific advancement of anatomy, such as Donatello (1386–1466), who is considered the first artist who dissected human bodies, Michelangelo (1475–1564), Eustachius (1500–1574), Vesalius (1514–1564), and Leonardo da Vinci (1452–1519). Leonardo is considered the founder of physiological anatomy.[3,4] The exponential development of medicine following the 18th century entailed the development of descriptive and functional anatomy, particularly in the study of the brain, including the most recent and amazing neuroscientific discoveries.

Here is a selective list of anatomists whose names are still associated with discoveries and theories in skull base anatomy and its related neurovascular structures:

- **Erasistratus** (304–250 BC): Egyptian physician who coined the word *meninges*.
- **Herophilus of Chalcedon** (ca. 335–280 BC): Greek physician considered to be the father of anatomy for his advocacy of animal and human dissections.[5,6] Founder, together with Erasistratus, of the medical school of Alexandria. His name is associated with the *torcular herophili* (torcular in Latin means "winepress"). The *torcular herophili* is the point at which the superior sagittal sinus, straight sinus, and occipital sinus meet at the inner side of the occipital protuberance[7,8] (although the precise definition of the torcular is not the convergence of the sinuses itself but the bony concavity where the dural convergence is located).
- **Galen of Pergamon** (129–200/216): Greek physician and philosopher, who served as the physician and surgeon to the gladiators of the Roman Empire. Among other descriptions, Galen identified seven pairs of cranial nerves, assigning each pair terminations and functions, but no names. According to Galen, the optic nerve was the first pair, and the facial and vestibulocochlear nerves were grouped together into the same pair. He failed to identify the glossopharyngeal, vagus, and accessory nerves as separate cranial nerves, instead grouping them together as well.[9] Among other identified structures that are credited to him is the *vein of Galen.*
- **Leonardo da Vinci** (1452–1519): Italian genius and polymath. In the field of skull base anatomy, Leonardo holds the distinction of being the first anatomist to produce anatomic diagrams showing the cranial nerves and optic chiasm.[4]
- **Berengario da Carpi** (ca. 1460–1530): Italian physician and author of the first modern textbook of neurotraumatology, *The Treatise on Fractures of the Calvaria or Cranium*, published in 1518. In his book, Berengario not only described an entire set of surgical instruments to be used for cranial operations to treat head traumas, but also systematically reviewed the existing literature and added many personal cases to explain the mechanisms, classification, and medical and surgical treatments.[10]
- **Bartolomeus Eustachius** (ca. 1500–1574): Italian anatomist who described several structures of the internal ear. The auditory or pharyngotympanic tube, the eustachian tube, is named for him.[11]
- **Andreas Vesalius** (1514–1564): Belgian anatomist and physician and professor of anatomy in Padua, Italy. He is very well known in the history of medicine as the author of *De Humani Corporis Fabrica* ("On the Fabric of the Human Body"), one of the most influential modern textbooks of human anatomy, published in 1543. In skull base anatomy, the *foramen of Vesalius*, that is, the sphenoidal emissary foramen, is named for him. This foramen is an anatomic variant (not always present, but consistently symmetrical when present) of an aperture of the great wing of the sphenoid bone, medial to the foramen ovale, crossed by a small vein (vein of Vesalius) that enables communication between the cavernous sinus and the pterygoid plexus.[12]

- **Gabriele Falloppio (Fallopius)** (1523–1562): Italian physician and anatomist who described the canal through which the facial nerve traverses the petrous part of the temporal bone, from the internal acoustic meatus to the stylomastoid foramen (facial canal, or *fallopian canal*).
- **Arcangelo Piccolomini** (1525–1586): Italian anatomist known for being the first to differentiate between the white and gray matter of the brain (in 1586) and for his description of the origins and terminations of some intracranial nerves, especially of the acoustic nerve.
- **Costanzo Varolio** (1543–1575): Italian anatomist and papal physician considered to be one of the first physicians to examine the base of the brain and the cranial nerves. The description of the formation of the pons (then defined as *pons Varolii*) is named for Varolio.[13]
- **Thomas Willis** (1621–1675): English anatomist and physician who described the physiological function of the arteries at the base of the brain and its anatomic connections. Also introduced the word *neurology*. His name is linked to one of the best known structures in anatomy, the *circle (or polygon) of Willis*, historically considered to be the first depiction of the brain arteries (published in 1664),[14] although several anatomists described the basal circle before Willis.[15] The first portrayal was provided more than 50 years earlier by Julius Casserius (1552–1616),[16] an Italian anatomist and one of the six great Vesalian anatomists. Casserius' engravings showing the first detailed circle of arteries at the base of the brain were published posthumously in 1627.
- **Johann Friedrich Meckel, the Elder** (1724–1774): German anatomist, physician, and botanist. *Meckel's cave* is named for him, as he wrote his undergraduate dissertation on the trigeminal nerve and the meningeal space containing the trigeminal ganglion over the petrous bone.[17]
- **Jacques-René Tenon** (1724–1816): French surgeon who provided the first description of the membrane enveloping the eyeball, the so-called *capsule of Tenon*.
- **Johann Gottfried Zinn** (1727–1759): German anatomist and botanist who provided detailed descriptions of the anatomy of the human eye. The *annulus of Zinn* (the annular tendon, called also the common tendinous ring, located at the apex of the orbit, surrounding the optic nerve and giving origin to the rectus inferior, superior, lateralis, and medialis extraocular muscles) bears his name, although this structure was described some decades before by Antonio Maria Valsalva (1666–1723),[18] the developer of the Valsalva maneuver and the first to use the term *eustachian tube*.
- **Domenico Cotugno** (1736–1822): Italian physician who provided the first systematic description of cerebrospinal fluid.[19] At the age of 25, he published a book on the anatomy of the inner ear (with the first descriptions of the acoustic and vestibular nerves, semicircular canals, scalae tympani and vestibuli, the oval and round windows, the vestibular aqueduct, and the helicotrema), and showed that the semicircular canals are filled with fluid. His

book also proposed theories concerning the physiology of hearing (later developed further and associated with Hermann von Helmholtz).

- **Henrich August Wrisberg** (1739–1808): German anatomist who described the sympathetic nervous system. His name is associated with the nervus intermedius.
- **Johann Friedrich Blumenbach** (1752–1840): German physician and naturalist, famous for his study of comparative anatomy and craniometry. The eponymous *clivus blumenbachii* is named for him.
- **Samuel Thomas von Sömmering** (1755–1830): German anatomist, physician, anthropologist, paleontologist, and inventor who studied the cranial nerves, publishing his findings in his doctoral work at age 23. Before him, Herophilus, Galen, Avicenna, Mondino de' Luzzi, Piccolomini, Willis, and others had published their own descriptions and classification systems of the cranial nerves. Von Sömmering enumerated the cranial nerves and created the numeration system, which is still in use today.[9]
- **Charles Bell** (1774–1842): Scottish anatomist and surgeon who described the facial nerve palsy bearing his name.
- **Friedrich Gustav Jacob Henle** (1809–1885): German physician and anatomist. In the field of skull anatomy, the eponymous *Henle's spine* is the suprameatal spine in the mastoid region.
- **Wenzel Leopold Gruber** (1814–1890): Bohemian anatomist who extensively studied the anatomy of the skull base. The eponymous *Gruber's ligament* is the petrosphenoidal ligament, which is continuous with the petrolingual ligament, running from the petrous apex to the lingual process of the sphenoid bone and covering the lacerum segment of the internal carotid artery (ICA).[20-22]
- **Moritz F. Trautmann** (1832–1902): German otologist who described the triangular area of the temporal bone delimited by the posterior semicircular canal, the superior petrosal sinus, and the sigmoid sinus (*triangle of Trautmann*).
- **Francesco Durante** (1844–1934): Considered to be the first surgeon to successfully remove a skull base meningioma (in 1884); it was in the region of the olfactory groove.[23]
- **Charles Labbé** (1851–1889): French physician and anatomist. In 1883, he published an article on the venous circulation of the brain and the development of Pacchioni's granulations, adding to the already known Trolard's vein the *greater anastomotic posterior cerebral vein,* later named the *vein of Labbé.*[24]
- **Charles Ballance** (1856–1936): English surgeon considered to be the first to perform a radical mastoidectomy (also performing a ligation of the jugular vein), one of the earliest facial nerve grafts, and one of the first acoustic neuroma resections.[4]

- **Giuseppe Gradenigo** (1859–1926): Italian otolaryngologist who described the inflammation of the petrous apex in relation to ear suppuration,[25] known as *Gradenigo syndrome.*
- **Hermann Schloffer** (1868–1937): Austrian surgeon considered to be the first to have successfully resected a pituitary adenoma by means of a nasal-transsphenoidal approach (in 1907).[26] His approach was based on previous anatomic experiences with a transglabellar-nasal approach suggested by the Italian physician Davide Giordano in 1897.[27]
- **Harvey William Cushing** (1869–1939): American neurosurgeon, pioneer of modern neurosurgery and of the studies and operations on the pituitary gland. He was professor of surgery at the Johns Hopkins Hospital (Baltimore, Maryland) and developed several surgical instruments and techniques that are still in use in brain and skull base surgery. In 1938, together with Eisenhardt, he published the most significant contribution to meningioma surgery: *Meningiomas: Their Classification, Regional Behavior, Life History, and Surgical End Results.* The eponymous *Cushing's syndrome, Cushing's disease,* and the *Cushing reflex* are named for him.[28]
- **Primo Dorello** (1872–1963): Italian anatomist who described the anatomy of the petroclival region and formulated some hypotheses relating to abducens paralysis. His name is attached to the *Dorello canal,* although some descriptions of this structure were already given by Gruber 50 years before.[21]
- **Thierry de Martel** (1875–1940): French surgeon who introduced surgical innovations in the treatment of trigeminal neuralgia, as well as the sitting position in posterior fossa surgery. He is also the designer of one of the first electric automatic trephines.[4]
- **Walter Edward Dandy** (1886–1946): American neurosurgeon, pioneer of several discoveries and innovations in neurosurgery. In the field of skull base anatomy, his name is associated with the lateral superior cerebellar veins, draining into the superior petrosal vein (*Dandy's vein*).
- **Lars Leksell** (1907–1986): Swedish neurosurgeon and professor at the Karolinska Institute (Stockholm, Sweden). He is considered the father of stereotaxis and radiosurgery, as well as a pioneer of functional neurosurgery.
- **Dwight Parkinson** (1916–2005): Canadian neurosurgeon and pioneer of cavernous sinus surgery, whose name is associated with the triangular space between cranial nerves IV and V_1 (*Parkinson's triangle*). He also described the meningohypophyseal trunk and introduced the concept of the extradural neuraxial compartment (EDNAC).
- **William Fouts House** (1923–2012): American otolaryngologist, pioneer of temporal bone surgery, and inventor of the cochlear implant. His name is related to *Bill's bar,* the bony component separating the two superior quadrants in the internal acoustic canal (see **Fig. 2.8** on page 24).

- **Vittorio L. Bernasconi** (1921–) and **Valentino Cassinari** (1926–2014): these two Italian physicians (radiologist and neurosurgeon, respectively) described a tentorial artery on angiographic imaging of tentorial meningiomas.[29] The medial tentorial artery, now called the *artery of Bernasconi-Cassinari*, usually arises from the meningohypophyseal trunk of the intracavernous segment of the ICA and mainly supplies the tentorium.[30]

■ References

Boldfaced references are of particular importance.

1. **Di Ieva A, Tschabitscher M, Prada F, et al. The neuroanatomical plates of Guido da Vigevano. Neurosurg Focus 2007;23:E15**
2. **Andrioli G, Trincia G. Padua: the renaissance of human anatomy and medicine. Neurosurgery 2004;55:746–754, discussion 755**
3. Hopstock H. Leonardo as an anatomist. In: Singer C, ed. Studies in the History of Medicine. Oxford: Clarendon Press; 1921:153–191
4. **Goodrich JT. A millennium review of skull base surgery. Childs Nerv Syst 2000; 16:669–685**
5. Bay NS, Bay BH. Greek anatomist Herophilus: the father of anatomy. Anat Cell Biol 2010;43:280–283
6. Moon K, Filis AK, Cohen AR. The birth and evolution of neuroscience through cadaveric dissection. Neurosurgery 2010;67:799–809, discussion 809–810
7. Pearce JM. The neuroanatomy of Herophilus. Eur Neurol 2013;69:292–295
8. **Acar F, Naderi S, Guvencer M, Türe U, Arda MN. Herophilus of Chalcedon: a pioneer in neuroscience. Neurosurgery 2005;56:861–867, discussion 861–867**
9. **Davis MC, Griessenauer CJ, Bosmia AN, Tubbs RS, Shoja MM. The naming of the cranial nerves: a historical review. Clin Anat 2014;27:14–19**
10. **Di Ieva A, Gaetani P, Matula C, Sherif C, Skopec M, Tschabitscher M. Berengario da Carpi: a pioneer in neurotraumatology. J Neurosurg 2011;114:1461–1470**
11. Simpson D. The papal anatomist: Eustachius in renaissance Rome. ANZ J Surg 2011; 81:905–910
12. Lanzieri CF, Duchesneau PM, Rosenbloom SA, Smith AS, Rosenbaum AE. The significance of asymmetry of the foramen of Vesalius. AJNR Am J Neuroradiol 1988;9:1201–1204
13. **Tubbs RS, Loukas M, Shoja MM, et al. Costanzo Varolio (Constantius Varolius 1543–1575) and the Pons Varolli. Neurosurgery 2008;62:734–737, discussion 734–737**
14. **Choudhari KA, Sharma D, Leyon JJ. Thomas Willis of the "circle of Willis". Neurosurgery 2008;63:1185–1190, discussion 1190–1191**
15. **Lo WB, Ellis H. The circle before Willis: a historical account of the intracranial anastomosis. Neurosurgery 2010;66:7–18, discussion 17–18**
16. **Bender M, Olivi A, Tamargo RJ. Iulius Casserius and the first anatomically correct depiction of the circulus arteriosus cerebri (of Willis). World Neurosurg 2013; 79:791–797**

17. Janjua RM, Schultka R, Goebbel L, Pait TG, Shields CB. The legacy of Johann Friedrich Meckel the Elder (1724–1774): a 4-generation dynasty of anatomists. Neurosurgery 2010;66:758–770, discussion 770–771
18. Zampieri F, Marrone D, Zanatta A. Should the annular tendon of the eye be named "annulus of Zinn" or "of Valsalva"? Acta Ophthalmol (Copenh) 2015;93:97–99
19. Di Ieva A, Yaşargil MG. Liquor cotunnii: the history of cerebrospinal fluid in Domenico Cotugno's work. Neurosurgery 2008;63:352–358, discussion 358
20. Ambekar S, Sonig A, Nanda A. Dorello's canal and Gruber's ligament: historical perspective. J Neurol Surg B Skull Base 2012;73:430–433
21. Kshettry VR, Lee JH, Ammirati M. The Dorello canal: historical development, controversies in microsurgical anatomy, and clinical implications. Neurosurg Focus 2013;34:E4
22. Iaconetta G, Fusco M, Cavallo LM, Cappabianca P, Samii M, Tschabitscher M. The abducens nerve: microanatomic and endoscopic study. Neurosurgery 2007; 61(3, Suppl):7–14, discussion 14
23. Tomasello F, Germanò A. Francesco Durante: the history of intracranial meningiomas and beyond. Neurosurgery 2006;59:389–396, discussion 389–396
24. Bartels RH, van Overbeeke JJ. Charles Labbé (1851–1889). J Neurosurg 1997;87:477–480
25. Felisati D, Sperati G. Gradenigo's syndrome and Dorello's canal. Acta Otorhinolaryngol Ital 2009;29:169–172
26. Liu JK, Das K, Weiss MH, Laws ER Jr, Couldwell WT. The history and evolution of transsphenoidal surgery. J Neurosurg 2001;95:1083–1096
27. Artico M, Pastore FS, Fraioli B, Giuffrè R. The contribution of Davide Giordano (1864–1954) to pituitary surgery: the transglabellar-nasal approach. Neurosurgery 1998;42:909–911, discussion 911–912
28. Bliss M. Harvey Cushing: A Life in Surgery. Oxford University Press; 2005.
29. Bernasconi V, Cassinari V. Un segno carotidografico tipico di meningioma del tentorio. Chirurgia (Milan) 1956;11:586–588
30. Tubbs RS, Nguyen HS, Shoja MM, Benninger B, Loukas M, Cohen-Gadol AA. The medial tentorial artery of Bernasconi-Cassinari: a comprehensive review of its anatomy and neurosurgical importance. Acta Neurochir (Wien) 2011;153:2485–2490

2 Anatomy of the Skull Base and Related Structures: Elements of Surgical Anatomy

■ Skull Definitions

The skull has two components:

Neurocranium ("braincase"): houses the brain.
Splanchnocranium (or *viscerocranium*): formed by the bones of the face.

The neurocranium has two components:

Calvaria ("skull cap")
Skull base (*basicranium*): the floor of the cranial cavity, on which the brain rests.

■ 2.1 Skull Base Anatomy—Anterior and Middle Skull Base

The skull base has two surfaces:

Endocranial (inner): the floor of the cranial cavity, on which the brain rests **(Fig. 2.1)**.
Exocranial (external) surface **(Fig. 2.2)**.

- The bones, which form the skull base, are the frontal, sphenoid, ethmoid, temporal, and occipital bones (the anterior part of the exocranial surface is also formed by the zygomatic, maxillary, and palatine bones).
- The inner surface of the skull base can be divided into three transverse parts (anterior, middle, and posterior fossae) **(Fig. 2.3a)** and in three sagittal parts (central and lateral parts) **(Fig. 2.3b)**.
- The median part of the anterior skull base covers the upper nasal cavity and the sphenoid sinus; the middle part contains the cavernous sinuses laterally, which house the carotid arteries (parasellar compartments); the posterior part includes the clivus, which reaches the anterior margin of the great occipital foramen.

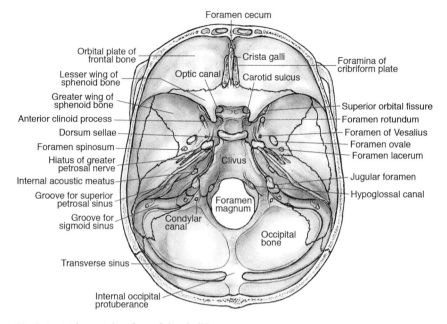

Fig. 2.1 Endocranial surface of the skull base.

Foramen cecum

Orbital plate of frontal bone
Lesser wing of sphenoid bone
Greater wing of sphenoid bone
Anterior clinoid process
Dorsum sellae
Foramen spinosum
Hiatus of greater petrosal nerve
Internal acoustic meatus
Groove for superior petrosal sinus
Groove for sigmoid sinus
Transverse sinus
Internal occipital protuberance

Crista galli
Optic canal
Carotid sulcus

Foramina of cribriform plate
Superior orbital fissure
Foramen rotundum
Foramen of Vesalius
Foramen ovale
Foramen lacerum
Jugular foramen
Hypoglossal canal

Clivus
Condylar canal
Foramen magnum
Occipital bone

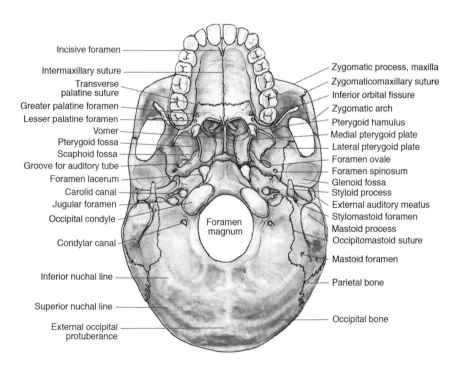

Fig. 2.2 Exocranial surface of the skull base.

Incisive foramen
Intermaxillary suture
Transverse palatine suture
Greater palatine foramen
Lesser palatine foramen
Vomer
Pterygoid fossa
Scaphoid fossa
Groove for auditory tube
Foramen lacerum
Carotid canal
Jugular foramen
Occipital condyle
Condylar canal
Inferior nuchal line
Superior nuchal line
External occipital protuberance

Zygomatic process, maxilla
Zygomaticomaxillary suture
Inferior orbital fissure
Zygomatic arch
Pterygoid hamulus
Medial pterygoid plate
Lateral pterygoid plate
Foramen ovale
Foramen spinosum
Glenoid fossa
Styloid process
External auditory meatus
Stylomastoid foramen
Mastoid process
Occipitomastoid suture
Mastoid foramen
Parietal bone
Occipital bone

Foramen magnum

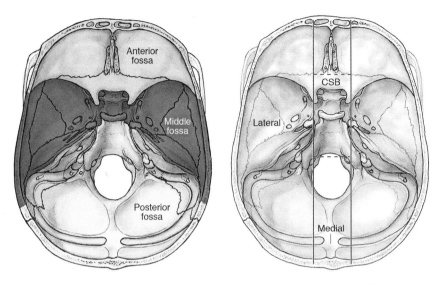

Fig. 2.3a,b **(a)** Skull base: anterior, middle, and posterior cranial fossae. **(b)** Lateral and median regions. CSB, central skull base (see also **Fig. 5.7** on page 114).

Osteology of the Cranial Fossae

- **Anterior skull base**: formed by one ethmoidal, two frontal, and one sphenoid bones. The anterior skull base (ASB) is delimited anteriorly by the frontal bone and the posterior wall of the frontal sinus, and posteriorly by the lesser wings of the sphenoid bone. The lateral parts of the anterior skull base form the roof of the orbits, on which the frontal lobes of the brain lie. The median (central) part is formed by the crista galli, the cribriform plate of the ethmoid bone, and the planum of the sphenoid bone.
- **Middle skull base:** formed by one sphenoid and two temporal bones. The middle skull base (MSB) is delimited anteriorly by the lesser wings of the sphenoid bones, and posteriorly by the surface of the petrous part of the temporal bone. The temporal lobe lies in the middle cranial fossa. The central part of the middle cranial fossa is defined as the sella turcica (part of the sphenoid bone).

The **sellar compartment** contains the hypophysis. It is separated from the suprasellar compartment (brain) by a meningeal sheet, the diaphragma sellae, which has an opening at the center called the ostium of the diaphragma sellae. The pituitary stalk crosses through this opening. The lateral parts of the sellar compartments are defined as "parasellar compartments." This is the location of the cavernous sinus, which is crossed by the cranial nerve (CN) VI and the inter-

---

Surgical Anatomy Pearl

For each skull base foramen, it is very important to remember its neurovascular relationships. **Tables 2.1** and **2.2** summarize the foramina of the endocranial surface and the exocranial surface of the skull base with its contents, respectively. **Table 2.3** summarizes the foramina and other structures visible on the splanchnocranium **(Fig. 2.4)**.

---

nal carotid artery (ICA). The lateral wall of the cavernous sinus is also lined by CN III, IV, V_1, and V_2.

- **Posterior skull base:** formed by the occipital and temporal bones. This fossa is delimited anteriorly by the posterior walls of the petrous bone and posteriorly by the grooves for the transverse sinuses. It contains the foramen magnum, in which the medulla oblongata continues downward into the spinal cord.

Sellar and Parasellar Compartments

- The pituitary fossa is in the central part of the sphenoid bone, at the center of the skull. The sellar region is delimitated anteriorly by the jugum sphenoidale, which is the most posterior border of the planum sphenoidale, anterolaterally by the extension of the lesser sphenoid wings (anterior clinoid processes, ACPs), laterally by the greater sphenoid wings, posterolaterally by the posterior clinoid processes (PCPs) and petrous apex, and posteriorly by the clivus.
- The ACP forms the anterolateral bony protuberance; the optic canal runs medial to it. The optic strut is the medial attachment of the ACP, forming part of the optic canal and separating the carotid sulcus from the optic canal.
- The portion of the ICA passing between the optic strut and the superior surface of the ACP is the clinoidal segment of the ICA.[1]
- Chiasmatic groove (sulcus): a depression between the tuberculum sellae, the planum sphenoidale, and the optic foramina.
- Anterolaterally to the sella and ACP lie the superior orbital fissures on each side. The cavernous sinus extends from the petrous apex to the superior orbital fissure (SOF).[2]
- The normal average size of the pituitary fossa is 13 × 17 × 15 mm, with an average volume of 1,100 mm^3.

Surgical Anatomy Pearl

An anatomic variant is the presence of the middle clinoid process, which can bridge the ACP. In such a situation, the carotid artery would run through a caroticoclinoid foramen.

Table 2.1   Foramina of the Skull Base: Endocranial Surface and Its Contents

Foramen cecum	Emissary vein from the superior sagittal sinus to frontal sinus and nose; eventually anterior falcine artery
Foramina of the cribriform plate	Olfactory nerve bundles from the nasal mucosa to the olfactory bulb
Anterior, middle (variable), and posterior ethmoidal foramina	Anterior, middle (whenever present the middle foramina) and posterior ethmoid arteries and veins
Optic canal	CN II and ophthalmic artery
Superior orbital fissure	CNs III, IV, VI, V_1, superior and inferior ophthalmic veins, orbital branches of the MMA, sympathetic fibers (that enter mainly with nasociliary nerve), parasymphathetic fibers (entering with CN III)
Inferior orbital fissure	Venous channels connecting orbital venous system with pterygoid plexus, small nameless arterial branches, branches from pterygopalatine ganglion and zygomatic nerve from infraorbital nerve
Foramen rotundum	CN V_2, accompanied by some emissary veins and an arterious branch from the internal maxillary artery
Foramen ovale	CN V_3, lesser superficial petrosal nerve, accessory meningeal artery branch from the maxillary artery
Foramen spinosum	Middle meningeal artery and vein, meningeal recurrent branch of V_3
Foramen lacerum	Meningeal branches from the ascending pharyngeal artery, as well as the nerve of pterygoid canal, cartilage
Vidian canal	Vidian nerve (formed by the GSPN and the deep petrosal nerve), veins, and two arteries
Hiatus for greater petrosal foramen	Greater superior petrosal nerve
Hiatus for lesser petrosal nerve	Lesser superior petrosal nerve
Internal acoustic canal	CNs VII–VIII, labyrinthine artery
Jugular foramen	CNs IX, X, XI, convergence of inferior petrosal sinus and sigmoid sinus into the internal jugular vein, Jacobson's nerve (tympanic branch of CN IX), Arnold's nerve (auricular branch of CN X), posterior meningeal artery (from the VA)
Hypoglossal canal	CN XII with meningeal artery
Foramen magnum	Medulla oblongata, vertebral arteries, spinal roots of CN XI, anterior spinal artery, posterior spinal arteries, and posterior meningeal arteries

Abbreviations: CN, cranial nerve; GSPN, greater superficial petrosal nerve; MMA, middle meningeal artery; VA, vertebral artery.

Table 2.2 Foramina of the Exocranial Surface of the Skull Base

Carotid canal	ICA surrounded by the sympathetic plexus
Greater palatine foramen	Greater palatine nerve (from V_2) and vessels
Lesser palatine foramen	Lesser palatine nerve (from V_2) and vessels
Sphenopalatine foramen	Nasopalatine nerve (from V_2), nasal nerve (from V_2), sphenopalatine artery
Stylomastoid foramen	CN VII
Foramen magnum	See Table 2.1
Petrotympanic fissure	Anterior tympanic branch of the internal maxillary artery

Abbreviation: ICA, internal carotid artery.

Table 2.3 Foramina of the Splanchnocranium

Supraorbital foramen/incisura	Supraorbital nerve (from V_1), supraorbital vein and artery
Infraorbital canal and foramen	Infraorbital nerve (from V_2), infraorbital vein and artery
Zygomaticotemporal foramen	Zygomaticotemporal nerve and vessels
Zygomaticofacial foramen	Zygomaticofacial nerve and vessels
Incisive foramen	Nasopalatine nerve (from V_2) and vessels
Mandibular foramen	Inferior alveolar nerve (from V_3)
Mental foramen	Mental nerve (from V_3)

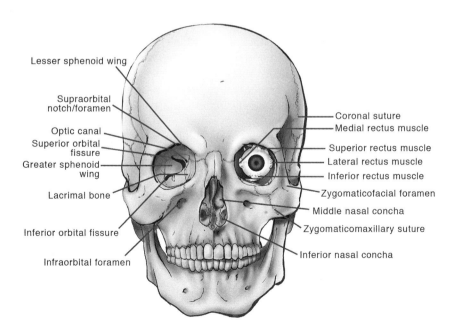

Fig. 2.4 Anatomic structures of the splanchnocranium and orbits.

> **Parasellar Region**
>
> The parasellar region encompasses the anatomic compartments around the sella:
>
> **Parasellar compartments**: cavernous sinuses
> **Suprasellar compartment**: region above the diaphragma sella, with the suprasellar cistern and its contents
> **Retrosellar compartment**: clivus

- The pituitary fossa contains the pituitary gland. The pituitary gland is formed by an anterior part (adenohypophysis), a more orange-colored posterior lobe (neurohypophysis), and an often cystic intermediate lobe.
  - The anterior lobe forms the pars tuberalis at the lower part of the pituitary stalk.
  - The inferior surface of the gland conforms to the shape of the sellar floor.
  - The superior part can be more flat or concave around the stalk. The stalk crosses the diaphragma into the ostium of the diaphragma sellae.

Cavernous Sinuses

The cavernous sinuses are lateral to the sphenoid sinus, sella turcica, and pituitary gland **(Fig. 2.5)**. Each cavernous sinus sits in the central aspect of the middle fossa and is lateral to the sella.

- Cavernous sinus (CS) is the historical definition of the lateral sellar compartment; it is part of the extradural neural axis compartment (EDNAC), which extends from the coccyx to the orbit.[2] The name incorrectly suggests that the CS is a "sinus," but it is not a sinus like the superior sagittal sinus; rather, it is a multiloculated network of lacunae on the lateral compartment of the sellar region.
- The CS is one component of the basal venous system, which consists of a valveless network of interconnected venous channels. Should an obstruction

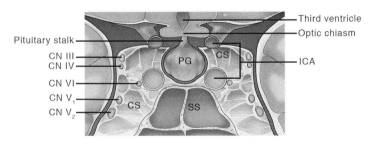

Fig. 2.5 Cavernous sinus (CS), coronal section. ICA, internal carotid artery; SS, sphenoidal sinus.

occur in one region, venous flow can decant into a collateral system and so allow venous drainage. These veins include anterior and posterior intercavernous sinuses, the petroclival plexus, the superior and inferior ophthalmic veins, the sphenoparietal sinus, the superior and inferior petrosal sinuses, a variety of emissary veins that can enlarge in the event of occlusion, and some variable veins from the brain (e.g., *vena Vasaliana*).

Anatomic Boundaries: Dural Layers of the Cavernous Sinus

- **Lateral wall:** A double layer of dural mater, the outer layer is continuous with the internal layer of the dura of the middle cranial fossa and tentorium, whereas the inner layer of the lateral wall is formed by the epineurium of CNs III, IV, and V. The outer layer of the middle fossa dura separates at the lateral margin of the cavernous sinus to continue as the periosteum and to form the floor and medial wall of the cavernous sinus. There is a cleavage plane between the medial and lateral layers, which may be dissected without entering the venous compartment of the CS[3] (see Chapter 21).
- **Medial wall:** layer of dura/periosteum.
- **Roof:** The third or distal ring of dura around the ICA forms the carotico-oculomotor membrane.[4,5] The clinoid and carotid triangles are part of the roof as well. The roof of the CS has the shape of a trapezium, extending from the diaphragma sellae medially, to the anterior petroclinoid ligament laterally, from the base of the anterior clinoid process anteriorly, and to the posterior petroclinoid ligament posteriorly.[3] It provides a base for the cistern of the CN III.
- **Posterior wall:** dura of the clivus.
- **Contents of the double layer of the lateral wall:** CNs III and IV and the branches of the trigeminal nerve run within the double layer.
- **Contents of the cavernous sinus:** venous lacunae, CN VI, fat, cavernous ICA surrounded by sympathetic plexus, with its branches:
  - **Meningohypophyseal trunk:** Branches of this trunk are variable, but in pure form consist of the tentorial artery (also known as the artery of Bernasconi-Cassinari), dorsal meningeal artery (also known as the clival artery), and the inferior hypophyseal artery.
  - **Inferolateral trunk:** branches supplying the intracavernous nerves.
  - **Capsular artery:** McConnel's artery, present in 30% of cases.[6,7]
  - **Ophthalmic artery:** generally extracavernous, but in 3 to 8% it originates from the infraclinoidal segment of the ICA.[8]

Cranial nerve VI runs from the posterior part of the CS, passing through the Dorello canal, medially to the Meckel's cave and medial to the trigeminal root,[9] to the SOF, medial and superior to V_1.

Triangles of the Skull Base

Specific anatomic landmarks create triangular-shaped corridors, which are useful in understanding the anatomy of the region and in planning/performing surgical approaches. Quantitative studies have shown size and shape variants of the triangles, but it should be emphasized that the normal geometry and shape of these spaces may be distorted by pathology or during surgery.[10,11] Different authors describe different triangles, so a lack of uniform nomenclature often impairs communication and limits the usefulness of these triangle terms in the anatomy of this region. Anatomic landmarks of such triangles are described in **Table 2.4**[10-21] and demonstrated in **Fig. 2.6**. According to Dolenc,[18,20] there are 10 triangles in three subregions of the skull base:

- **Parasellar subregion:** anteromedial triangle, paramedial triangle, oculomotor trigone, Parkinson's triangle
- **Middle cranial fossa subregion:** anterolateral triangle, lateral triangle, posterolateral (also called Glasscock's triangle), posteromedial (also called Kawase's triangle)
- **Paraclival subregion:** inferomedial triangle, inferolateral (trigeminal triangle)

■ 2.2 Temporal Bone Anatomy

The temporal bone is a complex structure that contributes to the cranial cavity, the sensory organs of hearing and vestibular balance, the temporomandibular joint (TMJ), and provides an intraosseous pathway for CNs VII and VIII. It connects with the parietal, occipital, sphenoid, and zygomatic bones.

Osteology

There are four distinct bony components based on the embryological development of the temporal bone:

- **Squamous:** contributes to the lateral wall of the middle fossa and has an anterior projection of bone called the zygomatic process that articulates with the zygomatic bone.
  - Inferior surface of the zygomatic root forms an articulating surface of the TMJ called the glenoid fossa.
  - Surgical landmark: temporal line or crest, a horizontal ridge of bone along the inferior-most aspect of the origin of the temporalis muscle, which signifies the level of the floor of the middle cranial fossa (approximately 5 mm). The spine of Henle is the suprameatal bony prominence located at the posterosuperior margin of the external acoustic meatus.

Table 2.4 Triangles of the Skull Base[10–21]

Definition/Position*	Borders	Contents
Parasellar Triangles		
Clinoidal (anteromedial)	1. Lateral border of the extradural CN II 2. Medial border of the CN III 3. Tentorial edge, with the posterior border on the dural ring	1. Clinoidal ICA (identifiable after ACP removal) 2. Venous channels of the anteromedial CS 3. Proximal dural ring Note: Exposure of this triangle requires extradural ACP removal
Supratrochlear (or paramedial, or superior)	1. CN III 2. CN IV 3. Tentorial edge (dura between the entry point of the CNs III and IV)	1. Horizontal segment of the intracavernous ICA 2. MHT 3. Inferolateral trunk branches 4. CN VI (proximal segment)
Oculomotor (or medial)	1. Anterior petroclinoid dural fold 2. Posterior petroclinoid dural fold 3. Interclinoid dural fold	1. CN III (from the porus oculomotorius) 2. Proximal siphon, horizontal segment of ICA
Infratrochlear Parkinson's triangle	1. CN IV 2. CN V$_1$ 3. Tentorial edge and anterior clival dura	1. Horizontal segment of the cavernous ICA 2. MHT 3. CN VI 4. Sympathetic fibers Note: Originally described as the main entry access to the CS
Middle Fossa Triangles		
Anteromedial[14] Anterolateral[18]	1. CN V$_1$ 2. CN V$_2$ (the apex of these two sides is on the GG) 3. A line connecting the SOF and the FR	1. Dura and floor of the MSB 2. Venous trabecular channels of the inferolateral CS 3. Superior ophthalmic vein 4. CN VI Note: Opening the floor of the triangle may lead into the sphenoid sinus

(continued)

Table 2.4 (*continued*)

Definition/Position*	Borders	Contents
Anterolateral[14] Lateral loop[18] Far lateral[17]	1. CN V_2 (anteromedial border) 2. CN V_3 (posterior side) 3. A line connecting the FR with the FO	1. Lateral sphenoid wing 2. Sphenoid emissary vein 3. Cavernous-pterygoid venous anastomosis
Posterolateral Glasscock's triangle	1. CN V_3 2. GSPN 3. A line between the FS and the arcuate eminence	1. FS 2. Posterior loop and horizontal petrous segment of the ICA 3. Labyrinthine branch of the MMA 4. GSPN and LSPN ✖ The opening of this triangular space, by drilling from the FS and medially along the posterior margin of CN V_3, exposes the horizontal intrapetrous ICA
Posteromedial Kawase's triangle Rhomboid area	1. Posterior border of the GG, CN V_3 2. GSPN 3. A line connecting the hiatus of the GSPN and the posterior aspect of the CN V, approximately at the arcuate eminence Note: The most posterior aspect of this triangle is the superior petrosal sinus	1. Petrous Apex 2. Posterior edge of the petrous ICA 3. Cochlea (laterally) Note: Bone removal from this area leads to anterior petrosectomy (Kawase approach); it connects the middle and posterior cranial fossae

Posterior Fossa Triangles

Inferomedial paraclival (or posteroinferior)[17,18,21]	1. Posterior dural fold of the dural entry of CN IV under the tentorium 2. A line from the dural entries of the CN VI and PCP 3. Petrous apex	1. Porous abducens (dural opening into Dorello's canal, where the CN VI enters the CS) 2. Gruber's ligament (posterior petroclinoid fold) 3. Basilar venous plexus
Trigeminal (inferolateral paraclival)[18]	1. Line between the entry point of the CN IV and VI 2. Line between the entry point of the CN VI and the superior petrosal vein, below the trigeminal nerve 3. Line between the entry point of the CN IV and the entry point of the petrosal vein into the SPV	The superior part of the trigeminal triangle is the tentorial part, where the petrous vein enters the superior petrosal vein, while the inferior part (osseous triangle) represents the posterior extension of Kawase's triangle in the MSB
Premeatal[21]	1. Medial lip of the IAC 2. Carotid genu 3. Geniculate ganglion	1. Cochlea
Postmeatal[21]	1. Geniculate ganglion 2. Lateral lip of the IAC 3. Intersection of the arcuate eminence with the petrous ridge	1. IAC Note: It defines the bone between the SSC and the IAC

Abbreviations: CS, cavernous sinus; FO, foramen ovale; FR, foramen rotundum; FS, foramen spinosum; GG, Gasser ganglion; GSPN, greater superficial petrosal nerve; IAC, internal auditory canal; ICA, internal carotid artery; LSPN, lesser superficial petrosal nerve; MHT, meningohypophyseal trunk; MMA, middle meningeal artery; MSB, middle skull base; PCP, posterior clinoid process; SOF, superior orbital fissure; SPV, superior petrosal vein; SSC, superior semicircular canal.

*Some definitions vary, according to different authors

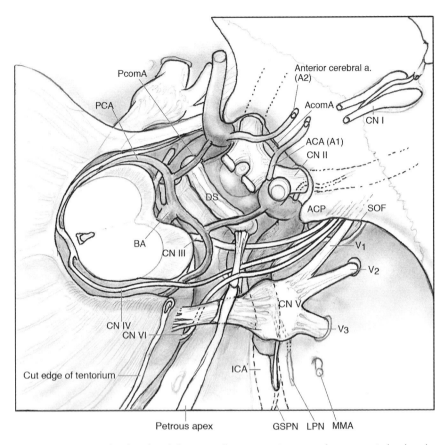

Fig. 2.6 Anatomic landmarks of the parasellar region. Compare the anatomic landmarks with the description of the skull base triangles in Table 2.4. ACA, anterior cerebral artery; AcomA, anterior communicating artery; ACP, anterior clinoid process; BA, basilar artery; CN, cranial nerve; DS, dorsum sellae; GSPN, greater superficial petrosal nerve; ICA, internal carotid artery; LPN, lesser petrosal nerve; MMA, middle meningeal artery; PcomA, posterior communicating artery; PCA, posterior cerebral artery; SOF, superior orbital fissure.

- **Mastoid:** a variably pneumatized bulbous bone (in the adult), the pneumatized cells of which are in direct communication with the middle ear via the aditus ad antrum (orifice of the mastoid antrum into the epitympanic recess).
  - Koerner septum: Formed by the petrosquamous lamina, it is a thin bony septum that travels posteriorly from the epitympanum, separating the mastoid cavity into medial and lateral compartments.
  - Muscular attachments:
    - Sternocleidomastoid at the mastoid tip.

- ▪ Posterior belly of the digastric muscle at a sulcus just posterior to the stylomastoid foramen, often called the "digastric groove."
- **Tympanic:** forms approximately three quarters of the bony external auditory canal in the adult (anterior wall, floor, and part of the posterior wall and roof).
  - ○ Surgical landmark: tympanomastoid suture line—the landmark for the exocranial facial nerve as the line curves inferiorly from the external auditory canal (EAC) in close proximity with the stylomastoid foramen.
  - ○ Anatomic landmark: petrotympanic suture—the chorda tympani exits from its intraosseous course through the suture/fissure.
- **Petrous:** forms the substrate of the middle and inner ear **(Fig. 2.7)** and has numerous surface landmarks as follows:
  - ○ Styloid process: a long bony process, 18 to 51 mm in length, that serves as an attachment point for muscles (stylohyoid, styloglossus, stylopharyngeus) and ligaments (stylohyoid, stylomandibular).[22]

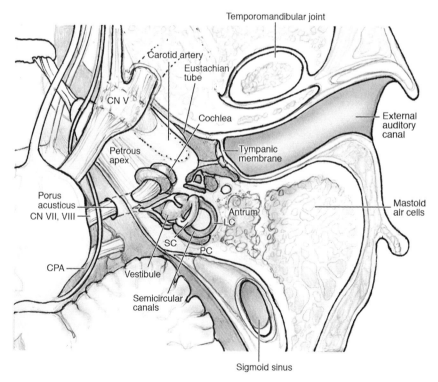

Fig. 2.7 Representation of the axial section of the petrous bone, showing the anatomic relationships with the middle fossa and cerebellopontine angle (CPA). Semicircular canals: SC, superior canal; PC, posterior canal; LC, lateral canal.

- ▪ Located anterior to the stylomastoid foramen (exit point of the facial nerve).
- ○ Jugular fossa: Located medial to the styloid process and inferior to the middle ear cavity, the fossa is occupied by the internal jugular vein and nerves.
- ○ Carotid canal: located directly anterior to the jugular fossa but is separated by a small wedge of bone. In the horizontal segment, the bone can be nonexistent on the superior surface.
- ○ Sigmoid sulcus: The sulcus of the sigmoid sinus lies on the posterior intracranial surface and along the anterior limit of the posterior fossa.
- ○ Arcuate eminence: Located superomedially on the intracranial surface, it signifies the superior semicircular canal, lateral to which is the roof of the middle ear and mastoid.
- ○ Subarcuate fossa: situated superiorly and just posterior to the IAC and sometimes transmits the subarcuate artery.
- ○ Depression of the trigeminal nerve (pars compacta): located on the superior surface of the petrous apex.
- ○ Internal auditory canal (IAC): located on the medial aspect of the petrous portion. The medial opening is termed the *porus acusticus internus*, whereas the lateral end is termed the *fundus*.
  - ▪ The fundus is divided into an upper and lower part by the horizontal crest **(Fig. 2.8)**. The upper part is divided in two quadrants by a vertical bar ("Bill's bar"). Considering four quadrants of the fundus (but anatomically the two lower ones are not separated by any bony structures), their contents are:
    - ▫ Anterosuperior: facial and intermedius nerves
    - ▫ Anteroinferior: cochlear division of CN VIII

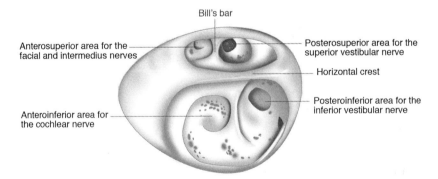

Bill's bar

Anterosuperior area for the facial and intermedius nerves

Posterosuperior area for the superior vestibular nerve

Horizontal crest

Anteroinferior area for the cochlear nerve

Posteroinferior area for the inferior vestibular nerve

Fig. 2.8 Fundus of the internal auditory canal (IAC), right side. (Adapted from Koos WT, Matula C, Lang J. Color Atlas of Microneurosurgery of Acoustic Neurinomas. New York: Thieme; 2002.)

- □ Posterosuperior: superior vestibular division of CN VIII
- □ Posteroinferior: inferior vestibular division of CN VIII
  - ○ Groove of the endolymphatic duct: located posterolateral to the IAC within the posterior fossa and houses the endolymphatic duct and sac.

The Ear

- **External ear:** includes the auricle, the EAC, and the tympanic membrane.
  - ○ EAC: in adults, lateral one third is fibrocartilage; medial two thirds are bony, composed of the tympanic portion (anterior wall, floor, and part of the posterior wall and roof) and the mastoid portion of the temporal bone (remainder of the posterior wall and roof).
  - ○ Tympanic membrane (TM): typically measures 10 mm in size and is anchored to the EAC via the tympanic sulcus.
- **Middle ear:** an air-filled, mucous membrane–lined cavity containing the ossicles. The middle ear directly communicates with the mastoid cavity via the aditus ad antrum posteriorly, and the nasopharynx via the pharyngotympanic tube anteriorly.
  - ○ Boundaries:
    - ▪ Anterior: pharyngotympanic tube (eustachian tube)
    - ▪ Posterior: mastoid cavity
    - ▪ Medial: otic capsule and promontory
    - ▪ Lateral: tympanic membrane
    - ▪ Superior: tegmen tympani (thin layer of bone separating the contents of the middle cranial fossa from the middle ear)
    - ▪ Inferior: jugular wall (floor)
  - ○ Divisions of the middle ear[23,24]
    - ▪ Epitympanum: also referred to as the attic and is the area superior to the level of the TM. The epitympanum communicates with the mastoid cavity via the aditus ad antrum
      - □ Prussak's space (superior recess): important region in acquired cholesteatoma.
        - ♦ Subtended by the *scutum* and *pars flaccida* laterally, the neck of the malleus medially, and the lateral malleolar ligament superiorly.
    - ▪ Mesotympanum: The area at the level of the TM and houses the majority of the ossicular chain.
      - □ Ossicles: responsible for conductive hearing within the middle ear and amplify oscillations between the TM and the oval window.
        - ♦ Malleus: composed of a head (articulates with incus), neck, anterior process, lateral process, and manubrium (attached to the TM).
        - ♦ Incus: composed of a body (articulates with malleus), short process, long process, and lenticular process (articulates with stapes).

- ▫ Stapes: composed of head/capitellum (articulates with incus), an anterior and posterior crus, and a footplate (attached to the oval window).
  - ▫ Suspensory ossicular ligaments: superior, lateral, and posterior malleal, and posterior incudal.
- ▪ Hypotympanum: area inferior to the level of the TM and contains the orifice of the pharyngotympanic tube (eustachian tube).
- **Inner ear:** consists of the bony labyrinth (otic capsule) and the membranous labyrinth that contains endolymph and is surrounded by perilymph. The bony labyrinth is very dense and represents the hardest bone in the body. The labyrinth consists of continuous subunits including the vestibule and three semicircular canals.
  - ○ Cochlea: Snail-shaped structure that tapers in width from base to apex during its 2½ to 2¾ turns; the basal, middle, and apical turns are separated by interscalar septa.
    - ▪ Communicates with the middle ear at the oval window, which is abutted by the stapes footplate, and the round window membrane at the basal end of the cochlea
    - ▪ Promontory: bulge of the basal turn of the cochlea that protrudes into the middle ear cavity that is visible on standard otoscopy through the TM.
      - ▫ Jacobson's nerve (branch of CN IX) runs over the middle ear surface of the promontory.
    - ▪ *Modiolus*: highly porous crown-shaped bone at the core of the cochlea that enables passage of the auditory nerve fibers from the cochlear nerve to the organ of Corti.
    - ▪ Cochlear aqueduct: a narrow bony passage that extends from the basal turn of the cochlea to the subarachnoid space in the posterior fossa that enables communication of perilymph and cerebrospinal fluid (CSF).
  - ○ Vestibule: ovoid-shaped structure that is situated posterior to the cochlea but is connected via the *ductus reuniens.*
    - ▪ Within the vestibule are two end organs termed maculae, one oriented in the horizontal plane (utricle) and the other in the vertical plane (saccule).
    - ▪ Relationships
      - ▫ Anterior: cochlea
      - ▫ Posterior: mastoid air cells
      - ▫ Medial: posterior cranial fossa, into which the endolymphatic duct and sac extend
      - ▫ Lateral: middle ear cavity (anterior) and mastoid air cells (posterior)
  - ○ Semicircular canals: three orthogonally oriented semicircular canals that project from the vestibule in a posterosuperior direction. Each semicircu-

lar canal has a dilated end, termed the ampulla, containing the receptors. The semicircular canals are the anterior (superior), posterior (dorsal), and horizontal (lateral).

- ○ The anterior and posterior semicircular canals are vertically oriented and share a common *crus*, which opens into the superomedial part of the vestibule. The horizontal semicircular canal, however, has two separate openings into the vestibule.

Contents

- **Musculature:** Both the tensor tympani and stapedius muscles contract reflexively in response to loud noises to reduce excessive oscillation at the tympanic membrane and oval window, respectively.
  - ○ Stapedius
    - ▪ Origin: within the pyramidal eminence (bony structure situated on posterior wall of middle ear)
    - ▪ Insertion: head of the stapes
    - ▪ Innervation: CN VII
  - ○ Tensor tympani
    - ▪ Origin: within the superior aspect of the cartilaginous part of the eustachian tube
    - ▪ Insertion: following a sharp turn at the terminus of the cochleariform process, inserts on the neck of the malleus
    - ▪ Innervation: CN V_3
- Neural Structures
  - ○ Sensory organs: anatomy described (see Inner Ear).
    - ▪ Cochlea: anatomic structure responsible for the sensation of hearing via the organ of Corti, the primary sensory structure containing both inner and outer hair cells.
    - ▪ Utricle and saccule: otolith organs within the vestibule responsible for the sensation of linear acceleration of the head in space.
    - ▪ Semicircular canals: three orthogonally oriented structures responsible for vestibular function, specifically for the sense of angular acceleration/velocity (head rotation).
  - ○ Auditory and vestibular nerves (CN VIII): course through the IAC from the *porus acusticus* to the *fundus* and abuts the labyrinth.
    - ▪ Cochlear nerve: traverses the modiolus to the cochlear end organ, the organ of Corti
    - ▪ Superior vestibular nerve: supplies the anterior and horizontal semicircular canals and the utricle
    - ▪ Inferior vestibular nerve: supplies the posterior semicircular canal and saccule
  - ○ Facial nerve (CN VII) (see Chapter 3, page 83).

- Greater superficial petrosal nerve: originates as the first branch of the facial nerve from the geniculate ganglion and carries presynaptic parasympathetic nerve fibers to the pterygopalatine fossa ganglion.
  - Travels anteriorly and medially within the petrous portion of the temporal bone and emerges on its anterior surface via the hiatus for the greater petrosal nerve.
- *Chorda tympani*: conveys special sensory innervation to the anterior two thirds of the tongue and to the soft palate along with parasympathetic innervation to all salivary glands below the level of the oral fissure.
  - Typically branches from the mastoid segment of the facial nerve just prior to its exit from the skull at the stylomastoid foramen.
  - Ascends through the posterior canaliculus (*canaliculus chordae tympani*), which opens into the middle ear, and then arcs upward to cross the pars flaccida of the TM and passes between the neck of the malleus and the long process of the incus to reach the entrance of the anterior canaliculus (canal of Huguier or Civinini) above the insertion of the *tensor tympani.*
  - The anterior canaliculus runs within the medial part of the petrotympanic fissure and exits into the infratemporal fossa.
- Nerve to stapedius: Innervates the stapedius muscle, as its name implies.
  - Branches early from the mastoid segment of the facial nerve.
- Vascular
  - External ear: arterial supply from the following branches of the ECA and venous drainage follows the arteries:
    - Anterior auricular branches of the superficial temporal artery
    - Posterior auricular artery
    - Occipital artery
  - Middle ear: primary arterial blood supply from the tympanic branch of the maxillary artery and the mastoid branch of either the posterior auricular or occipital arteries.
    - Other arterial contributions from smaller branches of the following:
      - Artery of the pterygoid canal
      - Ascending pharyngeal artery
      - Middle meningeal artery
      - Tympanic branch of the ICA and rami caroticotympanici, whenever present
    - Venous drainage into the pterygoid plexus and the superior and inferior petrosal sinuses.
  - Inner ear: arterial supply is divided into vessels providing blood to the bony labyrinth and the membranous labyrinth, and venous drainage follows the arteries primarily into the inferior petrosal or sigmoid sinuses.
    - Bony
      - Anterior tympanic branch of the maxillary artery

- Stylomastoid branch of the posterior auricular artery
- Petrosal branch of the middle meningeal artery
  - Membranous: Supplied by the labyrinthine artery which divides into:
    - Cochlear branch
    - Vestibular branch

■ 2.3 Topographic Anatomy of the Posterior Skull Base

Cerebellopontine Angle

The cerebellopontine angle (CPA) is the anatomic space between the petrous bone and the petrosal cerebellar surface folding around the pons and middle cerebellar peduncle, containing the posterior cranial fossa nerves (**Figs. 2.7** and **2.9**).[25] The structures in the CPA can be summarized as follows:

- **Upper neurovascular complex:** formed by the trochlear and trigeminal nerves, superior cerebellar artery (SCA) and its branches, and the petrosal veins complex.
  - The motor root of the trigeminal nerve arises rostral to the sensory root. There are diffuse anastomoses between the sensory and motor component of the nerve, posteriorly to the ganglion of Gasser.
  - The veins of the cerebellopontine fissure draining into the superior petrosal sinus are generally lateral to the trigeminal nerve.
  - The superior petrosal veins drain into the superior petrosal sinus[26,27]: above and lateral to the IAC (type I), between the lateral limit of the trigeminal nerve and the medial limit of the facial nerve at the IAC (type II), and above and medial to Meckel's cave (type III). Type II is the commonest arrangement, and type III is related to the best outcome in most retrosigmoid approaches that do not need to access regions medial to the entrance to Meckel's cave.[27]
- **Middle neurovascular complex:** It includes the pons, middle cerebellar peduncle, cerebellopontine fissure, cerebellar petrosal surface, anterior inferior cerebellar artery (AICA), and CNs VI to VIII.
- **Lower neurovascular complex:** It includes the medulla, inferior cerebellar peduncle, cerebellomedullary fissure, vertebral artery and posterior inferior cerebellar artery (PICA), and glossopharyngeal, vagus, and spinal accessory nerves converging into the jugular foramen. The hypoglossal nerve is more medial and reaches the hypoglossal canal posteriorly to the vertebral artery.

> **Surgical Anatomy Pearl**
>
> All the inferior cranial nerves arise from rootlets exiting the brainstem in the post-olivary sulcus.

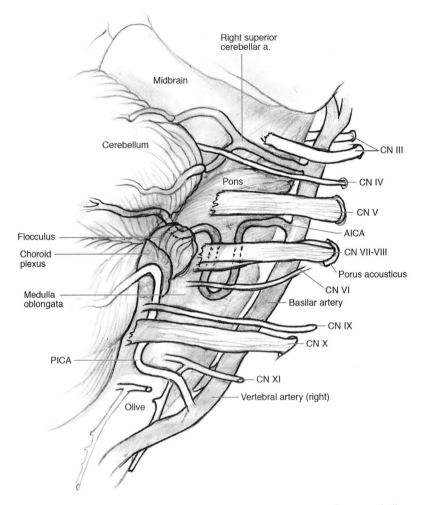

Fig. 2.9 Cerebellopontine angle anatomy (right side). AICA, anterior inferior cerebellar artery; CN, cranial nerve; PICA, posterior inferior cerebellar artery.

Foramen Magnum

The foramen magnum (FM) is oval-shaped and is delimited anteriorly by the clivus, laterally by the occipital condyles, and posteriorly by the anterior border of the occipital bone. The region of the FM includes the following:

- Cerebellar tonsils and inferior vermis
- Brainstem and rostral aspect of spinal cord
- CNs IX to XII

- Upper cervical nerves (C1 and C2)
- C1-C2 complex
- Vertebral arteries
- Posterior inferior cerebellar arteries
- Anterior and posterior spinal arteries
- Meningeal branches of the vertebral, external and internal carotid arteries
- Veins and dural sinuses of the craniovertebral junction
- Dentate ligaments

The hypoglossal canal is located above the occipital condyle.

Jugular Foramen

The jugular foramen is located on the floor of the posterior fossa, bordered anterolaterally and posteromedially, by the petrous bone and occipital bone, respectively. It is often morphometrically described as a triangular canal with exo- and endocranial openings that are located medial to the mastoid tip and tympanomastoid suture. The jugular spine or process splits the jugular foramen into the following two parts:

- **Pars nervosa:** smaller, anteromedial part that contains the CN IX and the inferior petrosal sinus.
- **Pars venosa (pars vascularis):** larger, posterolateral part that contains the internal jugular vein, jugular bulb, CNs X and XI, and the posterior meningeal branch of the ascending pharyngeal artery.

■ 2.4 Meningeal Folds

Anatomy of the Tentorium Cerebelli

The tentorium is a fold of dura mater forming the roof of the posterior fossa that separates the cerebellum from the cerebrum. Its free margin is the incisura, which is crossed by the brainstem and the cerebral peduncles. It slopes downward, like a tent, from its apex at the level of the posterior side of the incisura, to its attachment to the bones.

- **Anterior borders:** at the level of the petrous ridge on the posterior aspects of the petrous bone, where a tentorial division encloses the superior petrosal sinus.

The attachments of the tentorium on the petrous bone and clinoid processes form the anterior and posterior petroclinoid and interclinoid folds, resulting in the oculomotor triangle.[28]

- **Lateral and posterior borders:** the tentorium attaches to the internal occipital protuberance and laterally to the temporal bone, to the edges of the osseous groove crossed by the transverse sinus.
  - The falx cerebri fuses perpendicularly to the tentorium over its midline. The falcotentorial junction encloses the straight sinus, which receives venous blood from the vein of Galen and the inferior sagittal sinus. The straight sinus terminates posteriorly into the convergence of the sinuses at the level of the torcular herophili.
  - The tentorial incisura has (a) anterior space, which is anterior to the brainstem, extending around the optic chiasm; (b) middle space, which is lateral to the brainstem, related to the hippocampal formation laterally; and (c) posterior space, which is posterior to the midbrain, in the region of the pineal gland and vein of Galen.[28]
  - The average width of the incisura is about 30 mm, and the anteroposterior diameter is an average of 52 mm.
  - The topographic neurovascular relationships of the tentorium and the tentorial incisura are with CNs III and IV, ICA, posterior cerebral artery (PCA), SCA, anterior choroidal artery, basal vein of Rosenthal, internal cerebral veins, vein of Galen, and straight sinus with the lateral and sagittal sinuses in the posterior part, at the level of the torcular.

Falx Cerebri (Cerebral Falx)

The falx cerebri is a thick fold of dura mater, attached anteriorly to the crista galli and posteriorly to the tentorium. Its superior margin is attached to the inner surface of the calvaria, and forms the superior sagittal sinus, whereas its inferior margin is free, containing the inferior sagittal sinus. The falx divides the two cerebral hemispheres.

Falx Cerebelli

The falx cerebelli is a dural fold below the tentorium cerebelli, projecting into the posterior cerebellar notch and into the vallecula of the cerebellum between the two cerebellar hemispheres.

Diaphragma Sellae

The diaphragma sellae is a horizontal meningeal fold attaching to the four clinoid processes, forming the roof of the sella turcica. It has an opening in the middle (ostium of the diaphragma sellae), crossed by the pituitary stalk (infundibulum). It separates the supradiaphragmatic space from the infradiaphragmatic space, where the pituitary gland lies.

■ 2.5 Veins and Dural Venous Sinuses

See **Fig. 2.10** and Chapter 26.

Transverse Sinus

The transverse sinus comprises symmetrical sinuses that drain blood from the superior sagittal sinus and from the straight sinus into the sigmoid sinuses. They begin at the internal occipital protuberance and, after a curvilinear course, reach the base of the petrous portion of the temporal bone.

Sigmoid Sinus

The sigmoid sinus is a paired sinus, beginning at the temporal bone, reaching the jugular foramen and draining into the internal jugular vein. It drains blood coming from the transverse sinus and petrosal sinuses, as well as from the vein of Labbé.

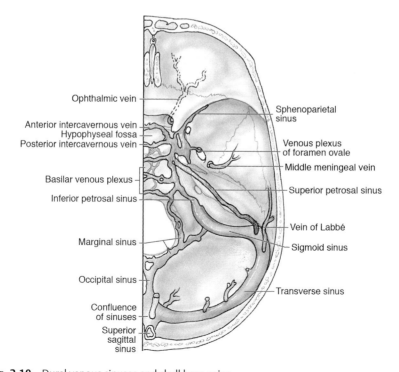

Fig. 2.10 Dural venous sinuses and skull base veins.

Superior Sagittal Sinus

The superior sagittal sinus (SSS) drains venous blood from the hemispheres, beginning above the foramen caecum, coursing in the midline from anterior to posterior to reach the confluence of sinuses. On either sides of the sinus there are several venous lacunae. The SSS is divided in an anterior third portion (from the foramen caecum to the coronal suture), a middle third portion (from the coronal suture to the lambdoid suture), and a posterior third portion (from the lambdoid suture to the confluence sinus).

Confluence of Sinuses

The confluence of sinuses is located beneath the internal occipital protuberance and it is the connecting point of the SSS, the straight sinus, and the occipital sinus, draining into the left and right transverse sinuses.

Superior Petrosal Sinus

The superior petrosal sinus comprises paired narrow channels running in a sulcus of the petrous bone dorsolaterally from the cavernous sinus into the transverse-sigmoid junction. It runs in the attachment of the tentorium cerebelli at the petrous bone, receiving blood from the cerebellum, inferior cerebral veins, and veins of the tympanic cavity.

Inferior Petrosal Sinus

This sinus is located in the inferior petrosal sulcus, between the pars petrosa of the temporal bone and the clivus, connecting the cavernous sinus to the jugular bulb at the level of the jugular foramen.

Vein of Labbé (Inferior Anastomotic Vein)

The vein of Labbé can be bilateral, is very rarely absent, and is generally predominant on the left side, and typically located at the entry point into the anterior third of the transverse sinus almost a third to halfway between the external occipital protuberance and the external acoustic meatus.[29–33]

■ 2.6 Exocranial Surface of the Skull Base

Anatomic Structures

The exocranial surface of the skull base does not have specific anatomic boundaries as does the intracranial surface; nevertheless, specific anatomic structures must be identified (**Fig. 2.2**).

- **Pterygoid processes**
  - Medial and lateral pterygoid plates descend perpendicularly (from the sphenoid bone).
  - The medial and lateral plates diverge, forming the pterygoid fossa, which contains the internal pterygoid muscle (for mastication) and the *tensor veli palatini* muscle (for tensing the soft palate).
- **Styloid process** of the temporal bone
  - Exocranial elongation of the temporal bone
  - Serves as an anchor point of three muscle and ligaments for the tongue and larynx
  - Topographic relationships: facial and glossopharyngeal nerves
- **Mastoid process**
  - Inferior and lateral prominence of the temporal bone, behind the external acoustic meatus
  - Point of attachment of the splenius capitis, posterior belly of the digastric, longissimus capitis, and sternocleidomastoid muscles
  - Topographic relationships: lateral to the styloid process, covering the sigmoid sinus
- **Occipital condyle**
  - Facets of the occipital bone articulating with the superior facets of the atlas
  - Attachments: atlanto-occipital articulations, alar ligaments
  - Topographic relationships: lateral to the foramen magnum; their anterior base contains the hypoglossal canal and the condylar emissary vein canal

Infratemporal Fossa

As the name implies, the infratemporal fossa (ITF) lies below the temporal fossa and represents an important anatomic region for lateral skull base surgery (**Fig. 2.11**). The ITF is important for both the spread of infection and neoplasm as it communicates with the following:

- Orbit (via the inferior orbital fissure and venous anastomoses to the ophthalmic veins)

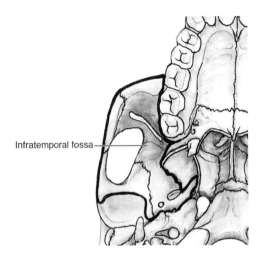

Fig. 2.11   Infratemporal fossa (see the anatomic structures in Fig. 2.2).

- Middle cranial fossa (via the foramen spinosum, foramen ovale, and foramen of Vesalius, whenever present, as well as the venous anastomoses to the cavernous sinus)
- Pterygopalatine fossa (via the pterygopalatine fissure)

There exists some debate as to the precise definition of the ITF. In general there are two definitions: traditional and surgical, the latter being more inclusive. The borders of each are described below.

Traditional Definition[34,35]

- Anterior
  - Posterior maxillary bone and tuberosity, inferior orbital fissure, and the pterygomandibular raphe
- Posterior
  - Styloid process of the temporal bone
- Medial
  - Pterygomaxillary fissure (anterior), lateral pterygoid plate and muscle, tensor and levator veli palatini muscles (posterior)
- Lateral
  - Ramus of the mandible
- Superior
  - Infratemporal surface of the greater wing of the sphenoid
- Inferior
  - Horizontal plane at the level of the angle of the mandible

Surgical Definition

This is a more inclusive definition: The ITF extends under the middle fossa, medial to the pterygoid plates and musculature, and more lateral to the extent of the skin. Within this definition, the ITF can be further subdivided into the pterygomandibular (anterolateral) and the maxillopharyngeal (posteromedial) regions.[36]

- Anterior
  - Posterior maxillary bone and tuberosity, inferior orbital fissure, and pterygomandibular raphe
- Posterior
  - Prevertebral fascia of the neck, mastoid and tympanic portions of the temporal bone
- Medial
  - Lateral wall of the pharynx
- Lateral
  - Skin overlying the parotid and masseter muscle
- Superior
  - Infratemporal surface of the greater wing of the sphenoid and exocranial part of the petrotympanic part of the temporal bone
- Inferior
  - Horizontal plane at the level of the angle of the mandible

Contents (Table 2.5)

- Musculature
  - Medial pterygoid
    - Origin: The deep head originates from the medial surface of the lateral pterygoid plate. The superficial head originates from the maxillary tuberosity.
    - Insertion: medial surface of the mandibular ramus, near the angle (tuberositas pterygoidea mandibulae).
    - Innervation: CN V_3.

Table 2.5   Fossae of the Exocranial Skull Base Fossae and Its Contents

Infratemporal fossa	CN V_3 and branches, chorda tympani, otic ganglion, maxillary artery, pterygoid venous plexus, temporalis, medial and lateral pterygoid muscles
Pterygopalatine fossa	CN V_2, pterygopalatine ganglion, vidian nerve, maxillary artery, vidian artery and vein
Jugular fossa	Internal jugular vein

- Relationships: Fibers descend obliquely and take on a more vertical orientation; muscle runs medial to the sphenomandibular ligament.
  - Lateral pterygoid
    - Origin: The superior part originates from the roof of the infratemporal fossa (inferior surface of the greater wing of the sphenoid and infratemporal crest). The inferior part originates from the lateral surface of the lateral pterygoid plate.
    - Insertion: anterior aspect of the temporomandibular joint (fovea pterygoidea mandibulae, capsula, and discus articularis).
    - Innervation: CN V_3.
    - Relationships: The lower aspect of the inferior part of the lateral pterygoid lies between the superficial and deep heads of the medial pterygoid.
  - Styloglossus
    - Origin: anterior border of the styloid process, near its tip
    - Insertion: lateral and inferior aspect of the tongue
    - Innervation: hypoglossal nerve (CN XII)
    - Relationships: situated medial and anterior to the stylohyoid
  - Stylopharyngeus
    - Origin: medial surface of the styloid process.
    - Insertion: courses between the superior and middle pharyngeal constrictor muscles to insert on the posterior and superior borders of the thyroid cartilage.
    - Innervation: CN IX.
    - Relationships: most medial muscle of the styloid muscle group and runs between the ICA and ECA. The glossopharyngeal nerve circles around the posterior border and passes along its lateral surface prior to innervating the pharynx.
  - Stylohyoid
    - Origin: posterior surface of the styloid process.
    - Insertion: body of the hyoid (*cornu majus ossis hyoidei*).
    - Innervation: CN VII.
    - Relationships: Its tendon forms a fibrous loop at the hyoid bone, through which the digastric muscle tendon courses.
  - Styloid diaphragm: An important concept for surgical anatomy, as its muscular component must be addressed when attempting exposure of the cervical ICA.
    - Components
      - The posterior belly of the digastric muscle
      - The styloid musculature (styloglossus, stylopharyngeus, stylohyoid)
      - The styloid ligaments (stylohyoid, stylomandibular)
      - The fascia spanning the digastric and sternocleidomastoid muscles, along with the stylopharyngeal fascia

- Divides the maxillopharyngeal region of the ITF into prestyloid and retrostyloid regions.
  - Prestyloid contents: external carotid artery, parotid gland, facial nerve (CN VII)
  - Retrostyloid contents: internal carotid artery, internal jugular vein, the proximal extracranial course of the glossopharyngeal nerve, vagus nerve, spinal accessory nerve, and hypoglossal nerve (CNs IX–XII)
- Vascular
  - Arterial
    - Maxillary artery: divided into first (between the neck of the mandible and sphenomandibular ligament), second (related to the lateral pterygoid muscle), and third (within the pterygopalatine fossa [PPF]) parts.
      - Branches of first part: middle meningeal, inferior alveolar, deep auricular, anterior tympanic, and accessory meningeal arteries
      - Branches of the second part: deep temporal, pterygoid, masseteric, and buccal arteries
      - Branches of the third part
  - Venous
    - Pterygoid plexus: drains anteriorly into the facial vein and posteriorly into the maxillary and retromandibular veins.
      - Forms anastomotic connections to the cavernous sinus, ophthalmic veins, and the pharyngeal venous plexus.
        - Specific risk of hematogenous spread of infection or tumor intracranially or to the orbit from an ITF source.
- Neural
  - Mandibular nerve (V_3): enters into the ITF via the foramen ovale.
    - Provides motor innervation to all muscles of mastication: the masseter (masseteric nerve), temporalis (deep temporal nerves), and the medial and lateral pterygoids (nerve to medial pterygoid and nerve to lateral pterygoid, respectively).
    - Provides sensory innervations via the alveolar, auriculotemporal, buccal, lingual, and meningeal nerves.
  - *Chorda tympani*: Branch of the *nervus intermedius* (Wrisberg nerve) that provides sensation to the anterior two thirds of the tongue.
    - Originates in the mastoid facial canal, travels through the middle ear, exits the temporal bone via the *canaliculus of the chorda tympani* (canal of Huguier) in the petrotympanic fissure to enter the ITF.
    - Passes medial to the lateral pterygoid muscle to join the lingual nerve.

Pterygopalatine Fossa[35,37–41]

The PPF is an inverted six-sided pyramidal space, located inferior to the orbital apex and the skull base (**Fig. 2.12**). It is an important anatomic site as it is a

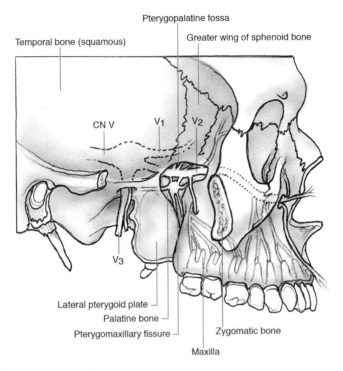

Fig. 2.12 Pterygopalatine fossa.

common area of neoplastic invasion and perineural spread because of its unique communications via the foramen and fissures with the orbit, middle cranial fossa, and nasal and oral cavities.[37]

Borders:

- Anterior
  - Posterior wall of the maxillary sinus (*facies infratemporalis* with *tuber maxillae*).
    - Anterosuperiorly communicates through the inferior orbital fissure with the orbit.
- Posterior
  - Vertical portion of the common root of the pterygoid plates.
    - Contains the opening of the foramen rotundum and the vidian (pterygoid) canal for communication with the middle cranial fossa.
- Medial
  - Vertical plate of the palatine bone and lateral wall of the nasal cavity.

- Contains the pterygopalatine foramen located in the superomedial aspect of the PPF for communication with the nasal cavity. The pterygopalatine foramen is vertically oriented, elliptical, and opens into a 4- to 7-mm-long canal into the nasal cavity.[38]
- Lateral
  - Pterygomaxillary fissure, lateral to which is the infratemporal fossa.
- Superior
  - Body of the sphenoid.
- Inferior
  - Pterygopalatine (greater palatine) canal.
    - Communicates with the oral cavity.

Contents (Table 2.5)

- Vascular
  - Arterial
    - Internal maxillary artery (IMAX)[38]
      - Third part of the IMAX resides in the pterygopalatine fossa.
      - Enters the fossa from the lateral aspect via the pterygomaxillary fissure.
      - Variable configuration within the fossa: single looped (less tightly packed, 18%); double looped (more tightly packed, 82%).[38]
      - Of the double looped configurations, 61% are oriented in an M shape and 39% are oriented in an E shape within the fossa.
    - Sphenopalatine artery
      - Terminal branch of the IMAX.
      - Major blood supply of the posterior nasal cavity and septum.
      - Exits the superomedial aspect of the pterygopalatine fossa via the sphenopalatine foramen.
        - Enters into the lateral nasal wall near the lower part of the superior meatus and the posterior aspect of the tail of the middle turbinate.
    - Descending palatine artery
      - Travels inferiorly with the palatine nerve into the palatine canal.
      - Provides two branches: greater and lesser palatine arteries.
      - Blood supply of the hard and soft palates, along with supply to the anterior nasal cavity and septum via the greater palatine artery.
    - Infraorbital artery
      - Travels anteriorly within the fossa along with the infraorbital nerve (from V_2) and exits the fossa via the inferior orbital fissure.
      - Blood supply
        - Orbital structures (inferior rectus and inferior oblique muscles, lacrimal sac)

- ◆ Face (as it exits the inferior orbital foramen)
- ◆ Maxilla, maxillary sinus, and the superior incisor and canine dentition (via the branch of the anterior superior alveolar arteries)
- Posterior-superior alveolar artery
  - □ Branches laterally from the maxillary artery near the pterygomaxillary palatine fissure.
  - □ Meets with the posterior-superior alveolar nerve and travels inferiorly to the alveolar foramen in the postero-lateral surface of the maxilla.
  - □ Blood supply of the premolar and molar dentition, gingival, and maxillary sinus.
- Pharyngeal branch
  - □ Passes posteriorly to exit the fossa via the palatovaginal foramen alongside the pharyngeal nerve.
  - □ Blood supply of the posterior aspect of the nasal cavity, the sphenoid sinus, and the eustachian tube.
- Arteries of the pterygoid canal (vidian canal)
  - □ Passes posteriorly to exit the fossa via the pterygoid canal, then through the cartilage of the foramen lacerum inferiorly to terminate in the nasal cavity.
  - □ Blood supply of the adjacent structures of the pterygoid canal and nasal cavity.
  - ○ Venous
    - Pterygopalatine vein (59% absent unilateral, 21% absent bilateral).[38]
      - □ Resides in the most superficial aspect of the pterygopalatine fossa.
      - □ Exits via the pterygopalatine fissure to enter the infratemporal fossa to form the pterygoid plexus of veins.
- Neural
  - ○ Pterygopalatine ganglion (PPG)
    - Largest of the four parasympathetic ganglia of the head.
    - Receives input from the pterygoid nerve (vidian) and ganglionic branches of the maxillary nerve.
    - Branches of the PPG include:
      - □ Nasal and pharyngeal branches of the maxillary nerve
      - □ Descending palatine nerve (greater and lesser palatine nerves)
      - □ Contribute postganglionic fibers to the maxillary nerve branches:
        - ◆ Zygomatic nerve (lacrimal gland innervation)
        - ◆ Infraorbital nerve
        - ◆ Posterior superior alveolar nerve
    - Dysfunction of the PPG is said to be linked to cluster headache and associated dysautonomia (hyperlacrimation, mucosal congestion, rhinorrhea, and conjunctival injection).[40]

- ○ Maxillary nerve (V$_2$)
    - ▪ Enters into the PPF via the foramen rotundum and runs superior to the PPG.
    - ▪ Branches of the maxillary nerve:
        - ▫ Infraorbital nerve
        - ▫ Descending palatine nerves
        - ▫ Superior posterior alveolar nerve
        - ▫ Zygomatic nerve (zygomaticofacial and zygomaticotemporal branches)
        - ▫ Pharyngeal nerve
        - ▫ Orbital nerves
- ○ Pterygoid nerve (vidian nerve)
    - ▪ Formed by the deep petrosal and greater superficial petrosal nerves in the foramen lacerum.
    - ▪ Travels through the pterygoid canal to enter into the posterior aspect of the PPF.

■ 2.7 Orbits

Bony orbital walls delineate a pear-shaped structure, widening anteriorly and narrowing at the apex **(Fig. 2.4)**.

- Total volume of the orbit: approximatively 30 cm^3. Anterior opening dimensions: 3.5 cm (height) × 4 cm (width). The orbital circumference expands behind the orbital rim. The lateral orbital walls form a 45-degree angle to their corresponding medial walls so the lateral walls of the orbit are more or less perpendicular to one another.[42,43]
- Four walls with four margins can be described:
    - ○ *Medial* wall is very thin and formed mainly by the lamina papyracea and, to a lesser extent, by the frontal and lacrimal bone. Posteriorly, the orbital apex is a part of the sphenoid bone. It houses the lacrimal fossa and the ethmoidal foramina.
    - ○ *Lateral* wall is formed by zygomatic and frontal bones anteriorly and the greater wing of the sphenoid posteriorly.
    - ○ *Superior* wall is very thin (sometimes dehiscent) and mainly formed by the frontal bone and, to a lesser extent, the lesser wing of the sphenoid.
    - ○ *Inferior* wall is mainly formed by the maxillary bone, although the orbital process of the palatine bone also contributes a small portion of the orbit.
- Relationships: The roof of the orbit (superior wall) is closely related to the anterior cranial fossa, whereas the lateral wall is related to the temporal fossa anteriorly and middle cranial fossa posteriorly **(Fig. 2.13)**. Inferior and lateral walls are related to the paranasal sinuses.

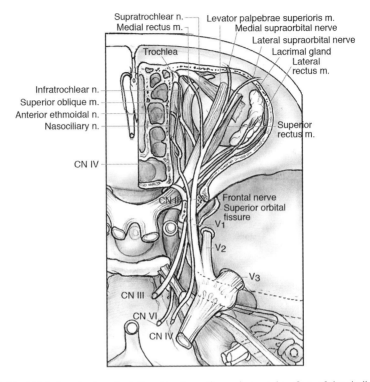

Fig. 2.13 Orbital content and relationships from the endocranial surface of the skull base.

- Two fissures, superior and inferior, connect the orbit with surrounding structures. The inferior orbital fissure connects the orbit with the infratemporal fossa, and the superior fissure creates a connection with the middle cranial fossa/cavernous sinus. The two fissures join each other posteriorly. See **Table 2.1** for contents of the fissures.

Surgical Anatomy Pearl

In rare cases the ophthalmic artery can also pass through the SOF.

- Orbital content can be divided into two regions: the anterior contains the eyeball (the "globe") and the posterior contains muscles, nerves, and vessels all included in a cellular fatty matrix (adipose body of the orbit). The orbital contents are surrounded by periorbita, which is firmly adhered to the bone at the orbital rim (*arcus marginalis*).
- The muscular cone (also called the "intraconal space") is bordered by the four rectus muscles (inferior, medial, lateral, and superior). Other extraocular muscles include the inferior and superior oblique and levator palpebrae muscles.

- Within the orbit, a complex reticular system of septa divides the fat into distinct lobules. These septa are very evident anteriorly, and they bridge together extraocular muscles, thus creating an intraconal and extraconal space. Posteriorly this division is less evident.

> **Surgical Anatomy Pearl**
>
> The four rectus muscles, the inferior and superior oblique and levator palpebrae muscles provide the most obvious anatomic landmarks for intraorbital dissection.

- The optic nerve runs within the orbit from the posterior surface of the eyeball to the optic chiasm and passes through the optic canal. Three major segments are the intraorbital, intracanalicular, and intracranial segments, respectively.
- The optic canal (average diameter 6 mm, average length 8 mm) is located superomedially with respect to the superior orbital fissure. It is formed by four walls: medial, lateral, inferior, and superior (roof).
  - The lateral wall is formed by the optic strut.
  - The medial wall of the optic canal corresponds to the lateral wall of the sphenoid sinus and is continuous with the inferior wall.
  - The roof is continuous with the planum sphenoidale, and it is more thick medially.
- The optic canal contains the intracanalicular part of the optic nerve. This segment of the nerve typically shares the canal with the ophthalmic artery. The artery enters the canal inferior and medial to the nerve and runs anteriorly, leaving the canal inferolaterally to the nerve.
- Annulus of Zinn: an elliptical fibrous ring just anterior to the optic canal and superior orbital fissure. It divides the superior orbital fissure into an intraconal and extraconal space.

> **Surgical Anatomy Pearl**
>
> Most extraocular muscles originate from the annulus.

- Neural structures: sensory and motor nerves. Main sensory nerves (nasociliary, frontal, and lacrimal) are branches of the ophthalmic division of the trigeminal nerve. Muscles motor innervation is provided by CNs III, IV, and VI (see chapter 3).
- The ciliary ganglion is located in the orbital apex, lateral to the optic nerve and measures 1 mm × 2 mm. The short ciliary nerves arise from the forepart of the ganglion.
- **Vascularization**: Orbital vasculature mainly originates from the ophthalmic artery. It presents a great number of anastomoses with the external carotid artery system (superficial temporal artery–supraorbital/

> **Surgical Anatomy Pearl**
>
> These anastomoses are so significant that in most patients the ophthalmic artery can be closed before it starts branching without major consequence.[43]

supratrochlear arteries; angular artery–dorsal nasal/palpebral arteries; sphenopalatine artery–anterior and posterior ethmoidal arteries; infraorbital artery–inferior palpebral artery; middle meningeal artery–lacrimal artery; deep temporal arteries–lacrimal artery).

- The central retinal artery and posterior ciliary arteries provide vasculature for the optic nerve. The ophthalmic artery, within the orbit, crosses from lateral to medial around the stem of the optic nerve (in most cases it passes above the nerve to get its final superomedial position).[42] Other important arteries within the orbit are the lacrimal artery and the supraorbital, ethmoidal, and muscular arteries.

- Venous system: The superior ophthalmic vein is the most constant and important vein of the orbit. It originates from supraorbital and angular veins close to the trochlea and runs posteriorly below the levator palpebrae-superior rectus muscle complex, in close relationship with the ophthalmic artery. It exits the orbit via the SOF, outside the annulus of Zinn. The inferior ophthalmic vein, when present, originates anteromedially, close to the orbital floor, and runs posteriorly in close relationship with the inferior rectus muscle to directly join either the cavernous sinus or the superior ophthalmic vein. Superior and inferior ophthalmic veins are generally linked by the medial collateral vein.

> **Surgical Anatomy Pearl**
>
> In the orbit, there is no direct correspondence between the arteries and the veins, except for the ophthalmic artery and the superior ophthalmic vein.

- Eyelids: **lower eyelid** has four layers, from anterior to posterior:
  1. Skin and subcutaneous tissue
  2. Orbicularis oculi muscle
  3. Tarsus above and septum below
  4. Conjunctiva

  The lower retractor (capsulopalpebral fascia) inserts in the lower tarsus and skin (it corresponds to Muller's muscle, superiorly).

  Superior eyelid: five layers, from anterior to posterior:
  1. Skin
  2. Orbicularis oculi muscle
  3. Orbital septum above and levator palpebrae aponeurosis below
  4. Muller muscle/tarsus complex
  5. Conjunctiva

- Lacrimal gland: two parts; orbital or upper part, and palpebral or inferior part. The orbital part is housed in the lacrimal fossa (frontal bone). It lies superolateral to the levator palpebrae muscle. Its anterior aspect is in contact with orbital septum. The inferior aspect is linked to the levator palpebrae fascial system. The small palpebral part of the lacrimal gland can be seen through the conjunctiva.

■ 2.8 Sinonasal Anatomy

Nasal Cavity

The function of the naval cavity is olfaction. It cleans, warms, and humidifies inspired air and acts as a conduit to the middle and lower respiratory tract.

- **(Internal) Nasal valve**: Having the smallest cross-sectional area of the respiratory tract, it is the anatomic region of greatest resistance to airflow and thus nasal obstruction (two thirds of total resistance of the entire respiratory tract).
  - Borders:
    - Superior: angle between the lower/caudal border of the upper lateral cartilage and the nasal septum (typically 10–15 degrees)
    - Inferior: floor of nasal cavity
    - Lateral: piriform aperture
    - Posterior: anterior face of the inferior turbinates (not always included in definition)
- **Septum**: Bony-cartilaginous midline structure separating the two halves of the nasal cavity.
  - Consists of the perpendicular plate of the ethmoid superoanteriorly, the vomer posteroinferiorly, and the quadrangular cartilage anteroinferiorly.
  - Lined primarily with ciliated respiratory epithelium with variable thickness depending on vascularity.
  - Superiorly the septum is lined with specialized olfactory epithelium and olfactory nerve fibers, which contribute to olfaction. This lining also extends to the superior turbinate and the superior element of the middle turbinate.

> **Surgical Anatomy Pearl**
>
> Often the septum is deviated, either from bony elements, cartilaginous elements, or both.

  - Bony deviation often involves the vomer and is represented by septal spurs.
  - Cartilaginous deviation may be secondary to uneven facial growth or trauma.

> **Pearl**
>
> Septal perforation may be present from varying etiologies: cocaine-induced, iatrogenic, traumatic, and/or systemic autoimmune disease (granulomatosis with polyangiitis, formerly known as Wegener's granulomatosis).

- **Turbinates and meatuses**: There are typically three paired turbinates (occasionally a fourth, supreme, pair of turbinates exists) with similarly named meatuses.
  - **Inferior turbinate**: It is an independent bone, the longest of the turbinates, spanning most of the length of the lateral nasal wall. More so than the other turbinates, the inferior turbinate is subject to significant variation in mucosal thickening throughout the day secondary to the nasal cycle (fluctuation in blood supply).
  - The inferior meatus houses the inferior ostium of the nasolacrimal duct, a conduit for tear outflow from the orbit into the nasal cavity. The ostium is most commonly situated in the anterior roof at the level of the first molar of the meatus (Hasner's valve).
  - **Middle turbinate:** Important surgical landmark with a complex sigmoid-shaped attachment to the lateral nasal wall and ethmoid roof/skull base.
    - Anteriorly it attaches to the superior aspect of the uncinate process and the medial wall of the agger nasi cell, in close proximity to the anterior skull base near the junction of the orbital plate of the frontal bone and the lateral lamella of the cribriform.
      - There is surgical risk of accidental penetration resulting in a CSF leak.
    - Posterior to the bulla ethmoidalis the attachment of the turbinate is termed the basal lamella of the ethmoid bone, which connects laterally with the thin lamina papyracea.
  - **Anatomic variants of the middle turbinate:**
    - **Concha bullosa**: anatomic variant of the middle turbinate occurring in 25% of individuals.
      - Pneumatization of the middle turbinate, lined with respiratory epithelium. It has variable ostia and drainage patterns.
      - Important potential to impair the drainage of the ostiomeatal complex (OMC).
    - **Paradoxic middle turbinate**: The curvature of the middle turbinate typically projects medially toward the midline, but in this anatomic variant it projects laterally instead.
      - Important potential to narrow the infundibulum and middle meatus, thus impairing the drainage of the OMC.
    - Duplication: True duplication is rare, but embryological remnants running longitudinally along the middle turbinate can exist resembling deep furrows or grooves.
  - **Middle meatus**: houses the hiatus semilunaris, a two-dimensional structure defined by the gap between the bulla ethmoidalis and the uncinate process connecting the middle meatus to the infundibulum.
    - **Uncinate process**: appears as a thin, J-shaped bone from a sagittal perspective that spans from its anterosuperior attachment on the lateral nasal wall to its posteroinferior attachment to the inferior turbinate.

- Variable attachment of the superior edge:
  1. Middle turbinate
  2. Directly to the skull base
  3. Laterally to the lamina papyracea
- The posterosuperior border is a free edge that defines the infundibulum (the air space connection of the maxillary sinus ostium to the middle meatus).
- Immediately posterior and lateral to the uncinate is the true maxillary sinus ostium.
- Where the uncinate process is deficient, the anterior and posterior fontanelles (covered with mucosa) separate the middle meatus from the maxillary sinus.
  - **Superior turbinate**: the most superior turbinate of the ethmoid bone (except in anatomic variants having supreme turbinates).
  - **Superior meatus**: smallest of the meatuses.
    - Drainage area of the posterior ethmoid sinuses.
    - Sphenopalatine foramen situated inferiorly, around the level of the middle turbinate tail.
      - Contents: sphenopalatine artery and venous drainage, posterior superior lateral nasal nerves, nasopalatine nerves.
- Drainage points
  - **Nasolacrimal duct**: Within the inferior meatus, it is a bony duct allowing for accessory drainage of tears into the nasal cavity from the orbit.
  - **Ostiomeatal complex/unit:** functional anatomic complex composed of the ethmoid infundibulum, the frontal recess, and the maxillary sinus.
    - No consensus on precise borders, but in general:
      - Medial: middle turbinate
      - Lateral: lamina papyracea
      - Superior: ethmoid roof
      - Posterior: basal lamella
    - Final common drainage point of the frontal, maxillary, and anterior ethmoid sinuses.
  - **Sphenoethmoidal recess**: located between the superior turbinate and the roof of the nasal cavity.
- **Eustachian tubes (pharyngotympanic tubes):** bony and cartilaginous conduit, the latter aspect being collapsible, connecting the middle ear to the nasopharynx; the opening is termed isthmus, with a diameter of ~1 mm.
  - Upon its opening the pressures between the middle ear and nasopharynx are equalized.
  - Bony part is the one third that is closest to the middle ear; cartilaginous part is the two thirds that are closest to the nasopharynx.
  - Its opening into the nasopharynx is posterior to the inferior turbinate, over the soft palate and behind the choana, and it creates a prominence anterior to the posterior nasopharyngeal wall.

Sinuses

Maxillary Sinus

- Pyramid-shaped, largest of the paranasal sinuses.
- Borders:
  - Anterior: facial surface of the maxilla
  - Posterior: infratemporal (tuber maxillae) and pterygopalatine fossae
  - Superior: orbital floor
  - Inferior: alveolar processes
  - Medial: uncinate process, nasolacrimal duct, fontanelles, and the inferior turbinate
  - Lateral: zygomatic process
- Drainage: Natural ostium is located within the superior aspect of the medial wall, in close proximity to the orbital floor.
  - Drains into the ethmoid infundibulum immediately posterior to the uncinate process.
  - Accessory ostium present in 15 to 40%.
- "Haller cell" (infraorbital ethmoid cell): laterally pneumatized ethmoid cell located between the orbital floor and the maxillary sinus.[44]
  - Important potential to impair maxillary sinus drainage flow.
- Anatomic variation
  - Hypoplasia: 3–10%
  - Aplasia: < 0.5%
  - True duplication: rare

> **Surgical Anatomy Pearl**
>
> The roof of the maxillary sinus is often a useful fixed landmark during endoscopic sinus and skull base surgery as a relative reference point to the skull base.

Ethmoid Sinuses

- Highly variable in both size and shape, the ethmoid sinuses line the roof of the nasal cavity with the cribriform plate medially.
- Anterior and posterior ethmoid sinuses are separated by the basal lamella.
- Borders:
  - Anterior: nasal bone
  - Posterior: sphenoid sinus
  - Superior: anterior cranial fossa
  - Inferior: nasal cavity
  - Medial: septum
  - Lateral: medial wall of orbit (lamina papyracea)
- Drainage:
  - Anterior ethmoid sinuses drain into the middle meatus.
  - Posterior ethmoid sinuses drain into the sphenoethmoidal recess and the superior meatus.

- **Bulla ethmoidalis**: Also known as the ethmoid bulla, it is the most consistent ethmoid air cell of the anterior ethmoid, forming the posterior edge of the *hiatus semilunaris.*
  - Three anatomic variants of the *bulla ethmoidalis*[45]:
    - Simple (47%): single large cavity with a single ostium draining either anterior to the basal lamella or directly into the infundibulum.
    - Complex (27%): two or three noncommunicating cavities draining into the hiatus semilunaris, infundibulum, and/or the superior meatus.
    - Compound (26%): two or three noncommunicating cavities draining anterior to the basal lamella and the hiatus semilunaris.
  - **Suprabullar recess** (also known as the suprabullar cell of Mouret): anatomic variant related to the bulla ethmoidalis.
    - Borders:
      - Anterior: *bulla lamella* (anatomic variant airspace located above the bulla ethmoidalis) or directly into the frontal sinus if the bulla lamella is not directly attached to the skull base
      - Posterior: basal lamella of the middle turbinate
      - Superior: ethmoid roof
      - Inferior: *bulla ethmoidalis*
      - Lateral: *lamina papyracea*
  - **Retrobullar recess** (also known as the lateral sinus of Grünwald): anatomic variant airspace located behind the bulla ethmoidalis
    - Borders:
      - Anterior: *bulla ethmoidalis*
      - Posterior: *basal lamella*
      - Superior: ethmoid roof if the bulla ethmoidalis is attached to the skull base; if not, the retrobullar recess can communicate directly with the suprabullar recess
- ***Agger nasi* cell**: It creates a prominence just anterior to the middle turbinate.
  - Forms the anterior border of the frontal recess, and, depending on the degree of pneumatization, can encroach on the drainage outflow of the frontal sinus.
- **Onodi cell**: originates as posterior ethmoid air cell that pneumatizes lateral and superior to the sphenoid sinus.
  - Potential risk factor for surgical injury to a dehiscent optic nerve.
- **Keros classification**: describes the length of the lateral lamella (bone connecting the cribriform plate to the roof of the ethmoid bone), which is variable.[46]
  - Class 1: 1–3 mm (lateral lamella is short or absent)
  - Class 2: 4–7 mm
  - Class 3: 8–16 mm (long lateral lamella that poses a risk for CSF leak during endoscopic sinus surgery)

Sphenoid Sinus

- Posterior-most sinus, of special significance for endoscopic transsphenoidal surgery (the central corridor for the skull base).
- Sphenoid sinus is the most medial superior and posterior airspace within the skull base; however, more laterally, the posterior ethmoid sinuses can assume this position (e.g., Onodi cell) with the sphenoid more inferior.
- Borders:
  - Anterior: posterior ethmoid sinuses, sphenoethmoidal recess (medially)
  - Posterior: clivus
  - Superior: optic nerves and chiasm, sella turcica, and pituitary
  - Inferior: roof of the choana and nasopharynx
  - Lateral: cavernous sinus, internal carotid artery, middle cranial fossa
- Drainage: Natural ostia are located within the anterior superomedial aspect of the anterior wall of the sinus and drain into the sphenoethmoidal recess along with the drainage of the posterior ethmoid sinuses.
  - Landmark for ostia: posteroinferior margin of the superior turbinates.[46]
    - Medial to turbinate (83%)
    - Lateral to turbinate (17%)
  - Best visualized in axial and sagittal planes on computed tomography (CT) imaging modalities.
- Anatomic variants are based on pneumatization patterns and have clinical relevance for the amount of bone that may need to be removed during endoscopic transsphenoidal skull base surgery (the latter two variants are more common in children with incomplete pneumatization)[47,48] (**Fig. 2.14**).
  - Sellar type: most common and occurs in 86% of individuals.
    - Pneumatizes inferior to the sella turcica and pituitary. In some cases, it pneumatizes into the clivus (post-sellar type)
  - Presellar type: occurs in 11% of individuals.
    - Pneumatizes only anterior to the sella turcica.
  - Conchal type: occurs in 3% of individuals.
    - Absent pneumatization of the sphenoid bone.
- Optic nerve: bony prominence in 40% of cases.[48]
    - 6% are dehiscent within the sphenoid sinus.

Surgical Anatomy Pearl

Internal carotid artery produces bony prominence within the sphenoid in 65% of cases[48]; 25% are partially dehiscent within the sphenoid sinus. The sphenoid sinus septations are often irregular and not midline. They may terminate at the internal carotid artery, so great care must be taken not to twist this bone during bony removal.

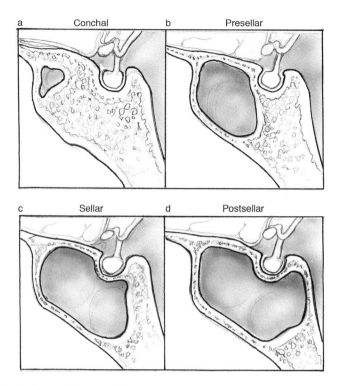

Fig. 2.14a–d Sphenoid sinus variations.

Frontal Sinuses

- Pyramid/funnel-shaped air cells within the frontal bones formed from extension of one or more anterosuperior ethmoid cells.
- Common to have an intersinus septum dividing frontal sinuses, and incomplete septa are frequent.
- Borders:
  - Anterior: anterior table of the vertical plate of the frontal bone (two times thicker than posterior table)
  - Posterior: posterior table of the vertical plate of the frontal bone, anterior ethmoid sinuses, frontal lobes
  - Superior: vertical plate of the frontal bone
  - Inferior: frontal recess, agger nasi cells
- Drainage: The floor of the sinus slopes toward the midline to reach the primary ostia and connect to the hourglass-shaped frontal recess.

Anatomical Landmarks of the Sphenoid Sinus from the Transsphenoidal Route[49]

- The bony depression into the medial part of the optic strut is visible as the opticocarotid recess, above which the optic nerve and the ophthalmic artery run in the dura of the optic canal, and inferolaterally to which it is possible to visualize the course of the ICA.
- By tracking two lines along the carotid arteries and two perpendicular lines at the level of the floor and roof of the sella, it is possible to divide the sellar/parasellar region into three sections: a central region, formed superiorly by the ethmoid-sphenoidal planum, in the middle by the pituitary fossa, and inferiorly by the clivus, and two lateral regions.
- By labeling regions with the same numbering as seen on a clock face, when viewed from the foot of the patient upward, the anatomic landmarks are (**Fig. 2.15**):
  - The planum between 11 and 1 o'clock
  - The opticocarotid recesses and optic nerves protuberances at 10 and 2 o'clock
  - The right cavernous ICA between 9 and 10 o'clock and the left between 2 and 3 o'clock
  - The right paraclival ICA at 8 to 9 o'clock and the left at 4 to 5 o'clock
  - The clivus at 6 o'clock

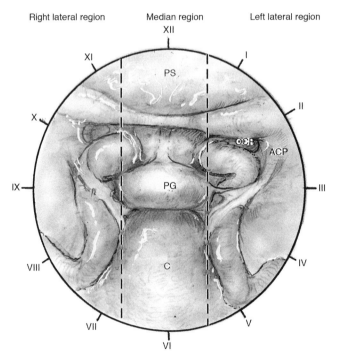

Fig. 2.15 Anatomic landmarks of the sphenoid sinus. The left-sided ICA is here shown unroofed. ACP, anterior clinoid process; C, clivus; OCR, opticocarotid recess; PG, pituitary gland; PS, planum sphenoidale.

- ○ Frontal recess connects the frontal sinus to the anterior aspect of the middle meatus.
  - ▪ Anterior ethmoid sinuses and the maxillary sinus also drain to the ostiomeatal complex.
- ○ Shape of the frontal recess is variable depending on the pneumatization pattern of the *agger nasi* cell and the *bulla ethmoidalis*, along with the position of the uncinate process.
- ○ **Frontal recess (Kuhn) cells**: four types, with prevalence ranging from 20 to 79%.[50]
  - ▪ Type I: single frontal cell above the agger nasi
  - ▪ Type II: vertical column of cells above the agger nasi within the frontal recess
  - ▪ Type III: large cell pneumatizing into the frontal sinus from the frontal recess
  - ▪ Type IV: totally isolated cell within the frontal sinus
- ○ Uncinate process position[45]
  - ▪ Anterosuperior attachment to the lamina papyracea (88%): the uncinate process separates the infundibulum from the frontal recess.
    - ▫ Frontal recess drains into the middle meatus between the middle turbinate and the uncinate (medial to the infundibulum).
  - ▪ Attachment to the ethmoid roof or the middle turbinate (12%).
    - ▫ Frontal recess drains into the infundibulum (potential for obstruction secondary to ethmoid inflammation).
- • Anatomic Variations
  - ○ Paired frontal sinuses (most common)
  - ○ Single unilateral sinus with unilateral aplasia/hypoplasia
  - ○ Third inter-sinus cell
  - ○ Complete aplasia/hypoplasia

Arterial Blood Supply

- • Branches of both the internal and external carotid arteries supply the nasal cavity. There are many anastomoses between the branches, the most prominent of which is Kiesselbach's plexus/Little's area, an area prone to anterior epistaxis.
  - ○ Kiesselbach's plexus: superior labial artery, anterior ethmoid artery, terminal part of the greater palatine artery, sphenopalatine artery, *rami posteriores septi.*
- • Internal carotid artery: runs in the lateral wall of the sphenoid sinus.
  - ○ Anterior ethmoid artery (AEA): branch of the ophthalmic artery, passes forward within a bony canal in the skull base/superior nasal cavity and enters the crista galli through the lateral lamella of the cribriform plate.

Surgical Anatomy Pearl

The AEA may cross the skull base in a pedicled mesentery in the superior nasal cavity and may be inadvertently injured during anterior ethmoid surgery (which can result in retraction of the artery into the orbit with resultant retrobulbar hematoma). Assess with preoperative coronal CT scan: the AEA is located at the junction between the medial rectus and the superior oblique muscle (looks like a tent).

Surgical Anatomy Pearl

The anterior ethmoidal artery must be endoscopically controlled (with either bipolar cautery or surgical clip) prior to an endoscopic transcribriform approach. The posterior ethmoidal artery passes through the cribriform plate and supplies the posterosuperior septum and lateral nasal wall. Both the ethmoidal arteries are branches of the ophthalmic artery.

- Continues anteriorly to supply the external nose and cutaneous structures as the external branch of the anterior ethmoidal artery.
- External carotid artery
  - Sphenopalatine artery: originates in the pterygopalatine fossa as a terminal branch from the maxillary artery.
    - The largest vessel supplying the nasal cavity, it is divided into posterior lateral nasal and posterior septal branches, both of which form extensive anastomoses with other arteries within the nasal cavity.
    - Posterior lateral nasal branches: supply the lateral nasal wall.
    - Posterior septal branches: cross the nasal cavity over the anterior face of the sphenoid sinus inferior to the ostia, and supply the nasal septum.
      - This is the main axial blood supply to the pedicled nasoseptal mucosal flap and must not be inadvertently injured while performing sphenoidotomy.
      - It has a direct anastomosis with the terminal part of the greater palatine artery in the anterior septum.
  - Greater palatine artery (terminal part): originates in the pterygopalatine fossa as a branch from the maxillary artery and descends through the palatine foramen to supply the roof of the oral cavity.
    - Enters the nasal cavity through the paired incisive foramina just lateral to the septum and anastomoses with the septal branches of the sphenopalatine artery.
      - Supplies the anterior septum and floor of the nasal cavity.
  - Superior branch of the labial artery: branch of the facial artery, also contributing to the upper lip, as its name implies.
    - Septal branches supply the anterior septum, and alar branches supply the lateral aspect of the naris.
  - Lateral nasal artery: branch of the facial artery.
    - Supplies the external nose and vestibule.

- In the nasal cavity, venous drainage generally follows the same path as the respective arterial counterparts.
- Anterior regions of the nasal cavity drain via the facial vein.
- Structures receiving vascular supply from the maxillary artery (sphenopalatine, greater palatine) drain via the pterygoid plexus into the infratemporal fossa.
- Emissary venous drainage (extracranial vein draining into an intracranial venous sinus):
  - Venous tributaries of structures supplied by the anterior and posterior ethmoid arteries drain into the superior ophthalmic vein and into the cavernous sinus.
  - Variable anatomy: There can be an additional nasal vein draining directly into the superior sagittal sinus via the foramen cecum (midline structure anterior to the crista galli) (Zuckerkandl's vein).
  - Clinical significance: Emissary veins pose potential risk of intranasal/peripheral infections seeding the intracranial cavity.

■ 2.9 Craniovertebral Junction

The craniovertebral junction (CVJ) (or occipitocervical, occipitovertebral) is the topographic region between the occipital bone and the upper cervical vertebrae, in relation to the foramen magnum, inferior brainstem, upper cervical spinal cord, and vertebral arteries.

- Osseous components: clivus, occipital condyles, hypoglossal canals, and C1-C2 complex. There is a tubercle for the attachment of the alar ligament of the odontoid located medially to the occipital condyles.
- Ligaments: cruciform, alar, accessory atlantoaxial, apical, and capsular ligaments, anterior and posterior atlanto-occipital membranes, and tectorial membrane.[51,52] The transverse ligament, which is part of the cruciform ligament, is one of the most important ligaments involved in the CVJ stability, and is responsible of the nearly half of the rotation of the joint.[51]
- The dentate (or denticulate) ligaments are paired meningeal extensions bending between the lateral aspects of the spinal cord and internal part of the surrounding dura mater. The first dentate ligament is intracranial, superior to the vertebral artery (VA), in relation to CN XI.[53]
- Neural relationships: caudal brainstem, cerebellum, fourth ventricle, lower cranial nerves, and upper cervical nerves.
- Vascular relationships: arteries—vertebral artery, PICA, spinal arteries, meningeal arteries; veins–intradural and extradural veins, dural venous sinuses.
- Neck muscles (**Fig. 2.16**):
  - 1st layer (superficial): trapezius and sternocleidomastoid

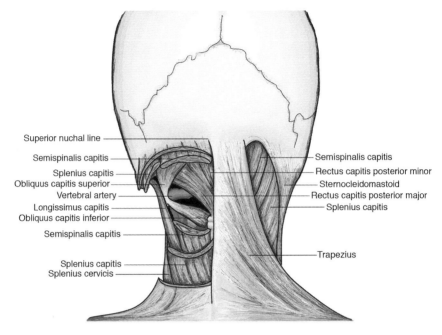

Superior nuchal line
Semispinalis capitis
Splenius capitis
Obliquus capitis superior
Vertebral artery
Longissimus capitis
Obliquus capitis inferior
Semispinalis capitis
Splenius capitis
Splenius cervicis

Semispinalis capitis
Rectus capitis posterior minor
Sternocleidomastoid
Rectus capitis posterior major
Splenius capitis
Trapezius

Fig. 2.16 Posterior muscles of the neck. Note the muscles forming the suboccipital triangle, in which the vertebral artery can be identified.

- ○ 2nd layer: splenius capitis
- ○ 3rd layer: semispinalis
- ○ 4th layer: rectus capitis posterior major, rectus capitis posterior minor, inferior and superior oblique muscles
- • Suboccipital triangle: located between the superior and inferior oblique muscles and the rectus capitis posterior major, in which the vertebral artery and the first cervical nerve can be identified within the fat of the triangle.

■ 2.10 Elements of Surgical Anatomy

Superficial Surgical Landmarks in Skull Base Surgery

Intraoperative neuronavigation, careful study of the preoperative radiological images, and three-dimensional (3D) neuroimaging reconstructions enable precisely localizing the projections of the intracranial structures to the external surface. Despite this, knowledge of anatomic landmarks is still of paramount importance in performing skull base surgical approaches (**Fig. 2.17**).

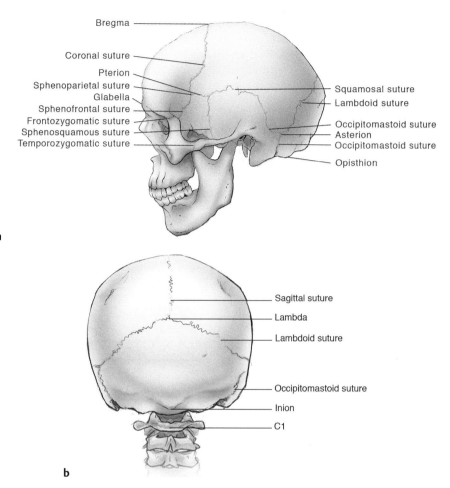

Fig. 2.17a,b   Anatomic landmarks of the **(a)** lateral and **(b)** posterior skull.

Relevant Craniometric Points in Skull Base Surgery

- **Asterion:** Its Greek root refers to the shape of a star. It is on the lateral surface of the skull, behind the ear, and it is the junction point of the lambdoid, occipitomastoid, and parietomastoid sutures. It is generally considered to be overlying the transverse and sigmoid sinus junction, although this is quite inconsistent, as it is not a very reliable landmark.[54]
- **Digastric point:** At the top of the mastoid notch, above the posterior belly of the digastric muscle, it marks the anterior curve of the sigmoid sinus toward the jugular bulb.[55]

- **Glabella:** Named from the Latin word for "smooth," it is above the nose, between the eyebrows, at the level of the supraorbital ridge.
- **Inion:** The name carries Greek origins, meaning "occipital bone." It is the most prominent external protuberance of the occipital bone. Generally its internal projection is inferior to the internal occipital protuberance and torcular herophili.[56]
- **Opisthion:** It is the midline posterior margin of the foramen magnum.
- **Pterion:** Named from the Greek word for wing, in anatomy it is the junction of the coronal, squamous, and sphenoparietal sutures, although in surgery it is generally considered like a region, marking the convergence point of the frontal, parietal, temporal, and sphenoid greater wing bones, behind the frontal process of the zygomatic bone.

Transverse-Sigmoid Sinus Complex Landmarks

- A line between the inion and the posterior root of the zygomatic process (which is on the same level of the superior nuchal line) generally overlies the transverse sinus area. An almost perpendicular line from the tip of the mastoid process to the squamosal/parietomastoid junction tracks the sigmoid sinus (**Fig. 2.18**).

> **Surgical Anatomy Pearl**
>
> The right transverse sinus is usually dominant, larger, and placed more inferiorly than the left one.[57,58]

- The junction of parietomastoid and squamous sutures marks the anterior border of the superior curve of the sigmoid sinus (SS).[59]

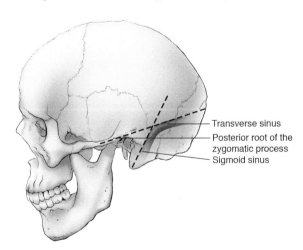

Transverse sinus
Posterior root of the zygomatic process
Sigmoid sinus

Fig. 2.18 Transverse and sigmoid sinuses: anatomic landmarks on the surface of the skull.

- The asterion is considered the landmark for the junction between the transverse and sigmoid sinuses,[59] although its position has been described to be over the complex in 61% of cases on the right and 66% on the left; over the posterior fossa dura in 32% of cases on the right and 25% on the left; above the complex in 7% of cases on the right and 9% on the left.[54] It is not a reliable landmark, then, and bur holes placed on the asterion may often directly expose the transverse sinus, or at least its inferior half,[60] with potential damage.[54]
- The occipitomastoid suture at the most superior aspect of the mastoid notch is an adequate site for the bur hole for performing a suboccipital craniectomy.[60]
- The superior nuchal line is considered the landmark for the internal location of the transverse sinus.[57] By placing the belly of your fingertip parallel with the superior nuchal line and running it carefully and gently from inferior to superior, you will feel a groove in most cases. This groove marks the insertion point of the nuchal musculature and signifies the superior nuchal line. On the deep surface of this line will be the transverse sinus. Checked properly, this landmark is reliable and useful for knowing the position of the underlying transverse sinus.

> **Surgical Anatomy Pearl**
>
> Staying at least 5 mm below the point of insertion of the musculus semispinalis capitis, the transverse sinus can be avoided.[56]

- Supramastoid crest: generally at the same level of the middle cranial fossa floor, very close to the transverse sinus and the vein of Labbé.[61]
- The emissary foramen, existing in 78% of cases,[62] is crossed by the mastoid emissary vein and has to be recognized and coagulated (with the patient in the sitting position, it can be the cause of air embolism). Whenever stripped out, it can cause a laceration of the sigmoid sinus.

Middle Fossa Landmarks

The point where the parietomastoid suture reaches the squamous suture is located at the level of the posterior part of the middle fossa floor.[60]

Foramen Magnum Landmarks

The foramen magnum is generally at the level of the tip of the mastoid.

Occipital Artery

The knowledge of the anatomy of the occipital artery is relevant for (1) performing a carotid endarterectomy, (2) avoiding excessive blood loss in the retrosigmoid paracerebellar approach, and, rarely, (3) performing bypasses between it and the posterior inferior cerebellar artery. The occipital artery originates from the ECA and runs below and medial to the digastric muscle, turning, at the level of the mastoid groove, posteromedially, toward the external occipital protuberance, terminating in one or two main trunks.[62]

Facial Nerve Landmarks

The facial nerve exits the skull base from the stylomastoid foramen, posterior to the styloid process and anterior to the mastoid notch, crossing the styloid process, the retromandibular vein, and the ECA, before dividing behind the neck of the mandible into its five terminal branches.

■ 2.11 Soft Tissues Relations in the Pterional Region

The anatomic complexity of the pterional region results from the existence and complex relations of different soft tissues. It is of paramount importance to use a univocal standardized nomenclature for the different structures, in order to avoid confusion and misunderstanding.

From superficial to deep, the soft tissues of the region are[63] (**Fig. 2.19**):

1. Temporoparietal fascia
2. Loose areolar tissue plan
3. Superficial leaflet of temporal fascia
4. Fat pad of temporal fascia
5. Deep leaflet of temporal fascia
6. Fat pad deep to temporal fascia
7. Temporal muscle
8. Pericranium

- The *temporoparietal fascia* is commonly called superficial temporal fascia, or galea, superficially related to the subcutaneous tissue, connected superiorly to the galea aponeurotica (which is the fibrous sheet connecting the occipital and auricular to the frontal muscles).
- The *loose areolar tissue* enables mobility of the skin and temporoparietal fascia in relation to the underlying structures.
- The *temporal fascia* is formed by the duplication of two leaflets (superficial and deep), which diverge to encompass a fat pad and the branches of the facial nerve. Below the zygomatic arch, the *superficial leaflet of the temporal fascia* is directly continuous with the fascia covering the parotid gland and masseter muscle.

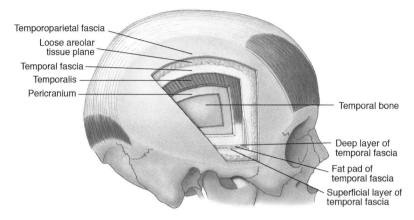

Temporoparietal fascia
Loose areolar tissue plane
Temporal fascia
Temporalis
Pericranium

Temporal bone

Deep layer of temporal fascia

Fat pad of temporal fascia

Superficial layer of temporal fascia

Fig. 2.19 Soft tissues layers of the temporoparietal region. [Adapted from Davidge KM, van Furth WR, Agur A, Cusimano M. Naming the soft tissue layers of the temporoparietal region: unifying anatomic terminology across surgical disciplines. Neurosurgery 2010;67(3, Suppl Operative):ons120–ons129, discussion ons129–ons130. Reprinted with permission].

- The *temporal muscle* is fan-shaped, extending inferiorly from the coronoid process and anterior ramus of the mandible to the superior temporal line, superiorly.
- Between the temporal muscle and the bone there is a thin layer of fascia, the *pericranium*, which has been often defined as deep temporal fascia, although this definition should be applied instead to the deep leaflet of the true temporal fascia. The branches of the superficial temporal artery supply the superficial soft tissues of the region, whereas the temporal muscle itself is more vascularized by deep arteries coming from the maxillary artery.
- The innervation of the temporal muscle comes mainly from the V_3 branches.
- The preservation of the pericranium during the mobilization of the temporal muscle enables preservation of its vascularization and innervation, reducing the chances of postoperative muscle atrophy.
- The presence and size of the fat pad can be variable, depending on individual characteristics. To summarize: in the anterior portion of the temporalis muscle, there are three fat pads: (1) in the subgaleal space, (2) between the two leaflets of the temporal fascia, and (3) beneath the superficial temporalis fascia.[64]
- The *temporal branch of the facial nerve* emerges at the anterosuperior aspect of the parotid gland, just caudal to the zygomatic arch. It initially runs in the subcutaneous tissue of the parotid-masseteric fascia, below the zygomatic arch, and, when it crosses the arch, runs in the subgaleal space (i.e., in the fat pad between the two leaflets of the temporoparietal fascia). In the parotid

fascia, the nerve divides into an anterior, middle (frontal), and posterior ramus. Several variable branches form the terminal twigs as the branches cross the zygomatic arch. A useful landmark to track the course of the nerve is an oblique line connecting the lateral canthus and the crus of the helix. The nerve innervates the frontalis, corrugator, and orbicularis oculi muscles.

■ 2.12 Classification of Intracranial Arteries

Review anatomy of the circle of Willis in **Fig. 2.20**. Knowledge of the segments of the ICA and VA is mandatory for decision making regarding the approach to the vascular pathology, and it is helpful for research purposes and communication among physicians. Different classification systems, each having their benefits and drawbacks, have been proposed in the literature and are discussed below.

- Current classification systems are based on anatomic landmarks.
- The most commonly used classification systems of the ICA consist of six or seven segments.
- Some segments are named identically in the two most commonly used classification systems, but do not refer to the same anatomic landmarks.
- The classification system of the VA consists of four segments.
- Digital subtraction angiography (DSA) and CT angiography (CTA) are most helpful to assess the segmentation of the ICA and VA, as the transitions between the segments are based on skull base landmarks and branching arteries.

Internal Carotid Artery

The first study proposing a classification system for the ICA was published by Fischer[65] in 1938. This system described five segments, based on the angiographic course of the ICA, but appeared to be inaccurate from the anatomic point of view. Therefore, new classification systems were developed that were based on microsurgical anatomy.[66,67] These systems classify the ICA into four (with three additional subclassifications) or seven segments. One has to be aware that these systems are not interchangeable, and some segments have identical names, although they do not refer to the same anatomic landmarks (**Table 2.6** and **Fig. 2.21a**).

Because these systems are less useful for the modern extended endonasal endoscopic approaches, some authors proposed a new system[68,69] of which the most recent is reviewed in **Table 2.7**.

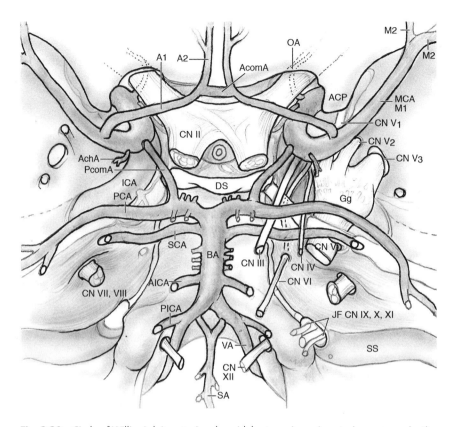

Fig. 2.20 Circle of Willis. AchA, anterior choroidal artery; AcomA, anterior communicating artery; ACP, anterior clinoid process; AICA, anterior inferior cerebellar artery; BA, basilar artery; CN, cranial nerve; DS, dorsum sellae; Gg, gasser ganglion; ICA, internal carotid artery; JF, jugular foramen; MCA, middle cerebral artery; OA, occipital artery; PCA, posterior cerebral artery; PcomA, posterior communicating artery; PICA, posterior inferior cerebellar artery; SA, anterior spinal artery; SCA, superior cerebellar artery; SS, sigmoid sinus; VA, vertebral artery.

Vertebral Artery

The VA is divided into four segments, which include an extradural and intradural part.[70] Knowledge of each segment and its anatomic variations is helpful in preventing vascular complications in a suboccipital craniotomy, far lateral approach, and instrumentation of the atlantoaxial and subaxial spine.[70-73] The paired vertebral arteries arise at the subclavian arteries and ascend along the cervical spine, through the foramen magnum and join to form the basilar artery. See **Table 2.8** and **Fig. 2.21b** for a description of each segment.

Table 2.6 Overview of Classification Systems of the Internal Carotid Artery, Based on Anatomic Landmarks

Anatomic Landmarks of Segment	Segment According to Gibo et al Classification[67]	Segment According to Bouthillier et al Classification[66]
Junction with CCA to entry into carotid canal, the first dural ring	C1 (cervical)	C1 (cervical)
Entry in carotid canal to entry in CS	C2 (petrous)	
Entry in carotid canal to posterior edge foramen lacerum		C2 (petrous)
Posterior edge foramen lacerum to superior margin of petrolingual ligament		C3 (lacerum)
Superior margin of petrolingual ligament to second dural ring surrounding ICA		C4 (cavernous)
Second dural ring at the inferior ACP to the third dural ring surrounding ICA at the superior surface of the ACP		C5 (clinoid)
Entry into cavernous sinus to distal or third dural ring surrounding ICA	C3 (cavernous)	
Distal dural ring surrounding ICA to bifurcation into MCA and ACA	C4 (supraclinoid)	
Distal dural ring surrounding ICA to origin of PcomA	C4 (ophthalmic)	C6 (ophthalmic)
PcomA to the origin of ant. choroidal artery	C4 (communicating)	
PcomA to bifurcation into MCA and ACA		C7 (communicating)
Anterior choroidal artery to bifurcation into MCA and ACA	C4 (choroidal)	

Abbreviations: ACA, anterior cerebral artery; ACP, anterior clinoid process; CCA, common carotid artery; CS, cavernous sinus; ICA, internal carotid artery; MCA, middle cerebral artery; PcomA, posterior communicating artery.

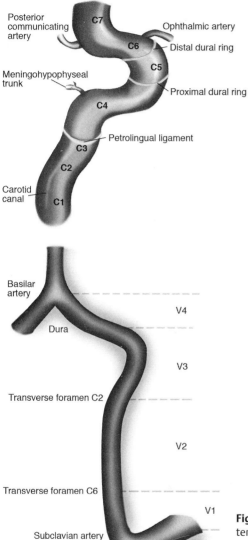

Posterior communicating artery

C7

Ophthalmic artery

C6

Distal dural ring

C5

Proximal dural ring

Meningohypophyseal trunk

C4

Petrolingual ligament

C3

C2

Carotid canal

C1

a

Basilar artery

V4

Dura

V3

Transverse foramen C2

V2

Transverse foramen C6

V1

Subclavian artery

b

Fig. 2.21a,b Segments of the **(a)** internal carotid artery and **(b)** vertebral artery.

Table 2.7   Overview of Classification System of the Internal Carotid Artery for the Endonasal Endoscopic Approach[69]

Anatomic Landmarks of Segment	Segment
Junction with CCA to entry into carotid canal	Parapharyngeal
Entry in carotid canal to posterior edge foramen lacerum	Petrous
Posterior edge foramen lacerum to superior margin of petroclival fissure	Paraclival
Superior margin of petroclival fissure to proximal dural ring surrounding ICA	Parasellar
Proximal dural surrounding ICA to distal ring surrounding ICA	Paraclinoid
Distal dural ring surrounding ICA to bifurcation into MCA and ACA	Intradural

Abbreviations: ACA, anterior cerebral artery; CCA, common carotid artery; ICA, internal carotid artery; MCA, middle cerebral artery.

Table 2.8   Overview of Classification System of the Vertebral Artery[70]

Anatomic Landmarks of Segment	Segment
Origin at subclavian artery to entrance into lowest transverse foramen (usually C6)	V1
Ascending part in transverse foramina to transverse foramen of C2	V2
Transverse foramen of C2 to entry into dura	V3
Intradural part of vertebral artery	V4
Entry into dura to preolivary sulcus	Lateral medullary
Preolivary sulcus to basilar artery	Medial medullary

■ References

Boldfaced references are of particular importance.

1. **Seoane E, Rhoton AL Jr, de Oliveira E. Microsurgical anatomy of the dural collar (carotid collar) and rings around the clinoid segment of the internal carotid artery. Neurosurgery 1998;42:869–884, discussion 884–886**
2. **Parkinson D. Extradural neural axis compartment. J Neurosurg 2000;92:585–588**
3. **Campero A, Campero AA, Martins C, Yasuda A, Rhoton AL Jr. Surgical anatomy of the dural walls of the cavernous sinus. J Clin Neurosci 2010;17:746–750**
4. Perneczky A, Knosp E, Vorkapic P, Czech T. Direct surgical approach to infraclinoidal aneurysms. Acta Neurochir (Wien) 1985;76:36–44
5. Reisch R, Vutskits L, Filippi R, Patonay L, Fries G, Perneczky A. Topographic microsurgical anatomy of the paraclinoid carotid artery. Neurosurg Rev 2002;25:177–183
6. Renn WH, Rhoton AL Jr. Microsurgical anatomy of the sellar region. J Neurosurg 1975; 43:288–298

7. Harris FS, Rhoton AL. Anatomy of the cavernous sinus. A microsurgical study. J Neurosurg 1976;45:169–180

8. Sekhar LN, Linskey ME, Sen CN, Altschuler EM. Surgical management of lesions within the cavernous sinus. Clin Neurosurg 1991;37:440–489

9. Lanzino G, Sekhar LN, Hirsch WL, Sen CN, Pomonis S, Snyderman CH. Chordomas and chondrosarcomas involving the cavernous sinus: review of surgical treatment and outcome in 31 patients. Surg Neurol 1993;40:359–371

10. Isolan GR, Krayenbühl N, de Oliveira E, Al-Mefty O. Microsurgical anatomy of the cavernous sinus: measurements of the triangles in and around it. Skull Base 2007;17: 357–367

11. Watanabe A, Nagaseki Y, Ohkubo S, et al. Anatomical variations of the ten triangles around the cavernous sinus. Clin Anat 2003;16:9–14

12. Parkinson D. A surgical approach to the cavernous portion of the carotid artery. Anatomical studies and case report. J Neurosurg 1965;23:474–483

13. Glasscock ME. Exposure of the intra-petrous portion of the carotid artery. In: Hamberger CA, Wersall J, eds. Disorders of the Skull Base Region: Proceedings of the 10th Nobel Symposium. Stockholm: Almqvist and Wicksell; 1969:135–143

14. Mullan S. Treatment of carotid-cavernous fistulas by cavernous sinus occlusion. J Neurosurg 1979;50:131–144

15. **Ono M, Ono M, Rhoton AL Jr, Barry M. Microsurgical anatomy of the region of the tentorial incisura. J Neurosurg 1984;60:365–399**

16. Kawase T, Toya S, Shiobara R, Mine T. Transpetrosal approach for aneurysms of the lower basilar artery. J Neurosurg 1985;63:857–861

17. Fukushima T. Direct operative approach to the vascular lesions in the cavernous sinus: summary of 27 cases. Mt Fuji Workshop Cerebrovasc Dis 1988:169–189

18. **Dolenc VV. Anatomy and Surgery of the Cavernous Sinus. New York: Springer-Verlag; 1989**

19. **Rhoton AL Jr. The cavernous sinus, the cavernous venous plexus, and the carotid collar. Neurosurgery 2002;51(4, Suppl):S375–S410**

20. **Dolenc VV. Microsurgical Anatomy and Surgery of the Central Skull Base. New York: Springer-Verlag; 2003**

21. **Friedman AH, Arango Alvarez G, Asaoka K, et al. Manual of Skull Base Dissection, 2nd ed. Raleigh, NC: AF-NeuroVideo; 2004**

22. Cullu N, Deveer M, Sahan M, Tetiker H, Yilmaz M. Radiological evaluation of the styloid process length in the normal population. Folia Morphol (Warsz) 2013;72:318–321

23. Fujii N, Inui Y, Katada K. Temporal bone anatomy: correlation of multiplanar reconstruction sections and three-dimensional computed tomography images. Jpn J Radiol 2010;28:637–648

24. Juliano AF, Ginat DT, Moonis G. Imaging review of the temporal bone: part I. Anatomy and inflammatory and neoplastic processes. Radiology 2013;269:17–33

25. **Rhoton AL Jr. The cerebellopontine angle and posterior fossa cranial nerves by the retrosigmoid approach. Neurosurgery 2000;47(3, Suppl):S93–S129**

26. Tanriover N, Abe H, Rhoton AL Jr, Kawashima M, Sanus GZ, Akar Z. Microsurgical anatomy of the superior petrosal venous complex: new classifications and implications for subtemporal transtentorial and retrosigmoid suprameatal approaches. J Neurosurg 2007;106:1041–1050

27. **Watanabe T, Igarashi T, Fukushima T, Yoshino A, Katayama Y. Anatomical variation of superior petrosal vein and its management during surgery for cerebellopontine angle meningiomas. Acta Neurochir (Wien) 2013;155:1871–1878**

28. Rhoton AL Jr. Tentorial incisura. Neurosurgery 2000;47(3, Suppl):S131–S153

29. Silva PS, Vilarinho A, Carvalho B, Vaz R. Anatomical variations of the vein of Labbé: an angiographic study. Surg Radiol Anat 2014;36:769–773

30. Avci E, Dagtekin A, Akture E, Uluc K, Baskaya MK. Microsurgical anatomy of the vein of Labbé. Surg Radiol Anat 2011;33:569–573

31. Lustig LR, Jackler RK. The vulnerability of the vein of Labbé during combined craniotomies of the middle and posterior fossae. Skull Base Surg 1998;8:1–9

32. **Koperna T, Tschabitscher M, Knosp E. The termination of the vein of "Labbé" and its microsurgical significance. Acta Neurochir (Wien) 1992;118:172–175**

33. Rhoton AL Jr. The cerebral veins. Neurosurgery 2002;51(4, Suppl):S159–S205

34. Cruz OLM. Surgical anatomy of the lateral skull base. In: Cummings Otolaryngology—Head and Neck Surgery, 5th ed. Philadelphia: Mosby, Elsevier; 2010:2434–2441

35. Drake RL, Vogl AW, Mitchell AWM. Gray's Anatomy for Students, 2nd ed. Philadelphia: Churchill Livingstone, Elsevier; 2010

36. Bejjani GK, Sullivan B, Salas-Lopez E, et al. Surgical anatomy of the infratemporal fossa: the styloid diaphragm revisited. Neurosurgery 1998;43:842–852, discussion 852–853

37. Ginsberg LE. Imaging of perineural tumor spread in head and neck cancer. Semin Ultrasound CT MR 1999;20:175–186

38. Chiu T. A study of the maxillary and sphenopalatine arteries in the pterygopalatine fossa and at the sphenopalatine foramen. Rhinology 2009;47:264–270

39. Cummings Otolaryngology—Head and Neck Surgery, 5th ed. Philadelphia: Mosby, Elsevier; 2010

40. Khonsary SA, Ma Q, Villablanca P, Emerson J, Malkasian D. Clinical functional anatomy of the pterygopalatine ganglion, cephalgia and related dysautonomias: a review. Surg Neurol Int 2013;4(Suppl 6):S422–S428

41. Bryant L, Goodmurphy CW, Han JK. Endoscopic and three-dimensional radiographic imaging of the pterygopalatine and infratemporal fossae: improving surgical landmarks. Ann Otol Rhinol Laryngol 2014;123:111–116

42. Hayreh SS. Orbital vascular anatomy. Eye (Lond) 2006;20:1130–1144

43. Rootman J. Orbital Surgery. A Conceptual Approach, 2nd ed. Philadelphia: Lippincott & Williams; 2014

44. Kainz J, Braun H, Genser P. [Haller's cells: morphologic evaluation and clinico-surgical relevance]. Laryngorhinootologie 1993;72:599–604

45. Youngs R, Evans K, Watson M. The paranasal sinuses. In: Youngs R, Evans K, Watson M, eds. A Handbook of Applied Surgical Anatomy. London: Taylor & Francis; 2006

46. Leung RM, Walsh WE, Kern RC. Sinonasal anatomy and physiology. In: Johnson JT, Rosen CA, eds. Bailey's Head and Neck Surgery—Otolaryngology, 5th ed. Baltimore: Lippincott Williams & Wilkins; 2014:359–370

47. **Lang J. Skull Base and Related Structures. Atlas of Clinical Anatomy. Stuttgart, New York: Schattauer Verlag; 2001**

48. Janfaza P, Montogomery WW, Salman SD. Nasal cavities and paranasal sinuses. In: Janfaza P, Nadol JB, Galla R, et al., eds. Surgical Anatomy of the Head and Neck. Philadelphia: Lippincott Williams & Wilkins; 2001:259–318

49. Di Ieva A. Anatomical study of the endoscopic endonasal transsphenoidal approach to the sellar region and planum sphenoidalis. [Degree experimental thesis.] Naples, Italy: University of Naples "Federico II"; July 2002

50. Eweiss AZ, Khalil HS. The prevalence of frontal cells and their relation to frontal sinusitis: a radiological study of the frontal recess area. ISRN Otolaryngol 2013;2013: 687582

51. Tubbs RS, Hallock JD, Radcliff V, et al. Ligaments of the craniocervical junction. J Neurosurg Spine 2011;14:697–709

52. Debernardi A, D'Aliberti G, Talamonti G, Villa F, Piparo M, Collice M. The craniovertebral junction area and the role of the ligaments and membranes. Neurosurgery 2011;68:291–301

53. Tubbs RS, Mortazavi MM, Loukas M, Shoja MM, Cohen-Gadol AA. The intracranial denticulate ligament: anatomical study with neurosurgical significance. J Neurosurg 2011;114:454–457

54. Day JD, Tschabitscher M. Anatomic position of the asterion. Neurosurgery 1998;42: 198–199

55. Raso JL, Gusmão SN. A new landmark for finding the sigmoid sinus in suboccipital craniotomies. Neurosurgery 2011;68(1, Suppl Operative):1–6, discussion 6

56. Tubbs RS, Salter G, Oakes WJ. Superficial surgical landmarks for the transverse sinus and torcular herophili. J Neurosurg 2000;93:279–281

57. Ebraheim NA, Lu J, Biyani A, Brown JA, Yeasting RA. An anatomic study of the thickness of the occipital bone. Implications for occipitocervical instrumentation. Spine 1996;21:1725–1729, discussion 1729–1730

58. Modic MT, Weinstein MA, Starnes DL, Kinney SE, Duchesneau PM. Intravenous digital subtraction angiography of the intracranial veins and dural sinuses. Radiology 1983; 146:383–389

59. Day JD, Kellogg JX, Tschabitscher M, Fukushima T. Surface and superficial surgical anatomy of the posterolateral cranial base: significance for surgical planning and approach. Neurosurgery 1996;38:1079–1083, discussion 1083–1084

60. Ribas GC, Rhoton AL Jr, Cruz OR, Peace D. Suboccipital burr holes and craniectomies. Neurosurg Focus 2005;19:E1

61. Duangthongpon P, Thanapaisal C, Kitkhuandee A, Chaiciwamongkol K, Morthong V. Supramastoid crest, safety landmark for craniotomy? J Med Assoc Thai 2013;96(Suppl 4):S138–S141

62. Lang J Jr, Samii A. Retrosigmoidal approach to the posterior cranial fossa. An anatomical study. Acta Neurochir (Wien) 1991;111:147–153

63. Davidge KM, van Furth WR, Agur A, Cusimano M. Naming the soft tissue layers of the temporoparietal region: unifying anatomic terminology across surgical disciplines. Neurosurgery 2010;67(3, Suppl Operative):ons120–ons129, discussion ons129–ons130

64. Ammirati M, Spallone A, Ma J, Cheatham M, Becker D. An anatomicosurgical study of the temporal branch of the facial nerve. Neurosurgery 1993;33:1038–1043, discussion 1044

65. Fischer E. Die Lageabweichungen der vorderen Hirnarterie im Gefässbild. Zentralbl Neurochir 1938;3:300–313

66. Bouthillier A, van Loveren HR, Keller JT. Segments of the internal carotid artery: a new classification. Neurosurgery 1996;38:425–432, discussion 432–433

67. **Gibo H, Lenkey C, Rhoton AL Jr. Microsurgical anatomy of the supraclinoid portion of the internal carotid artery. J Neurosurg 1981;55:560–574**

68. Alfieri A, Jho HD, Schettino R, Tschabitscher M. Endoscopic endonasal approach to the pterygopalatine fossa: anatomic study. Neurosurgery 2003;52:374–378, discussion 378–380

69. **Labib MA, Prevedello DM, Carrau R, et al. A road map to the internal carotid artery in expanded endoscopic endonasal approaches to the ventral cranial base. Neurosurgery 2014;10(Suppl 3):448–471, discussion 471**

70. **Rhoton AL Jr. The foramen magnum. Neurosurgery 2000;47(3, Suppl):S155–S193**

71. Rhoton AL Jr. The far-lateral approach and its transcondylar, supracondylar, and paracondylar extensions. Neurosurgery 2000;47(3, Suppl):S195–S209

72. Ozgen S, Pait TG, Cağlar YS. The V2 segment of the vertebral artery and its branches. J Neurosurg Spine 2004;1:299–305

73. Ulm AJ, Quiroga M, Russo A, et al. Normal anatomical variations of the V_3 segment of the vertebral artery: surgical implications. J Neurosurg Spine 2010;13:451–460

3 Functional Anatomy of the Cranial Nerves

■ Twelve Pairs of Cranial Nerves

Review the anatomic relationship of the 12 pairs of cranial nerves (CNs) that pertain to the skull base as shown in **Fig. 3.1**.

Cranial Nerve I: Olfactory Nerve

The olfactory nerve is formed by about 20 olfactory filaments, which collect the olfactory fibers coming from the olfactory epithelium in the nasal mucosa. They cross the foramina of the cribriform plate of the ethmoid bone, reaching the olfactory bulb.

- The **olfactory bulb** is the rostral enlargement of the olfactory tract, where mitral cells project their axons to the olfactory cortex via the medial and lateral (and intermediate) olfactory striae in the region of the olfactory trigone at the anterior perforated substance.
  - **Lesions:** anosmia/hyposmia

> **Surgical Anatomy Pearl**
>
> Fractures of the anterior skull base with the involvement of the cribriform plate may give rise to cerebrospinal fluid (CSF) leakage with associated anosmia.

Typical tumors giving rise to anosmia are cribriform plate meningiomas, nasal/paranasal tumors, and esthesioneuroblastoma.

Cranial Nerve II: Optic Nerve

The optic nerve is composed of a bundle of nervous fibers (almost one million fibers) carrying visual information, which leave the retina posteriorly to reach the optic chiasm. It passes through the optic canal, joining the contralateral optic nerve in the optic chiasm, where approximately 50% of the axons coming from the nasal retina cross the midline. The posterior limbs of the chiasm are the optic tracts.

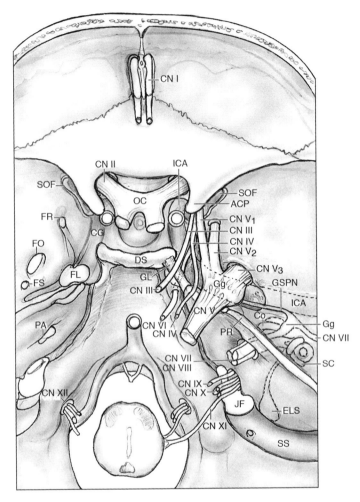

Fig. 3.1 Relationships of the cranial nerves with the endocranial surface of the skull base. ACP, anterior clinoid process; CG, Carotid Groove; CN, cranial nerve; Co, cochlea; DS, dorsum sellae; ELS, endolymphatic sac; FL, foramen lacerum; FO, foramen ovale; FR, foramen rotundum; FS, foramen spinosum; Gg, gasser ganglion; GL, Gruber's ligament; GSPN, greater superficial petrosal nerve; ICA, internal carotid artery; JF, jugular foramen; PA, porus acusticus; PR, petrous ridge; SC, semicircular canals; SOF, superior orbital fissure; SS, sigmoid sinus.

The optic nerve is ~ 50 mm long, formed by four segments:

- *Intraocular,* the head of the optic nerve, 1 mm long
- *Intraorbital,* between the globe and the optic canal, ~ 25 mm long
- *Intracanalicular,* within the optic canal, together with the ophthalmic artery and sympathetic plexus, ~ 9 mm long
- *Intracranial,* reaching the optic chiasm in the perioptic and chiasmatic cisterns, 4 to 16 mm long

The optic chiasm may have three different positions (**Fig. 3.2**), in relation to the surrounding structures[1,2]:

- Above the diaphragma sellae (~ 70%)
- Above the tuberculum sellae (prefixed, ~ 15%)
- Above the dorsum sellae (postfixed, ~ 15%)

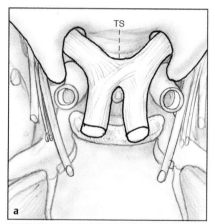

Fig. 3.2a–c Optic chiasm types. **(a)** The optic chiasm is above the diaphragm sellae, which is the most typical type. **(b)** Prefixed type, with a shorter distance between the tuberculum sellae (TS) and the anterior margin of the optic chiasm. **(c)** Postfixed type, with the optic chiasm above the dorsum sellae.

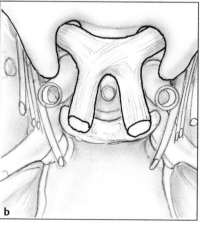

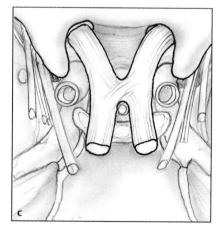

Vascularization

Vascularization occurs mainly from the ophthalmic artery, whereas the optic chiasm is vascularized by perforators from the internal carotid artery, anterior communicating artery, posterior communicating artery, and posterior cerebral artery.

The optic nerve also carries some fibers involved in the pupillary reflexes: retinopretectal tract and retinocollicular tract.

Lesions

The pathophysiological spectrum of the nerve opticus is wide. The visual field deficits associated with skull base pathologies are:

- Blindness, in cases of involvement of the entire nerve
- Bitemporal hemianopsia, due to the compression of the optic chiasm caused by pituitary tumors extending cranially
- Junctional scotoma: monocular central scotoma with contralateral superotemporal field loss, due to a lesion at the optic nerve/chiasm border (see **Fig. 10.2** on page 259).

Pupillary reflexes: see **Table 3.1**.

Typical skull base pathologies involving the optic nerve are pituitary adenomas, craniopharyngiomas, meningiomas, and trauma. The nerves involved in oculomotion are CNs III, IV, and VI (innervating the six extraocular muscles) (see also Chapter 2, **Figs. 2.6** on page 22 and **2.13** on page 44).

Cranial Nerve III: Oculomotor Nerve

The oculomotor nerve has the following functions and attributes:

- It innervates all the extrinsic muscles of the eye, except the lateral rectus and the superior oblique muscles:
  - Inferior rectus: depresses the eye
  - Superior rectus: elevates the eye
  - Medial rectus: adducts the eye
  - Inferior oblique: elevates the eye during eyeball adduction, or rotates it laterally when the eye is abducted
  - Levator palpebrae superioris: raises the eyelid
- It leaves the mesencephalon medially to the cerebral peduncle
- It crosses the roof of the cavernous sinus and enters the orbit via the superior orbital fissure, where it divides into the following:
  - Superior branch: supplying the superior rectus muscle and the levator palpebrae superioris

○ Inferior branch: supplying the medial rectus, inferior rectus, and inferior oblique muscles, as well as some parasympathetic fibers for the ciliary ganglion

Additional information about the oculomotor nerve:

- The parasympathetic fibers originate from the Edinger-Westphal nucleus (in the mesencephalon), innervating the constrictor muscle of the iris, causing miosis, and the ciliary muscles, involved in the control of the shape of the lens (accommodation reflex).
- Five segments of the nerve can be topographically defined: cisternal, petro-clinoid, cavernous, fissural, and orbital.[3]
- The cavernous segment begins at the oculomotor triangle and runs to the superolateral wall of the cavernous sinus, where it reaches the superior orbital fissure.

> **Surgical Anatomy Pearl**
>
> The cisternal segment of the CN III, in the posterior fossa, *always* passes between the superior cerebellar artery and posterior cerebral artery.

Lesions

In the specific innervated extraocular muscles, with associated strabismus or diplopia, the following conditions can occur:

- Lid drop (eyelid ptosis) and mydriasis.
- Oculomotor palsies, which can be isolated or associated with other neuropathies (complex), can be complete or incomplete, and can have varying pupil involvement.
- Complete oculomotor palsy: eye "down-and-out."
- Compressive lesions: sellar region and cavernous sinus tumors; cerebellopontine angle (CPA) tumors (meningioma, schwannoma) or aneurysms (of the posterior cerebral artery [PCA]), giving rise to compression of the parasympathetic fibers, which run peripherally to the nerve and can lead to ipsilateral fixed and dilated pupil.
- Schwannomas of the oculomotor nerve have been described but are very rare.

Cranial Nerve IV: Trochlear Nerve

The trochlear nerve is the only nerve that originates dorsally to the brainstem.

- The trochlear nerve is the smallest cranial nerve, with only 2,400 axons.
- It runs into the lateral wall of the cavernous sinus and enters the orbit via the superior orbital fissure, above the annulus of Zinn, to innervate the superior oblique muscle. This muscle has a tendon that curves around on the

Table 3.1   Anatomic Basis of the Cranial Nerve Reflexes

Function/Reflex	Anatomic Basis
Emotional response to odors	CN I to medial olfactory stria to septal area/subcallosal gyrus
Salivation with odors	CN I to lateral olfactory stria to piriform cortex to amygdala then via stria terminalis to hypothalamus then to superior and inferior salivatory nuclei (medulla)
Accelerated peristalsis and increased gastric secretion with odors ("cephalic" phase of digestion or "gastrocolic" reflex)	CN I to lateral olfactory stria to piriform cortex to amygdala, then via stria terminalis to hypothalamus, then to dorsal motor nucleus of CN X (medulla) to CN X to GI tract
Pupillary light reflex	CN II to retinopretectal tract to pretectum then via pretecto-oculomotor tract to bilateral Edinger-Westphal nuclei to CN III (parasympathetic) to ciliary ganglion to sphincter pupillae muscle
Light-induced circadian rhythms	CN II to retinohypothalamic tract to suprachiasmatic nucleus (SCN) of hypothalamus
"Near" reflex	1. *Pupillary constriction (miosis)*—via bilateral Edinger-Westphal nuclei to CN III (parasympathetic) to ciliary ganglion to sphincter pupillae muscle 2. *Lens accommodation*—via bilateral Edinger-Westphal nuclei to CN III (parasympathetic) to ciliary ganglion to ciliary muscles (contraction causes lens to bulge, increasing diopter power) 3. *Ocular convergence*—via superior colliculus to bilateral CN III (medial rectus)
Corneal reflex	CN V₁ to principal sensory nucleus of CN V to CN VII to orbicularis oculi
Jaw jerk (masseter reflex)	CN V₃ sensory to mesencephalic nucleus of CN V to motor nucleus of CN V to masseter and temporalis
Tearing	CN V₁ to superior salivatory nucleus (medulla) to GSPN parasympathetics (initially in nervus intermedius) to pterygopalatine ganglion to lacrimal gland and mucosa of nose and mouth (palatal and nasal glands)
Crying	Limbic system to hypothalamus to superior salivatory nucleus and lacrimal nucleus (medulla) to GSPN parasympathetics (initially in nervus intermedius) to pterygopalatine ganglion to lacrimal gland and mucosa of nose and mouth (palatal and nasal glands)

Salivation with taste stimulation	Anterior two thirds of tongue to chorda tympani nerve (of CN VII) to geniculate ganglion to rostral nucleus solitarius to superior and inferior salivatory nuclei or posterior one third of tongue to CN IX to rostral nucleus solitarius to superior and inferior salivatory nuclei
Salivation	Superior salivatory nucleus to chorda tympani parasympathetics to submandibular ganglion to submandibular and sublingual glands; inferior salivatory nucleus to CN IX parasympathetics via tympanic nerve (Jacobson's nerve) to LSPN to otic ganglion to parotid gland
Sneezing	CN V sensory to the nucleus ambiguus to the respiratory center of the reticular formation, phrenic nerves, and intercostal muscles
Acoustic reflexes	Mediated by CN VIII (cochlear nerve) to spiral ganglion to ventral cochlear nucleus to *superior olivary complex* to (1) both motor CN VII nuclei to the stapedius muscles to decrease amplitude of sound waves by reducing ossicle movement; and (2) both motor CN V nuclei to the tensor tympani muscles to decrease sensitivity of tympanic membrane by pulling it taut; reflex activated during loud sounds to protect cochlea and during speech production to decrease hearing of one's own speech.
Vestibulo-ocular reflex (VOR)	Keeps visual image still by compensating for horizontal eye movements; left head movement increases activity in left horizontal semicircular canal to CN VIII (vestibular nerve) to superior and medial vestibular nuclei to contralateral CN VI (stimulate right lateral rectus) and via medial longitudinal fasciculus to ipsilateral CN III (stimulate left medial rectus)
Gag reflex	CN IX sensory to caudal nucleus solitarius to nucleus ambiguus to CN X to pharyngeal muscles
Cough reflex	CN X sensory (usually larynx, trachea, or bronchial tree) to caudal nucleus solitarius to medullary respiratory center for forced expiration and to nucleus ambiguus to CN X to muscles of larynx and pharynx for cough
Vomiting reflex	CN X sensory to caudal nucleus solitarius to nucleus ambiguus to CN X to close glottis and also to reticulospinal tract to cause contraction of diaphragm and abdominal muscles; may be stimulated also by increased intracranial pressure and by emetics stimulating the area postrema of caudal medulla

Abbreviations: CN, cranial nerve; GI, gastrointestinal; GSPN, greater superficial petrosal nerve; LSPN, lesser superficial petrosal nerve.
Source: From Binder, Sonne, Fischbein. Cranial Nerves: Anatomy, Pathology, Imaging. New York: Thieme; 2010.

trochlea of the orbit (hence the name of the nerve) to reach the superior part of the eye.

- The contraction of the superior oblique muscle causes the inward rotation as well as the downward and lateral movement of the bulb.
- The cisternal segment runs under the free edge of the tentorium, reaching the cavernous sinus below the petroclinoid ligament.

Lesions

Weakness of the downward movement of the eyeball and vertical diplopia can occur. Trochlear lesions are the most common cause of vertical strabismus. Excyclodeviation, the outer rotation of the globe, can be corrected by instructing the patient to tilt the head to the side opposite the paretic muscle. This paresis makes it very difficult to descend a staircase, for example, or read a newspaper.

- Lesions causing trochlear nerve palsy: trauma (especially orbit trauma), vascular compression, tumors (tentorial meningiomas, or the very rare trochlear schwannoma, which is generally cystic), and iatrogenic causes.

Cranial Nerve V: Trigeminal Nerve

At its origin is on the ventral surface of the pons, the trigeminal nerve has a major branch (portio major, which is sensory) and a minor radix (portio minor, which is motor). Both branches reach the semilunar ganglion (of Gasser), from which the nerve splits mediolaterally into three branches: the ophthalmic nerve (V_1), the maxillary nerve (V_2) and the mandibular nerve (V_3). After exiting the lateral mid-pons level, the trigeminal nerve has a cisternal segment, a Meckel's cave segment, and three peripheral divisions.

Segments

Cisternal Segment

The cisternal segment is a large sensory root (receiving somatosensory sensation from the entire face, except the angle of the jaw innervated by the cervical plexus) called the *portio major* and a smaller motor root called the *portio minor*. The trigeminal cistern surrounds the nerve; the superior petrosal vein complex lies in the cistern's posterolateral space.[4]

Meckel's Cave Segment

Meckel's cave segment passes below the tentorial edge and superior petrosal sinus to reach the interdural layer of Meckel's cave. The abducens nerve is inferomedial to the porus trigeminus. The cave is situated on the trigeminal impression of the bone at the petrous apex and is formed by a dural cleft from the posterior fossa to the posteromedial middle fossa. The arachnoid extends within the cave, forming a pocket along the rootlets of the nerve and the trigeminal ganglion (cistern around the ganglion). The greater superficial nerve is posterolateral to the Meckel's cave.

Divisions

- V_1 enters the lateral wall of the cavernous sinus running in the wall inferior to the trochlear nerve and into the orbit, via the superior orbital fissure, where further divisions occur:
  - **Lacrimal:** It enters the orbit above the annulus of Zinn, innervating the lateral conjunctiva and skin near the lacrimal gland, as well as receiving postganglionic parasympathetic fibers (via the zygomatic and greater superficial petrosal nerve) for lacrimation.
  - **Frontal:** It reaches the orbit above the annulus of Zinn, dividing into the supraorbital nerve (for frontal sinuses, forehead) and supratrochlear nerve (forehead, side of the nose, medial conjunctiva, medial upper lid).
  - **Nasociliary:** It enters the orbit through the annulus of Zinn, branching into the infratrochlear nerve, anterior and posterior ethmoidal nerves, internal and external nasal nerves, long ciliary nerves (which also carry the sympathetic fibers from the internal carotid artery [ICA] to the dilator pupillae muscle), and short ciliary nerves (sensation for the globe, also carrying postganglionic parasympathetic fibers from the oculomotor nerve and ciliary ganglion to the sphincter pupillae and ciliary muscle).
  - **Meningeal branches**: for the dura of the anterior and middle cranial fossae, tentorium cerebelli, and cavernous sinus.
- V_2 runs in the inferolateral wall of the cavernous sinus, enters the pterygopalatine fossa via the foramen rotundum, and reaches the orbit via the inferior orbital fissure (infraorbital nerve).
  - Branches in the pterygopalatine fossa (see **Fig. 2.12**)
    - **Infraorbital nerve**: It enters the orbit via the inferior orbital fissure, travels in a canal to exit on the splanchnocranium via the infraorbital foramen, where it innervates the midportion of the face. Branches of the infraorbital nerve are: alveolar nerves, inferior palpebral nerves, external nasal branches, and superior labial branches to the upper lip.
    - **Zygomatic nerve:** It enters the orbit via the inferior orbital fissure (IOF), to give rise to the zygomaticotemporal nerve (running in the lateral wall of the orbit and exiting through the zygomaticotemporal foramen). It innervates the lateral side of the forehead and the angle of the orbit. The zygomaticofacial nerve exits the zygomaticofacial foramen (which is a landmark in the orbitozygomatic approaches) to innervate the skin of the cheek and has postganglionic parasympathetic fibers for lacrimation.

- Palatine nerves, posterior superior nasal nerve (to the septum and lateral wall of the nasal fossa, via the sphenopalatine foramen), orbital branches, pharyngeal branches.
- V_3 carries a sensory component and the motor component of the minor branch of CN V, exiting the base of the skull via the oval foramen. V_3 gives rise to branches innervating the tensor muscle of velum palatinum and the tensor of the tympanum (the latter involved in the regulation of sound intensity).
  - Meningeal recurrent branch, medial pterygoid nerve, masseteric nerve, deep temporal nerves, buccal nerve, lateral pterygoid nerve, auriculotemporal nerve, lingual nerve (for innervation of the mucosa of the mouth, gums, and anterior two thirds of the tongue, joined by the chorda tympani from the facial nerve, which also provides parasympathetic innervation to the submandibular gland), inferior alveolar nerve.
- The motor component innervates the chewing muscles (masseter; temporal, medial, and lateral pterygoid muscles; tensor tympani, involved in the acoustic reflexes; tensor veli palatini, involved in the mechanism of control of the pressure in the middle ear; mylohyoid; anterior belly of the digastric muscle).

Functions

The sensory branches of the trigeminal nerve carry touch, pain, thermal, and proprioceptive information from the whole face, conjunctiva, cornea, orbit, frontal sinuses, nasal cavity, palate, nasopharynx, and meninges.

Lesions

Hypo-anesthesia in somatic sensations, such as light touch, pain, or temperature, and paresthesias/dysesthesias can occur. The most common neurologic condition associated with the trigeminal nerve is trigeminal neuralgia, a lancinating pain in the specific territories innervated by the branches of CN V. The condition can be idiopathic, secondary to neurovascular compression (see Section 22.8, page 615), or secondary to tumors.

Motor Evaluation

With the mouth open, the jaw deviates toward the paralyzed side (due to the contralateral pterygoid muscle action).

Pathology

In the posterior fossa, tumors can affect the cisternal segments of the trigeminal nerve. In the middle cranial fossa, and extracranially, the nerve may be compressed/injured by tumors or trauma.

Cranial Nerve VI: Abducens Nerve

The abducens nerve innervates the lateral rectus muscle, which makes "abduction" (lateral movement) of the eye possible. The abducens nerve has the following attributes:

- It emerges from the lateroventral side of the brainstem, between the pons and medulla, medial to the facial nerve, therefore entering the cavernous sinus via the dura/periosteum on the lateral clivus and the Dorello's canal in the petrous apex.
- In the cavernous sinus, it runs free, unlike the other intracavernous nerves, which are included in the meningeal lateral wall.
- It enters the orbit via the superior orbital fissure.
- Topographically, five segments can be identified: cisternal, gulfar, cavernous, fissural, and intraconal.[5]

> **Surgical Anatomy Pearl**
>
> The abducens nerve is therefore the only true intracavernous nerve! In the cavernous sinus it is lateral to the ICA and medial to V_1.

Lesions

- Impaired lateral gaze and paralysis of the abduction of the eye, which can be a sign of increased intracranial pressure.

Skull base pathologies causing CN VI palsy: CPA tumors, clival meningioma, or chordoma.

Cranial Nerve VII: Facial Nerve

The facial nerve emerges from the brainstem in two distinct bundles: the motor branch and the nerve intermedius (it is "intermedius" between the motor CNs VII and VIII, carrying sensory and parasympathetic fibers). The facial nerve crosses the petrous bone (via the internal auditory canal) to reach the geniculate ganglion (neurons involved in taste). It leaves the skull base, emerging from the stylomastoid foramen, to cross the parotid gland and innervate facial muscles involved in facial mimicking, and the stapedial muscle involved in the control of sound intensity (like the muscle tensor tympani, innervated by CN V). Sensory fibers also innervate the external part of the tympanic membrane.

Functions

The facial nerve innervates the muscles of facial expression, including the orbicularis oculi, orbicularis oris, zygomaticus major, levator and depressor anguli oris muscles, risorius, mentalis, buccinators, frontalis, occipitalis, corrugator supercilii, platysma, as well as the stapedius, stylohyoid, and the posterior belly of the digastric muscle. It has the following functions:

- Provides parasympathetic innervation to the lacrimal gland (via greater superficial petrosal nerve [GSPN]), oral and nasal mucosa (via GSPN), submandibular and sublingual glands (via chorda tympani).
- Supplies somatosensory information from the auricle and retroauricular area, and external auditory meatus.
- Provides taste information for the anterior two thirds of the tongue, and sensory information for the hard and soft palate (chorda tympani).

The nervus intermedius is the sensory and parasympathetic component of CN VII. It is involved in the sensation of taste (anterior two thirds of the tongue), via the chorda tympani, and also the cutaneous sensation of the external auditory canal. The parasympathetic component of CN VII is responsible for control of the salivary glands (except the parotid gland, which is innervated by CN IX via the otic ganglion) via the superior petrous nerve.

Segments

Cisternal Segment

The cisternal segment goes from the ventrolateral pons to the internal auditory canal, together with the statoacoustic nerves and the labyrinthine artery and vein.

Intracanalicular (Meatal) Segment

The meatus is divided into four quadrants. The meatal segment is located in the anterosuperior quadrant.

Labyrinthine Segment

The labyrinthine segment comes from the fundus of the internal auditory canal (IAC), and courses through the petrous bone superior and anterior to the cochlea to reach the geniculate ganglion, which gives rise to the anteromedially directed greater superficial petrosal nerve at the first (or anterior) genu of the facial nerve. At the genu the nerve takes an acute turn (ranging from 40 to 86 degrees) posteriorly toward the medial aspect of the middle ear cavity into the tympanic segment of the facial nerve.

Tympanic Segment

Following the first genu, the tympanic segment travels behind the cochleariform process and tensor tympani muscle and continues its course inferior to the lateral semicircular canal and superolateral to the oval window. The course of the tympanic segment can be visualized as the prominence of the facial canal within the middle ear.

Mastoid Segment

The second (or posterior) genu marks the beginning of the mastoid segment of the facial nerve. Once the facial nerve reaches the posterior wall of the middle ear cavity at the pyramidal eminence, it turns inferiorly at the second genu (ranging from 92 to 125 degrees) and continues to course through the medial aspect of the mastoid bone to exit the skull through the stylomastoid foramen. From this segment, three branches emerge:

- Nerve of the stapedius muscle
- Chorda tympani (in ~ 5% of the cases it can arise distally to the stylomastoid foramen)
- Sensory auricular branch

This segment leaves the skull base at the level of the stylomastoid foramen, entering the parotid gland, where it divides into the peripheral divisions (temporal, zygomatic, buccal, marginal mandibular, and cervical branches).

Lesions

Ipsilateral facial palsy, loss of taste of the anterior two thirds of the tongue, and hyperacusia can occur (see also Bell's palsy in Chapter 8).

The CPA lesions are tumors such as vestibular schwannoma, epidermoid, or meningioma.

> **Surgical Anatomy Pearl**
>
> Facial schwannoma is very rare, and greater petrosal nerve schwannomas are even rarer.

- Hemifacial spasm may be due to neurovascular compression.
- Geniculate neuralgia: Hunt's neuralgia, affecting the nervus intermedius, with paroxysmal otalgia.
- Posttraumatic, parotid-facial malignancies.

Cranial Nerve VIII: Vestibulocochlear Nerve

The vestibulocochlear nerve is formed by two distinct nerves, the vestibular nerve (providing balance information, formed by a superior and an inferior branch) and the cochlear nerve (hearing). The nerve crosses the skull base at the IAC, and is formed by axons originating from sensory receptors of the vestibulocochlear organ (cochlea, labyrinth, and semicircular canals) in the internal ear. The nerve enters the brainstem posteriorly to the facial nerve at the lateral

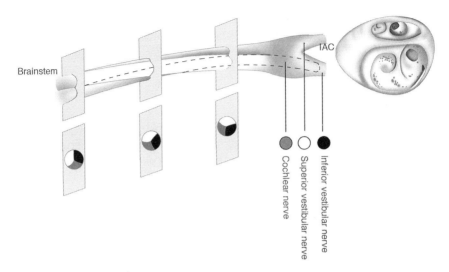

Fig. 3.3 Right-sided vestibulocochlear complex. Note the changed relationship of the nerves from the brainstem to the internal auditory canal (IAC). (Adapted from Koos WT, Matula C, Lang J. Color Atlas of Microneurosurgery of Acoustic Neurinomas. New York, Stuttgart: Georg Thieme Verlag; 2002.)

recess of the fourth ventricle, at the pontomedullary junctions. The relationships of the vestibular and cochlear components of CN VIII change from the brainstem to the IAC, twisting clockwise on the right side and counterclockwise on the left side[6,7] (**Fig. 3.3**).

Lesions

Damage to the cochlear component gives rise to tinnitus or hearing loss, whereas dysfunction of the vestibular apparatus results in dizziness and abnormal eye movements (nystagmus), oscillopsia, and vertigo (see also Chapter 8).

Cranial Nerve IX: Glossopharyngeal Nerve

The glossopharyngeal nerve is formed by several rootlets emerging laterally from the medulla of the brainstem, from the postolivary sulcus (between the olive and the inferior cerebellar peduncle), converging together in the nerve, which exits the skull base through the jugular foramen. The cisternal part is 15 mm long, and before exiting it releases the Jacobson's nerve (tympanic nerve) to the middle ear. At the level of the jugular foramen, the superior and inferior petrosal ganglia can be found.

Functions

- The glossopharyngeal nerve provides sensation to the posterior part of the tongue (general sensation and taste), in addition to some parts of the skin around the ear, and to the internal part of the tympanic membrane, pharynx, and carotid glomus (the latter structure is involved in monitoring the oxygen tension in blood).
- The Jacobson's nerve has parasympathetic innervation to the parotid gland and sensory information from the tympanic membrane and eustachian tube. It also provides the nerve to the carotid sinus (Hering's nerve).
- The glossopharyngeal nerve provides motor function to the stylopharyngeus muscle and part of the superior pharyngeal constrictor.
  - Parasympathetic to the parotid gland (via the lesser superficial petrosal nerve).
  - Sensory information from the posterior external ear, tragus, posterior one third of the tongue (also taste in this part of the tongue), soft palate, nasopharynx, tympanic membrane, eustachian tube, and mastoid region.
  - Visceral sensory information from the carotid body and carotid sinus.

Lesions

Mild dysphagia; loss of taste over the posterior part of the tongue; loss of sensation of the palate, and the posterior part of the tongue; and sometimes otalgia can occur.

Posterior Fossa Lesions

Schwannoma, meningiomas, trauma, or neurovascular compression can occur, causing glossopharyngeal neuralgia (see page 618).

Cranial Nerve X: Vagus Nerve

The vagus nerve "wanders" within the body, due to the long course of the nerve from the brainstem to the colon, reaching several organs in the thorax and abdomen.

- Several roots exit the medulla, from the postolivary sulcus, converging into the nerve, which leaves the skull through the jugular foramen. In the foramen, the nerve lies in the posterior part of the foramen (pars vascularis), with CN XI.
- The superior jugular ganglion in the jugular foramen is also joined by CN XI, giving rise to a meningeal branch and Arnold's nerve (auricular branch).
- The inferior ganglion conveys visceral and special sensory information.

Functions

The vagus nerve provides motor function to the pharyngeal and laryngeal muscles and palatoglossus.

- Parasympathetic fibers to the smooth muscles and glands of the pharynx, larynx, heart, esophagus, stomach, and colon
- Somatic sensory information from the external auditory meatus, tympanic membrane (external surface), dura of the posterior fossa, and larynx
- Visceral afferent from several abdominal/thorax organs
- Sensory for taste from epiglottis, hard and soft palate, and pharynx

Lesions

Paralysis of the vocal fold can occur, resulting in dysphonia.

Skull Base Lesions

Posterior fossa tumors (e.g., meningioma, schwannoma, paraganglioma) can cause CN X dysfunction.

Cranial Nerve XI: Accessory Nerve

The accessory nerve is formed by axons coming from the upper cervical spinal cord, ascending into the cranium through the foramen magnum, and converging into the nerve, which leaves the skull through the jugular foramen. The cranial radices of CN XI (pars vagalis) come from the nucleus of the vagus nerve, which is why the nerve is defined as the accessory nerve of the vagus. The accessory nerve innervates the sternocleidomastoid and trapezius muscles.

Lesions

Drop of the shoulder, with downward and lateral rotation of the scapula, can occur, in addition to weakness in the rotation of the head.

Cranial Nerve XII: Hypoglossal Nerve

From the hypoglossal nerve's nucleus in the medulla oblongata, the axons emerge from the brainstem from the preolivary sulcus (between the inferior olive and the pyramid) in several rootlets, which, after a cisternal course of about 15 mm, converge in two bundles, which then run into the hypoglossal canal, anteriorly to the occipital condylus. The hypoglossal nerve innervates all the extrinsic muscles of the tongue (except the palatoglossus muscle, which is innervated by the vagus nerve).

Examination Pearl

For the contralateral innervation of the muscles of the tongue, a peripheral lesion of the nerve causes deviation of the tongue toward the side of the inactive muscle (because of the action of the contralateral functioning muscles).

Typical Signs of Hypoglossal Dysfunction

Paresis, atrophy, and fibrillations can occur, as can fasciculations of the affected half tongue, which leads to dysarthria (especially with lingual consonants like D, T, and L).

Cranial Nerve Reflexes

See **Box 3.1** and **Table 3.1.**

Box 3.1   Summary of Cranial Nerve Reflexes

CN	Reflex
I	Odor-induced salivation, emotional response, gastric secretion
II–III	Miosis, accommodation, ocular convergence
V–VII	Corneal, glabellar, masseter reflexes, tearing
VIII–	–VII and –V: acoustic reflexes
	–III and –VI: vestibulo-ocular reflex
IX–X	Gag, cough, vomiting reflexes

◼ Intraoperative Neuromonitoring of the Cranial Nerves

- Intraoperative nerve monitoring aims to minimize iatrogenic injury with subsequent nerve dysfunction,[8] and provides prognostic information on the functional outcome by assessing the nerve integrity after the surgical dissection.[9]
- Various monitors provide simultaneous monitoring of several cranial nerves as well as monopolar/bipolar stimulation.
- Monopolar and bipolar stimulation provide a useful aid in nerve localization. Bipolar stimulation provides more precise localization (greater spatial

selectivity), but it has a lower sensitivity compared with monopolar mapping, and is used only during differentiation of adjacent nerves.[9]

Cranial Nerve II

Flash stimulation by means of fiber optic cables can be used during surgery for monitoring of visual evoked potentials (VEPs). Electroretinograms are another tool for intraoperative electrophysiological monitoring.

- Generally, the dominating peak of the VEP is P100 (positive 75–100 ms), with an inconstant N70 (negative ~ 70 ms), both generated in the visual cortex. However, false-positives (intraoperative VEP changes with no postoperative deficits) and false-negatives (normal VEP with postoperative deficits) have been shown; therefore, VEP is not very useful in skull base surgery and optic nerve decompression.

Motor Cranial Nerve Monitoring

There are several types of intraoperative techniques, with electromyographic (EMG) monitoring being the most used.[10-12]

Electromyograms of specific muscles/muscles-groups are generated by means of transdermal intramuscular electrodes.[10] The responses can be monitored on an oscilloscope and heard by a loudspeaker[11] equipped with circuitry for stimulus artifact suppression

Surgical Pearls

- The pair of electrodes needed should be placed deep in the muscle, parallel to each other at a distance of ~ 2 mm. Remember to position the ground electrode and the anode of the monopolar stimulator (shoulder, on the clavicle, etc.).
- Avoid muscle relaxant use!

Cranial Nerves III, IV, and VI

Monitoring of the extraocular muscle and the intracavernous cranial nerves can be performed during surgery in the parasellar space.[13] The muscles monitored are the medial and inferior rectus muscles (CN III), superior oblique (CN IV), and lateral rectus (CN VI).

- The needle electrode or wire hooks (or even small ring electrodes placed under the eyelids[14]) have to be placed percutaneously in or at least very close to the muscles, taking care so as not to injure the eyeball.

- Stimulation parameters may be slightly higher than the ones used for facial nerve stimulation (1–1.5 V at impulses of 100 μs). The recorded potentials amplitudes are in the range of 0.2 to 1 mV.

Cranial Nerve V

In surgery of the CPA, it may be useful to monitor the function of the portio minor of the trigeminal nerve. The muscles monitored are the digastricus and masseter.

- Trigeminal evoked potentials are part of the somatosensory evoked potentials (SSEPs), but are rarely used in intraoperative monitoring, and due to a lack of standardization on the interpretation of the values, have minimal value in skull base surgery, except for some limited applications in trigeminal rhizotomy in patients with trigeminal neuralgia.[15]

Cranial Nerve VII

Recording of the facial EMG is one of the most often used intracranial nerve monitoring techniques, especially in CPA surgery. The muscles monitored include the orbicularis oculi/superior frontalis, orbicularis oris muscles, and mentalis.

- Parameters of stimulation: 4 Hz, pulse 100 μs, intensities vary between 0.01 and 1 mA.
- Stimulation creates a typical "pulse response" and a synchronous compound muscle action potential. The mechanical evoked responses can be seen as a "burst" or "train" responses.[11] Surgical manipulation of the facial nerve may trigger a synchronous compound muscle action potential.
- After surgical removal of the tumor, a potential unresponsive to electric stimulation of the facial nerve may suggest the need to perform a graft.
- Direct electrical stimulation and evoked muscular responses are not only used for localization and confirmation of the functional integrity of the nerve, but also for prognostication. The proximal (root entry zone) and distal portion (at the fundus of the IAC) of the nerve can be stimulated. A facial nerve response elicited by a proximal stimulation in the range of 0.05 to 0.1 mA is an indicator of good postoperative function. Amplitudes of the responses from the proximal and distal stimulations > 200 mV are also good indicators. When a threshold > 0.3 mA has to be used for eliciting nerve function, the functional prognosis is generally worse. One of the parameters used for prognostication is the percent maximum (%max), where the evoked response of each patient is compared to the supramaximal response.[16] The increase in the intraoperative percent maximum responses has been associated with a good facial outcome.[17]

Hearing and Auditory Evoked Potentials Monitoring

Among the different potentials generated within the auditory system, the auditory brainstem-evoked response (ABR, also called brainstem auditory evoked potential [BAEP]), the electrocochleographic (ECoG or EcochG) potentials, and the nerve direct potentials (NAPs) are the most often used measures.

Lower Cranial Nerves Monitoring

The muscles monitored include the stylopharyngeus muscle (CN IX), vocalis (CN X), trapezius and sternocleidomastoid muscles (CN XI), hypoglossus, and genioglossus (CN XII).

- The recording electrodes for monitoring the stylopharyngeus muscle can be placed in the soft palate ipsilateral to the side of the operation.
- The electrodes for monitoring the recurrent nerve (branch of the vagus nerve) may be placed in the laryngeal musculature via a laryngoscope, or can be coupled with the endotracheal tube (see Chapter 11, page 280). A percutaneous placement in the criocothyroid muscle is also feasible.[18] Vagus nerve stimulation is generally not advisable due to the possible heart block and blood pressure interaction.
- Stimulation of CN XI may cause intense contractions of the neck, which can be dangerous in patients with their head fixed in the clamp.
- CN XII monitoring may be advisable in cases of surgery in the foramen magnum and clivus regions.[19]

■ References

Boldfaced references are of particular importance.

1. Renn WH, Rhoton AL Jr. Microsurgical anatomy of the sellar region. J Neurosurg 1975;43:288–298
2. Rhoton ALJ. Anatomy of the pituitary gland and sellar region. In: Thapar K, Kovacs K, Scheithauer BW, Lloyd RV, eds. Diagnosis and Management of Pituitary Tumors. Totowa, NJ: Humana Press; 2000:13–40
3. **Iaconetta G, de Notaris M, Cavallo LM, et al. The oculomotor nerve: microanatomical and endoscopic study. Neurosurgery 2010;66:593–601, discussion 601**
4. **Joo W, Yoshioka F, Funaki T, Mizokami K, Rhoton AL Jr. Microsurgical anatomy of the trigeminal nerve. Clin Anat 2014;27:61–88**
5. **Iaconetta G, Fusco M, Cavallo LM, Cappabianca P, Samii M, Tschabitscher M. The abducens nerve: microanatomic and endoscopic study. Neurosurgery 2007;61(3, Suppl):7–14, discussion 14**
6. Day JD, Tschabitscher M. Microsurgical Dissection of the Cranial Base. New York: Churchill Livingstone; 1996
7. **Koos WT, Matula C, Lang J. Color Atlas of Microneurosurgery of Acoustic Neurinomas. New York, Stuttgart: Georg Thieme Verlag; 2002**

8. Maurer J, Pelster H, Amedee RG, Mann WJ. Intraoperative monitoring of motor cranial nerves in skull base surgery. Skull Base Surg 1995;5:169–175

9. Kartush JM, Larouere MJ, Graham MD, Bouchard KR, Audet BV. Intraoperative cranial nerve monitoring during posterior skull base surgery. Skull Base Surg 1991;1:85–92

10. Møller AR, Jannetta PJ. Preservation of facial function during removal of acoustic neuromas. Use of monopolar constant-voltage stimulation and EMG. J Neurosurg 1984; 61:757–760

11. Prass RL, Lüders H. Acoustic (loudspeaker) facial electromyographic monitoring: Part 1. Evoked electromyographic activity during acoustic neuroma resection. Neurosurgery 1986;19:392–400

12. Harner SG, Daube JR, Ebersold MJ, Beatty CW. Improved preservation of facial nerve function with use of electrical monitoring during removal of acoustic neuromas. Mayo Clin Proc 1987;62:92–102

13. Sekhar LN, Pomeranz S, Sen CN. Management of tumours involving the cavernous sinus. Acta Neurochir Suppl (Wien) 1991;53:101–112

14. Sekiya T, Hatayama T, Iwabuchi T, Maeda S. A ring electrode to record extraocular muscle activities during skull base surgery. Acta Neurochir (Wien) 1992;117:66–69

15. Stechison MT, Kralick FJ. The trigeminal evoked potential: part I. Long-latency responses in awake or anesthetized subjects. Neurosurgery 1993;33:633–638

16. Lin VY, Houlden D, Bethune A, et al. A novel method in predicting immediate postoperative facial nerve function post acoustic neuroma excision. Otol Neurotol 2006; 27:1017–1022

17. Arnoldner C, Mick P, Pirouzmand F, et al. Facial nerve prognostication in vestibular schwannoma surgery: the concept of percent maximum and its predictability. Laryngoscope 2013;123:2533–2538

18. Stechison MT. Vagus nerve monitoring: percutaneous versus vocal fold electrode recording. Am J Otol 1995;16:703–706

19. Møller AR. Intraoperative Neurophysiological Monitoring. 3rd Edition. Springer, 2011

4 Skull Base Embryology

■ Development of the Skull Base[1-17]:

- The skull base undergoes a complex sequence of developmental stages, especially in the first 12 weeks of fetal development.[1-4]
- The rostral neural crest cells form the whole viscerocranium and the rostral part of the neurocranium.[1,2]
- Migration of neural crest cells around the embryonic pharynx leads to formation of six pairs of embryonic arches.

> **Pearl**
>
> Skull base development failure is associated with anencephaly.[5]

- Neural crest cells of the first two branchial arches form the bones and connective tissue of the skull.
- Chondrification occurs for condensation of neural crest-derived mesenchyme.
- Endochondral ossification of the skull base is predominant.
- First skeletal structures to differentiate: viscerocranium, occipital bone, and cartilage of the skull base.
- Skull base foramina develop as cartilage condensation around cranial nerves and blood vessels *before* bones are formed.[2]
- The chorda dorsalis is the rostral tip of the notochord, at the caudal level of the hypophysis, and represents the beginning of the skull base development.

> **Pearl**
>
> Both mesoderm and ectoderm give rise to skull base development.[2,6,7]

- Multiple centers of chondrification form chondroblasts around week 7: presphenoid cartilage, basisphenoid cartilage, nasal capsule, orbitosphenoid, alisphenoid, otic capsule, parachordal cartilage, occipital somites.
- The ossification of the chondrobasicranium (basal plate) begins at week 8, and it is perforated by the preexisting cranial nerves and blood vessels[8] (**Fig. 4.1** and **Table 4.1**).
- The parachordal cartilage forms the basioccipital elements (occipital bone and foramen magnum) at the 7th week. Exo-occipital somitic components contribute to the formation of the occipital bone and its elements, which is

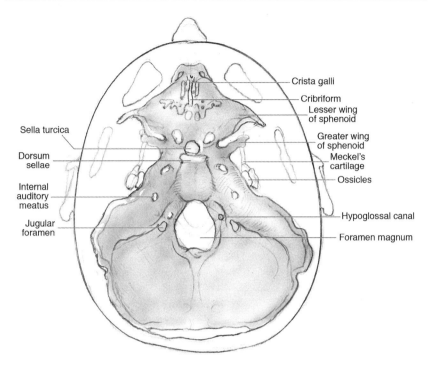

Crista galli

Cribriform

Lesser wing
of sphenoid

Sella turcica

Greater wing
of sphenoid

Dorsum
sellae

Meckel's
cartilage

Ossicles

Internal
auditory
meatus

Jugular
foramen

Hypoglossal canal

Foramen magnum

Fig. 4.1   Ossification of the chondrobasicranium (seventh to eighth weeks).

why the occipital bone represents a vertebral element that has expanded to support the brain.[6,7,9-11]

- During formation of the basioccipital elements, different developmental variants of the occipital condyles and craniovertebral ligaments may cause anatomic variants in the craniovertebral junction (e.g., "occipitalization" of the atlas, caused by ossification of the atlanto-occipital joint).[12]
- The ossification of the occipital bone also occurs around the hypoglossal nerves, giving rise to the formation of the hypoglossal canals.
- During the formation of the skull base cartilage, the adenohypophysial pouch remains connected to the roof of the oral cavity (Rathke's pouch). After further differentiation, the sella turcica and the sellar fossa are formed.
- The presphenoid cartilages, the cartilaginous basis for the jugum of the sphenoid body, differentiate last within the medial aspect of the cranial base and bridge the gap between the postsphenoid and the cartilaginous nasal capsule (already developed by the third month of fetal development).

Pearl

The persistence of this communication gives rise to the craniopharyngeal canal.

Table 4.1   Summary of the Primary Centers of Ossification of the Skull Base[26]

Anatomic Part	Appearance Period of the Primary Ossification Center	Time of Fusion
Occipital bone (basioccipital and exo-occipital parts)	3rd embryonic month	1–4 years of life
Sphenoidal bone (wing, basisphenoidal and presphenoidal parts, lingula, hamulus pterygoideus)	2nd–3rd embryonic months	From the 4th fetal month to the end of the 1st year of life
Ethmoidal bone	5th–6th fetal months	6–16 years of life
Temporal bone		
Pars petrosa	5th–6th fetal months	1st year of life
Pars squamosa	3rd embryonic month	
Pars tympanica	4th fetal month	
Inner ear ossicles		
Malleus	2nd–6th embryonic months	6th fetal month
Incus	6th fetal month	
Stapes	6th fetal month	
Nasal bone	10th–11th months of life	
Lacrimal bone	End of the 3rd embryonic month	
Zygomatic bone	3rd month of life	
Palatal bone	8th–9th month of life	
Vomer	3rd embryonic month	

- The foramen cecum represents a transient opening of the anterior skull base. At this stage, a temporary fontanel, the fonticulus frontalis, divides the inferior frontal bone from the nasal bone.[13] All these structures regress during development, persisting in some pathological variants.
- The ossification of a cartilaginous bridge between the orbit and the presphenoid cartilage gives rise to the lesser wing of the sphenoid bone. Ossification of the cartilage around the optic nerve forms the optic canal.
- Around the otocyst, mesenchymal condensation leads to formation of the cochlea and semicircular canals followed by chondrogenesis around the vestibulocochlear nerve to create the internal acoustic meatus. Adjacent chondrogenesis around the carotid arteries forms the carotid canals.
- Skeletogenesis and apoptosis are important during the final process of skull development.
- In rare cases, fibrous dysplasia alters ossification of the skull resulting in replacement of the bone structure with fibrous tissue.[14,15]

- Because of its central position and regulation of adjacent differentiation during ongoing craniofacial development, malformations like craniosynostosis commonly manifest within the spheno-occipital synchondrosis.[16] In normal conditions, this synchondrosis closes between the ages of 13 and 18 years.[17]

■ Nasal Embryology

The developmental stages of the nose are described as follows[18–22]:

- Nasal structures are derived from the frontonasal process, an ectodermal structure that develops over the forebrain, and from the maxillary process, a structure from the first branchial arch, which contributes to the floor of the nasal cavity and the septum.[18]
- At 4 to 8 weeks' gestation, the frontonasal process contributes to the olfactory placodes induced by the olfactory bulb.
  - Medial and lateral nasal prominences develop around the placodes to eventually become nares.
  - Nasal placodes deepen, leading to the development of the nasal pit and the nasal sac.
- Intranasally, the frontonasal process contributes to the nasal capsule, which has two portions:
  - Mesethmoid: precursor of the nasal septum.
  - Lateral ectethmoid: precursor of the lateral nasal wall and the turbinates.
- The nasal septum develops from the posterior frontonasal process in a superior to inferior direction and from extensions of mesodermal tissues from the maxillary processes.
  - Simultaneously, the palate is created by both primary and secondary palatal shelves merging in the midline within the axial plane, which merges with the septum.
- Sixth week: The lateral nasal wall is formed by mesenchymal tissue.
- Seventh week: The turbinates begin to form from furrows within the lateral nasal wall.
  - First ethmoturbinal: The ascending portion forms the agger nasi, whereas the descending portion forms the uncinate process.
  - Second ethmoturbinal: middle turbinate.
  - Third ethmoturbinal: superior turbinate.
  - Fourth and fifth ethmoturbinal: fuse to form the variably present supreme turbinate.
- Tenth week: Within the lateral nasal wall, invagination of the middle meatus immediately posterior to uncinate process results in the formation of the maxillary sinus (first sinus to develop).

- Week 14: Further invagination of the middle meatus results in the formation of the anterior ethmoid sinuses.
  - Invagination of the floor of the superior meatus results in the formation of the posterior ethmoid sinuses.
- Weeks 17 to 21 (fourth fetal month):
  - Frontal sinus begins to develop at this time, most commonly from either an ethmoid cell within the infundibulum or a laterally placed ethmoid cell within the frontal recess.
    - The frontal sinus remains small at birth and is essentially undetectable, but is often distinguishable at age 1.
    - At age 5 years, pneumatization of the vertical portion of the frontal bone occurs.
  - Sphenoid sinus arises from an evagination of the posterior nasal capsule and is represented as such at birth.
    - It remains small until the age of 3 years, when it begins to pneumatize the sphenoid bone proper.
    - At age 7 years, the sinus pneumatizes to the level of the sella turcica.
- Week 36: The nasal cavity is developed to adult proportions, but sinuses continue to develop well into adolescence.
- Order of developmental completion: ethmoid, maxillary, sphenoid, frontal sinuses.

■ Embryology of the Meninges

Precursors are derived from the neural crest and mesodermal cells. A single layer of cells surrounds the neural tube at 22 to 24 days of gestation, later covered by a thicker layer of mesenchymal cells (24–28 days), which envelop the brain at 33 to 41 days. These layers are the substrate of the primary meninx,[19,20] which is clearly divided into two distinct layers at 34 to 48 days: the ectomeninx, which is the external layer and gives rise to the dura mater; and the endomeninx, which forms the pia mater at 45 to 55 days. The arachnoidal layer appears much later during fetal development. Skull base meninges may arise from the cephalic mesoderm, having different origins of the telencephalic meninges, which come from the neural crest cells.[21,22]

■ Embryology of the Craniovertebral Junction

At the fourth week of gestation, four occipital sclerotomes give rise to the basioocciput (first and second sclerotome), the jugular tubercles (third sclerotome), and the exoccipital structures, concurring together to be in line with the foramen magnum. The fourth sclerotome gives rise to the proatlas, with its three components (the hypocentrum, the centrum, and the neural arch) forming the anterior tubercle of the clivus, the occipital condyles, the posterior arch of C1, and the lateral atlantal masses. The first two spinal sclerotomes give rise to the other portions of C1 and C2. The formation of these structures concurs at the lining of the foramen magnum.[23–25]

- At birth, the odontoid process is separated from the body of C2 by the neural central synchondrosis (vestigial disk), which is present in most children younger than 4 years of age but disappears by 8 years of age. The tip of the odontoid is not ossified at birth; its ossification center fuses with the other centers at about 12 years of age.
- The expansion of the posterior fossa is mediated by a balance of endocranial reabsorption, sutural growth, and bony accretion. Deficits in this process may give rise to different pathologies, such as the Chiari malformation.

■ References

Boldfaced references are of particular importance.

1. Nie X. Cranial base in craniofacial development: developmental features, influence on facial growth, anomaly, and molecular basis. Acta Odontol Scand 2005;63:127–135
2. **McBratney-Owen B, Iseki S, Bamforth SD, Olsen BR, Morriss-Kay GM. Development and tissue origins of the mammalian cranial base. Dev Biol 2008;322:121–132**
3. Santaolalla-Montoya F, Martinez-Ibargüen A, Sánchez-Fernández JM, Sánchez-del-Rey A. Principles of cranial base ossification in humans and rats. Acta Otolaryngol 2012;132:349–354
4. **Di Ieva A, Bruner E, Haider T, et al. Skull base embryology: a multidisciplinary review. Childs Nerv Syst 2014;30:991–1000**
5. Lomholt JF, Fischer-Hansen B, Keeling JW, Reintoft I, Kjaer I. Subclassification of anencephalic human fetuses according to morphology of the posterior cranial fossa. Pediatr Dev Pathol 2004;7:601–606
6. Balczerski B, Zakaria S, Tucker AS, et al. Distinct spatiotemporal roles of hedgehog signalling during chick and mouse cranial base and axial skeleton development. Dev Biol 2012;371:203–214
7. Couly GF, Coltey PM, Le Douarin NM. The triple origin of skull in higher vertebrates: a study in quail-chick chimeras. Development 1993;117:409–429
8. **Ricciardelli EJ. Embryology and anatomy of the cranial base. Clin Plast Surg 1995; 22:361–372**
9. Evans DJ, Noden DM. Spatial relations between avian craniofacial neural crest and paraxial mesoderm cells. Dev Dyn 2006;235:1310–1325
10. Couly GF, Coltey PM, Le Douarin NM. The developmental fate of the cephalic mesoderm in quail-chick chimeras. Development 1992;114:1–15

11. Kuratani S. Craniofacial development and the evolution of the vertebrates: the old problems on a new background. Zoolog Sci 2005;22:1–19
12. Al-Motabagani MA, Surendra M. Total occipitalization of the atlas. Anat Sci Int 2006; 81:173–180
13. Hedlund G. Congenital frontonasal masses: developmental anatomy, malformations, and MR imaging. Pediatr Radiol 2006;36:647–662, quiz 726–727
14. Davies ML, Macpherson P. Fibrous dysplasia of the skull: disease activity in relation to age. Br J Radiol 1991;64:576–579
15. Bowers CA, Taussky P, Couldwell WT. Surgical treatment of craniofacial fibrous dysplasia in adults. Neurosurg Rev 2014;37:47–53
16. Smartt JM Jr, Karmacharya J, Gannon FH, et al. Intrauterine fetal constraint induces chondrocyte apoptosis and premature ossification of the cranial base. Plast Reconstr Surg 2005;116:1363–1369
17. Scheuer L. Application of osteology to forensic medicine. Clin Anat 2002;15:297–312
18. Halewyck S, Louryan S, Van Der Veken P, Gordts F. Craniofacial embryology and postnatal development of relevant parts of the upper respiratory system. B-ENT 2012; 8(Suppl 19):5–11
19. Barshes N, Demopoulos A, Engelhard HH. Anatomy and physiology of the leptomeninges and CSF space. Cancer Treat Res 2005;125:1–16
20. **Mack J, Squier W, Eastman JT. Anatomy and development of the meninges: implications for subdural collections and CSF circulation. Pediatr Radiol 2009;39:200–210**
21. Catala M. Embryonic and fetal development of structures associated with the cerebro-spinal fluid in man and other species. Part I: The ventricular system, meninges and choroid plexuses. Arch Anat Cytol Pathol 1998;46:153–169
22. **Perry A, Gutmann DH, Reifenberger G. Molecular pathogenesis of meningiomas. J Neurooncol 2004;70:183–202**
23. Ganguly DN, Roy KK. A study on the craniovertebral joint in man. Anat Anz 1964; 114:433–452
24. **Pang D, Thompson DN. Embryology and bony malformations of the craniovertebral junction. Childs Nerv Syst 2011;27:523–564**
25. Hita-Contreras F, Roda O, Martínez-Amat A, Cruz-Díaz D, Mérida-Velasco JA, Sánchez-Montesinos I. Embryonic and early fetal period development and morphogenesis of human craniovertebral junction. Clin Anat 2014;27:337–345
26. Scammon RE. Growth and development of the child. part II, anatomy and physiology. The central nervous system. In: White House Conference on Child Health and Protection. New York, London: Century; 1933:176–190

5 Skull Base Imaging

■ Interaction of the Radiologist and Surgeon

- The radiologist is an active member of the skull base team and has a very important role in the outcome of the patient.
- Surgeons should treat every request they make for imaging in the same way as making a request for a consultation from a clinical specialist. Requests and responses should be tailored to the patient's symptoms and signs, and should provide the radiologist with clinical information that will aid in diagnosis. This is critical for optimum patient care (**Fig. 5.1**).

> **Radiology Pearl**
>
> Good communication with the radiologist is essential to good outcomes.

■ Role of Neuroimaging in Skull Base Surgery

Diagnosis

Final diagnosis comes from the pathologist. However, a radiologist's opinion regarding diagnosis is extremely helpful to the team making management decisions. A purely descriptive report that skirts or avoids a working diagnosis is of much less value.

Location

Information regarding the location of the tumor should also specify the origin and extent of the tumor and relationships to critical structures.

- Determining the origin can provide a clue to pathology (**Fig. 5.2**). The origin can be ascertained in many ways: by the epicenter of the lesion, by focal

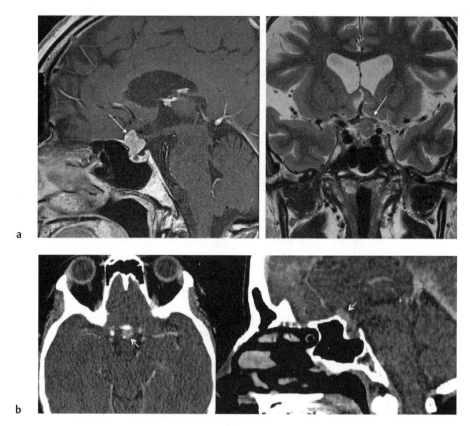

a

b

Fig. 5.1a,b **(a)** A tuberculum sellae meningioma *(arrow)* elevating the chiasm is readily apparent on the appropriate magnetic resonance imaging (MRI) sequences: sagittal post-gadolinium T1 *(left)*, coronal T2 *(right)*. Note an incidental microadenoma within the pituitary gland *(arrow)*. **(b)** A small tuberculum sellae meningioma, however, may be difficult to diagnose on axial computed tomography (CT) unless the appropriate technique is used (thin axial sections and a sagittal reformat in this example). The radiologist cannot plan the appropriate CT technique or MRI protocol without adequate clinical information on the requisition.

hyperostosis or erosion in certain lesions, and by the way the surrounding structures are displaced.

- Extent: Information about patterns of growth is important in understanding pathology **(Figs. 5.3** and **5.4)**. Extension into foramina and fissures, across bone and dura, in proximity to and with encasement of vessels and nerves can alter management and help determine the surgical plan.[1]
- Understanding the extent also helps to determine the stage and volume of the tumor. The determination of volume and any change in volume, signify-

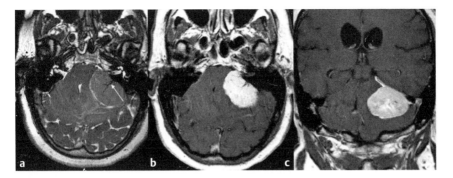

Fig. 5.2a–c A cerebellopontine angle meningioma on axial T2 **(a)**, postgadolinium T1 axial **(b)**, and coronal **(c)** views. The eccentric relationship to the internal auditory canal (IAC), the broad base on the dura, an obtuse angle of contact, and the enhancing dural tail are obvious clues to the diagnosis. In addition, a converging leash of vessels **(a**, *arrow)* and focal hyperostosis (if present) can provide additional clues to the exact site of origin.

ing growth, is critical in deciding on the management of benign tumors such as meningiomas.

- Relationships: Three-dimensional (3D) rendering can help in understanding in detail the relationships among bone, soft tissue, and vessels. Because 3D images can be rotated, sectioned, and viewed at any desired angle to simulate the surgical approach, they can help guide management **(Fig. 5.5)**.

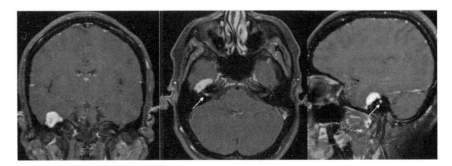

Fig. 5.3 Facial schwannoma presenting as an enhancing extra-axial mass in the middle fossa. Such a lesion can be mistaken for a meningioma; enhancement of the facial nerve is the clue to the diagnosis *(arrow)*. Careful inspection of all possible pathways of spread is an essential step in skull base imaging. Note fat suppression used on these postgadolinium T1 images.

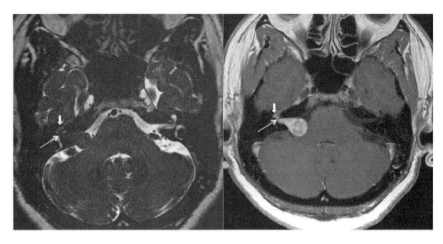

a   b

Fig. 5.4a,b Facial schwannoma on a heavily T2-weighted sequence (T2 DRIVE) **(a)** and corresponding postgadolinium T1 section **(b)**. The enhancing "ice-cream cone"–like cisternal and IAC component of the mass is similar to a vestibular schwannoma. The distinguishing feature is the involvement of the labyrinthine segment of the facial nerve *(thin arrow)* and the geniculate ganglion *(thick arrow)*.

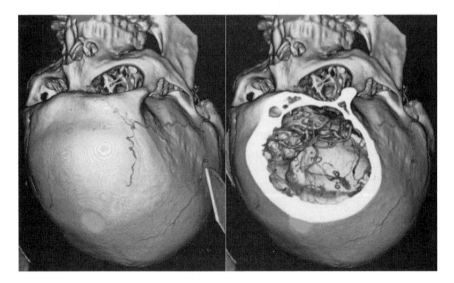

Fig. 5.5 A volume-rendered 3D image can be rotated and sectioned to simulate the surgical approach.

Resectability and Risk Assessment

By understanding the location and extent of the tumor, an understanding of resectability and the risks of resection are possible. Thus, with a proper and careful diagnosis, it is useful to determine which treatment approach—observation, surgery, radiation, or palliation—can achieve the goals desired for the patient. Proper diagnosis can help to plan the surgical approach or the radiation plan, determine the prognosis, and decide on a follow-up schedule.[2]

Surgical Navigation

Good-quality imaging data transferred to the operating room are essential and routinely used for safe surgical navigation.[3] The surgeon must understand not only the location of the tumor and the pathology but also where normal structures are expected to be found. For example, does the meningioma originate medial to or lateral to the entrance of cranial nerve (CN) V into Meckel's cave? If medial, CN V will be on the superficial side of the tumor when accessed by a retrosigmoid or petrosal approach, meaning that the surgeon will encounter the trigeminal nerve at the beginning of the tumor resection. If the origin is lateral, then the surgeon accessing the tumor from any posterolateral approach will encounter the nerve at the end of the tumor resection, preferably deep to the arachnoid of the trigeminal cistern. The same principles can be enunciated for the arteries and veins around the tumor and along the pathway of access. Understanding these relationships is important for optimal surgical outcomes. Understanding these navigational issues requires close communication between radiologists and surgeons.

Adjunctive Treatment

Preoperative embolization is the most common adjunctive treatment. Intra-arterial chemotherapy and procedures to open the blood–brain barrier are more recent additions to the role of interventional neuroradiologists (see Chapter 12).[4]

■ Imaging Choices

The complementary role of computed tomography (CT) and magnetic resonance imaging (MRI) is long known and well established, but cannot be overemphasized.[5] Each technique has advantages, but most skull base pathology requires both modalities for a complete evaluation.

Computed Tomography

- Computed tomography is the obvious choice in evaluating the bony skull base (bone tumors, erosion of bone by soft tissue tumors and infection, fractures, cerebrospinal fluid [CSF] leaks).
- It provides exquisite bony detail, high spatial resolution vascular imaging, and excellent 3D images, and enables detection of calcium and acute blood.
- It is superior in detecting subtle erosions of cortical margins and foramina, and in demonstrating reactive changes in bone (e.g., hyperostosis and pneumosinus dilatans around meningiomas) or tiny areas of calcification within lesions.[5,6]
- A thin-section axial helical CT data set is initially acquired usually with contrast; 64-slice scanners are standard in most skull base centers, but some centers have access to 256-slice or higher scanners with better computed tomography angiography (CTA) and 3D reconstructions, although there is no clear clinical advantage in the skull base.[7]
- Axial images of desired thickness are then generated, and high-quality coronal and sagittal images are reconstructed, using soft tissue and bone algorithms.
- It is important to use the correct "bone algorithm" images, which are generated from the same data set with edge enhancement to evaluate bone in sharp detail. Looking at the routine soft tissue images using a bone window setting is suboptimal.
- Intravenous contrast is necessary to look for intracranial or extracranial disease, to evaluate the vessels and cavernous sinus, and to help characterize the lesion. Contrast provides an initial assessment of tumor vascularity and may determine the need for dedicated vascular imaging [CTA/magnetic resonance angiography (MRA) or digital subtraction angiography (DSA)]. CT and MR perfusion studies have been used for grading the tumor, determining the prognosis, assessing the treatment response, and differentiating treatment/radiation effects and nonneoplastic lesions from neoplasms.[8]
- Contrast may be omitted on follow-up CT of osseous tumors with no soft tissue components, of sinonasal lesions clearly without intracranial extension, or if there is a contraindication.
- An unenhanced CT should be performed first if intracranial hemorrhage (or calcification) is a concern; contrast images can follow.
- Patients known to be at higher risk for contrast allergy may be premedicated using the following regimen (all three medications) to reduce the frequency or severity of reactions, after obtaining informed consent[9]:
  - Prednisone 50 mg PO at 13 hours, 7 hours, and 1 hour before
  - Diphenhydramine PO 50 mg at 13 hours, 7 hours, and 1 hour before
  - Ranitidine PO at 1 hour before contrast administration

Computed Tomography Angiography

- Computed tomography angiography (CTA) is invaluable in preoperative planning, particularly when intracranial disease is in close proximity to arteries, the cavernous sinus, or the dural sinuses. It is also important to recognize variant vascular anatomy such as a persistent trigeminal artery or unexpected vascular lesions such as aneurysms.[10]
- Three-dimensional images can be postprocessed from the CTA source data set **(Fig. 5.5)**.
- A "less is more" approach is advocated when ordering CTA studies. A focused region of interest (ROI) should be clearly defined in the radiology request.
- Coverage beyond the ROI results in unnecessary radiation, redundant images, and lower quality images at the region of interest. One study quotes an effective dose of 0.67 millisievert (mSv) for CTA of the cerebral vessels and 4.85 mSv for the cervicocerebral vessels.[11] No radiation risk is acceptable, however small, without benefit to the patient.[12] As an example, a CTA covering from C2 to the circle of Willis will provide high-quality vascular imaging at the skull base. This advantage is lost on a CTA covering the aortic arch to the vertex.
- Computed tomography angiography will show vascular variants of surgical importance[10,13]:
  - The internal carotid artery (ICA) medially positioned, bulging into sphenoid sinus. The bony wall may be thin or deficient, putting the ICA at risk during transsphenoidal surgery. Manipulation of a septum attached to this thin wall may also jeopardize the ICA.
  - A persistent trigeminal artery may also bulge into the sphenoid sinus.
  - A persistent hypoglossal artery traverses the hypoglossal canal (which may be enlarged). This rare variant may be the major or sole contributor to the basilar system. Another rare variant is the proatlantal artery, an ICA or external carotid artery (ECA) branch that supplies the vertebral artery.
  - A high-riding jugular bulb may be at risk during translabyrinthine surgery; often visible on coronal CTA images; best seen on computed tomography venography (CTV).
  - Venous varix at the basiocciput can occasionally be mistaken for a bony lesion.

Computed Tomography Venography

- Computed tomography venography is done by acquiring a similar axial data set following intravenous contrast, but later in the venous phase.
- Performing both CTA and CTV involves twice the amount of radiation.[11] The second acquisition may be difficult to achieve, resulting in suboptimal CTV images, particularly in patients with cardiac dysfunction.

Cisternography

- Cisternography is occasionally indicated for detection or confirmation of the site of a CSF leak along the skull base. It is usually performed if unenhanced high-resolution CT of the skull base and/or MR cisternography fail to show the site of CSF leakage.[14,15]
- Ideally, to have maximum sensitivity, the patient should be actively leaking at the time of the test.
- The procedure involves intrathecal administration of *nonionic* iodinated myelographic contrast medium under fluoroscopy, usually by lumbar puncture, occasionally by lateral C1-C2 puncture. The usual adult doses are 10 to 15 mL of nonionic contrast at concentrations not exceeding 300 mg/mL, and up to a maximum dose of 3 g. Strict adherence to safe practice guidelines is mandatory, as inadvertent use of ionic contrast can cause seizures and death.[16]
- The contrast column is gravitated cranially by tilting the fluoroscopy table, followed by high-resolution CT of the skull base with coronal reconstructions. Direct coronal CT with the patient in the prone position may be attempted in CSF rhinorrhea.
- Also see Magnetic Resonance Cisternography, below.

Magnetic Resonance Imaging

- Magnetic resonance imaging is clearly superior in evaluating the soft tissues, particularly neoplastic intracranial extension, dural integrity, leptomeningeal spread, and brain invasion.[17,18]
- The same applies to perineural spread, orbital extension, cavernous sinus involvement, and extension into fissures and foramina.[19]
- Routine brain sequences are insufficient; dedicated skull base protocols are required. These commonly include T1, fat-suppressed T2, or short tau inversion recovery (STIR) in appropriate planes, focused on the ROI and not the whole brain (**Tables 5.1** and **5.2**).
- Specifying anterior, middle, or posterior skull base, and specifying regions of interest such as orbital apex, cavernous sinus, cerebellopontine angle (CPA), sella, clivus, foramen magnum, etc., will prompt a protocol dedicated to that region by the radiologist. Without this information, studies cannot be tailored to the ROI (**Fig. 5.1**).
- Gadolinium is required for the detection of intracranial disease, cavernous sinus involvement, and meningeal and perineural spread, usually with fat suppression. Documenting enhanced scans in the three primary orthogonal planes is very helpful in tumor surgery planning.
- Bright signal from fat and marrow may mask a lesion or make enhancement unappreciable. Fat-suppression techniques (**Figs. 5.3** and **5.6**) are therefore invaluable, but can be a double-edged sword, as they are prone to susceptibility

Table 5.1   Common Magnetic Resonance Imaging (MRI) Sequences Used in the Skull Base

MRI Sequence	Appearance/Role
T1	• Fat is T1 bright (marrow, extracranial fat, dermoid, lipoma). Displacement of fat planes can help detect skull base lesions ("fat is a friend"). Replacement of marrow fat can help detect bone involvement. • Methemoglobin (subacute hematoma), melanin, and highly proteinaceous fluids (e.g., Rathke's) are also T1 bright. • Water and cerebrospinal fluid (CSF) are T1 dark. Most pathologies are relatively dark on T1 unless fatty, hemorrhagic, or proteinaceous.
T2	• Water, CSF, cystic and necrotic areas, fluid collections, and edema are T2 bright. Most tumors are bright and stand out on T2, but not all tumors. • Tumors with tightly packed cells and high nuclear cytoplasmic ratio are relatively T2 dark (lymphoma, primitive neuroectodermal tumor, germinoma), and so are meningiomas (variable). Calcium and hemosiderin are dark on T2. Fungal hyphae are very dark on T2. Flowing blood causes signal dropout (flow voids) often better seen on T2
Fluid-attenuated inversion recovery (FLAIR)	• Useful for evaluating effect on the adjacent brain (edema, gliosis). Epidermoids appear bright on FLAIR and stand out against dark CSF signal
Diffusion-weighted imaging (DWI)	• Acute infarction, abscess, and epidermoids show restricted diffusion (bright on DWI, dark on apparent diffusion coefficient [ADC]). Make sure it is not T2 shine-through (bright on both).
Fat suppression (FS), FS T2/T2 short-tau inversion recovery (STIR), FS T1 postgadolinium	• Fat signal can mask bright pathology on T2. • Fat is very bright on T1, and can mask enhancement. • Suppression of fat signal in marrow, subcranial soft tissues, orbit and craniovertebral junction (for ligamentous injury) is therefore invaluable in skull base imaging.

Radiology Pearl

Fat suppression techniques are prone to artifacts and are highly sensitive to motion; inhomogeneous fat suppression can make interpretation difficult.

Table 5.2   Magnetic Resonance Imaging Appearance of Intracranial Hematoma

Hyperacute blood	Isointense to dark on T1	Bright on T2
Acute hematoma	Dark on T1	Dark on T2
Early subacute	Bright on T1	Dark on T2
Late subacute	Bright on T1	Bright on T2
Chronic	Dark on T1	Dark on T2 (from periphery to center)

artifacts. Artifacts from dental hardware, clips, and implants are markedly exaggerated on fat-suppressed sequences.

- Fat-suppressed and non–fat-suppressed images may be complementary, but acquiring them will take double the time. Every choice has a trade-off in MRI. MR sequences and planes of section therefore need to be carefully chosen.

> **Radiology Pearl**
>
> A "one-size-fits-all" approach does not apply.

- The protocol needs to be tailored so that the best planes of section and the most appropriate sequences are applied, every time. As an example, a clival lesion may be best seen on a midsagittal thin-section T2 sequence, but this may not be part of the "routine" protocol.
- Once established, the same protocol should be used on follow-up imaging to facilitate comparisons. This may be requested on follow-up requisitions.
- "Less is more" makes for better MR image quality. A smaller field of view (more focused imaging) translates into higher resolution images in the same amount of time. A rough sketch on the requisition can be very effective.

> **Radiology Pearl**
>
> Ordering too many scans during one sitting may be counterproductive.

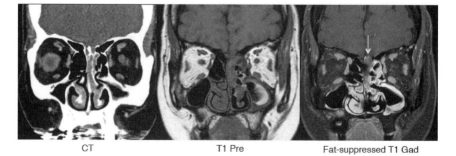

CT   T1 Pre   Fat-suppressed T1 Gad

Fig. 5.6 Sinonasal mass (esthesioneuroblastoma) with intracranial extension that is best identified on the fat-suppressed postgadolinium coronal T1 image on right *(arrow)*. Fat-suppressed sequences are invaluable in the skull base and orbit.

- Patients tolerate shorter scans better. Long studies are often degraded by patient motion.

Magnetic Resonance Cisternography

This is performed using highly T2-weighted 3D thin-section "myelographic" sequences. These can be reconstructed in multiple planes. Intrathecal injection of gadolinium is also an option, but is not widely used as of yet.[20]

Cerebrospinal Fluid Flow Studies

Cerebrospinal fluid flow studies traditionally use the phase contrast technique; newer techniques, which use variations of arterial spin labeling, are now available.[21] These techniques can demonstrate the presence or absence of CSF flow across the foramen magnum in a Chiari malformation, across the aqueduct of Sylvius, within an obstructed ventricular system (such as posterior fossa tumor), across a third-ventriculocisternostomy, and across a fenestrated arachnoid cyst. A series of images are acquired over short periods of time, which are then viewed as a cine sequence.

Magnetic Resonance Tractography

Advanced diffusion tensor imaging methods on 3-tesla or higher systems can map the facial nerve preoperatively in patients with large CPA tumors.[22] Similarly, preoperative mapping of CNs II, III, V, and VIII has been achieved and its clinical utility is being examined.[23]

Magnetic Resonance Angiography

- Magnetic resonance angiography is usually performed using gadolinium. If vascular imaging is not a high priority and gadolinium is not otherwise indicated, or the patient has an allergy to gadolinium, time of flight (TOF) MRA may be considered.
- If a CTA has already been performed, MRA is usually unnecessary. Exceptions include suspected dissection at the skull base with a negative CTA, or the presence of metal artifact on the CTA from coils.

Magnetic Resonance Venography

- Magnetic resonance venography (MRV) is best achieved using gadolinium, as TOF MRV is prone to artifacts. A common indication is to look for encroachment of a dural sinus by a skull base meningioma.

Digital Subtraction Angiography

- The development of high-quality cross-sectional vascular imaging (CTA, MRA) has mostly obviated the need for DSA using catheter techniques, except as part of interventional procedures. Additional indications are as follows:
  - Patients with severe artifacts from implants on CTA and MRA, or artifacts on CTA with a contraindication to MR; for example, a patient with an aneurysm clip that is unsafe for MRA and obscures the area of interest on CTA will need a DSA.
  - Digital subtraction angiography remains the gold standard and serves as a problem-solving tool when findings are not fully clarified on CTA or MRA (such as suspicion of subtle vascular injury or confirming patency of a small encased branch).
  - Occasionally, a patient with renal failure can undergo a limited DSA using less contrast than a CTA requires.
- Digital subtraction angiography can demonstrate vascular displacement, stretching, encasement, stenosis, occlusion, collaterals, tumor vascularity, angiogenesis, and vascular injury.
- It assesses the lumen only and cannot demonstrate extraluminal pathology the way MR or CT can (except indirectly by studying the effect on the lumen and tumor vascularity).
- Digital subtraction angiography, on the other hand, provides temporal resolution with arterial, capillary and venous phase images not available on MRA or CTA. DSA is therefore indicated for evaluating arteriovenous shunting lesions, such as dural arteriovenous fistula (DAVF) and arteriovenous malformation (AVM); for determining the timing and adequacy of collateral flow when an artery is stenosed or occluded; and for assessing venous drainage when a dural sinus is compromised, such as by a meningioma.
- Time-resolved MRA techniques [such as Time-Resolved Imaging of Contrast KineticS (TRICKS), 4D Time-Resolved Angiography using Keyhole (4D TRAK), and Time-resolved angiography WIth Stochastic Trajectories (TWIST)] are a promising tool that can occasionally obviate the need for a catheter angiogram, but they cannot match the spatial or the temporal resolution of conventional angiography as of yet.[24,25]
- Neurologic complications occur in 1.3% of catheter angiographies, of which some are transient or reversible, but 0.5% of deficits are permanent.[26]
- Additional complications include hematoma around the puncture site (4.2%), nausea/vomiting and transient hypotension (1.2%), and headache, chest pain, arrhythmia, urticaria, anaphylaxis, circulatory failure, and acute renal failure (each below 1%). Risk of death from all complications is 0.06%, mostly related to neurologic complications.[27]
- Relative contraindications to catheter cerebral angiography include hypotension, coagulopathy, clinically significant sensitivity to contrast material,

renal insufficiency, and congestive heart failure. The patient can be optimized prior to angiography (for example, with premedication for contrast allergy), provided that the benefits outweigh the risks. Planning and prior discussion with the radiologist is essential.[28]

Nuclear Medicine

- Thallium-201 and technetium-99m (Tc-99m) glucoheptonate in conventional nuclear imaging, as well as sugar analogues such as fluorodeoxyglucose (FDG), radiolabeled amino acids, and cell membrane analogues in positron emission tomography (PET) are available to distinguish viable tumor from edema and necrosis in the skull base.[29,30]
- Osteomyelitis imaging in the skull base is best performed with tagged white blood cells, which is commonly achieved with either a Tc-99m or indium-111 (In-111) label rather than gallium-67, as the latter often fails to accumulate in marrow-rich bone such as skull.[31–33]
- Shunt studies are frequently performed via injection of 0.1 to 0.5 cc of pyrogen-free Tc-99m diethylenetriamine pentaacetic acid (DTPA) into the reservoir using sterile technique.[34] Delay in tracer migration beyond an hour with ambulation and shunt pumping is highly suspicious for obstruction.
- Tumors of the skull base including meningiomas and pituitary adenomas can be assessed by both somatostatin analogues such as In-111 octreotide and norepinephrine analogues such as iodinated meta-iodo-benzyl-guanosine.[35–38]
- Phosphorus-32 is an electron emitter with a 14.3-day half-life, usually prepared as a colloid, that has gained acceptance for the control of craniopharyngioma usually via direct transnasal injection, with some authors reporting a 70% tumor control rate at 10 years.[39–42]

Plain X-Rays

- Plain radiography has a very limited role in modern skull base imaging, except in the initial evaluation of the craniovertebral junction anomalies, basilar invagination, and ligamentous instability.[43]
- Lines and measurements can be used in the assessment of basilar invagination (digastric line and bimastoid line on the anteroposterior radiograph, and McRae, Chamberlain, and McGregor lines on the lateral radiograph).[44] CT or MRI can provide the same information and also demonstrate any mass effect on neural structures.[45]
- Useful information may still be obtained from plain X-rays in a low-resource environment. Lytic or sclerotic bone involvement, focal hyperostosis, enlargement of skull base foramina, vascular grooves (especially in the presence of occluded venous sinuses), opacification, enlargement or destruction

of a paranasal sinus, displacement of soft tissue planes, and soft tissue calcifications can provide evidence of an underlying lesion.[46]

■ Radiology of Selected Skull Base Pathologies

See boundaries of the skull base fossae in Chapter 2, **Fig. 2.3,** and in **Fig. 5.7.** **Tables 5.3** and **5.4** summarize the imaging choice criteria and main radiological findings of skull base pathologies. **Table 5.5** summarizes anterior skull base (ASB) pathologies.

Meningioma

Radiology Pearl

In most instances, specifying anterior, middle, or posterior skull base location on the requisition is sufficient. A diagram on the requisition can be invaluable to the radiologist for planning the appropriate protocol.

- Small tuberculum sellae meningiomas can be missed on routine axial CT unless suspected clinically and appropriate techniques are used **(Fig. 5.1)**. MRI sella sequences, particularly sagittal postgadolinium, are preferred; contrast

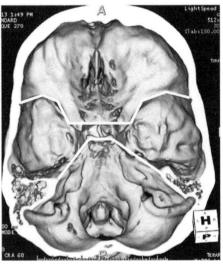

Fig. 5.7   Boundaries of the skull base fossae.

Table 5.3   Imaging Choices

Modality	Role/Comments
Computed tomography (CT)	Bone tumors, bone destruction, subtle cortical/foraminal erosions, hyperostosis, calcification
Computed tomography angiography (CTA)	Vascular relationship to lesion, encasement, caliber change, occlusion, collaterals, variants, and anomalous anatomy
CT-3D models	Surgical planning, can simulate surgical approach
CT cisternography	CSF leaks not detected on MR cisternography (needs intrathecal contrast administration)
Magnetic resonance (MR)	
Magnetic resonance angiography (MRA)	Similar to CTA, better maximum intensity projection (MIP) reconstructions at skull base, choice of time of flight (TOF), contrast-enhanced MR angiography (CEMRA), and time-resolved techniques
MR cisternography	Uses heavily T2-weighted sequences (no contrast needed) to detect leakage; intrathecal gadolinium technique also described but not widely used
Cerebrospinal fluid (CSF) flow studies	CSF flow across foramen magnum in Chiari malformation
Tractography	Advanced techniques such as diffusion tensor imaging hold promise in mapping cranial nerves and white matter tracts preoperatively
CT and MR	Complementary role, both required in most cases
Plain films	Limited role in craniovertebral anomalies, flexion extension studies, and in low resource situations
Diagnostic cerebral angiography (DSA)	Limited role in select cases

CT with sagittal and coronal reconstructions is also satisfactory. Small olfactory groove and planum sphenoidale meningiomas are less likely to be missed on routine brain CT.

- Preoperatively, MRI is used to assess the lesion's relationship to the optic nerves and anterior cerebral arteries, transgression of the skull base, involvement of the optic canals, and mass effect on frontal lobe. Dedicated MR fat-suppressed orbit sequences are required.
- Disproportionate edema and irregular interfaces with brain on the postgadolinium images are suspicious for atypical or aggressive meningiomas or dural-based metastases such as breast or lung carcinoma.

Table 5.4 Typical Radiological Findings of Skull Base Pathologies

Pathology	CT	MRI
Meningioma (differentials include dural metastases, schwannoma, hemangiopericytoma, lymphoma, sarcoid, infection, tuberculosis)	• Usually hyperdense to isodense, only occasionally hypodense, one quarter show variable patterns of calcification • Look for adjacent bone changes: hyperostosis, cortical irregularities, overt invasion, rarely enlargement of adjacent sinus (pneumosinus dilatans) • Closely examine adjacent foramina/fissures on bone windows; hyperostotic bone can occasionally compress neurovascular structures even if the soft tissue component does not	• Relatively T2 dark, iso- to hypointense on T1 • Often show converging flow voids toward dural attachment, best seen on T2 • Most enhance brightly and homogeneously with a "dural tail" • Irregular interface with brain, disproportionate brain edema on FLAIR, enhancement across tissue planes, low ADC raises concern about atypical or malignant varieties • The angle that the lesion makes with bone is more obtuse than schwannoma, especially at the cerebellopontine angle (CPA) • Closely look for extension along fissures, foramina and cranial nerves on fat-suppressed (FS) T1 postgadolinium (requires appropriate cranial nerve protocols) • Encasement of artery, vein, encroachment of dural sinuses on MRA/MRV • Determining encasement versus invagination of neurovascular structures is of surgical importance because determining the positions of displaced cranial nerves in relation to the tumor is critical
Dural metastases	• Enhancing mass along skull base that can mimic meningioma, particularly en plaque pattern • Lytic or sclerotic destruction of adjacent bone • Multifocal and permeative destruction are helpful signs	• Focal areas of marrow replacement on T1, bright on FS T2 or STIR, enhancement on FS T1 postgadolinium • Dural-based enhancement may be indistinguishable from atypical or malignant meningioma; multifocality, nodularity, and multiple lobulations are helpful signs

Lesion	Imaging features	
Schwannoma	• Usually isodense, does not calcify, difficult to detect on CT when small • Subtle asymmetry of the cavernous sinus or cerebellopontine angle cisterns important clue on noncontrast CT, may lead to incidental detection in asymptomatic patients • Larger lesions cause smooth expansion of respective bony canal (foramen ovale, rotundum, superior orbital fissure, internal auditory canal [IAC])	• Generally more bright and more heterogeneous than meningioma on T2, particularly when large • Isointense on T1 (unless there is blood) • Strong, heterogeneous enhancement with cystic/necrotic areas commonly seen (homogeneous in small lesions) • Long axis of lesion along the respective cranial nerve: heavily T2-weighted 3D sequences helpful in tracing the nerve (but not good for assessing signal within the lesion) • The angle the tumor makes with the adjacent bone is usually more acute (e.g., CPA)
Hemangiopericytoma	• Skull base not typical location • Relatively dense on CT but does not calcify • Can erode bone, but does not cause hyperostosis • Strong enhancement	• Mimics meningioma including "dural tail," may be indistinguishable • Intense enhancement and prominent flow voids raise suspicion, but difficult to predict with certainty • Can encroach and occlude dural sinuses
Chordoma (differentials include metastases, fibrous dysplasia, chondrosarcoma)	• Midline clival, well-defined lytic lesion, may have a sclerotic margin • Usually expansive and destructive when detected • Relatively hyperdense soft tissue component with calcifications • Enhances heterogeneously	• Very bright and heterogeneous on T2 (except poorly differentiated variant in children, which can be dark on T2) • Sagittal T2 most useful sequence • Low to intermediate signal on T1 (unless blood present) • Moderate to strong heterogeneous enhancement

(continued)

Table 5.4 (continued)

Pathology	CT	MRI
Chondrosarcoma	• Majority off-midline lytic lesions, petro-occipital synchondrosis is the most common site of origin • Popcorn or rings and arcs pattern of calcification are helpful when present • Midline location particularly difficult to differentiate from chordoma	• Low to intermediate signal on T1, heterogeneously bright on T2, heterogeneous enhancement, similar to chordoma • Measurement of ADC values can help differentiate; chondrosarcoma demonstrates significantly higher ADC values than chordoma
Pituitary macroadenoma (differentials include meningioma, hyperplasia, aneurysm, lymphocytic hypophysitis)	• Isodense to slightly hyperdense intrasellar lesion bulging into suprasellar cistern on routine axial CT • Dedicated CT of sella may be done if MRI is contraindicated, but MRI of sella is the modality of choice • Preoperative CTA for vascular variants, sinonasal anatomy • Expansion of bony sella, thinning of floor, extension into sphenoid sinus • Rarely bone destruction (floor, clivus, planum) by aggressive adenoma • Pituitary apoplexy: well-defined high-density material within macroadenoma; overt subarachnoid hemorrhage (SAH) and retroclival subdural hematoma (SDH) occasionally	• Usually isointense on T1 and T2 (unless blood present) • Enhances strongly, except cystic/necrotic areas; no glandular tissue visible separate from mass • Suprasellar extension, compression, elevation of chiasm ±T2 hyperintensity, stretching, thinning, bulge into third ventricle • Cavernous sinus extension, encasement of internal carotid artery (ICA) (usually without caliber change) • Occasionally ectopic adenoma in clivus, infrasellar and suprasellar locations • Rare giant adenoma may cause skull base destruction • Pituitary apoplexy: usually subacute blood within the mass when imaged (bright on T1, dark on T2) but variable depending on age; retroclival blood or subarachnoid blood occasionally (look on FLAIR)

Craniopharyngioma	• Usually large suprasellar cystic mass with variable solid components • CT particularly useful to demonstrate calcifications (90% of pediatric adamantinomatous type calcify) • Papillary type seen in adults is more solid, and calcification is rare	• T1 and T2 signal varies with cell type and cyst content • Wall and solid components enhance • Majority are suprasellar (if so, sella is usually of normal size); occasional intrasellar component and rare purely intrasellar lesion better seen on MR • Location is of surgical importance: prechiasmal can distort visual pathway, retrochiasmal can compress midbrain and cause hydrocephalus; location and relationship to chiasm is best demonstrated on sagittal T1 and coronal T2 sequences using sella protocols • MRA is indicated to examine relationship to the anterior cerebral artery (ACA), anterior communicating artery (AcomA), and posterior communicating artery (PcomA)
Rathke's cleft cyst	• Typically does not calcify or enhance (infrequent faint smooth wall calcification may be seen) • Relatively small compared to the typical craniopharyngioma • Classic Rathke's cysts are not difficult to differentiate from craniopharyngioma, suprasellar arachnoid cyst, epidermoid, cystic adenoma, empty sella, etc., but when in doubt follow-up imaging is indicated	• Intrasellar or intra-suprasellar ovoid cyst with smooth, well-demarcated margins • Small intracystic nodule may be seen, but no other solid components • Variable signal on T1 and T2 depending on cyst contents; occasional fluid level • No enhancement within cyst

Table 5.5   Pathologies of the Anterior Skull Base

Sinonasal	Skull Base and Intracranial
Mucocele/mucopyocele	Meningioma
Esthesioneuroblastoma	Fibrous dysplasia
Squamous cell carcinoma	Metastasis, direct extension, perineural extension
Non-Hodgkin's lymphoma	Frontoethmoid cephalocele, osteoma of the sinus
Miscellaneous: Osteoma, adenoid cystic carcinoma, juvenile angiofibroma, sinonasal undifferentiated carcinoma, melanoma, schwannoma, hemangiopericytoma, nasal dermal sinus, juvenile angio-fibroma, metastasis	

- Computed tomography is superior at confirming the integrity of the skull base and detecting hyperostosis, skull base erosion, and pneumosinus dilatans. CTA may show vascular supply if feeders are hypertrophied or tortuous.[47–49]

Sinonasal Tumors

- The role of radiology is to provide an accurate definition of tumor extent rather than to predict histology. From a surgical perspective, skull base, orbital, and brain extension is critical information. Equally critical from a head and neck surgical perspective is pterygopalatine fossa and palate involvement in addition to nodal spread.
- Intracranial extension may not be obvious; look carefully for perineural spread and subtle bony invasion (**Fig. 5.6**).
- Distinguishing a sinonasal tumor from inflammatory changes is challenging on CT; MRI is superior for this purpose.
- T2-weighted MRI is the most useful sequence. Most tumors are darkish on T2 (exceptions: salivary rest tumors, schwannomas, inverted papillomas). Most trapped secretions remain bright on T2.
- Defining extent is therefore better achieved on MRI; CT is better at detecting bone destruction and remodeling.
- Look for tumor spread to adjacent sinuses, alveolar buccal sulcus, pterygoid muscles, skin, and lymph nodes.
- Radiological patterns may not be specific enough to predict histology; small tumors are particularly difficult to differentiate from inflammatory changes unless bone is involved.

- Bone destruction is most commonly associated with squamous cell carcinomas. Mucoceles and polyps cause bone remodeling, as do inverted papillomas.[50,51]

Fibro-Osseous Lesions of the Skull Base

- Fibrous dysplasia and ossifying fibroma show characteristic dense expanded bone on CT.
- Paget's disease appears similar to osteoblastic metastases, but characteristic calvarial involvement in Paget's enables differentiation.
- Magnetic resonance appearances of fibro-osseous lesions can be confusing, but the diagnosis may be straightforward on CT.

Inflammatory Sinus Disease

- Acute bacterial sinusitis can rapidly spread intracranially without bone destruction, particularly from the frontal sinus (infection spreading through emissary veins). The intervening bone may be intact radiologically and the extension unsuspected unless contrast studies (CT or MRI) with coronal or sagittal views are obtained.
- *Fungal sinusitis* is a collective term encompassing noninvasive fungal colonization as well as invasive forms such as *Aspergillus* species (typically in neutropenic patients), mucormycosis, and others. High-density material within the sinus on CT and T2 dark areas on MRI raises suspicion. Thick secretions can have a similar appearance; recognizing invasion is the key. Look for thickening, remodeling, thinning, and erosion of surrounding bone, expansion of the sinus, and stranding of fat in the masticator space, pterygopalatine fossa, and orbit.
- Intracranially, look for edema, epidural abscess, enhancing granulomas, and leptomeningeal enhancement. Intracranial spread of fungal infection can occur without obvious bone erosion.
- Mucocele is an obstructed, expanded sinus. The frontal sinus is most commonly affected with remodeling of its posterior wall and mass effect on the frontal lobe. The bone may be thinned out and not radiologically visible, but this appearance does not necessarily mean bone erosion or destruction.
- When infection (mucopyocele) is suspected, contrast CT or better MRI with gadolinium is indicated to look for intracranial spread.[52]

■ The Central Skull Base

- The central skull base may be divided into three regions: central or midsagittal, off-midline or parasagittal, and lateral. Vertical lines medial to the

Table 5.6   Pathologies of the Central Skull Base and Its Compartments

Midline	Parasagittal	Lateral
Chordoma, ecchordosis physaliphora	Chondrosarcoma	
Meningioma	Meningioma	Meningioma
Fibrous dysplasia	Fibrous dysplasia	Fibrous dysplasia
Metastasis, myeloma	Metastasis, myeloma	Metastasis, myeloma
Intrasellar/suprasellar lesions (pituitary adenoma, Rathke's cyst, craniopharyngioma, meningioma, arachnoid cyst, dermoid, epidermoid, teratoma, sarcoid, opticochiasmatic and hypothalamic glioma, lymphocytic hypophysitis)	Nerve sheath tumors	
	Aneurysms	
Chondrosarcoma	Juvenile angiofibroma	
Cephalocele	Cephalocele	

petroclival fissure and lateral to the foramen ovale demarcate the regions (Chapter 2, **Fig. 2.3**).

- The pathology found in each region reflects these anatomical differences to some degree (**Table 5.6**).

The role of radiology is as follows:

- To localize the origin of the tumor to one of the above three regions, and eliminate possible diagnoses from the differential diagnosis. Radiology is often insufficient in making a precise diagnosis of aggressive-appearing lesions. However, an opinion can be offered when clinical data are also available. Ultimately, the diagnosis, as always, requires histological examination.
- To identify benign disease that may be followed up on imaging.
- To identify direct encroachment into dura and bone, invasion of orbital apex and cavernous sinus, and perineural invasion.

Accurate definition of tumor extent and recognition of perineural invasion requires detailed understanding of the foramina, fissures, cranial nerve anatomy, and soft tissue detail (**Table 5.7**. See also Chapter 2, pages 14–15). Methodical inspection of important imaging landmarks is crucial (**Fig. 5.8**).

Perineural Spread

- Most head and neck malignancies can demonstrate retrograde spread along nerves across the skull base. Adenoid cystic carcinoma, squamous cell

Table 5.7 Important Landmarks of the Central/Paracentral Skull Base (also see Fig. 5.8 and Fig, 2.1 and Fig. 2.2, on page 11)

• Optic canal	• Foramen ovale
• Superior orbital fissure	• Foramen spinosum
• Inferior orbital fissure	• Foramen lacerum
• Pterygopalatine fossa	• Jugular foramen
• Pterygomaxillary fissure	• Hypoglossal canal
• Foramen rotundum	• Cavernous sinus
• Vidian canal	

carcinoma, and melanoma are the more frequent causes of perineural tumor spread.[53]

- Perineural spread may also be seen in lymphoma, sarcoid, and other autoimmune diseases. Meningiomas may also extend across neural foramina.[54]
- Magnetic resonance imaging is the modality of choice for its multiplanar capability, superior soft tissue detail, and fewer dental artifacts. Fat-suppressed sequences are best at detecting enhancement along nerves. Non-fat-suppressed images are also useful to detect obliteration of fat planes at foraminal openings.
- Other signs to look for are denervation atrophy of affected muscles, cavernous sinus enlargement, and soft tissue within Meckel's cave.
- Nerve enlargement causing expansion and destruction of foramina and fissures is best detected on CT.
- Fluorodeoxyglucose (FDG) PET/CT may also demonstrate focal or linear uptake along pathways of perineural spread.[55]
- Perineural spread may not be associated with clinical deficits, and radiology may provide the only clue. Knowledge of the pathways of perineural spread is therefore imperative in preoperative evaluation and radiation planning.
- Some of the most commonly involved pathways are along the trigeminal divisions and the facial nerve.

Posterior Skull Base (Tables 5.8 and 5.9)

- The posterior surfaces of the clivus and petrous temporal bones form the anterior and lateral boundaries, respectively. Clival pathology can therefore extend into the posterior skull base.
- Approximately 90% of CPA schwannomas are vestibular, but look out for the odd facial schwannoma. CPA facial schwannomas are indistinguishable from vestibular schwannomas if they do not enter the labyrinthine segment. Enlargement (on CT) and enhancement (on MRI) of the labyrinthine segment are important clues, in the absence of which differentiation may be difficult.

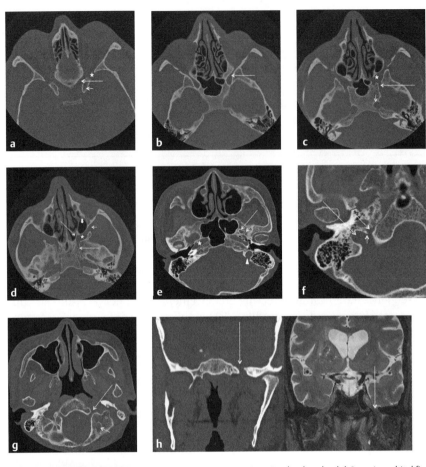

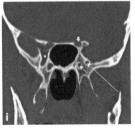

Fig. 5.8a–i Important imaging landmarks. **(a)** Superior orbital fissure *(asterisk)*, optic canal *(long arrow)*, and anterior clinoid process *(short arrow)*. **(b)** Inferior orbital fissure *(arrow)*, which communicates with the pterygopalatine fossa and the foramen rotundum. **(c)** Foramen rotundum *(long arrow)*, pterygopalatine fossa *(asterisk)*, and carotid canal, vertical portion *(vertical arrow)*. **(d)** Vidian canal *(long horizontal arrow)*, pterygopalatine fossa *(asterisk)*, pterygomaxillary fissure *(short thin arrow)*, sphenopalatine foramen *(diagonal arrow)*, and maxillary sinus *(short thick arrow)*. **(e)** Foramen ovale *(long arrow)*, foramen spinosum *(short arrow)*, carotid canal *(asterisk)*, and jugular foramen *(arrowhead)*. **(f)** Jugular fossa: pars vascularis *(long arrow)*, pars nervosa *(short diagonal arrow)*, and jugular spine *(vertical arrow)*. **(g)** Hypoglossal canal *(long arrow)* and condylar canal *(short arrow)*. **(h)** Foramen ovale *(arrows)* on CT (coronal reformat viewed on bone window) and MRI (T2 fat-suppressed coronal) showing cranial nerve (CN) V₃ traversing the foramen. **(i)** Foramen rotundum *(long arrow)* and the vidian canal *(short arrow)* on coronal CT. Note these structures on the contralateral side, showing the relationship of the foramen rotundum to the inferior orbital fissure *(asterisk)*. The *vertical solid arrow* points to the optic canal.

Table 5.8   Posterior Skull Base Pathologies

Cerebellopontine Angle	Jugular Foramen	Foramen Magnum Region	Clivus
Schwannoma, vestibular (90%), facial, lower cranial nerve	Paraganglioma	Meningioma	Chordoma
Meningioma	Schwannoma CN IX–XI	Schwannoma CN XII	Meningioma
Epidermoid Arachnoid cyst Aneurysm Metastasis Lipoma	Meningioma Metastasis	Metastasis Basilar invagination Rheumatoid pannus Degenerative pseudopannus Congenital and developmental (Chiari, Dandy-Walker continuum, mega cisterna magna, arachnoid cyst, Blake's pouch cyst)	Metastasis

Facial schwannomas centered on the geniculate ganglion are classically tubular, but may present as a round mass expanding the geniculate fossa. Extending along the greater superficial petrosal nerve, it may also present as a round extra-axial mass in the middle fossa. Tympanic segment involvement may be initially tubular, but may later lobulate into the middle ear cavity. Mastoid segment involvement may expand the stylomastoid foramen, and later break through into mastoid air cells resulting in an aggressive-appearing mass.

- A thin-section 3D heavily T2-weighted sequence such as Driven Equilibrium (DRIVE; Philips), constructive interference steady state (CISS; Siemens), or fast imaging employing steady-state acquisition (FIESTA; GE) shows the cisternal and intracanalicular segments of CNs VII and VIII in detail so that small schwannomas can be detected even without gadolinium. Small vascular loops can be demonstrated in detail, often better than MRA sequences. All cranial nerve segments within the CSF cisterns are well demonstrated on this sequence, and their relationship to intracranial lesions can be evaluated.
- It is important to differentiate whether nerves or vessels invaginate into a CPA mass or are truly encased, information that may determine resectability. Determination of the positions of displaced cranial nerves in relation to the

Table 5.9 Cerebellopontine Angle (CPA) Pathologies and Radiological Findings

Pathology	CT	MRI
Vestibular schwannoma (differential: meningioma)	• Thin-section contrast-enhanced CT if MRI contraindicated • Enhancing ovoid cisternal component and conical IAC component constitute the typical "ice-cream cone" lesion • Widening of bony IAC • Small intracanalicular lesions may be entirely missed on CT	• 3D T2-weighted sequences show the CN VII–VIII complex and the lesion as dark signal against bright CSF • Inherent signal is better assessed on routine T2 on which schwannomas are typically brighter than meningiomas, and more heterogeneous when large • Enhances strongly but more heterogeneously compared to meningioma; dural tail uncommon; tiny intracanalicular lesions can be picked up with gadolinium
Meningioma	• Typically not centered on the IAC • Often more dense than schwannomas and may calcify, unlike schwannomas • Hyperostosis may be seen • Can enter IAC and even cause mild flaring, but not to the extent seen with schwannoma	• Eccentric to IAC, broad base on dura, relatively dark on T2, more homogeneous enhancement often with a dural tail • Converging vessels and focal hyperostosis may indicate the site of origin, which in turn may help determine in which direction cranial nerves and vessels are displaced by the tumor • The angle of contact of the tumor to the bone is more obtuse than in schwannomas
Epidermoid	• Slightly grayish and spotty in relation to dark CSF • Insinuate into CSF spaces • Scalloped interface with surrounding brain • Does not calcify	• Shows restricted diffusion (very bright on DWI, dark on ADC); this may be less marked or absent in postoperative residual epidermoid • Bright on FLAIR • Does not enhance

tumor is also critical. MRI tractography has a promising role in preoperative mapping of cranial nerves.

- Also assess the level of the jugular bulb, the dominance of the sinuses, the entry and size of the vein of Labbé, and the size of clival plexus and the superior petrosal sinuses. These factors are important in deciding on the approach.
- The relation of the tumor to the arteries and how the tumor displaces or encases arteries, both large and small, are critical in planning and executing tumor resection.
- The status of the fourth ventricle and other ventricles is important pre- and postoperatively.
- Whether the cerebellar tonsils are herniated and the status of the cisterna magna and any CSF space that the surgeon can drain are important for planning surgery.
- In the jugular foramen region, look out for vascular variants of surgical importance (high-riding and dehiscent jugular bulb) and vascular pseudolesions (thrombus, or merely slow flow mimicking a lesion). MRV or CTV may be required.
- The intrinsic imaging characteristics are best assessed by MRI/MRV with gadolinium. Paragangliomas (glomus tumors) enhance like a lightbulb and show a characteristic "salt and pepper" appearance on T2-weighted images (occasionally also seen in hypervascular metastasis).[56]
- The bony margins are best assessed on high-resolution CT: paraganglioma cause a moth-eaten pattern of bone destruction, whereas schwannomas cause a scalloped, well-corticated expansion.
- Glomus tumors show intense vascularity on catheter angiography, a feature earlier used to make the diagnosis; currently, angiography is performed for preoperative embolization and only rarely for purely diagnostic purposes.

■ References

Boldfaced references are of particular importance.

1. **Curtin HD. Embryology, anatomy, and imaging of the central skull base. In: Som PM, Curtin HD, eds. Head and Neck Imaging, 5th ed. St. Louis: Mosby; 2011**
2. de Almeida JR, Witterick IJ, Gullane PJ, et al. Physical morbidity by surgical approach and tumor location in skull base surgery. Head Neck 2013;35:493–499
3. **Sure U, Alberti O, Petermeyer M, Becker R, Bertalanffy H. Advanced image-guided skull base surgery. Surg Neurol 2000;53:563–572, discussion 572**
4. Guillaume DJ, Doolittle ND, Gahramanov S, Hedrick NA, Delashaw JB, Neuwelt EA. Intra-arterial chemotherapy with osmotic blood-brain barrier disruption for aggressive oligodendroglial tumors: results of a phase I study. Neurosurgery 2010;66:48–58, discussion 58

5. Kraus DH, Lanzieri CF, Wanamaker JR, Little JR, Lavertu P. Complementary use of computed tomography and magnetic resonance imaging in assessing skull base lesions. Laryngoscope 1992;102:623–629

6. Parizel PM, Carpentier K, Van Marck V, et al. Pneumosinus dilatans in anterior skull base meningiomas. Neuroradiology 2013;55:307–311

7. Siebert E, Bohner G, Dewey M, et al. 320-slice CT neuroimaging: initial clinical experience and image quality evaluation. Br J Radiol 2009;82:561–570

8. **Jain R. Perfusion CT imaging of brain tumors: an overview. AJNR Am J Neuroradiol 2011;32:1570–1577**

9. Baerlocher MO, Asch M, Myers A. Allergic-type reactions to radiographic contrast media. CMAJ 2010;182:1328

10. Dimmick SJ, Faulder KC. Normal variants of the cerebral circulation at multidetector CT angiography. Radiographics 2009;29:1027–1043

11. Manninen AL, Isokangas JM, Karttunen A, Siniluoto T, Nieminen MT. A comparison of radiation exposure between diagnostic CTA and DSA examinations of cerebral and cervicocerebral vessels. AJNR Am J Neuroradiol 2012;33:2038–2042

12. Verdun FR, Bochud F, Gundinchet F, Aroua A, Schnyder P, Meuli R. Quality initiatives radiation risk: what you should know to tell your patient. Radiographics 2008;28:1807–1816

13. **Hamid O, El Fiky L, Hassan O, Kotb A, El Fiky S. Anatomic variations of the sphenoid sinus and their impact on trans-sphenoid pituitary surgery. Skull Base 2008;18:9–15**

14. Stone JA, Castillo M, Neelon B, Mukherji SK. Evaluation of CSF leaks: high-resolution CT compared with contrast-enhanced CT and radionuclide cisternography. AJNR Am J Neuroradiol 1999;20:706–712

15. **Lloyd KM, DelGaudio JM, Hudgins PA. Imaging of skull base cerebrospinal fluid leaks in adults. Radiology 2008;248:725–736**

16. American College of Radiology (ACR)/American Society of Neuroradiology (ASNR)/ Society for Pediatric Radiology (SNR). Practice guideline for the performance of myelography and cisternography. Available at: http://www.acr.org/~/media/f4c49aa 1834d46a081f5f0ff20e1e26b.pdf. Accessed August 4, 2014

17. **Borges A. Imaging of the central skull base. Neuroimaging Clin N Am 2009;19:669–696**

18. **Parmar H, Gujar S, Shah G, Mukherji SK. Imaging of the anterior skull base. Neuroimaging Clin N Am 2009;19:427–439**

19. Ginsberg LE. Perineural tumor spread associated with head and neck malignancies. In: Som PM, Curtin HD, eds. Head and Neck Imaging, 5th ed. St. Louis: Mosby; 2011

20. Algin O, Turkbey B. Intrathecal gadolinium-enhanced MR cisternography: a comprehensive review. AJNR Am J Neuroradiol 2013;34:14–22

21. Yamada S, Tsuchiya K, Bradley WG, et al. Current and emerging MR imaging techniques for the diagnosis and management of CSF flow disorders: a review of phase-contrast and time-spatial labeling inversion pulse. AJNR Am J Neuroradiol 2014

22. Roundy N, Delashaw JB, Cetas JS. Preoperative identification of the facial nerve in patients with large cerebellopontine angle tumors using high-density diffusion tensor imaging. J Neurosurg 2012;116:697–702

23. Garcíaa LC, Alonsoa PA, Cardarellia A, Martinoa AP, Rimoldi J, Figari A. Diffusion tensor technique as a preoperative identification of cranial nerves in skull base tumors. Rev Argent Radiol 2013;77:197–201

24. Lim RP, Shapiro M, Wang EY, et al. 3D time-resolved MR angiography (MRA) of the carotid arteries with time-resolved imaging with stochastic trajectories: comparison with 3D contrast-enhanced Bolus-Chase MRA and 3D time-of-flight MRA. AJNR Am J Neuroradiol 2008;29:1847–1854

25. Farb RI, Agid R, Willinsky RA, Johnstone DM, Terbrugge KG. Cranial dural arteriovenous fistula: diagnosis and classification with time-resolved MR angiography at 3T. AJNR Am J Neuroradiol 2009;30:1546–1551

26. Willinsky RA, Taylor SM, TerBrugge K, Farb RI, Tomlinson G, Montanera W. Neurologic complications of cerebral angiography: prospective analysis of 2,899 procedures and review of the literature. Radiology 2003;227:522–528

27. Kaufmann TJ, Huston J III, Mandrekar JN, Schleck CD, Thielen KR, Kallmes DF. Complications of diagnostic cerebral angiography: evaluation of 19,826 consecutive patients. Radiology 2007;243:812–819

28. American College of Radiology (ACR)/American Society of Neuroradiology (ASNR)/ Society for Pediatric Radiology (SNR)/Society of Neurointerventional Surgery (SNIS). Practice guideline for the performance of diagnostic cervicocerebral catheter angiography in adults. Available at: http://www.acr.org/Quality-Safety/Standards-Guidelines/Practice-Guidelines-by-Modality/~/media/ACR/Documents/PGTS/guidelines/Cervicocerebral_Catheter_Angio.pdf. Accessed August 4, 2014

29. Siepmann DB, Siegel A, Lewis PJ. Tl-201 SPECT and F-18 FDG PET for assessment of glioma recurrence versus radiation necrosis. Clin Nucl Med 2005;30:199–200

30. Heiss WD, Raab P, Lanfermann H. Multimodality assessment of brain tumors and tumor recurrence. J Nucl Med 2011;52:1585–1600

31. Noyek AM, Kirsh JC, Greyson ND, et al. The clinical significance of radionuclide bone and gallium scanning in osteomyelitis of the head and neck. Laryngoscope 1984;94(5 Pt 2, Suppl 34):1–21

32. Gupta NC, Prezio JA. Radionuclide imaging in osteomyelitis. Semin Nucl Med 1988;18: 287–299

33. Sharma P, Agarwal KK, Kumar S, et al. Utility of (99m)Tc-MDP hybrid SPECT-CT for diagnosis of skull base osteomyelitis: comparison with planar bone scintigraphy, SPECT, and CT. Jpn J Radiol 2013;31:81–88

34. Graham P, Howman-Giles R, Johnston I, Besser M. Evaluation of CSF shunt patency by means of technetium-99m DTPA. J Neurosurg 1982;57:262–266

35. Tumiati MN, Facchi E, Gatti C, Bossi A, Longari V. Scintigraphic assessment of pituitary adenomas and several diseases by indium-111-pentetreotide. Q J Nucl Med 1995;39(4, Suppl 1):98–100

36. Maini CL, Sciuto R, Tofani A, et al. Somatostatin receptor imaging in CNS tumours using ^{111}In-octreotide. Nucl Med Commun 1995;16:756–766

37. Rieger A, Rainov NG, Elfrich C, et al. Somatostatin receptor scintigraphy in patients with pituitary adenoma. Neurosurg Rev 1997;20:7–12

38. Sasajima T, Kinouchi H, Naitoh Y, Tomura N, Watarai J, Mizoi K. ^{123}I-metaiodobenzylguanidine single-photon emission computerized tomography in brain tumors—a preliminary study. J Neurooncol 2006;77:185–191

39. Voges J, Sturm V, Lehrke R, Treuer H, Gauss C, Berthold F. Cystic craniopharyngioma: long-term results after intracavitary irradiation with stereotactically applied colloidal beta-emitting radioactive sources. Neurosurgery 1997;40:263–269, discussion 269–270

40. Hasegawa T, Kondziolka D, Hadjipanayis CG, Lunsford LD. Management of cystic craniopharyngiomas with phosphorus-32 intracavitary irradiation. Neurosurgery 2004; 54:813–820, discussion 820–822

41. Barriger RB, Chang A, Lo SS, et al. Phosphorus-32 therapy for cystic craniopharyngiomas. Radiother Oncol 2011;98:207–212

42. Kickingereder P, Maarouf M, El Majdoub F, et al. Intracavitary brachytherapy using stereotactically applied phosphorus-32 colloid for treatment of cystic craniopharyngiomas in 53 patients. J Neurooncol 2012;109:365–374

43. **Menezes AH. Abnormalities of the craniocervical junction. In: Fessler RG, Sekhar L, eds. Atlas of Neurosurgical Techniques. Spine and Peripheral Nerves. New York: Thieme; 2006:3–11**

44. **Smoker WR, Khanna G. Imaging the craniocervical junction. Childs Nerv Syst 2008;24:1123–1145**

45. Rojas CA, Bertozzi JC, Martinez CR, Whitlow J. Reassessment of the craniocervical junction: normal values on CT. AJNR Am J Neuroradiol 2007;28:1819–1823

46. Newton TH, Potts DG. Radiology of the Skull and Brain. St. Louis: Mosby; 1977

47. Ginsberg LE. Radiology of meningiomas. J Neurooncol 1996;29:229–238

48. **Lee JH. Meningiomas, Diagnosis, Treatment, and Outcome. New York: Springer-Verlag; 2009**

49. Smith AB, Horkanyne-Szakaly I, Schroeder JW, Rushing EJ. From the radiologic pathology archives: mass lesions of the dura: beyond meningioma-radiologic-pathologic correlation. Radiographics 2014;34:295–312

50. Madani G, Beale TJ, Lund VJ. Imaging of sinonasal tumors. Semin Ultrasound CT MR 2009;30:25–38

51. Som PM, Brandwein-Genslar MS, Kassel EE, Genden EM. Tumors and tumor-like conditions of the sinonasal cavities. In: Som PM, Curtin HD, eds. Head and Neck Imaging, 5th ed. St. Louis: Mosby; 2011

52. Aribandi M, McCoy VA, Bazan C III. Imaging features of invasive and noninvasive fungal sinusitis: a review. Radiographics 2007;27:1283–1296

53. Caldemeyer KS, Mathews VP, Righi PD, Smith RR. Imaging features and clinical significance of perineural spread or extension of head and neck tumors. Radiographics 1998;18:97–110, quiz 147

54. **Pieper DR, Al-Mefty O. Management of intracranial meningiomas secondarily involving the infratemporal fossa: radiographic characteristics, pattern of tumor invasion, and surgical implications. Neurosurgery 1999;45:231–237, discussion 237–238**

55. Paes FM, Singer AD, Checkver AN, Palmquist RA, De La Vega G, Sidani C. Perineural spread in head and neck malignancies: clinical significance and evaluation with 18F-FDG PET/CT. Radiographics 2013;33:1717–1736

56. Vogl TJ, Mack MG, Juergens M, et al. Skull base tumors: gadodiamide injection—enhanced MR imaging—drop-out effect in the early enhancement pattern of paragangliomas versus different tumors. Radiology 1993;188:339–346

6 Pathology of the Skull Base Tumors

■ Key Points

Definition

- Skull base tumors are a diverse group of neoplasms with different clinical, biological, and pathological features.
- They vary from benign, clinically indolent lesions to very aggressive malignancies that have a dismal prognosis.
- Both the biological behavior and anatomic location of the tumor have to be considered.

Classification

- Tumors of the skull base can arise from a wide array of tissues and may originate intracranially, extracranially, or from the skull base itself. The skull base can also be involved with systemic neoplasms (hematologic malignancies and metastases) and benign cysts.
- Despite this heterogeneity, the differential diagnoses can often be narrowed based on the location of the lesion (**Table 6.1**).
- Immunohistochemistry is a useful tool for differentiating tumors that have a similar morphological appearance (**Table 6.2**).

■ Intracranial Tumors: Tumors of the Nervous System

Pilocytic Astrocytoma (Optic Pathway Glioma)

Pilocytic astrocytoma is a relatively slow-growing, well-circumscribed tumor, World Health Organization (WHO) grade I[1], likely of astrocytic origin occurring anywhere along the neuraxis.

Table 6.1 Anatomically Based Classification of Skull Base Tumors

Anterior Skull Base	
Intracranial	Meningioma, optic pathway glioma
Sinonasal tract	Inverted papilloma, nasopharyngeal angiofibroma, squamous cell carcinoma, adenocarcinoma, adenoid cystic carcinoma, sinonasal undifferentiated carcinoma, esthesioneuroblastoma, mucosal melanoma, sinonasal lymphoma
Orbit	Cavernous hemangioma, capillary hemangioma, lymphangioma, melanoma, retinoblastoma, lymphoma, optic pathway glioma, optic nerve sheath meningioma, osteoma, orbital rhabdomyosarcoma
Middle Skull Base	
Sellar/suprasellar	Pituitary adenoma, meningioma, craniopharyngioma, germ cell tumors, pilocytic astrocytoma/optic pathway glioma, nasopharyngeal carcinoma, sinonasal carcinomas, (epi)dermoid cyst, Rathke cleft cyst, arachnoid cyst
Pterygopalatine/infratemporal fossae	Meningioma, schwannoma, lymphoma, ameloblastoma, adenoid cystic carcinoma, juvenile nasopharyngeal angiofibroma, hemangioma, squamous cell carcinoma, chondrosarcoma
Posterior Skull Base	
Petrous apex	Chondrosarcoma, meningioma, chordoma, plasmacytoma, paraganglioma, endolymphatic sac tumor, schwannoma, cholesterol granuloma, mucocele, epidermoid cyst
Cerebellopontine angle	Schwannoma, meningioma, epidermoid cyst, arachnoid cyst
Jugular foramen	Paraganglioma, schwannoma, meningioma
Clivus	Chordoma, chondrosarcoma, meningioma, plasmacytoma
Foramen magnum	Meningioma, schwannoma, chordoma, chondrosarcoma, fibrous dysplasia
Craniocervical junction	Meningioma, neurofibroma, chordoma, bone tumors

Table 6.2   Common Antibodies in Skull Base Tumors[168]

Antibody	Tumor(s)
Brain, Neuroendocrine, Meninges	
Glial fibrillary acid protein (GFAP)	Astrocytoma, nasal glial heterotopia, schwannoma (variable), esthesioneuroblastoma (variable), endolymphatic sac tumor (variable)
Synaptophysin	Paraganglioma, esthesioneuroblastoma
Chromogranin	Paraganglioma, esthesioneuroblastoma
S100	Schwannoma, neurofibroma, astrocytoma, chordoma, melanoma, paraganglioma (sustentacular cells), esthesioneuroblastoma (sustentacular cells), meningioma (variable)
EMA	Meningioma, chordoma, nasopharyngeal carcinoma, adenocarcinoma, sinonasal undifferentiated carcinoma, squamous cell carcinoma (variable), arachnoid cyst
GH, PRL, TSH, ACTH, LH, FSH, α-subunit	Pituitary adenoma (see text)
Germ cells	
α-fetoprotein	Yolk sac tumor, teratoma (variable)
β-HCG	Choriocarcinoma
Human placental lactogen (HPL)	Choriocarcinoma
Placental alkaline phosphatase (PLAP)	Germinoma, embryonal carcinoma, yolk sac tumor (variable), choriocarcinoma (variable)
C-kit	Germinoma, teratoma (variable)
OCT4	Germinoma, embryonal carcinoma
Cytokeratins	
AE1/AE3	Wide panel that stains most epithelium (does not include cytokeratins [CK] 8 and 18)
CAM5.2	Panel that includes CKs 8, 18, and 19; used with AE1/AE3 in screening panel
CK5/6	Low molecular weight keratins that are positive in squamous cell carcinoma (not adenocarcinoma)
Soft tissue	
CD34	Hemangiopericytoma, normal endothelium
Desmin	Muscle differentiation, including rhabdomyosarcoma
Vimentin	Most mesenchymal cells; soft tissue tumors, meningioma
Myogenin	Rhabdomyosarcoma
CD99	Chondrosarcoma, Ewing's sarcoma

(continued)

Table 6.2 (*continued*)

Antibody	Tumor(s)
Hematopoietic	
CD45	Lymphocytes but not plasma cells
CD20	B-cells (and related lymphomas)
CD3	T-cells (and related lymphomas)
CD56	NK cells, NK/T-cell lymphoma
CD79a	B cells (and lymphomas) and plasma cells (and myeloma)
CD138	Plasma cells, myeloma/plasmacytoma
Melanocytic	
HMB-45	Melanoma
Melan-A	Melanoma

Abbreviations: ACTH, adrenocorticotropic hormone; EMA, epithelial membrane antigen; FSH, follicle-stimulating hormone; GH, growth hormone; HCG, human chorionic gonadotropin; LH, luteinizing hormone; NK, natural killer; PRL, prolactin; TSH, thyroid-stimulating hormone.

- Relevant to the skull base, pilocytic astrocytomas commonly occur along the optic pathway (optic nerve, chiasm, hypothalamic region), and hence are termed optic pathway gliomas (OPGs).
- In children, the optic pathway is the most common supratentorial site. Overall, 25% involve only the optic disk and nerve, but 40 to 75% involve the chiasm. Of these, 33 to 60% also involve the hypothalamus or third ventricle.[2]

Epidemiology

Pilocytic astrocytomas account for 3 to 5% of childhood intracranial tumors.[3]

- Typically, the mean age of onset is 9 years, but OPGs have been reported in patients up to 79 years of age; males and females are affected equally.[4]
- Optic pathway gliomas are seen in 11 to 30% of individuals with neurofibromatosis type 1 (NF1).[5]

Pathology

Pilocytic astrocytomas are soft, gray, and generally well circumscribed; often they are cystic.[1] OPGs involving the optic nerve show fusiform enlargement and kinking. Microscopically, the tumor shows a biphasic pattern of growth, consisting of compacted bipolar cells with Rosenthal fibers and looser multipolar cells with microcysts and eosinophilic granular bodies. Tumors exhibit either perineural or intraneural growth, with sporadic cases favoring the latter and NF1 patients the former.[4]

Diagnostic Criteria for Neurofibromatosis Type 1[6]

Two or more of the following:

- Six or more café-au-lait spots ≥ 5 mm in diameter in prepubertal individuals and ≥ 15 mm in postpubertal individuals
- Axillary or inguinal freckles
- Two or more typical neurofibromas or one plexiform neurofibroma
- Optic pathway glioma
- Two or more iris hamartomas (Lisch nodules)
- A distinctive osseous lesion such as sphenoid dysplasia or thinning of long bone cortex, with or without pseudarthrosis
- First-degree relative with NF1 by above criteria

Prognosis

Generally, the prognosis is favorable, as OPGs are slow growing and low grade.

- The presence of NF1 and an anterior location are favorable factors, whereas younger age at presentation confers a poorer prognosis.[7]
- Optic pathway gliomas involving the chiasm, hypothalamus, or third ventricle fare worse than those involving the anterior visual pathway or the optic nerve alone and tend to have higher rates of recurrence.[8]

Schwannoma

Schwannoma is a benign encapsulated tumor, WHO grade I[9], arising from the Schwann cells that support peripheral nerves.

- Schwannomas are the main peripheral nerve sheath tumor that should be considered in the skull base, usually from the vestibular divisions of cranial nerve (CN) VIII (90%).[10]
- Less commonly, they can also be associated with the CNs V (second most common),[11] VII (third most common),[12] IX, X, XI, and XII. Very rare localizations are CN IV (probable origin of some of the described tentorial schwannomas), greater superficial petrosal nerve, ethmoidal nerves (the latter as the probable cause of the "anterior skull base" schwannomas).
- Terms such as *acoustic neurinoma* or *neuroma* are incorrect.

Epidemiology

Schwannomas represent 8% of intracranial tumors and 85% of cerebellopontine angle (CPA) tumors.[10]

- Approximately 4% are in the setting of neurofibromatosis type 2 (NF2) and in 5% are multiple but not associated with NF2.[13] Men and women are affected equally, usually in the fourth to sixth decades.[9]

Pathology

Schwannomas appear as globoid masses measuring a few centimeters in size, sometimes with cystic or hemorrhagic components.

- Microscopically, neoplastic cells have a characteristic histology that falls into two intermixed patterns:
  - Antoni A pattern is composed of compact, elongated cells with occasional nuclear palisading (Verocay bodies), although this is less common with intracranial schwannomas.
  - Antoni B areas are less cellular, with loosely textured cells, indistinct process, and variable lipidization (the most typical in the CPA schwannomas).[9]
- Cystic and hemorrhagic degeneration may be present.
- A bizarre nuclear appearance, cytoplasmic-nuclear inclusions, and occasional mitotic figures are known as "ancient" changes and are not features associated with malignancy.
- Thick-walled, hyalinized blood vessels may be present.
- Variants of the classic morphology include cellular (hypercellular with predominant Antoni A tissue), plexiform (plexiform or multinodular growth pattern, which is not common in intracranial schwannomas as this usually involves a nerve plexus), and melanotic (pigmented cells containing melanosomes).
- Immunohistochemistry: tumor cells strongly express S100 and may focally express glial fibrillary acid protein (GFAP). All tumor cells possess a surface basal lamina, which can be stained using collagen IV or visualized by electron microscopy.
- Malignant change in schwannoma is exceptionally rare[14]

Treatment and Prognosis

Schwannomas are benign and slow-growing tumors. Cellular schwannomas tend to recur more commonly (30–40%).[15]

Neurofibroma

Neurofibroma is a tumor consisting of a mixture of cell types (Schwann cells, perineurial-like cells, fibroblasts) either growing in a well-circumscribed intraneural or diffusely infiltrative extraneural fashion. It occurs in peripheral nerves/plexus, skin, and, more rarely, orbit, spinal roots, or cranial nerves.

Schwannomas and Neurofibromatosis Type 2

- Schwannomas are one of the tumors associated with NF2, an autosomal-dominant syndrome that occurs much less frequently than NF1, with a prevalence of 1 in 50,000.[16]
- NF2 is a tumor suppressor and its mutation results in loss of expression of its protein product merlin.[17,18]
- Patients may have benign and hamartomatous lesions of Schwann and meningothelial cells.
- The presence of bilateral vestibular schwannomas is a diagnostic feature of this syndrome.
- NF2-associated schwannomas are similar to their sporadic counterparts, but there are some special features: earlier presentation, higher proliferative indices, and increased entrapped facial nerve fibers

Diagnostic Criteria for Neurofibromatosis Type 2[16]

- Bilateral vestibular schwannomas
- A first-degree relative with NF2 AND
  - Unilateral vestibular schwannoma OR
  - Any two of: meningioma, schwannoma, glioma, neurofibroma, posterior subcapsular lenticular opacities
- Unilateral vestibular schwannoma AND
  - Any two of: meningioma, schwannoma, glioma, neurofibroma, posterior subcapsular lenticular opacities
- Multiple meningiomas AND
  - Unilateral vestibular schwannoma OR
  - Any two of: schwannoma, glioma, neurofibroma, cataract

- Multiple or plexiform neurofibromas are associated with the neurofibromatosis type.

Epidemiology

Neurofibroma is sporadic or associated with NF1. It has no sex predilection, and all ages are affected.

Pathology

Solitary neurofibromas are well circumscribed and fusiform.

- Plexiform neurofibromas have a "bag of worms" appearance (NF1).
- Microscopically, neurofibromas are composed mostly of Schwann cells with spindled nuclei and fibroblasts, on a background of collagen and myxoid material that may appear in bundles ("shredded carrots").
- Immunohistochemistry: invariably positive for S100.

Prognosis

Tumors of major nerves or of a plexiform pattern may transform to malignant peripheral nerve sheath tumors.

■ Meningothelial and Dural-Based Tumors

Meningioma

Meningiomas arise from arachnoid cap cells and usually appear grossly as a well-demarcated solid mass with broad dural attachment.[19]

- Invasion of the dura is common, sometimes with hyperostotic changes in the overlying skull.
- In 2 to 9% of cases, the meningioma appears en plaque, showing flat, plate-like growth.[20]
- Multiple meningiomas occur in less than 10% of cases, often in association with NF2.[21]

Epidemiology

Overall, meningiomas are the most common primary intracranial tumor with an incidence of 13 per 100,000 and occur mainly in middle-aged to elderly patients.[19] They are more common in women (2:1).

Location

Intracranial meningiomas occur most commonly over the convexities, sometimes parasagittal in association with the falx. Other common sites include the anterior skull base (olfactory groove, planum sphenoidale), sphenoid wing, sellar/suprasellar region, optic nerve sheath, petrous ridge (CPA), tentorium, and posterior fossa.

- Higher grade meningiomas may metastasize outside the central nervous system (CNS), with the most common sites of involvement being the lung, pleura, bone, and liver.[22]

Pathology

Microscopically, meningiomas have diverse histological appearances and can fall into WHO grades I to III.[19]

- 80% grade I; 15–18% grade II; 2–5% grade III.[19,23]
- Common immunohistochemical markers for meningiomas include epithelial membrane antigen (EMA), vimentin, and progesterone receptor.
- Proliferative marker Ki-67 is also a useful indicator of aggressiveness but currently not part of the WHO grading criteria. A proliferative index < 5% is generally seen in grade I tumors, but there are no specific cut-offs delineating the different grades.
- Cytokeratins and S100 are variably positive.
- On electron microscopy, interdigitating cell membranes with desmosomes are a characteristic feature.

Meningioma Subtypes by Grade (2007 WHO Classification)[19]

WHO Grade I
- Meningothelial
- Fibrous (fibroblastic)
- Transitional (mixed)
- Psammomatous
- Angiomatous
- Microcystic
- Secretory
- Lymphoplasmacyte-rich
- Metaplastic

WHO Grade II
- Atypical
- Chordoid
- Clear cell
- Any WHO grade I histology with brain invasion

WHO Grade III
- Anaplastic
- Papillary
- Rhabdoid

WHO Grade I

- *Meningothelial:* lobules and whorls formed by largely uniform tumor cells (closely resembling the normal arachnoid cap cells) with oval nuclei that occasionally show clearing or "pseudoinclusions." Lobules are demarcated by thin collagenous septa.
- *Fibrous* (or *fibroblastic*): spindle cells forming a network of bundles and fascicles in a collagen-rich matrix.
- *Transitional* (or *mixed*): coexistence of the features of the two previous patterns.

These first three subtypes are the most common.

- *Psammomatous:* predominance of psammoma bodies, which are round collections of calcium. Tumor cells usually have a transitional appearance with whorl-formation.
- *Angiomatous:* predominance of blood vessels of variable size and wall thickness. Vessel walls usually show marked hyalinization. The differential diagnosis includes vascular malformations and hemangioblastomas. Cerebral edema may be seen on imaging.
- *Microcystic:* tumor cells with long thin processes and intercellular microcysts containing eosinophilic mucinous fluid. This can result in edema.
- *Secretory:* Focal epithelial differentiation results in formation of pseudopsammoma bodies, which contain periodic acid-Schiff (PAS)-positive, eosinophilic fluid. These structures stain for carcinoembryonic antigen (CEA).[24] Due to its secretory nature, significant peritumoral edema can be seen on imaging.[25]
- *Lymphoplasmacyte-rich:* the rarest variant, characterized by extensive inflammatory infiltration that may leave the meningothelial component difficult to appreciate. Abnormal systemic hematology may be a clinical finding.[26]
- *Metaplastic:* Mesenchymal components (bone, cartilage, fat) may be present. Care must be taken to distinguish these from meningiomas exhibiting bone and/or soft tissue invasion.

WHO Grade II

- Higher grades are more likely to recur and take a more aggressive clinical course. They are also more likely to metastasize.
  - *Chordoid:* cords or trabeculae of eosinophilic and often vacuolated cells in mucoid matrix, similar to chordomas. These areas are often contained with more meningothelial elements.[27]
  - *Clear cell:* Growing in no specific pattern, there is abundant glycogen in tumor cell cytoplasm, giving it a clear appearance, and abundant interstitial and perivascular collagen deposition. The glycogen-rich cytoplasm is PAS positive. Most commonly, clear cell meningiomas occur in the CPA and cauda equina, which can result in cerebrospinal fluid (CSF) seeding.
  - *Atypical:* Tumors can meet criteria for the "atypical" category independent of morphological subtype. The criteria, which correlate with an eightfold increase in recurrence rate, are increased mitotic activity (≥ 4 mitoses/10 high-power fields) or three or

> **Pathology Pearl**
>
> The presence of brain invasion in a tumor with grade I histology is associated with increased rate of recurrence, and so this feature is sufficient to warrant classification as grade II.[19]

more of the following: increased cellularity, small cell morphology with high nuclear/cytoplasmic ratio, prominent nucleoli, patternless or sheet-like growth, and foci of "spontaneous" or "geographic" necrosis.

WHO Grade III

- These highest grade meningiomas are rare, with an incidence of 0.17 per 100 000 persons[10] and a median survival time of < 2 years.[28]
  - *Rhabdoid:* Sheets of rhabdoid (muscle-like) cells, with eccentric nuclei, prominent nucleoli, and prominent eosinophilic cytoplasm, are present. They are highly proliferative and often contain another histological hallmark of malignancy.
  - *Papillary:* A perivascular pseudopapillary (finger-like) pattern composes most of the tumor. This tends to occur mainly in younger patients, and local and/or brain invasion is present in the majority of cases.
  - *Anaplastic* (or *malignant*): These tumors demonstrate the histological features of malignancy in excess of what is seen in atypical meningiomas. These features include obvious malignant cytology resembling carcinoma, melanoma, or high-grade sarcoma, or a highly elevated mitotic index, i.e., ≥ 20 mitoses/10 high-power fields.

Meningioma Metastasis

Metastases to outside the CNS can be seen in an estimated 0.15 to 0.76% of all meningiomas,[29,30] usually in higher grades. Lungs/pleura (37%), bones (16.5%), intraspinal (15%), and liver (9%)[22] are the most common sites, with sporadic reports in other locations as well.

- Metastases *into* meningiomas by systemic neoplasms have also been reported. In cases with a high index of suspicion, even benign-appearing meningioma specimens should be submitted *in toto* and examined carefully because the presence of a systemic micrometastasis would significantly alter the prognosis.[31]

Meningioma Mimics[32]

Neoplastic
- Dural-based metastasis
- Schwannoma (CPA)
- Hemangiopericytoma/solitary fibrous tumor
- Lymphoma, plasmacytoma
- Melanocytic neoplasms

Nonneoplastic
- Rosai-Dorfman disease
- Neurosarcoidosis
- Hypertrophic pachymeningitis

Hemangiopericytoma/Solitary Fibrous Tumor

Recent evidence suggests that hemangiopericytoma (HPC) and solitary fibrous tumor (SFT) represent morphological variants of the same tumor type, with HPC being the cellular variant and SFT the less cellular variant.[33]

- Classically, HPC is a very cellular and vascularized mesenchymal tumor, with dural attachment and high tendency to recur (almost invariably) or to metastasize (bones, lung, liver).[34]
- Hemangiopericytoma is WHO grade II, with an anaplastic variant that is WHO grade III.
- Hemangiopericytomas are usually solitary and generally radiologically indistinguishable from meningioma. However, edema is usually present in the underlying brain parenchyma and it lacks the calcifications sometimes seen in meningiomas.

Epidemiology

Hemangiopericytomas are rare, accounting for 0.4% of all primary brain tumors, and they are more frequent in men than in women, with mean age of onset in the fifth decade.[35]

Pathology

Grossly, HPCs are solid and well-demarcated tumors that have a tendency to bleed.

- Microscopically, tumor cells are monomorphous and closely packed, arranged randomly, and with little intervening collagen.
- Nuclei are round to oval and sometimes spindled.
- There is a rich vasculature with slit-like vessels lined by flattened endothelium and thin-walled branching vascular spaces known as "stag-horn" vessels.
- Infiltration into adjacent brain or bone (without hyperostosis seen in meningiomas) can occur.
- Anaplastic (grade III) tumors show high mitotic activity ($\geq$ 5 mitoses/10 high-power field) or necrosis, and two or more of the following: hemorrhage, moderate to high nuclear atypia, and cellularity.[34]
- Immunohistochemistry: HPCs stain for vimentin and CD34. They are negative for EMA, progesterone receptor (usually positive in meningioma), and CD31.
- As mentioned previously, HPC and SFT exist on a spectrum as they share a genetic mutation that results in a STAT6-NAB2 fusion protein. This results in constitutive activation of STAT6 and its aberrant localization to the nucleus,

which can be detected by immunohistochemistry and distinguishes it from histological mimics.[36,37]

Prognosis

The median survival for grade II hemangioperycitomas is 216 months versus 142 months for grade III tumors.[38]

■ Pituitary Tumors

Pituitary Adenoma

Pituitary adenoma accounts for 10 to 15% of all intracranial tumors, and have been found in almost 20% of the general population at autopsy.[39]

- They are rare in the pediatric population, accounting for 2% of pituitary tumors.
- Although considered benign, as many as 25 to 55% of pituitary adenomas are invasive[40–42] and may have clinically aggressive behavior.[43,44]

Classification

Adenomas can be classified by size as microadenomas (diameter < 10 mm), macroadenomas (≥ 10 mm), or giant adenomas (> 4 cm).

- Clinically, they are also divided into functional (two thirds of cases) and nonfunctional (or silent) by the presence of symptomatic endocrinopathy or elevated serum levels of a circulating hormone.[45]
- In contrast, the histological classification of pituitary adenomas is based on the cell of origin (somatotroph, lactotroph, corticotroph, thyrotroph, gonadotroph), mainly by the use of immunohistochemistry for hormone(s) and specific transcription factors expressed. Each cell type can give rise to a tumor that is either clinically functional or nonfunctional.[46]

Functional Adenomas

Growth Hormone–Producing Adenoma[47]

Growth hormone–producing adenoma accounts for 25 to 30% of surgically removed pituitary adenomas but 11 to 13% in clinical series (due to medical management),[48] and it manifests as growth hormone (GH)/insulin-like growth factor (IGF)-1 excess, mass effect, or tumor-induced adenohypophyseal dysfunction.

- Microadenomas are well circumscribed, but macroadenomas have been known to invade the meninges, cavernous sinus, bone, and sphenoid sinus.

- The pseudocapsule, composed mainly of fibroblasts and collagen, distinguishes adenoma from a normal pituitary gland. It may contain tumor cells, and its resection may result in higher rates of remission.[49]
- Growth hormone–producing adenomas can be monohormonal somatotroph adenomas, bihormonal mammosomatotroph adenomas, or plurihormonal adenomas that produce thyroid-stimulating hormone (TSH) and α-subunit of glycoprotein as well.
- Somatotroph adenomas can be densely granulated or sparsely granulated.
    - Densely granulated somatotroph adenoma is characterized by medium-size, round acidophilic cells with granular cytoplasm. It stains for GH in a strong, uniform, and diffuse manner. Half of these tumors also stain for α-subunit of glycoprotein hormones.
    - The sparsely granulated somatotroph adenomas are cellular chromophobic tumors composed of small, round irregular cells with a round nucleus and prominent nucleolus. The cytoplasm often contains a "fibrous body" that causes peripheral displacement of the nucleus. Immunoreactivity for GH is often scant or negative. Fibrous bodies are reactive for low molecular weight keratins (e.g., CAM 5.2).
    - The electron microscopic characterization in densely and sparsely granulated tumors is clinically relevant. Sparsely granulated GH-adenomas may show resistance to long-acting somatostatin analogues (54% acute GH reduction and 7% long-term IGF-1 reduction vs 87% and 52%, respectively, for densely granulated).[50,51]
- Mammosomatroph adenoma is a rarer entity, containing both GH and prolactin.
- Plurihormonal adenomas can produce β-TSH, and sometimes β-follicle-stimulating hormone (FSH) and β-luteinizing hormone (LH), in addition to GH, prolactin (PRL), and α-subunit.
- Pit-1 transcription factor, localized in somatotrophs, lactotrophs, and thyrotrophs, is expressed in all these tumors.[46]
- Pituitary tumor transforming gene (PTTG) has been found to have highest expression in GH-producing adenomas[52]; in other studies, it is an emerging biomarker for aggressive behavior.[53,54]

Prolactin-Producing Adenoma[55]

Prolactin-producing adenoma accounts for 11 to 26% of pituitary adenomas in surgical series, but represents ~ 50% of all adenomas. Medical management is the mainstay of treatment.[48] Onset usually occurs in young adulthood, with a female predominance.

- Prolactin-producing adenomas fall into either sparsely granulated (most common) or densely granulated lactotroph categories. A rarer entity known as acidophil stem cell adenoma is variably classified as a subtype of either GH-producing adenoma or PRL-producing adenoma.

- Sparsely granulated lactotroph adenomas have a diffuse or rarely papillary growth pattern and contain relatively large and elongated tumor cells. The cytoplasm is chromophobic or slightly acidophilic. PRL is positive in the cytoplasm exhibiting an extremely rare paranuclear pattern, and α-subunit is usually negative.
- Densely granulated lactotroph adenoma is distinguished by stronger cytoplasmic acidophilia and strong, diffuse PRL staining.
- The transcription factors Pit-1 and Estrogen Receptor (ER) are positive in PRL-producing adenoma.[46]

Thyroid-Stimulating Hormone–Producing Adenoma[56]

Thyroid-stimulating hormone–producing adenomas are rare tumors accounting for about 1% of pituitary adenomas, the rarest cause of hyperthyroidism. Age of onset was found to be 20s to 60s with a female predominance in a small series.

- At the time of presentation, most tumors are macroadenomas.
- Thyrotroph adenoma is composed of chromophobic cells with indistinct cell borders, growing in a solid or sinusoidal pattern. Stromal fibrosis is a common finding. Cytoplasmic globules representing lysosomes stain strongly with PAS. Tumor cells are immunoreactive for α-subunit and β-TSH.

Adrenocorticotropic Hormone (ACTH)-Producing Adenoma[57]

Adrenocorticotropic hormone (ACTH)-producing adenoma is the cause of Cushing's disease and occurs at a rate of 1 to 10 cases per million per year; it accounts for 10 to 15% of pituitary adenomas. The peak incidence is in the fourth decade and is much more prevalent in women (8:1).

- Corticotroph adenomas contain monomorphic round cells in a diffuse pattern with a characteristic sinusoidal pattern around capillaries. The cells are basophilic and PAS-positive. Immunoreactivity is positive for ACTH, β-lipotropic pituitary hormone (LPH), and β-endorphin, which are cleavage products of the precursor molecule pro-opiomelanocortin.
- Crooke cell adenoma is another subtype that may produce ACTH. It is clinically aggressive and distinguished by prominent cytoplasmic cytokeratin filaments.[58–60]
- Crooke's hyaline change refers to nonadenomatous corticotrophs with a zone of glassy agranular cytoplasm (accumulation of keratin filaments) around its nucleus and is indicative of glucocorticoid excess (corticotroph adenoma, ectopic ACTH secretion, adrenocortical hyperplasia, or exogenous source)[46]

Plurihormonal Adenoma[61]

These tumors are defined as those having immunoreactivities for more than one pituitary hormone, which are not explained by normal developmental mechanisms. Hence, they do not include combinations of GH, PRL, and TSH or of FSH and LH.

- Microscopically, these tumors tend to be chromophobic and negative for PAS.
- Combinations of hormone reactivities commonly found include TSH, FSH, and GH or PRL and TSH, although any combination is possible.[62]

Nonfunctional Adenomas

Nonfunctional adenomas are those that do not present with clinical or biochemical evidence of a hormone excess syndrome. Most commonly, these are gonadotroph adenomas.[46,63]

Gonadotropin-Producing Adenoma[63]

Functional gonadotropin (FSH, LH)-producing adenomas are uncommon and are usually diagnosed in men more than in women.

- Gonadotroph adenomas are usually clinically silent.[46]
- At the time of diagnosis, the tumor is often a macroadenoma and can show significant sellar/suprasellar invasion.
- The tumor can grow in several histological patterns, which can occur in combination.
- The majority consists of uniform, tall, polar cells forming a sinusoidal pattern with perivascular pseudorosettes. Papillary growth is another pattern, although less common. A minority shows diffuse growth. This histological variability is also reflected in its immunohistochemical profile. There is often patchy, uneven staining with α-subunit, β-FSH, and β-LH.
- These tumors are also positive for the transcription factor Steroidogenic Factor 1 (SF1).[46]

α-Subunit of Glycoprotein Hormones[64]

The hormones human chorionic gonadotropin (HCG), LH, FSH, and TSH consist of an α- and β-subunit. The α-subunits of these hormones (expressed in certain pituitary adenomas) are nearly identical, whereas the β-subunits confer specificity.

Silent Corticotroph Adenomas

There are two types of silent corticotroph adenomas: subtype 1 and subtype 2.[57]

- Subtype 1 very closely resembles functional corticotroph adenomas seen in Cushing disease.
- Subtype 2 has smaller than average polyhedral cells and sparse, irregular secretory granules on electron microscopy. It resembles sparse corticotrophs.

Silent Subtype 3 Adenoma[65]

A nonfunctional *plurihormonal adenoma*, the silent subtype 3 adenoma tends to occur in women between 20 and 35 years of age, but it has no age predilection in men.[66] Often, it is a macroadenoma at the time of diagnosis. It is composed of spindle cells and fibrous stroma and may show positivity for GH, PRL, and TSH, and other hormones.

Null Cell Adenoma[67]

These tumors have no hormone immunoreactivity or any other markers of differentiation along a particular adenohypophysial lineage. They occur often in elderly individuals. They are immunopositive for synaptophysin and chromogranin, providing evidence that they are pituitary tumors.

- Microscopically, tumor cells are usually chromophobic and round or polyhedral in shape. There is usually diffuse or papillary growth pattern, with pseudorosette formation.
- These tumors are PAS negative, and they stain for adenohypophyseal hormones and transcription factors.

> **Pathology Pearl**
>
> Pituitary adenomas are defined as "atypical" when they show high mitotic activity, Ki-67 labeling ≥ 3% of cells, and extensive p53 immunoreactivity.

Pituitary Carcinoma

It is defined as a tumor of adenohypophyseal cells that exhibits cerebrospinal and/or systematic metastasis.[68] It accounts for 0.2% of pituitary tumors.

- More than 75% of pituitary carcinomas are functional, with PRL and ACTH as the most common tumors.[69]

Other Tumors of the Pituitary

- Spindle cell oncocytoma of the adenohypophysis is a benign sellar tumor, WHO grade I,[70] consisting of granular, mitochondria-rich spindle cells.
- Pituicytoma is a rare neurohypophyseal tumor, WHO grade I,[71] composed of spindle cells arranged in fascicles.
- Granular cell tumor is a sellar/suprasellar tumor of the neurohypophysis or infundibulum, WHO grade I.[72] It is composed of large, eosinophilic, lysosome-rich cells.

- Spindle cell oncocytoma consists of a folliculostellate mass. Other findings suggest that these tumors are all derived from pituicytes, the modified glial cells of the neurohypophysis.[73]
- Pituitary blastoma is a rare embryonal pituitary tumor affecting children < 2 years of age. Microscopically, it shows glandular structures resembling Rathke epithelium, clusters of large secretory pituitary cells, and small undifferentiated cells.[74]

Craniopharyngioma

Craniopharyngiomas are benign, often totally or partially cystic, epithelial tumors, WHO grade I,[75] purported to arise from Rathke's pouch. They occur almost exclusively in the suprasellar region with a minor intrasellar component.

Epidemiology

Craniopharyngiomas account for 1.2 to 4.6% of all intracranial tumors, with an incidence of 0.5 to 2.5 cases per 1 million.[75] They are the most common non-neuroepithelial brain tumor in children (5–10%)[76]. Men and women are affected equally.

Classification

There are two subtypes of craniopharyngioma: adamantinomatous and papillary.

- Although adamantinomatous craniopharyngiomas have a bimodal age distribution with peaks at the ages 5 to 15 and 45 to 60,[77] the papillary subtype occurs nearly exclusively in adults.[76,78]

Adamantinomatous Craniopharyngioma

Adamantinomatous craniopharyngioma appears as a lobulated solid mass with a variable cystic component that contains a dark green-brown liquid resembling machinery oil. Calcification is common.

- Microscopically, it is composed of squamous epithelium organized in cords and lobules, bordered by palisaded columnar epithelium. These dense areas merge with looser areas of squamous cells known as stellate reticulum. "Wet keratin" nodules are another feature, composed of remnants of pale nuclei embedded within an eosinophilic keratinous mass. Flattened epithelium lines the cystic cavities and is filled with squamous debris.[79]

- At the brain–tumor interface, piloid gliosis with Rosenthal fibers is commonly seen and may be mistaken for pilocytic astrocytoma at frozen section or in small biopsies.[75]

Papillary Craniopharyngioma

Papillary craniopharyngioma is generally a solid tumor, without or with scarce cysts, and without cholesterol-rich machinery oil. Calcifications are uncommon.

- Microscopically, it consists of well-differentiated squamous epithelium arranged in pseudopapillae or papillae around a fibrovascular core.[80]

Prognosis

Approximately 60 to 90% of patients are recurrence-free at 10 years; the overall 10-year survival is likewise about 60 to 90%.[78,81,82] The most important factor in determining the risk of recurrence is the extent of resection.[75]

■ Germ Cell Tumors of the Central Nervous System

General

There are two different theories regarding the histogenesis of homologues of gonadal germ cell tumors: aberrant migration of primordial germ cells versus displaced embryonic tissues incorporated into neural tube.[83]

- Germ cell tumors preferentially occur in the midline, with the pineal region being the most common site affected, followed by the suprasellar location.

Epidemiology

Germ cell tumors are rare in Western countries, accounting for only 0.3 to 0.6% of intracranial neoplasms.[84] The peak age of onset is 10 to 14 years old, and 80 to 90% occur in patients under 25 years.[85]

- Pineal region germ cell tumors have a male predominance while suprasellar ones have a female predominance.[83]

Classification

Germ cell tumors have multiple subtypes: germinoma, teratoma (mature, immature), yolk sac tumor, embryonal carcinoma, and choriocarcinoma. With the exception of germinoma and teratoma, most germ cell tumors are of mixed histology.[86]

Germinoma

Germinoma grossly appears as a solid tumor with small foci of cystic change.

- Microscopically, they are large tumor cells with round nuclei and prominent nucleoli, growing in sheets or lobules. Lymphoid or lymphoplasmacytic infiltrate may be striking. Granulomatous response may be present.
- Immunohistochemistry: strong membranous positivity for c-kit and nuclear staining for OCT4. Placental alkaline phosphatase (PLAP) positivity (cytoplasmic and membranous) is less common.[87]
- A minority contain a syncytiotrophoblastic component that stains for β-HCG (also detected in serum/CSF[88]) and human placental lactogen (HPL).

Teratoma

Teratoma differentiates along three embryonic germ layers and can be mature (containing fully differentiated, adult tissues), immature (incompletely differentiated, fetal tissues), or a malignant transformation (teratoma with an additional malignant neoplasm of a conventional somatic type).

- Immunohistochemistry: expresses antigens appropriate to component parts, e.g., α-fetoprotein (AFP) in glandular epithelium.[87]

Yolk Sac Tumor

Yolk sac tumor contains primitive epithelial cells growing in a reticular pattern or sheets, representing yolk sac endoderm, set in a loose, variably cellular myxoid matrix resembling extra-embryonic mesoblast.

- Immunohistochemistry: AFP positive; OCT4 and c-kit negative[87]; serum/CSF marker: AFP.[88]

Embryonal Carcinoma

Embryonal carcinoma contains large cells growing in nests and sheets, with large nucleoli, a high mitotic rate, and zones of necrosis. It also may form irregular papillae or may line gland-like spaces.

- Immunohistochemistry: PLAP, OCT4, cytokeratins, and AFP (sometimes) are positive; serum/CSF: AFP ± β-HCG.[88]

Choriocarcinoma

Choriocarcinoma differentiates along extra-embryonic trophoblastic lines with cytotrophoblastic (large mononucleated cells) and syncytiotrophoblastic (multinucleate giant cells) components.

- Immunohistochemistry: syncytiotrophoblastic cells stain for β-HCG and HPL[87]; serum/CSF: β-HCG.[88]

Prognosis

- Mature teratomas can be cured by complete resection.
- Germinomas (pure) are very sensitive to radiation and have a 10-year survival rate > 85%.[83,89]
- Immature teratoma and mixed tumors with teratoma- or germinoma-dominant composition have an intermediate prognosis.[84]
- Yolk sac tumors, embryonal carcinoma, choriocarcinoma, and mixed tumors dominated by these components have a poor prognosis.[84]

■ Paraganglioma

Paraganglioma is a neuroendocrine tumor of neural crest origin arising from the paraganglionic system. It is a collection of specialized cells that are in close association with cranial nerves, large blood vessels, and autonomic nerves and ganglia. This system is widely distributed throughout the body and is divided into sympathetic/adrenal and parasympathetic paraganglia.[90]

- Paragangliomas of the head and neck (related to the parasympathetic nervous system) are commonly found at the bifurcation of the carotid artery (carotid body paraganglioma), in the middle ear/temporal bone, along the vagus nerve (jugulotympanic paraganglioma), and, rarely, in the orbit, nasal cavity, paranasal sinuses, nasopharynx, larynx, trachea, and thyroid.[91]
- Of relevance to the skull base, jugulotympanic paragangliomas are most commonly encountered. More than half of them are in relation to the jugular bulb and are termed glomus jugulare tumors; the ones related to the mucosa of the middle ear in the region of the medial promontory wall are termed glomus tympanicum.
- Pheochromocytoma is an intra-adrenal sympathetic paraganglioma.

Epidemiology

The mean age of onset is 50 years, with a range of 13 to 85 years.[92]

- The sporadic, solitary form and the familial form are due to mutations in succinate dehydrogenase subunits B, C, or D, which have a younger age of onset and are more likely present with multiple tumors.[93]

Pathology

Paraganglioma presents with an irregular reddish mass, which can invade the adjacent petrous temporal bone.

- Microscopically, small, uniform neoplastic cells with fine granular cytoplasm are organized into nests or lobules with surrounding sustentacular cells (i.e., cells associated with a structural support function). Generally, there is a rich vasculature.[94]
- Immunohistochemistry: positive for synaptophysin and chromogranin A, whereas sustentacular cells are positive for S100. Negative for keratins, thyroid transcription factor, renal cell carcinoma antigen, and human melanoma black (HMB)-45.

Prognosis

Jugulotympanic paragangliomas are slow growing but may infiltrate the petrous bone. Distant metastasis, however, is rare.[95]

■ Melanocytic Neoplasms of the Central Nervous System

Primary melanocytic neoplasms of the CNS are rare, arising from leptomeningeal melanocytes, and are usually dural-based lesions that can occur anywhere in the neuraxis; CPA localization is not uncommonly reported.[96]

- **Melanocytoma:** solitary, noninvasive tumor with oval-to-spindled tumor cells arranged in nests or whorls that may resemble a meningioma. Pigmented cells may be patchy or abundant. Cytological atypia, mitoses, and necrosis are not seen.[97]
- **Malignant melanoma:** variable morphology of epithelioid, spindled, plasmacytoid, rhabdoid, and/or multinucleated cells[97]; generally, medium to large tumor cells with atypia, high nuclear/cytoplasmic ratio, and pleomorphism that contain eosinophilic nucleoli and mitoses. Metastatic melanoma (arising from systemic site) is distinguished clinically.
- Immunohistochemistry: S-100, HMB-45, melan-A, and vimentin positive; cytokeratins, EMA, and muscle markers are negative.

■ Benign Cysts

Epidermoid and Dermoid Cyst

Epidermoid and dermoid cysts develop from ectodermal inclusions occurring during the closure from the neural tube.[98] The overall incidence is 1% of all intracranial masses.

Epidermoid Cyst

Epidermoids are extra-axial and can be located throughout the CNS.

- Also known as pearl tumors for their mother-of-pearl sheen forming its irregular nodules.
- Typically, they are located in the CPA.[99]
- Microscopically, they are composed of a layer of keratinized, stratified, differentiated squamous epithelium. There is no dermis or adnexa.
- Cystic contents include keratin and epithelium debris and cholesterol crystals.
- If ruptured, cyst contents can cause granulomatous inflammation.[100]

Dermoid Cyst

Dermoids are typically midline and can be found in the sellar/suprasellar region.[101]

- They are lined by stratified squamous epithelium but also contain dermis with adnexal skin structures (hair follicles, sebaceous glands, fibroadipose tissue).
- The cystic liquid is thick and sebaceous.

Rathke Cleft Cyst

Rathke cleft cyst is a benign cyst of the sella, derived from remnants of the embryological Rathke pouch.[102]

- Cysts that are large enough may cause symptoms through mass effect or hypopituitarism.
- The cyst is well circumscribed, and is lined by simple or pseudostratified ciliated columnar epithelium with goblet cells in some cases. The cyst contents are mucoid.

Arachnoid Cyst

Arachnoid cyst is benign and usually congenital, occurring mainly in the supratentorial compartment but also in the middle skull base (suprasellar) and CPA.[103]

- Is it lined by single layer of mature arachnoid cells that are positive for EMA.

■ Extracranial Tumors: Benign

Extracranial tumors appear in the nasal cavity, paranasal sinuses, and nasopharynx.

Schneiderian Papillomas

- The ectodermally derived mucosa that lines the nasal cavity and paranasal sinuses is known as the schneiderian membrane, which can give rise to three types of papillomas: inverted, oncocytic, and exophytic.
- Together, they are uncommon and account for < 5% of sinonasal tumors.[104]

Inverted Papilloma

Inverted papilloma is usually found in adults of ages 40 to 70, with a higher prevalence in men.[104]

- Although a viral etiology (human papilloma virus [HPV], Epstein-Barr virus [EBV]) has been suspected, to date there has been no definitive evidence demonstrating their causal role.[105]
- Inverted papillomas are usually located in the lateral nasal wall (89%) but can extend into sinuses, including the maxillary (54%), ethmoid (32%), frontal (6.5%), and sphenoid sinus (3.9%).[106,107]
- The tumors have an opaque yellow-tan polypoid appearance.
- Microscopically, they are composed of ribbons of basement-membrane enclosed epithelium that grows into (endophytically) the underlying stroma, hence the term *inverted*. The epithelium is stratified and composed of squamous or ciliated columnar cells, as well as mucocytes. The epithelium is usually nonkeratinizing.
- Malignant change is observed in inverted papillomas in approximately 11% of cases,[108] with squamous cell carcinoma being the most common histology.
- With the advent of endoscopic sinonasal surgery, the risk of recurrence is 6 to 15%.[107]

Oncocytic Papilloma

Oncocytic papilloma is usually localized to the nasal cavity or maxillary and ethmoid sinuses. It may extend into the orbit or cranial cavity if patients present late in the clinical course.

- The tumor grows both exophytically and endophytically, with an epithelium composed of multiple layers of columnar cells with oncocytic features.

Exophytic Papilloma

Exophytic papilloma forms papillary fronds with fibrovascular cores but almost never extends into the paranasal sinuses or skull base.

Juvenile Nasopharyngeal Angiofibroma

Juvenile nasopharyngeal angiofibroma is a rare, benign, highly vascularized mesenchymal tumor accounting for 0.05% of all head and neck tumors.[107] It occurs almost exclusively in adolescent boys, typically aged 15 to 18, as tumor growth is testosterone-dependent.[109]

- The tumor originates in the pterygopalatine fossa but grows to involve adjacent sinonasal cavity and possibly the skull base.
- Characteristically, it bulges into the posterior wall of the maxillary sinus on imaging.
- The main blood supply is usually from the internal maxillary artery, with possible contributions from the ascending pharyngeal artery and internal carotid artery.[110]

Pathology

Grossly, the tumor appears as a smooth, gray-red, polypoid mass with an average size of 4 cm at diagnosis.

- Microscopically, there is a thin-walled vascular network surrounded by a fibrous stroma with collagen fibers. The vessels have been described as slit-like, "staghorn," or dilated, with calibers ranging from the size of a capillary to much larger; the muscular layer may be absent. Stromal cells are generally cytologically bland and spindle, round, angular, or stellate in shape.[109]
- Immunohistochemistry: vessel wall cells are positive for vimentin, smooth muscle actin, and occasionally elastin, whereas stromal cells are positive for vimentin only. Desmin may be positive in larger vessels. Androgen, estrogen, and progesterone receptor may be positive. CD34 and CD31 are positive in vascular endothelium.

Prognosis

Although benign, nasopharyngeal angiofibroma is characterized by aggressive local growth, with 20% of patients experiencing recurrence. It tends to occur intracranially.[109]

Ameloblastoma

Ameloblastoma is a benign odontogenic tumor of the jaw that may spread to the pterygopalatine or infratemporal fossa.[111] It is rare, and onset usually occurs between 30 and 60 years of age.

- Microscopically, the solid/multicystic type appears as islands of odontogenic epithelium in a fibrous background or in a plexiform pattern with epithelium in anastomosing strands.
- Extraosseous, desmoplastic, and unicystic types also exist.

■ Extracranial Tumors: Malignant

General

- Nasal cavity and paranasal sinus carcinomas account for about 3% of head and neck malignancies.[112]
- The majority of sinonasal tumors arise in the maxillary sinus (60%), although they also frequently occur in the nasal cavity (20–30%) and ethmoid sinus (10–15%). The sphenoid and frontal sinus account for 1%.[113]

Epidemiology

Collectively, these tumors are rare, with an incidence of < 1.5 per 100,000; there is a slight male predominance[114] (higher in some countries, such as China, India, and Japan).[113]

- Occupational exposure to wood dust and other carcinogens is the main risk factor; smoking shows a weaker but consistent association.[113]

Squamous Cell Carcinoma

Squamous cell carcinoma is the most common malignant tumor of the sinonasal tract,[115] with a peak incidence in the sixth to seventh decades and a male predominance of 2:1.

- Maxillary sinus involvement is most common (60–70%) followed by nasal cavity (12–25%), ethmoid (10–15%), and frontal and sphenoid sinus (1%).[116]
- Advanced disease may involve the orbit, oral cavity, or skull base and intracranial contents.
- Known occupational risk factors include nickel, chromium, isopropyl alcohol, and radium exposure.[117]

Pathology

Grossly, the tumor appears as a friable, exophytic mass that may be ulcerated and necrotic.

- Microscopically, there is a proliferation of malignant epithelial cells with squamous differentiation, identical to those found at other sites.
- The *keratinizing* subtype forms extracellular or intracellular keratin, and tumor cells are apposed against each other in a mosaic arrangement. It may be well, moderately, or poorly differentiated.
- The *nonkeratinizing* subtype shows plexiform or ribbon-like growth and invades into the stroma with a well-delineated border. It is usually moderately to poorly differentiated.
- Immunohistochemistry: rarely required but cells stain positive to cytokeratin (CK5/6, CK8, and CK13).

Prognosis

The overall 5-year survival rate is 60%, and prognosis correlates with stage. The nonkeratinizing subtype tends to do better.[107]

Adenocarcinoma

Adenocarcinoma is a glandular carcinoma of the sinonasal tract, excluding that of the salivary type (see below).

- It is divided into two categories: intestinal type and nonintestinal type.
- Together, adenocarcinomas, including the salivary type, account for 10 to 20% of sinonasal tract malignant tumors.[117]

Intestinal-Type Adenocarcinoma

Intestinal-type adenocarcinoma most commonly occurs in the fifth to sixth decades with a male predominance.[118]

- Occupational risk factors include wood and leather dust exposure.[117]
- Usually, the tumor is unilateral, but an advanced presentation can have orbital or intracranial involvement.
- The more common sites of involvement are the ethmoid sinus (40%), nasal cavity (20%), and maxillary sinus (20%).[119]
- Grossly, the tumor appears as an irregular, bulging, exophytic pink or white mass. Often, it is friable and necrotic.
- Microscopically, there are five subtypes in the Barnes classification: papillary, colonic, solid, mucinous, and mixed.[118]

- ∘ The most common subtype is colonic (40%), which shows a tubuloglandular architecture.
- ∘ The solid subtype (20%) shows a trabecular or solid growth, representing a loss of differentiation.
- ∘ Papillary architecture dominates its named subtype (18%).
- ∘ Abundant mucus, analogous to colonic adenocarcinoma, is the feature of the mucinous subtype.
- ∘ The mixed subtype is composed of two or more patterns.
- Immunohistochemistry: intestinal-type adenocarcinomas stain for pancytokeratin, EMA, usually for CK20, and variably for CK7. CDX-2, usually found in intestinal adenocarcinomas, is positive here as well.
- The overall 5-year survival rate is 40 to 60%.[118,120]

Nonintestinal-Type Adenocarcinoma

Nonintestinal-type adenocarcinoma does not have intestinal-type differentiation and is divided into low- and high-grade subtypes.

- The average age at presentation is in the sixth decade, and there is a male predominance.[119]
- Low-grade tumors have a slower clinical presentation with a unilateral nasal mass, whereas high-grade tumors can present with locally advanced disease involving the orbit, infratemporal fossa, or intracranial contents.
- Tumors have an exophytic, papillary gross appearance.
- Microscopically, there is glandular and papillary growth, with glands lined by a single layer of cuboid to columnar epithelium in the low-grade subtype. Solid growth with high pleomorphism, mitotic activity, and necrosis mark the high-grade subtype.
- Low-grade tumors have a good prognosis with 5-year survival of 85%. High-grade tumors have a dismal 3-year survival of 20%.[118,119]

Salivary Gland–Type Carcinomas

There are several malignant salivary gland–type carcinomas of the sinonasal tract, the most common being *adenoid cystic carcinoma*.[121]

- Other types include acinic cell, mucoepidermoid, clear cell, and epithelial-myoepithelial carcinoma, all of which are rare in the sinonasal tract.
- Adenoid cystic carcinoma is most commonly found in the maxillary sinus (60%) and nasal cavity (25%), although the extent of tumor spread is often underestimated by radiology due to its propensity for perineural invasion. Osseous destruction is often present as well.[122]
- The tumor is composed of epithelial and myoepithelial cells often growing in tubular, cribriform, or solid patterns.

- Patients typically die from local spread/recurrence, and 10-year survival is only 7%.[121]

Sinonasal Undifferentiated Carcinoma

Sinonasal undifferentiated carcinoma is a rare (< 200 reported cases[123,124]) but highly aggressive tumor of uncertain histogenesis.[125] The median age at onset is in the sixth decade, with a male predominance.

- The tumor usually starts in the nasal cavity, maxillary, or ethmoid sinus, but local invasion of bone and surrounding structures soon follows. Invasion into the cranium is frequent.

Pathology

Grossly, tumors are typically very large (> 4 cm) on presentation, with poorly defined margins.[126]

- Microscopically, the tumor cells are arranged into nests, lobules, and sheets without squamous or glandular differentiation. The nuclear/cytoplasmic ratio is high, with frequent mitoses. Necrosis and lymphovascular invasion are also common findings.
- Immunohistochemistry is positive for cytokeratins (CK7, CK8, CK19) and may be positive for EMA, neuron-specific enolase (NSE), and p53. The tumor is negative for CEA and usually negative for synaptophysin, chromogranin, and S100.

Prognosis

Prognosis is poor, with a 5-year survival rate of 20% and median survival time of less than 18 months.[126]

Nasopharyngeal Carcinoma

Nasopharyngeal carcinoma (NPC) arises from the nasopharyngeal mucosa and shows squamous differentiation.

- The current WHO classification includes three subtypes: squamous cell carcinoma, nonkeratinizing carcinoma (differentiated or undifferentiated), and basaloid squamous cell carcinoma.[127]
- The most common site for NPC is the lateral wall of the nasopharynx.
- Extensive local/regional infiltration, early lymphatic spread, and hematogenous dissemination are hallmarks of NPC behavior.

- Erosion of the skull base and paranasal sinuses, cranial nerve involvement, and extension into the infratemporal fossa or orbit occur in advanced disease.
- Distant metastases to bone, lung, and liver is common.

Epidemiology

Nasopharyngeal carcinoma is rare in most parts of the world, making up 0.6% of all cancers, but its incidence is remarkably higher in Southeast Asia, North Africa, and among indigenous peoples of the Arctic. In Hong Kong, 1 in 40 men develop NPC by age 75.[128] The peak age of onset is in the fifth to seventh decades, with a male predominance.

- Nasopharyngeal carcinoma is almost always associated with EBV, regardless of ethnicity. EBV DNA or RNA is present in virtually all tumor cells and very likely plays a role in oncogenesis.[129]
- A diet high in volatile nitrosamines (found in preserved foods) has also been implicated as a carcinogen with respect to NPC, especially the salted fish commonly consumed in southern China.[130]

Squamous Cell Carcinoma

Squamous cell carcinoma (SCC) shows obvious squamous differentiation, and there is keratinization over most of the tumor. It resembles keratinizing SCC in other body areas.

- The tumor grows as irregular islands with a desmoplastic stroma that contains lymphocytes, plasma cells, neutrophils, and eosinophils.
- Tumor cells themselves are polygonal and stratified with distinct cell borders and hyperchromatic nuclei.
- The degree of differentiation is graded as well, moderately, or poorly differentiated.
- Immunohistochemistry: positivity of pan-cytokeratin (AE1/AE3), high molecular weight cytokeratin (CK5/6), and occasionally EMA. Unlike nonkeratinizing carcinoma (below), EBV is not invariably positive by in-situ hybridization.[127]

Nonkeratinizing Carcinoma

Nonkeratinizing carcinoma appears as solid sheets with irregular islands and trabeculae, intermixed with lymphocytes and plasma cells.

- It is further subclassified into differentiated and undifferentiated, although these two types are similar both clinically and prognostically.[127]

- The undifferentiated subtype is more common and is characterized by syncytial-like large tumor cells with indistinct cell borders, round to oval nuclei, and prominent central nucleoli. Often the cells are crowded together or even overlapping.
- The differentiated subtype appears as smaller tumor cells with more distinct cell borders and the nucleoli are not as prominent.
- All tumor cells typically stain for pan-cytokeratin (AE1/AE3), and staining for high molecular weight keratins (CK5/6) is strong. Low molecular weight keratins (CAM5.2) is weaker, whereas CK7 and 20 are negative.
- Epstein-Barr virus can detected in virtually all tumor nuclei via in-situ hybridization.

Basaloid Squamous Cell Carcinoma

As a primary tumor of the nasopharynx, basaloid squamous cell carcinoma is extremely rare and is characterized by rounded nests of atypical-appearing basaloid epithelial cells that frequently contain mitotic figures. The nuclear/cytoplasmic ratio is high.

- These tumors show lower aggressiveness than their morphological counterparts in other locations.
- Epstein-Barr virus was positive in three of four cases in one study.[131]

Prognosis

Although the prognosis for NPC has traditionally been poor, recent advances in radiation therapy has improved the overall 5-year survival rate to 75%.[127]

Esthesioneuroblastoma

Also known as olfactory neuroblastoma, esthesioneuroblastoma arises from neuroectodermal olfactory cells found in the upper nasal cavity (i.e., cribriform plate, superior nasal septum, and superior aspect of the middle and superior turbinate).[132] However, it can expand into the adjacent paranasal sinuses, orbit, or cranial vault.

Epidemiology

Esthesioneuroblastoma accounts for 1 to 6% of all intranasal/skull base malignancies, with an incidence of about 0.4 per million; it has a bimodal age distribution (second and sixth decades) with equal gender distribution.[107,132]

Pathology

Esthesioneuroblastoma appears as a glistening, mucosa-covered, polypoid, vascular appearing mass. Microscopically, it has a lobular architecture composed of circumscribed nests of small cells below intact mucosa with a rich fibrovascular stroma.[133] The tumor is composed of small, round, blue cells with a high nuclear/cytoplasmic ratio and "salt and pepper" chromatin.

- Two types of rosette patterns can be seen: Homer Wright in 30% and Flexner-Wintersteiner in 5%.[134]
- Esthesioneuroblastoma is histologically graded from I to IV based on the degree of differentiation, mitotic figures, presence of neural stroma, and necrosis.
- Immunohistochemistry: stains positively for markers of neuronal differentiation, such as synaptophysin, chromogranin, and neurofilament. S100 labels the sustentacular cells at the periphery of the lobules. There may also be reactivity for GFAP. Cytokeratin is usually negative, as are epithelial markers EMA and CEA. CD99 staining is absent. The Ki-67 proliferative index is high, at 10 to 50%.[134]

Prognosis

The overall 5-year survival rate is 80 to 90%.[134]

- Local recurrence and distant metastasis can occur years following the initial diagnosis.
- Histological grade also correlates with survival, and tumors of all grades have the capacity to metastasize.

Mucosal Melanoma

Mucosal melanoma is a rare tumor of the melanocytes either in surface epithelium or stroma,[133] most commonly arising de novo and not from preexisting nevi or from skin metastases.[135] It accounts for 0.3 to 2% of all malignant melanomas, and it can occur at any age.[107]

- More commonly found in the nasal cavity as opposed to paranasal sinuses, and can extend to involve a significant portion of the skull base.

Pathology

Mucosal melanoma grossly appears as a polypoid fleshy mass.

- Microscopically, variable morphology of epithelioid, spindled, plasmacytoid, rhabdoid, and/or multinucleated cells.

- Medium to large tumor cells with a high nuclear/cytoplasmic ratio and pleomorphism that contain eosinophilic nucleoli.
- Immunohistochemistry: S-100, HMB-45, melan-A, and vimentin positive; cytokeratins, EMA, and muscle markers are negative.

Treatment and Prognosis

Surgical excision with wide margins and postoperative radiation are indicated for advanced diseased; chemotherapy is indicated for distant metastases.

- Local recurrence is common (67–92%), and the 5-year survival rate is 17 to 47%.[134,136]

Heterotopic Central Nervous System Tissue

Sometimes called nasal glioma, this entity is actually heterotopic or ectopic neuroglial tissue, without connection to the brain (otherwise it would be an encephalocele).

- It is composed of a disorganized mixture of neuroglia and fibrovascular tissue, which can occur in the nasal cavity, nasopharynx, and other unusual regions of the head.[137]

■ Tumors of the Skull and Soft Tissues: Benign

Osteochondroma

Osteochondroma is likely the most common bone tumor (85%) but rarely is associated with the skull base.[138] It is made up of a cartilaginous cap and an underlying osseous component (sphenoid, ethmoid, or occipital bones).[139]

Osteoma

Osteoma is a bone-forming tumor composed of cortical, and less frequently, cancellous bone.[140]

- It affects 1 to 3% of the adult population and often is an incidental finding.
- Craniofacial skeleton and commonly sinuses are involved.
- Usually solitary, but multiple in Gardner's syndrome (also known as familial colorectal polyposis).
- Microscopically, cortical-like bone with vascular channels similar to haversian systems are seen. The cancellous variant appears as interconnecting broad trabeculae of bone surrounded by fatty marrow.
- Osteomas are indolent; malignant transformation does not occur.

Fibrous Dysplasia

Fibrous dysplasia is a fibro-osseous lesion leading to extreme thickening of bone. It can be monostotic or polyostotic.[141]

- The jaw is the most common site overall, and the skull can be a favored site in men.
- In the monostotic form, 35% of cases involve the head.[142]
- Microscopically, well-circumscribed fibrous (bland spindle cells) and osseous components (trabeculae of bone) are seen.
- Rarely, malignant transformation can occur.

■ Tumors of the Skull and Soft Tissues: Malignant

Chondrosarcoma

Chondrosarcoma is a slow-growing malignancy arising from cartilage, characterized by malignant chondrocytes cells.[143]

- Skull base chondrosarcomas arise from remnants of cartilage after ossification.
- They can affect the alveolar portion of the maxilla, the septum, the maxillary sinus, the sphenopetrous region, and the clivus.
- Unlike chordoma (see below), they occur in a paramedian position (typically, at the petrosphenoclival junction).

Epidemiology

Chondrosarcoma accounts for 6% of all skull base tumors and affects men and women equally.[107]

- Peak age of onset is between 30 and 50 years.

Pathology

There is a heterogeneous range of histological subtypes, from cartilaginous lesions appearing benign to highly cellular and malignant sarcoma, generally classified in three grades—(1) well-differentiated, (2) intermediate differentiated, and (3) poorly differentiated—based on cellularity, mitotic activity, atypia, and nuclear size.

- Low-grade chondrosarcoma has minimal metastatic potential.
- Different subtypes: myxoid, clear cell, dedifferentiated, mesenchymal.
- Immunohistochemistry: CD99 and SOX9 positive. Negative for epithelial markers and oncofetal antigens, which are important features that differentiate chondrosarcoma from chordoma.

Treatment and Prognosis

Treatment involves surgical excision, but en-bloc resection typically is not possible for extensive skull base lesions. Chondrosarcoma is relatively radioresistant; thus, high doses of radiation are required for incomplete resection.

- The 5-year survival rate is 80 to 90%, depending on the grade of the tumor.[144]

Chordoma

Chordoma is a rare tumor arising from remnants of the notochord.

- Benign notochord remnants can be found also in the intradural clival area (known as ecchordosis physaliphora), with an incidence of ~ 2% in autopsies.[145]
- Chordoma can arise from the entire axis, but commonly (35%) involving the skull base (spheno-occipital).[146]
- Usually extradural, with rare intradural cases that should not be confused with ecchordosis physaliphora.[147]

Epidemiology

Chordoma has an incidence of 0.8 cases per million,[148] accounting for 1 to 4% of primary malignant bone tumors. Age of onset most commonly is the sixth decade.

Pathology

Microscopically characterized by physaliphorous ("bubbly," vacuolated) cells containing intracellular mucin. The presence of abundant extracellular mucoid tissue is noted. Classic architecture consists of lobulated growth with cords and islands of tumor cells in myxomucoid substance.

- Variants include chondroid (characterized by areas of hyaline cartilaginous tissue) and dedifferentiated (marked atypia, high cellularity, high-grade sarcoma).
- Dedifferentiated subtypes account for < 5% of all chordomas.[149]
- Immunohistochemistry: cytokeratins, S-100, EMA, and AFP positive.

Treatment and Prognosis

Chordoma is generally slow growing, locally aggressive, and highly osteolytic, with a metastatic rate of 5 to 20% and a recurrence rate of 85% following surgery.[150] It has been noted to have an unusually rapid proliferation (Ki67 60% and recurrence within 2 months).[151]

Osteosarcoma

Osteosarcoma is a rare tumor, characterized by osteoid bone formation and malignant cellular proliferation.[152]

- Microscopically, this is a highly anaplastic tumor with cells that may appear as spindled (typical of sarcomas) or epithelioid, plasmacytoid, fusiform, small round cells.
- The presence of osteoid—a dense, pink, amorphous intercellular material—is important diagnostically.

Rhabdomyosarcoma

Rhabdomyosarcoma more frequently occurs in children and young adults, and there are embryonal (most common) and alveolar subtypes.[133,153]

- Rhabdomyosarcoma accounts for 75% of all childhood sarcomas and 1% of all sinonasal malignancy in adults.
- Microscopically, small round cells with scant eosinophilic cytoplasm are seen.
- Immunohistochemistry: positive for desmin, myogenin, myo-D1, myoglobulin, vimentin (usually), CD56 (usually), myosin (variable).

Ewing's Sarcoma[154]

Ewing's sarcoma is a rare bone tumor of childhood that has been reported to occur at the skull base.[155] It appears microscopically as a small, round, blue cell tumor.

- Rosettes (Homer Wright type) are another histological feature; their presence originally led to the designation (peripheral) primitive neuroectodermal tumor (PNET), but Ewing's sarcoma and PNET are today recognized as histological variants of the same tumor.
- Immunohistochemistry: positive for CD99; negative for CD45 (hematopoietic lineage).
- Characteristic chromosomal translocation between 22q and another chromosome, most commonly t(11:22)(q24; q12), resulting in the EWS/FLI-1 fusion gene (detected cytogenetically).

■ Vascular Tumors

Hemangioma and Lymphangioma

Hemangioma and lymphangioma account for 0.2% of all bone neoplasms and 10% of skull tumors.[156]

- A mass of thin-walled sinusoidal channels lined with endothelial cells and filled with blood is seen.[157]
- Hemangiomas are classified as cavernous, capillary, or venous, according to the dominant vascular component.
- Lymphangiomas are a related entity, but less frequent.[158]

Cavernous Hemangioma

Cavernous hemangioma is a common vascular lesion of the orbit, accounting for ~ 9% of orbital tumors.[159]

- Well-circumscribed masses bound by fibrous pseudocapsule are seen.
- Microscopically, dilated large vascular channels are lined by flattened endothelial cells.

■ Hematological Malignancies: Lymphoma

Skull base primary CNS lymphomas are rare, with reports of sporadic cases and small case series.[160,161]

- Involvement of the skull base may occur by extension from *sinonasal lymphomas*, which are the second most common malignancy of the sinonasal tract, after squamous cell carcinoma.[162]
  - Extranodal natural killer (NK)/T-cell lymphomas are the main form of lymphoma in the nasal cavity, and they are especially prevalent in Asian patients.[163]
  - B-cell lymphomas predominate in the skull base and paranasal sinuses, with diffuse large B-cell lymphoma (DLBCL) being the most common type.[164]

NK/T-Cell Lymphoma

A male predilection has been noted, and the tumor presents at a median age of 53 years. It is strongly associated with EBV.[162,165]

- Diffuse lymphocytic infiltrate is noted, with necrosis and apoptotic bodies in an angiocentric growth pattern (around blood vessels). Small to medium-sized lymphoma cells are seen, with irregular nuclei and a moderate amount of cytoplasm.

Diffuse Large B-Cell Lymphoma

The average age at presentation of DLBCL is in the 60s, and it affects both sexes about equally. DLBCL tends to be EBV negative.[162]

- Diffuse lymphocytic infiltrate is noted, with variable necrosis and angio-invasion; large or medium-sized lymphoid cells with round, multilobulated, or irregular nuclei are seen, with multiple small nucleoli or a single large nucleolus.

Treatment and Prognosis

Treatment consists of radiotherapy and/or systemic chemotherapy.

- NK/T-cell lymphoma: 30 to 50% overall survival rate, with a 33 to 50% local relapse rate.[162]
- DLBCL: 35 to 60% overall survival rate.[162]

■ Hematological Malignancies: Multiple Myeloma/Plasmacytoma

Multiple myeloma/plasmacytoma entails disseminated malignancy of plasma cells, rarely localized at the level of the skull base, with involvement of the neural foramina.

- Multiple myeloma/plasmacytoma consists of solitary plasmacytoma of bone, a localized bone tumor of monoclonal plasma cells, and no evidence of systemic disease; it accounts for 3 to 5% of plasma cell neoplasms and may present in the skull.[166]
- Extraosseous plasmacytoma occurs in tissues other than bone, including the CNS.

Pathology

Diffuse infiltrate of plasma cells is noted, accompanied by scant vascular stroma.

- The well-differentiated phenotype is characterized by normal to mildly atypical plasma cells; the moderately differentiated is characterized by moderately atypical plasma cells; the poorly differentiated is characterized by anaplastic large cells.

Treatment and Prognosis

Generally, radiotherapy is the favored modality.

- Progression to (diffuse) myeloma is common in solitary plasmacytoma (67%) but less frequent in extraosseous plasmacytoma (15%).[166]

■ Skull Base Metastases

Metastases isolated to the skull base are rare, occurring in 4% of cancer patients.[167] The most common sites of origin of metastatic neoplasms to the skull base are, in decreasing order, prostate, lung, kidney, bone (in men) and breast, genitourinary system, and thyroid (in women).

- In general, skull base metastases occur in an advanced stage of disease, when patients already have involvement of other sites, although they can also be the first presenting sign of cancer, with an overall median survival of 31 months.[167]
- Based on the source, metastases can be osteoblastic or osteoclastic (i.e., lytic, which are more frequent), or mixed.
- Osteoclastic metastases destroy only the inner or outer table.
- Pure blastic lesions (typically from breast, prostate, colon, or bone) expand the diploe symmetrically.

■ References

Boldfaced references are of particular importance.

1. Scheithauer BW, Hawkins C, Tihan T, VandenBerg SR, Burger PC. Pilocytic astrocytoma. In: Louis DN, Ohgaki H, Wiestler OD, Cavenee WK, eds. World Health Organization Classification of Tumours, 4th ed. Lyon: International Agency for Research on Cancer; 2007:14–20
2. **Binning MJ, Liu JK, Kestle JR, Brockmeyer DL, Walker ML. Optic pathway gliomas: a review. Neurosurg Focus 2007;23:E2**
3. Czyzyk E, Jóźwiak S, Roszkowski M, Schwartz RA. Optic pathway gliomas in children with and without neurofibromatosis 1. J Child Neurol 2003;18:471–478
4. Dutton JJ. Gliomas of the anterior visual pathway. Surv Ophthalmol 1994;38:427–452
5. Sylvester CL, Drohan LA, Sergott RC. Optic-nerve gliomas, chiasmal gliomas and neurofibromatosis type 1. Curr Opin Ophthalmol 2006;17:7–11
6. **Ferner RE, Huson SM, Thomas N, et al. Guidelines for the diagnosis and management of individuals with neurofibromatosis 1. J Med Genet 2007;44:81–88**
7. Tow SL, Chandela S, Miller NR, Avellino AM. Long-term outcome in children with gliomas of the anterior visual pathway. Pediatr Neurol 2003;28:262–270
8. Pepin SM, Lessell S. Anterior visual pathway gliomas: The last 30 years. Semin Ophthalmol 2006;21:117–124
9. **Scheithauer BW, Louis DN, Hunter S, Woodruff JM, Antonescu CR. Schwannoma. In: Louis DN, Ohgaki H, Wiestler OD, Cavenee WK, eds. World Health Organization Classification of Tumours, 4th ed. Lyon: International Agency for Research on Cancer; 2007:152–155**

10. Russell DS, Rubinstein LJ. Pathology of Tumours of the Nervous System, 5th ed. Baltimore: Williams & Wilkins; 1989

11. Wanibuchi M, Fukushima T, Zomordi AR, Nonaka Y, Friedman AH. Trigeminal schwannomas: skull base approaches and operative results in 105 patients. Neurosurgery 2012;70(1, Suppl Operative):132–143, discussion 143–144

12. Wiggins RH III, Harnsberger HR, Salzman KL, Shelton C, Kertesz TR, Glastonbury CM. The many faces of facial nerve schwannoma. AJNR Am J Neuroradiol 2006;27:694–699

13. Antinheimo J, Sankila R, Carpén O, Pukkala E, Sainio M, Jääskeläinen J. Population-based analysis of sporadic and type 2 neurofibromatosis-associated meningiomas and schwannomas. Neurology 2000;54:71–76

14. Woodruff JM, Selig AM, Crowley K, Allen PW. Schwannoma (neurilemoma) with malignant transformation. A rare, distinctive peripheral nerve tumor. Am J Surg Pathol 1994;18:882–895

15. Casadei GP, Scheithauer BW, Hirose T, Manfrini M, Van Houton C, Wood MB. Cellular schwannoma. A clinicopathologic, DNA flow cytometric, and proliferation marker study of 70 patients. Cancer 1995;75:1109–1119

16. Evans DG. Neurofibromatosis 2 [Bilateral acoustic neurofibromatosis, central neurofibromatosis, NF2, neurofibromatosis type II]. Genet Med 2009;11:599–610

17. Jacoby LB, MacCollin M, Louis DN, et al. Exon scanning for mutation of the NF2 gene in schwannomas. Hum Mol Genet 1994;3:413–419

18. Seizinger BR, Martuza RL, Gusella JF. Loss of genes on chromosome 22 in tumorigenesis of human acoustic neuroma. Nature 1986;322:644–647

19. **Perry A, Louis DN, Scheithauer BW, Budka H, von Deimling A. Meningiomas. In: Louis DN, Ohgaki H, Wiestler OD, Cavenee WK, eds. World Health Organization Classification of Tumours, 4th ed. Lyon: International Agency for Research on Cancer; 2007:164–172**

20. Simas NM, Farias JP. Sphenoid wing en plaque meningiomas: surgical results and recurrence rates. Surg Neurol Int 2013;4:86

21. Heinrich B, Hartmann C, Stemmer-Rachamimov AO, Louis DN, MacCollin M. Multiple meningiomas: Investigating the molecular basis of sporadic and familial forms. Int J Cancer 2003;103:483–488

22. Surov A, Gottschling S, Bolz J, et al. Distant metastases in meningioma: an underestimated problem. J Neurooncol 2013;112:323–327

23. Willis J, Smith C, Ironside JW, Erridge S, Whittle IR, Everington D. The accuracy of meningioma grading: a 10-year retrospective audit. Neuropathol Appl Neurobiol 2005; 31:141–149

24. Kepes JJ. The fine structure of hyaline inclusions (pseudopsammoma bodies) in meningiomas. J Neuropathol Exp Neurol 1975;34:282–294

25. Tirakotai W, Mennel HD, Celik I, Hellwig D, Bertalanffy H, Riegel T. Secretory meningioma: immunohistochemical findings and evaluation of mast cell infiltration. Neurosurg Rev 2006;29:41–48

26. Gi H, Nagao S, Yoshizumi H, et al. Meningioma with hypergammaglobulinemia. Case report. J Neurosurg 1990;73:628–629

27. **Di Ieva A, Laiq S, Nejad R, et al. Chordoid meningiomas: Incidence and clinico-pathological features of a case series over 18 years. Neuropathology 2015;35:137–147**

28. Perry A, Scheithauer BW, Stafford SL, Lohse CM, Wollan PC. "Malignancy" in meningiomas: a clinicopathologic study of 116 patients, with grading implications. Cancer 1999;85:2046–2056
29. Enam SA, Abdulrauf S, Mehta B, Malik GM, Mahmood A. Metastasis in meningioma. Acta Neurochir (Wien) 1996;138:1172–1177, discussion 1177–1178
30. Adlakha A, Rao K, Adlakha H, et al. Meningioma metastatic to the lung. Mayo Clin Proc 1999;74:1129–1133
31. Erdogan H, Aydin MV, Tasdemiroglu E. Tumor-to-tumor metastasis of the central nervous system. Turk Neurosurg 2014;24:151–162
32. Chourmouzi D, Potsi S, Moumtzouoglou A, et al. Dural lesions mimicking meningiomas: a pictorial essay. World J Radiol 2012;4:75–82
33. Penel N, Amela EY, Decanter G, Robin YM, Marec-Berard P. Solitary fibrous tumors and so-called hemangiopericytoma. Sarcoma 2012;2012:690251
34. Giannini C, Rushing EJ, Hainfellner JA. Haemangiopericytoma. In: Louis DN, Ohgaki H, Wiestler OD, Cavenee WK, eds. World Health Organization Classification of Tumours, 4th ed. Lyon: International Agency for Research on Cancer; 2007:178–180
35. Guthrie BL, Ebersold MJ, Scheithauer BW, Shaw EG. Meningeal hemangiopericytoma: histopathological features, treatment, and long-term follow-up of 44 cases. Neurosurgery 1989;25:514–522
36. Schweizer L, Koelsche C, Sahm F, et al. Meningeal hemangiopericytoma and solitary fibrous tumors carry the NAB2-STAT6 fusion and can be diagnosed by nuclear expression of STAT6 protein. Acta Neuropathol 2013;125:651–658
37. Doyle LA, Vivero M, Fletcher CD, Mertens F, Hornick JL. Nuclear expression of STAT6 distinguishes solitary fibrous tumor from histologic mimics. Mod Pathol 2014;27:390–395
38. Damodaran O, Robbins P, Knuckey N, Bynevelt M, Wong G, Lee G. Primary intracranial haemangiopericytoma: comparison of survival outcomes and metastatic potential in WHO grade II and III variants. J Clin Neurosci 2014;21:1310–1314
39. Aflorei ED, Korbonits M. Epidemiology and etiopathogenesis of pituitary adenomas. J Neurooncol 2014;117:379–394
40. Scheithauer BW, Kovacs KT, Laws ER Jr, Randall RV. Pathology of invasive pituitary tumors with special reference to functional classification. J Neurosurg 1986;65:733–744
41. Thapar K, Kovacs K, Scheithauer BW, et al. Proliferative activity and invasiveness among pituitary adenomas and carcinomas: an analysis using the MIB-1 antibody. Neurosurgery 1996;38:99–106, discussion 106–107
42. Meij BP, Lopes MB, Ellegala DB, Alden TD, Laws ER Jr. The long-term significance of microscopic dural invasion in 354 patients with pituitary adenomas treated with transsphenoidal surgery. J Neurosurg 2002;96:195–208
43. Buchfelder M. Management of aggressive pituitary adenomas: current treatment strategies. Pituitary 2009;12:256–260
44. Di Ieva A, Rotondo F, Syro LV, Cusimano MD, Kovacs K. Aggressive pituitary adenomas—diagnosis and emerging treatments. Nat Rev Endocrinol 2014;10:423–435
45. Dworakowska D, Korbonits M, Aylwin S, McGregor A, Grossman AB. The pathology of pituitary adenomas from a clinical perspective. Front Biosci (Schol Ed) 2011;3:105–116

46. Asa SL. Practical pituitary pathology: what does the pathologist need to know? Arch Pathol Lab Med 2008;132:1231–1240
47. Kontogeorgos G, Watson RE, Lindell EP, Barkan AL, Farrell WE, Lloyd RV. Growth hormone producing adenoma. In: DeLellis RA, Lloyd RV, Heitz PU, Eng C, eds. World Health Organization Classification of Tumours: Pathology and Genetics of Tumours of Endocrine Organs. Lyon: IARC Press; 2004:14–19
48. Lake MG, Krook LS, Cruz SV. Pituitary adenomas: an overview. Am Fam Physician 2013;88:319–327
49. Lee EJ, Ahn JY, Noh T, Kim SH, Kim TS, Kim SH. Tumor tissue identification in the pseudocapsule of pituitary adenoma: should the pseudocapsule be removed for total resection of pituitary adenoma? Neurosurgery 2009;64(3, Suppl):ons62–ons69, discussion ons69–ons70
50. Fougner SL, Casar-Borota O, Heck A, Berg JP, Bollerslev J. Adenoma granulation pattern correlates with clinical variables and effect of somatostatin analogue treatment in a large series of patients with acromegaly. Clin Endocrinol (Oxf) 2012;76:96–102
51. Kato M, Inoshita N, Sugiyama T, et al. Differential expression of genes related to drug responsiveness between sparsely and densely granulated somatotroph adenomas. Endocr J 2012;59:221–228
52. Salehi F, Kovacs K, Scheithauer BW, et al. Immunohistochemical expression of pituitary tumor transforming gene (PTTG) in pituitary adenomas: a correlative study of tumor subtypes. Int J Surg Pathol 2010;18:5–13
53. Mete O, Ezzat S, Asa SL. Biomarkers of aggressive pituitary adenomas. J Mol Endocrinol 2012;49:R69–R78
54. Salehi F, Agur A, Scheithauer BW, Kovacs K, Lloyd RV, Cusimano M. Biomarkers of pituitary neoplasms: a review (Part II). Neurosurgery 2010;67:1790–1798, discussion 1798
55. Saeger W, Horvath E, Kovacs K, et al. Prolactin producing adenoma. In: DeLellis RA, Lloyd RV, Heitz PU, Eng C, eds. World Health Organization Classification of Tumours: Pathology and Genetics of Tumours of Endocrine Organs. Lyon: IARC Press; 2004:20–23
56. Osamura RY, Sano T, Ezzat S, et al. TSH producing adenoma. In: DeLellis RA, Lloyd RV, Heitz PU, Eng C, eds. World Health Organization Classification of Tumours: Pathology and Genetics of Tumours of Endocrine Organs. Lyon: IARC Press; 2004:24–25
57. Trouillas J, Barkan AL, Watson RE, Lindell EP, Farrell WE, Lloyd RV. ACTH producing adenoma. In: DeLellis RA, Lloyd RV, Heitz PU, Eng C, eds. World Health Organization Classification of Tumours: Pathology and Genetics of Tumours of Endocrine Organs. Lyon: IARC Press; 2004:26–29
58. Kovács GL, Góth M, Rotondo F, et al. ACTH-secreting Crooke cell carcinoma of the pituitary. Eur J Clin Invest 2013;43:20–26
59. Rotondo F, Cusimano M, Scheithauer BW, Coire C, Horvath E, Kovacs K. Atypical, invasive, recurring Crooke cell adenoma of the pituitary. Hormones (Athens) 2012;11:94–100
60. Kovacs K, Diep CC, Horvath E, et al. Prognostic indicators in an aggressive pituitary Crooke's cell adenoma. Can J Neurol Sci 2005;32:540–545
61. Horvath E, Lloyd RV, Kovacs K, et al. Plurihormonal adenoma. In: DeLellis RA, Lloyd RV, Heitz PU, Eng C, eds. World Health Organization Classification of Tumours: Pathology and Genetics of Tumours of Endocrine Organs. Lyon: IARC Press; 2004:35

62. Luk CT, Kovacs K, Rotondo F, Horvath E, Cusimano M, Booth GL. Plurihormonal pituitary adenoma immunoreactive for thyroid-stimulating hormone, growth hormone, follicle-stimulating hormone, and prolactin. Endocr Pract 2012;18:e121–e126

63. Asa SL, Ezzat S, Watson RE, Lindell EP, Horvath E. Gonadotropin producing adenoma. In: DeLellis RA, Lloyd RV, Heitz PU, Eng C, eds. World Health Organization Classification of Tumours: Pathology and Genetics of Tumours of Endocrine Organs. Lyon: IARC Press; 2004:30–32

64. Fiddes JC, Goodman HM. The gene encoding the common alpha subunit of the four human glycoprotein hormones. J Mol Appl Genet 1981;1:3–18

65. Horvath E, Kovacs K, Smyth HS, Cusimano M, Singer W. Silent adenoma subtype 3 of the pituitary—immunohistochemical and ultrastructural classification: a review of 29 cases. Ultrastruct Pathol 2005;29:511–524

66. Yamaguchi-Okada M, Inoshita N, Nishioka H, Fukuhara N, Yamada S. Clinicopathological analysis of nonfunctioning pituitary adenomas in patients younger than 25 years of age. J Neurosurg Pediatr 2012;9:511–516

67. Sano T, Yamada S, Watson RE, Lindell EP, Ezzat S, Asa SL. Null cell adenoma. In: DeLellis RA, Lloyd RV, Heitz PU, Eng C, eds. World Health Organization Classification of Tumours: Pathology and Genetics of Tumours of Endocrine Organs. Lyon: IARC Press; 2004:33–34

68. Heaney AP. Clinical review: pituitary carcinoma: difficult diagnosis and treatment. J Clin Endocrinol Metab 2011;96:3649–3660

69. Scheihauer BW, Kovacs K, Horvath E, et al. Pituitary carcinoma. In: DeLellis RA, Lloyd RV, Heitz PU, Eng C, eds. World Health Organization Classification of Tumours: Pathology and Genetics of Tumours of Endocrine Organs. Lyon: IARC Press; 2004:36–39

70. Fuller GN, Wesseling P. Granular cell tumour of the neurohypophysis. In: Louis DN, Ohgaki H, Wiestler OD, Cavenee WK, eds. World Health Organization Classification of Tumours, 4th ed. Lyon: International Agency for Research on Cancer; 2007:241–242

71. Wesseling P, Brat DJ, Fuller GN. Pituicytoma. In: Louis DN, Ohgaki H, Wiestler OD, Cavenee WK, eds. World Health Organization Classification of Tumours, 4th ed. Lyon: International Agency for Research on Cancer; 2007:243–244

72. Louis DN, Perry A, Burger P, et al. International Society of Neuropathology—Haarlem consensus guidelines for nervous system tumor classification and grading. Brain Pathol 2014;24:429–435

73. Mete O, Lopes MB, Asa SL. Spindle cell oncocytomas and granular cell tumors of the pituitary are variants of pituicytoma. Am J Surg Pathol 2013;37:1694–1699

74. Scheithauer BW, Horvath E, Abel TW, et al. Pituitary blastoma: a unique embryonal tumor. Pituitary 2012;15:365–373

75. Rushing EJ, Giangaspero F, Paulus W, Burger PC. Craniopharyngioma In: Louis DN, Ohgaki H, Wiestler OD, Cavenee WK, eds. World Health Organization Classification of Tumours, 4th ed. Lyon: International Agency for Research on Cancer; 2007:238–240

76. Adamson TE, Wiestler OD, Kleihues P, Yaşargil MG. Correlation of clinical and pathological features in surgically treated craniopharyngiomas. J Neurosurg 1990;73:12–17

77. Bunin GR, Surawicz TS, Witman PA, Preston-Martin S, Davis F, Bruner JM. The descriptive epidemiology of craniopharyngioma. J Neurosurg 1998;89:547–551

78. Crotty TB, Scheithauer BW, Young WF Jr, et al. Papillary craniopharyngioma: a clinicopathological study of 48 cases. J Neurosurg 1995;83:206–214

79. Miller DC. Pathology of craniopharyngiomas: clinical import of pathological findings. Pediatr Neurosurg 1994;21(Suppl 1):11–17

80. Al-Brahim NY, Asa SL. My approach to pathology of the pituitary gland. J Clin Pathol 2006;59:1245–1253

81. Rajan B, Ashley S, Gorman C, et al. Craniopharyngioma—a long-term results following limited surgery and radiotherapy. Radiother Oncol 1993;26:1–10

82. **Yaşargil MG, Curcic M, Kis M, Siegenthaler G, Teddy PJ, Roth P. Total removal of craniopharyngiomas. Approaches and long-term results in 144 patients. J Neurosurg 1990;73:3–11**

83. Rosenblum MK, Nakazato Y, Matsutani M. CNS germ cell tumours. In: Louis DN, Ohgaki H, Wiestler OD, Cavenee WK, eds. World Health Organization Classification of Tumours, 4th ed. Lyon: International Agency for Research on Cancer; 2007:198–204

84. Thakkar JP, Chew L, Villano JL. Primary CNS germ cell tumors: current epidemiology and update on treatment. Med Oncol 2013;30:496

85. Goodwin TL, Sainani K, Fisher PG. Incidence patterns of central nervous system germ cell tumors: a SEER Study. J Pediatr Hematol Oncol 2009;31:541–544

86. Echevarría ME, Fangusaro J, Goldman S. Pediatric central nervous system germ cell tumors: a review. Oncologist 2008;13:690–699

87. Sato K, Takeuchi H, Kubota T. Pathology of intracranial germ cell tumors. Prog Neurol Surg 2009;23:59–75

88. Packer RJ, Cohen BH, Cooney K. Intracranial germ cell tumors. Oncologist 2000;5:312–320

89. McCarthy BJ, Shibui S, Kayama T, et al. Primary CNS germ cell tumors in Japan and the United States: an analysis of 4 tumor registries. Neuro-oncol 2012;14:1194–1200

90. Barnes L, Tse LLY, Hunt JL, Michaels L. Tumours of the paraganglionic system: introduction. In: Barnes L, Eveson JW, Reichart P, Sidransky D, eds. World Health Organization Classification of Tumours: Pathology and Genetics of Head and Neck Tumours. Lyon: IARC Press; 2005:362–363

91. Martin TP, Irving RM, Maher ER. The genetics of paragangliomas: a review. Clin Otolaryngol 2007;32:7–11

92. Mendenhall WM, Amdur RJ, Vaysberg M, Mendenhall CM, Werning JW. Head and neck paragangliomas. Head Neck 2011;33:1530–1534

93. Neumann HP, Pawlu C, Peczkowska M, et al; European-American Paraganglioma Study Group. Distinct clinical features of paraganglioma syndromes associated with SDHB and SDHD gene mutations. JAMA 2004;292:943–951

94. Michaels L, Soucek S, Beale T, Sandison A. Jugulotympanic paraganglioma. In: Barnes L, Eveson JW, Reichart P, Sidransky D, eds. World Health Organization Classification of Tumours: Pathology and Genetics of Head and Neck Tumours. Lyon: IARC Press; 2005: 366–367

95. **Kupferman ME, Hanna EY. Paragangliomas of the head and neck. Curr Oncol Rep 2008;10:156–161**

96. Kan P, Shelton C, Townsend J, Jensen R. Primary malignant cerebellopontine angle melanoma presenting as a presumed meningioma: case report and review of the literature. Skull Base 2003;13:159–166

97. Brat DJ, Perry A. Melanocytic lesions. In: Louis DN, Ohgaki H, Wiestler OD, Cavenee WK, eds. World Health Organization Classification of Tumours, 4th ed. Lyon: International Agency for Research on Cancer; 2007:181–183

98. Rubin G, Scienza R, Pasqualin A, Rosta L, Da Pian R. Craniocerebral epidermoids and dermoids. A review of 44 cases. Acta Neurochir (Wien) 1989;97:1–16
99. Miller ME, Mastrodimos B, Cueva RA. Hearing preservation in management of epidermoids of the cerebellopontine angle: CPA epidermoids and hearing preservation. Otol Neurotol 2012;33:1599–1603
100. Velamati R, Hageman JR, Bartlett A. Meningitis secondary to ruptured epidermoid cyst: case-based review. Pediatr Ann 2013;42:248–251
101. Zada G, Lin N, Ojerholm E, Ramkissoon S, Laws ER. Craniopharyngioma and other cystic epithelial lesions of the sellar region: a review of clinical, imaging, and histopathological relationships. Neurosurg Focus 2010;28:E4
102. Kucharczyk W, Peck WW, Kelly WM, Norman D, Newton TH. Rathke cleft cysts: CT, MR imaging, and pathologic features. Radiology 1987;165:491–495
103. Pradilla G, Jallo G. Arachnoid cysts: case series and review of the literature. Neurosurg Focus 2007;22:E7
104. Barnes L, Tse LLY, Hunt JL. Schneiderian papillomas. In: Barnes L, Eveson JW, Reichart P, Sidransky D, eds. World Health Organization Classification of Tumours: Pathology and Genetics of Head and Neck Tumours. Lyon: IARC Press; 2005:28–32
105. Gaffey MJ, Frierson HF, Weiss LM, Barber CM, Baber GB, Stoler MH. Human papillomavirus and Epstein-Barr virus in sinonasal Schneiderian papillomas. An in situ hybridization and polymerase chain reaction study. Am J Clin Pathol 1996;106:475–482
106. Hennessey PT, Reh DD. Benign sinonasal neoplasms. Am J Rhinol Allergy 2013; 27(Suppl 1):S31–34
107. Lund VJ, Stammberger H, Nicolai P, et al; European Rhinologic Society Advisory Board on Endoscopic Techniques in the Management of Nose, Paranasal Sinus and Skull Base Tumours. European position paper on endoscopic management of tumours of the nose, paranasal sinuses and skull base. Rhinol Suppl 2010; 22:1–143
108. Strojan P, Ferlito A, Lund VJ, et al. Sinonasal inverted papilloma associated with malignancy: the role of human papillomavirus infection and its implications for radiotherapy. Oral Oncol 2012;48:216–218
109. Thompson LDR, Fanburg-Smith JC. Nasopharyngeal angiofibroma. In: Barnes L, Eveson JW, Reichart P, Sidransky D, eds. World Health Organization Classification of Tumours: Pathology and Genetics of Head and Neck Tumours. Lyon: IARC Press; 2005:102–103
110. Chan KH, Gao D, Fernandez PG, Kingdom TT, Kumpe DA. Juvenile nasopharyngeal angiofibroma: vascular determinates for operative complications and tumor recurrence. Laryngoscope 2014;124:672–677
111. Gardner DG, Heikinheimo K, Shear M, Philipsen HP, Coleman H. Ameloblastomas. In: Barnes L, Eveson JW, Reichart P, Sidransky D, eds. World Health Organization Classification of Tumours: Pathology and Genetics of Head and Neck Tumours. Lyon: IARC Press; 2005:296–300
112. Morokoff AP, Danks RA, Kaye AH. Carcinoma of the paranasal sinuses. In: Kaye AH, Laws ER, eds. Brain Tumors: an Encyclopedic Approach, 3rd ed. New York: Saunders/ Elsevier; 2012:750–766
113. Barnes L, Tse LLY, Hunt JL, Brandwein-Gensler M, Curtin HD, Boffretta P. Tumours of the nasal cavity and paranasal sinuses: Introduction. In: Barnes L, Eveson JW, Reich-

art P, Sidransky D, eds. World Health Organization Classification of Tumours: Pathology and Genetics of Head and Neck Tumours. Lyon: IARC Press; 2005:12–14

114. Haerle SK, Gullane PJ, Witterick IJ, Zweifel C, Gentili F. Sinonasal carcinomas: epidemiology, pathology, and management. Neurosurg Clin N Am 2013;24:39–49

115. Slootweg PJ, Ferlito A, Cardesa A, et al. Sinonasal tumors: a clinicopathologic update of selected tumors. Eur Arch Otorhinolaryngol 2013;270:5–20

116. Pilch BZ, Bouquot J, Thompson LDR. Squamous cell carcinoma. In: Barnes L, Eveson JW, Reichart P, Sidransky D, eds. World Health Organization Classification of Tumours: Pathology and Genetics of Head and Neck Tumours. Lyon: IARC Press; 2005: 15–17

117. Harvey RJ, Dalgorf DM. Sinonasal malignancies. Am J Rhinol Allergy 2013;27(Suppl 1):S35–38

118. Franchi A, Santucci M, Wenig BM. Adenocarcinoma. In: Barnes L, Eveson JW, Reichart P, Sidransky D, eds. World Health Organization Classification of Tumours: Pathology and Genetics of Head and Neck Tumours. Lyon: IARC Press; 2005:20–23

119. Bhayani MK, Yilmaz T, Sweeney A, et al. Sinonasal adenocarcinoma: a 16-year experience at a single institution. Head Neck 2014;36:1490–1496

120. D'Aguillo CM, Kanumuri VV, Khan MN, et al. Demographics and survival trends of sinonasal adenocarcinoma from 1973 to 2009. Int Forum Allergy Rhinol 2014;4: 771–776

121. Thompson LD, Penner C, Ho NJ, et al. Sinonasal tract and nasopharyngeal adenoid cystic carcinoma: a clinicopathologic and immunophenotypic study of 86 cases. Head Neck Pathol 2014;8:88–109

122. Eveson JW. Salivary gland-type carcinomas. In: Barnes L, Eveson JW, Reichart P, Sidransky D, eds. World Health Organization Classification of Tumours: Pathology and Genetics of Head and Neck Tumours. Lyon: IARC Press; 2005:24–25

123. Reiersen DA, Pahilan ME, Devaiah AK. Meta-analysis of treatment outcomes for sinonasal undifferentiated carcinoma. Otolaryngol Head Neck Surg 2012;147: 7–14

124. Xu CC, Dziegielewski PT, McGaw WT, Seikaly H. Sinonasal undifferentiated carcinoma (SNUC): the Alberta experience and literature review. J Otolaryngol Head Neck Surg 2013;42:2

125. Gray ST, Herr MW, Sethi RK, et al. Treatment outcomes and prognostic factors, including human papillomavirus, for sinonasal undifferentiated carcinoma: A retrospective review. Head Neck 2015;37: 366–374

126. Frierson HF. Sinonasal undifferentiated carcinoma. In: Barnes L, Eveson JW, Reichart P, Sidransky D, eds. World Health Organization Classification of Tumours: Pathology and Genetics of Head and Neck Tumours. Lyon: IARC Press; 2005:19

127. Chan JKC, Bray F, McCarron P, et al. Nasopharyngeal carcinoma. In: Barnes L, Eveson JW, Reichart P, Sidransky D, eds. World Health Organization Classification of Tumours: Pathology and Genetics of Head and Neck Tumours. Lyon: IARC Press; 2005: 85–97

128. Yu MC, Yuan JM. Epidemiology of nasopharyngeal carcinoma. Semin Cancer Biol 2002;12:421–429

129. Tsao SW, Yip YL, Tsang CM, et al. Etiological factors of nasopharyngeal carcinoma. Oral Oncol 2014;50:330–338

130. Yu MC. Nasopharyngeal carcinoma: epidemiology and dietary factors. IARC Sci Publ 1991;105:39–47

131. Wan SK, Chan JK, Lau WH, Yip TT. Basaloid-squamous carcinoma of the nasopharynx. An Epstein-Barr virus-associated neoplasm compared with morphologically identical tumors occurring in other sites. Cancer 1995;76:1689–1693

132. Thompson LD. Olfactory neuroblastoma. Head Neck Pathol 2009;3:252–259

133. Bridge JA, Bowen JM, Smith RB. The small round blue cell tumors of the sinonasal area. Head Neck Pathol 2010;4:84–93

134. Wenig BM, Dulguerov P, Kapadia SB, Prasad ML, Fanburg-Smith JC, Thompson LDR. Neuroectodermal tumours. In: Barnes L, Eveson JW, Reichart P, Sidransky D, eds. World Health Organization Classification of Tumours: Pathology and Genetics of Head and Neck Tumours. Lyon: IARC Press; 2005:65–75

135. Thompson LD, Wieneke JA, Miettinen M. Sinonasal tract and nasopharyngeal melanomas: a clinicopathologic study of 115 cases with a proposed staging system. Am J Surg Pathol 2003;27:594–611

136. Gavriel H, McArthur G, Sizeland A, Henderson M. Review: mucosal melanoma of the head and neck. Melanoma Res 2011;21:257–266

137. Penner CR, Thompson L. Nasal glial heterotopia: a clinicopathologic and immunophenotypic analysis of 10 cases with a review of the literature. Ann Diagn Pathol 2003;7:354–359

138. Khurana J, Abdul-Karim F, Bovee JVMG. Osteochondroma. In: Fletcher CDM, Unni KK, Mertens F, eds. World Health Organization Classification of Tumours: Pathology and Genetics of Tumours of Soft Tissue and Bone. Lyon: IARC Press; 2002:234–236

139. Sato K, Kodera T, Kitai R, Kubota T. Osteochondroma of the skull base: MRI and histological correlation. Neuroradiology 1996;38:41–43

140. Georgalas C, Goudakos J, Fokkens WJ. Osteoma of the skull base and sinuses. Otolaryngol Clin North Am 2011;44:875–890, vii

141. Schreiber A, Villaret AB, Maroldi R, Nicolai P. Fibrous dysplasia of the sinonasal tract and adjacent skull base. Curr Opin Otolaryngol Head Neck Surg 2012;20:45–52

142. Kerr RSC, Milford CA. Skull base tumors. In: Moore AJ, Newell DW, eds. Neurosurgery Principles and Practice. New York: Springer; 2012:263–280

143. Harsh GR. Chordomas and chondrosarcomas of the skull base. In: Kaye AH, Laws ER, eds. Brain Tumors: an Encyclopedic Approach, 3rd ed. New York: Saunders/Elsevier; 2012:723–742

144. Bloch OG, Jian BJ, Yang I, et al. A systematic review of intracranial chondrosarcoma and survival. J Clin Neurosci 2009;16:1547–1551

145. Wolfe JT III, Scheithauer BW. "Intradural chordoma" or "giant ecchordosis physaliphora"? Report of two cases. Clin Neuropathol 1987;6:98–103

146. O'Neill P, Bell BA, Miller JD, Jacobson I, Guthrie W. Fifty years of experience with chordomas in southeast Scotland. Neurosurgery 1985;16:166–170

147. Nishigaya K, Kaneko M, Ohashi Y, Nukui H. Intradural retroclival chordoma without bone involvement: no tumor regrowth 5 years after operation. Case report. J Neurosurg 1998;88:764–768

148. Walcott BP, Nahed BV, Mohyeldin A, Coumans JV, Kahle KT, Ferreira MJ. Chordoma: current concepts, management, and future directions. Lancet Oncol 2012; 13:e69–e76

149. Mirra JM, Nelson SD, Rocca CD, Mertens F. Chordoma. In: Fletcher CDM, Unni KK, Mertens F, eds. World Health Organization Classification of Tumours: Pathology and Genetics of Tumours of Soft Tissue and Bone. Lyon: IARC Press; 2002:316–317

150. Hug EB, Loredo LN, Slater JD, et al. Proton radiation therapy for chordomas and chondrosarcomas of the skull base. J Neurosurg 1999;91:432–439

151. Karamchandani J, Wu MY, Das S, et al. Highly proliferative sellar chordoma with unusually rapid recurrence. Neuropathology 2013;33:424–430

152. Ottaviani G, Jaffe N. The epidemiology of osteosarcoma. Cancer Treat Res 2009;152:3–13

153. Newton WA Jr, Gehan EA, Webber BL, et al. Classification of rhabdomyosarcomas and related sarcomas. Pathologic aspects and proposal for a new classification—an Intergroup Rhabdomyosarcoma Study. Cancer 1995;76:1073–1085

154. Choi EY, Gardner JM, Lucas DR, McHugh JB, Patel RM. Ewing sarcoma. Semin Diagn Pathol 2014;31:39–47

155. Nakane T, Hashizume Y, Tachibana E, et al. Primary Ewing's sarcoma of the skull base with intracerebral extension—case report. Neurol Med Chir (Tokyo) 1994;34:628–630

156. Tyagi DK, Balasubramaniam S, Sawant HV. Giant primary ossified cavernous hemangioma of the skull in an adult: A rare calvarial tumor. J Neurosci Rural Pract 2011;2:174–177

157. Wold LE, Swee RG, Sim FH. Vascular lesions of bone. Pathol Annu 1985;20(Pt 2):101–137

158. Ito E, Saito K, Nagatani T, et al. Lymphangioma of the skull base bones leading to cerebrospinal fluid rhinorrhea. J Neurosurg Pediatr 2008;2:273–276

159. Bonavolontà G, Strianese D, Grassi P, et al. An analysis of 2,480 space-occupying lesions of the orbit from 1976 to 2011. Ophthal Plast Reconstr Surg 2013;29:79–86

160. Hans FJ, Reinges MH, Nolte K, Reipke P, Krings T. Primary lymphoma of the skull base. Neuroradiology 2005;47:539–542

161. Roman-Goldstein SM, Jones A, Delashaw JB, McMenomey S, Neuwelt EA. Atypical central nervous system lymphoma at the cranial base: report of four cases. Neurosurgery 1998;43:613–615, discussion 615–616

162. Chan ACL, Chan JKC, Cheung MMC, Kapadia SB. Haematolymphoid tumours. In: Barnes L, Eveson JW, Reichart P, Sidransky D, eds. World Health Organization Classification of Tumours: Pathology and Genetics of Head and Neck Tumours. Lyon: IARC Press; 2005:58–64

163. Suzuki R. Pathogenesis and treatment of extranodal natural killer/T-cell lymphoma. Semin Hematol 2014;51:42–51

164. Logsdon MD, Ha CS, Kavadi VS, Cabanillas F, Hess MA, Cox JD. Lymphoma of the nasal cavity and paranasal sinuses: improved outcome and altered prognostic factors with combined modality therapy. Cancer 1997;80:477–488

165. Suzuki R, Takeuchi K, Ohshima K, Nakamura S. Extranodal NK/T-cell lymphoma: diagnosis and treatment cues. Hematol Oncol 2008;26:66–72

166. McKenna RW, Kyle RA, Kuehl WM, Grogan TM, Harris NL, Coupland RW. Plasma cell neoplasms. In: Swerdlow S, Campo E, Harris NL, et al., eds. WHO Classification of Tumours of Haematopoietic and Lymphoid tissues, 4th ed. Lyon: International Agency for Research on Cancer; 2008:200–213

167. Laigle-Donadey F, Taillibert S, Martin-Duverneuil N, Hildebrand J, Delattre JY. Skull-base metastases. J Neurooncol 2005;75:63–69
168. Molavi D. A primer on immunostains. In: Molavi D, ed. The Practice of Surgical Pathology: A Beginner's Guide to the Diagnostic Process. New York: Springer; 2008: 308–315

7 Clinical and Neurologic Findings in Skull Base Pathology

A complete clinical and neurologic examination should be done in each patient affected by skull base pathologies.

■ Brain Involvement

Tumoral compression or infiltration of the brain, hemorrhages, and contusions/lacerations should be investigated, as they can affect frontal, temporal, and occipital lobe function. The long pathways (motor and sensory system), cranial nerves and brainstem reflexes should be carefully examined.

■ Clinical Features

The main clinical features of skull base pathology are related to the anatomic localization demonstrated in **Fig. 7.1.**

Anterior Skull Base

- Anosmia, frontal lobe syndrome (check neuropsychological testing as well), visual changes.
- Check for involvement of the nasal/paranasal cavities (obstruction, epistaxis), orbits (diplopia, blindness, visual field loss, ophthalmoparesis, ophthalmodynia, dyschromatopsia), face (splanchnocranium fractures with skull base involvement, as in Le Fort III fractures).

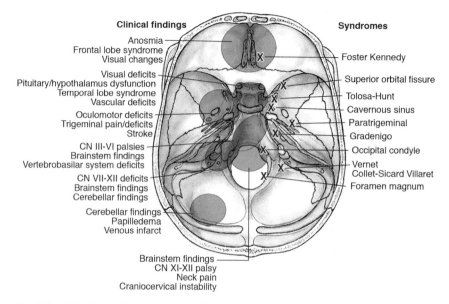

Fig. 7.1 Main clinical features and syndromes related to the anatomic localization of skull base pathologies.

Middle Skull Base

Central/Paracentral

- Optic neuropathy (check for optic nerve and chiasm dysfunctions), cavernous sinus syndromes (ophthalmoparesis, trigeminal pain, etc.).
- Check for pituitary/hypothalamus involvement.
- Check for vascular involvement (arterial dissection, traumatic aneurysms, iatrogenic pseudoaneurysms, carotid-cavernous fistula).

Lateral

- Trigeminal dysfunctions (dysesthesia, pain, anesthesia), chewing deficits trismus
- Proptosis, epistaxis

Posterior Skull Base

Cerebellopontine Angle/Jugular Foramen

- Cranial nerve involvement: all the neurologic deficits related to dysfunction of cranial nerves (CNs) III to XII
- Brainstem corticospinal findings
- Cerebellar findings

Clivus

- Uni/bilateral cranial neuropathies (e.g., CNs III to VI palsies)
- Vertebrobasilar system-related deficits

Foramen Magnum

- Brainstem findings (e.g., rotating and progressive weakness, alternate syndromes)
- CNs XI and XII palsies.
- Suboccipital neck pain

> **Examination Pearl**
>
> Look for wasting of the trapezius (especially in slowly progressive lesions).

Craniocervical Junction

- Brainstem/spinal cord findings
- Craniocervical instability, occipital/suboccipital pain

> **Examination Pearl**
>
> Horner syndrome (also called Bernard-Horner syndrome), consisting of ptosis, miosis, enophthalmos, and anhidrosis, may be caused by several conditions affecting the skull base **(Table 7.1)**.

Table 7.1   Skull Base Conditions Causing Horner Syndrome

- Skull base/nasopharyngeal/orbit tumors/carcinomas
- Skull base/middle ear infections
- Skull base fractures
- Internal carotid dissection (e.g., in trauma)
- Endovascular procedures

■ Skull Base Syndromes

Anterior Skull Base

- **Foster Kennedy syndrome**: due to tumors compressing the olfactory bulb/ tract, frontal lobes, and optic nerve, and giving rise to raised intracranial pressure, which leads to ipsilateral anosmia, ipsilateral optic atrophy, contralateral papilledema

Middle Skull Base/Orbit

- **Complete cavernous sinus syndrome:** CNs III, IV, VI, V_1, and V_2 involvement, and the sympathetic plexus around the internal carotid artery (ICA), which leads to total unilateral ophthalmoplegia, V_1 and V_2 pain/paresthesia/sensory loss, and pupil fixed and at midposition (tumors, ICA aneurysms).
- **Complete superior orbital fissure syndrome (sphenoidal fissure syndrome or Rochon-Duvigneaud's) syndrome):** total ophthalmoplegia, V_1 pain/ paresthesia, sensory loss, proptosis/chemosis/lid edema, exophthalmos, and ptosis, caused by tumors, bony lesions, e.g., fibrous dysplasia, or trauma. In pure superior orbital fissure (SOF) syndrome, the optic nerve is spared. For lesions involving the SOF and optic canal, see next entry.
- **Orbital apex syndrome (Jacod's syndrome)**: CNs II, III, IV, and V_1 involvement, with ophthalmoplegia and V_1 hypoesthesia, caused by tumors around the apex of the orbit.
- **Tolosa-Hunt syndrome**: inflammation of the lateral wall of the cavernous sinus or superior orbital fissure (requires magnetic resonance imaging [MRI] or biopsy proof of granuloma),[1] which leads to acute onset of severe ocular or retro-orbital pain, ophthalmoparesis with diplopia (typically with pupillary sparing), V_1 sensory loss/paresthesia, loss of ipsilateral corneal reflex, possible Horner syndrome.
- **Paratrigeminal (Raeder's) syndrome:** also called oculopupillary sympathetic paresis, due to a lesion in the middle cranial fossa, around Meckel's cave, or related to ICA dissection, giving rise to Horner syndrome with unilateral oculosympathetic paresis and ipsilateral trigeminal involvement.[2]
- **Gradenigo syndrome**: petrous apicitis (caused by inflammatory lesions of the apex, often as a complication of otitis media and mastoiditis), inflammation with trigeminal and abducens nerve involvement, which leads to facial pain/numbness (retro-orbital pain) and ipsilateral lateral rectus palsy, otorrhea.
- **Superior semicircular canal dehiscence syndrome**: pressure- or sound-induced oscillopsia.[3]

Posterior Skull Base

- **Jugular foramen syndrome (Vernet syndrome)**: caused by tumors/trauma around the jugular foramen, which leads to trapezius and sternocleidomastoid muscle paresis, dysphonia, dysphagia, vocal cord paresis, loss of sensation and taste from the posterior one third of the tongue, loss of gag reflex, and loss of sensation from the ipsilateral palate, uvula, pharynx, and larynx.
- **Collet-Sicard syndrome**: paresis of CNs IX, X, XI, and XII, caused by skull base neoplasms or trauma.
- **Villaret syndrome**: paresis of CNs IX, X, XI, and XII with Horner syndrome ± CN VII; essentially it is like a Collett-Sicard syndrome + Horner syndrome.
- **Foramen magnum syndrome**: spastic weakness or numbness/tingling of the extremities, craniocervical pain, dissociated sensory loss/reduction of pain/temperature contralateral to the lesion (tactile sensation preserved), loss of position and vibratory sense (more so in the upper extremities). Typically, the sensory loss begins in one arm, then the ipsilateral leg, then the contralateral leg, and finally the contralateral arm. There may also be paradoxical wasting of the intrinsics muscles of the hands in the presence of upper motor neuron lesions.
- **Occipital condyle syndrome**: severe and unilateral occipital pain with ipsilateral CN XII palsy, due to tumors or trauma.
- **Chiari syndrome**: In Chiari malformation, the typical symptoms are pain (headache, cervical pain), limb weakness/numbness, loss of temperature sensation, and unsteadiness. In some cases, dysphagia, tinnitus, vomiting, and other less common symptoms are seen. Among other signs, hyperactivity of the lower extremity reflexes, nystagmus, gait disturbances, and hand atrophy are the most common.[4]
- **Garcin syndrome**: unilateral paralysis ("half-base" syndrome) of all (global paralysis) or most of all the cranial nerves. This syndrome is very rare, and generally due to skull base metastases.[5,6]

Exocranial Skull Base

- **Eagle syndrome**: an elongated styloid process (SP) that may cause neurovascular compression and ICA compression at the neck, which leads to pain in the ear, neck, pharynx, and tongue (aggravated by swallowing), often in conjunction with rotation/tilting of the head or extension of the tongue.[7] Other symptoms: tinnitus, dysphonia, dysphagia, trismus, vertigo, taste alterations, due to compression of lower cranial nerves.
  - Carotidynia with irritation of the sympathetic nerve plexus, pain of the face, head, eye.
  - Internal carotid artery compression with neurologic symptoms; stroke-related.

- ○ A subset of patients with Eagle syndrome may have ICA stenosis/occlusion without elongation of the SP, due to compression by the stylopharyngeus muscle.[8]
- **Godtfredsen's Syndrome**: trigeminal neuralgia with ophthalmoplegia, CNs III and XII palsy, caused by nasopharyngeal tumors involving the skull base.

■ References

Boldfaced references are of particular importance.

1. **La Mantia L, Curone M, Rapoport AM, Bussone G; International Headache Society. Tolosa-Hunt syndrome: critical literature review based on IHS 2004 criteria. Cephalalgia 2006;26:772–781**
2. Shoja MM, Tubbs RS, Ghabili K, Loukas M, Oakes WJ, Cohen-Gadol AA. Johan Georg Raeder (1889–1959) and paratrigeminal sympathetic paresis. Childs Nerv Syst 2010; 26:373–376
3. da Cunha Ferreira S, de Melo Tavares de Lima MA. Superior canal dehiscence syndrome. Braz J Otorhinolaryngol 2006;72:414–418
4. **Greenberg MS. Chiari malformation. In: Greenberg MS, ed. Handbook of Neurosurgery, 7th ed. New York: Thieme; 2010:233–240**
5. Abe K, Mezaki T, Hirono N, Udaka F, Kameyama M, Kitahara Y. Garcin syndrome with hypopituitarhythm. MR imaging. Neuroradiology 1988;30:447–448
6. Greulich W, Sackmann A, Schlichting P. [Garcin syndrome. Clinical aspects and diagnosis of a rare cranial nerve syndrome with special reference to computerized tomography and nuclear magnetic resonance image findings]. Nervenarzt 1992;63:228–233
7. Woolery WA. The diagnostic challenge of styloid elongation (Eagle's syndrome). J Am Osteopath Assoc 1990;90:88–89
8. Tubbs RS, Loukas M, Dixon J, Cohen-Gadol AA. Compression of the cervical internal carotid artery by the stylopharyngeus muscle: an anatomical study with potential clinical significance. Laboratory investigation. J Neurosurg 2010;113:881–884

8 Otorhinolaryngology and Principles of Neurotology in Skull Base Surgery

Neurotology is the study of the neurology associated with the ear, including hearing and balance function.

- Common symptoms associated with skull base pathology such as hearing loss, tinnitus, imbalance, dysphagia, and nasal obstruction/epistaxis often prompt referral to otorhinolaryngology for assessment.

> **Diagnostic Pearl**
>
> A detailed history in a patient complaining of hearing and balance symptoms is the most valuable diagnostic information.

■ History

A detailed history should address the presenting complaint as well as related symptoms such as hearing loss, tinnitus, aural pressure, imbalance, vertigo (hallucination of circling movement), diplopia, vision loss, altered facial sensation or weakness and nasal symptoms.

Symptoms

- Lateral skull base
  - Diplopia, dizziness (imbalance), vertigo, hearing loss, unilateral tinnitus, aural fullness
  - Cranial nerve deficits causing dysphonia, dysphagia, dysarthria, facial weakness, and altered sensation to face
  - Shoulder weakness
  - Headache, otalgia
  - Midline lesions
  - Anosmia, epistaxis, nasal obstruction, unilateral hearing loss (conductive), headache, facial/sinus pain

- Signs
  - Hitselberger sign: decreased sensation in the external auditory canal from the sensory auricular branch of cranial nerve [CN] VII), often found in cerebellopontine angle (CPA) tumors.
  - Cranial nerve testing
    - Facial weakness
    - Facial numbness or reduced sensation, loss of corneal reflex
    - Palate symmetry with movement, gag reflex
    - Shoulder movement, strength, and head rotation
    - Tongue movement
- Local anatomy examination (including endoscopy)
  - Oral cavity inspection, palpation
  - Nasal examination including upper airway endoscopy (also examine vocal fold movement and constrictor muscle movement)
- Eye movements
  - Abnormal eye movements (asymmetric movement, saccadic pursuit)
  - Nystagmus: Vertical nystagmus represents central pathology, horizontal nystagmus may be peripheral or central pathology.
  - Careful observation of eye movements with four-direction lateral gaze as well as smooth pursuit testing
  - Horizontal nystagmus: etiology can be peripheral or central pathology
  - Vertical nystagmus: etiology is central

■ Testing

Halmagyi Head Thrust Test[1]

The Halmagyi head thrust is a test for unilateral peripheral vestibular weakness. The patient is asked to look at a target straight ahead, usually the nose of the examiner, while the examiner turns the patient's head rapidly to the side.

Interpretation

Normal: The patient's gaze stays fixed on the target.
Abnormal: A corrective saccadic eye movement occurs toward the target at the end of the head thrust, indicative of a peripheral vestibular weakness on the side that the head was moved toward.

- **Cerebellar testing**
  - Dysmetria, dysdiadochokinesis
  - Romberg test

- ○ Finger nose, assess for tremor
- ○ Alternative rapid movements, hand, foot
- **Gait**
  - ○ Spontaneous gait
  - ○ Tandem gait, eyes open/closed (normal: 10 steps without side stepping in patients < age 70)
- **Special tests**
  - ○ Tuning fork tests are very useful bedside tests for rapidly distinguishing between conductive and sensorineural hearing loss.
  - ○ A 512-Hz tuning fork is most useful, and both Rinne and Weber tests should be done for accurate diagnostic information.

Rinne Test

The Rinne test is useful to diagnose a conductive hearing loss and should be done along with the Weber test. A tuning fork is held firmly on the mastoid bone (bone conduction hearing) until patients report they can no longer hear the sound. Then the tuning fork is held adjacent to the external ear canal (air conduction). Patient are then asked if they can hear the tuning fork.

Interpretation

Normal: a positive test. The patient can hear the tuning fork held beside ear canal (air conduction is greater than bone conduction).

Abnormal: a negative test. The patient reports that the sound is not audible adjacent to the ear canal (bone conduction is greater than air conduction), which indicates a conductive hearing loss.

Weber Test

A tuning fork is held on the vertex of the head or on the midline of the forehead, and the patient identifies where the sound is loudest: central (equal in both ears) or lateralized to one side.

Interpretation

Normal: the sound is equal in both ears, or central.
Abnormal: the sound is louder or "lateralizes" to one ear.

In unilateral *conductive hearing loss*, sound is louder in, or lateralizes to, the *ipsilateral* ear. In unilateral *sensorineural hearing loss*, sound is louder in, or lateralizes to, the *contralateral* ear.

Dix Hallpike Position Test

Position testing is done with the patient in the sitting position, with the head turned 45 degrees to one side, and then rapid movement onto supine position and head hanging (neck in extension and supported by the examiner). The eyes are observed for nystagmus. Rotational geotropic nystagmus (toward the ground) is the classic diagnostic finding in benign positional vertigo. The test is repeated on the other side and with the head in the center position.

Audiometric Testing

Audiometric testing includes pure tone audiometry (PTA), which is standardized to assess the threshold of hearing between 250 and 8,000 Hz using a pure tone (sinusoidal) test frequencies. Normal threshold hearing levels are between 0 and 20 dB. Air conduction testing evaluates the entire hearing system, whereas bone conduction testing stimulates the cochlea, thereby bypassing the conduction mechanism. Both air and bone conduction hearing is tested using different headsets; air conduction headset is either an ear canal insert or a standard headset and the bone conduction headset is held against the mastoid bone.

Comparison of the air and bone conduction threshold levels is useful to diagnose the etiology of hearing loss.

- *Conductive hearing loss*: Air conduction threshold levels are elevated with normal bone conduction testing.
- *Air–bone gap:* There is a difference in threshold levels between air and bone conduction.
- *Sensorineural hearing loss*: Both the air and bone conduction thresholds levels are elevated (abnormal) to the same degree.
- *Mixed loss*: Bone conduction thresholds are abnormal and air conduction levels are elevated relative to the bone levels.
- *Speech tests:* each ear tested separately.

Speech Reception Threshold

The speech reception threshold (SRT) is the sound level (in dB) at which a patient can detect the presence of speech 50% of the time.

Speech Discrimination Testing

- The percentage of words correctly repeated by a patient that were presented at a comfortable hearing level with a headset.

- Important evaluation of hearing, because retrocochlear pathology (skull base lesions) affects speech discrimination early.
- Relevant test to evaluate surgical approach options that put hearing at risk and for rehabilitation (e.g., hearing aid). If the speech discrimination score is markedly abnormal, then a hearing aid would not be useful.

Pearl

Unilateral reduction in hearing, especially in speech discrimination or distortion of language perception, is a classic finding of central pathology.

Impedance Testing

Impedance testing is done with a probe inserted into the ear canal, which generates a sound pressure level tone high enough to assess middle ear pressure, and the mobility/integrity of the tympanic membrane as well as the ossicular chain. The peak of the tympanogram shows the pressure of the middle ear space, which has a normal range. The most common abnormality found in impedance testing is related to underlying eustachian tube (ET) dysfunction. Chronic ET dysfunction can cause middle ear fluid (serous otitis media [SOM]) and lead to chronic otitis media with or without a tympanic membrane perforation.

Most ET disorders are developmental (common in children) or due to an inflammatory process (viral upper respiratory tract infection being the most common). However, tumors of the skull base can also cause similar symptoms (hearing loss, ear pressure, tinnitus) due to either direct tumor extension or secondary ET obstruction.

Interpretation

Abnormal: A negative middle each pressure or middle ear fluid is often found when the ET is not ventilating the middle ear adequately.

Stapedial Reflex

The stapedial reflex is a bilateral protective mechanism mediated via CN VII that stimulates the stapedial muscle/tendon to tense, thereby stabilizing the stapes from excessive movement under loud sound conditions. The test records changes in tympanic membrane compliance with sound exposure.

- *Acoustic stapedial reflex threshold:* lowest level of sound pressure that stimulates contraction of the stapedial tendon as measured by changes in tympanic membrane compliance
- Normal: bilateral responses at 70- to 100-dB hearing level
- The reflex is absent if there is a conductive hearing loss in the test ear.
- *Acoustic reflex decay:* Assess if the stapedius muscle can sustain contraction in response to a test sound at 10 dB above the acoustic reflex threshold for 10 seconds.

Interpretation

Abnormal: the response decreases to half or less within 5 seconds (usually tested at 500 and 1,000 Hz).

Retrocochlear (Central) Pathology

Retrocochlear (central) pathology is an abnormal reflex decay or absent stapedial reflex without evidence of conductive hearing loss (ipsilateral ear).

Audiometric Brainstem Response

Auditory brainstem response (ABR, also termed brainstem auditory evoked potential [BAEP]) is an auditory evoked electrical potential of the auditory system. The ABR is measured using surface electrodes and a headset or in the ear canal insert probe presenting repeated tone or click stimuli. This test can be used to objectively determine auditory thresholds, diagnose auditory pathway pathology, and as an intraoperative monitoring tool.

This is an objective test that does not require patient participation and is not affected by anesthesia or central nervous system suppressants. A normal ABR is recorded 8 to 10 ms after a transient sound (click or tone), which generates five to seven electrical peaks or waves within 10 ms that represent an afferent auditory system response from the cochlear nerve through to the midbrain.

Prior to performing an ABR, a PTA is done to determine appropriate ABR test parameters.

Interpretation

Abnormal: sensorineural hearing loss most often in retrocochlear pathology with reduced, delayed, or absent peak potentials.

The ABR/BAEP waveform is generated by:

- I and II: cochlea and extra-intracranial component of the auditory nerve (the average distance from the ear to the brainstem is 2.6 cm; this distance is traversed by the impulse in ~1 ms)
- III: cochlear nucleus
- IV: superior olivary complex
- V: lateral lemniscus

Waves I,III, and V are most consistent, but the wave peaks associated with VI and VII are inconsistent, and they are maybe generated by inferior colliculus neurons.[2-5]

The ABR/BAEP should also be performed preoperatively for baseline evaluation.

Intraoperative Auditory Monitoring

Auditory evoked potential monitoring intraoperatively is most often done by ABR/BAEP, electrocochleography (ECochG) and/or compound action potential or CAP.

Pearls

- The ABR is affected by body temperature, traction, and ischemia. However, preservation of the ABR waveform is highly predictive of hearing preservation postsurgery.[6,7]
- Rapid loss of the ABR may be due to ischemic injury of the cochlear nerve.[7]
- Auditory waves give rise to a complex waveform that does not provide real-time feedback to the surgeon, as is the case in with facial nerve monitoring.[7,8]

Compound Action Potential

The compound action potential or CAP can be recorded either using a probe on the promontory or by direct auditory nerve monitoring at the internal auditory canal. The CAP is the depolarization of the distal end of the auditory/cochlear nerve, stimulated by means of a click via an earphone as in an ABR,[4] and registered by means of a wick electrode made from a Teflon-insulated silver wire. The CAP appears as a large (25–30 µV) triphasic response that can be reduced by surgical manipulation of the nerve. The main limitation of the technique is that the exposure of the nerve is often possible only at the end of the tumor resection, when the nerve may already be dysfunctional. Moreover, cerebrospinal fluid (CSF) may create impedance changes at the electrode–nerve interface.[7]

Electrocochleography (ECochG)

The ECochG consists of the electrical response to stimuli (i.e. clicks or tone bursts) from the cochlea and the distal auditory/cochlear nerve. The ECochG includes the cochlear microphonic (generated from the hair cells in the cochlea), the cochlear summating potential (also generated from within the cochlea) and the compound action potential. Near-field technique entails placing an electrode on the promontory of the inner ear through the tympanic membrane, or a ball-tip electrode on the round window membrane via a tympanomeatal flap or facial recess approach.[7,8] The generated potentials originate from the organ of Corti within the cochlea. A latency shift in the recording is generally associated with neural hearing loss,[9] and it can be useful for intraoperative monitoring.

> **Surgical Anatomy Pearl**
>
> Comparing ABR, recorded with a subdermal needle electrode at the mastoid, with ECochG, recorded by a ball electrode attached to the tympanic membrane or on the promontory, it has been shown that ECochG is more reliable in terms of clinical outcome, and it may replace ABR recording in CPA surgery.[10]

- The first wave of the ABR corresponds to the action potential of the cochlear/auditory nerve in response to the sound stimulus. The possible elicited responses include the cochlear microphonic, the summating potential (SP), and the whole nerve action potential (AP) depending on the type of sound stimulus presented. ECochG is primarily used to diagnose Meniere's disease (endolymphatic hydrops) with an abnormal ratio of the SP and AP.[11]

Otoacoustic Emissions

The outer hair cells of the cochlea are able to amplify movement of the cochlear membranous partition of the labyrinth, which results in extremely low intensity acoustic emissions measurable in the ear canal.

These otoacoustic emissions (OAEs) are classified as *spontaneous* (without any sound stimulus) or as *evoked* (in response to specific test sounds). OAEs are detectable in normal hearing and are reduced or absent in hearing loss of > 35 dB. The test uses an ear canal probe with a speaker and microphone and has become a standard of care to screen for hearing loss in newborn infants. Outer hair cells (and therefore OAEs) are particular sensitive to ototoxicity, hypoxia, and noise exposure.

■ Hearing Loss

Hearing loss is described according to the etiology as conductive, sensorineural, or mixed (both).

- **Conductive hearing loss: common causes**
  - Acute otitis media (serous otitis media or purulent)
  - Chronic otitis media
  - Otitis externa
  - Obstruction in canal (wax, debris, foreign body)
  - Tympanic membrane (TM) perforation
  - Otosclerosis (stapes fixation with abnormal bone growth at stapes footplate)
  - Trauma (temporal bone fracture, ossicular discontinuity, TM perforation)
  - Neoplasm in external canal, middle ear
- **Sensorineural hearing loss: common causes**
  - Presbycusis (aging)
  - Congenital/familial
  - Ototoxicity (e.g., aminoglycoside exposure, loop diuretics, nonsteroidal anti-inflammatory drugs)
  - Noise induced
  - Trauma (temporal bone fracture involving otic capsule)
  - Infectious (viral, bacterial [e.g., meningitis, herpes zoster oticus, syphilis])
  - Autoimmune (rare [e.g., Wegener's granulomatosis, Cogan's syndrome])

Management depends on the etiology, but workup will involve a complete physical examination, otoscopy (with microscope if there is an external/middle ear abnormality), and an audiogram including pure tone audiogram and speech discrimination testing.

Surgical Anatomy Pearls

- Most hearing loss and tinnitus symptoms are bilateral unless related to otitis media or trauma (identifiable from the history).
- Unilateral sensorineural hearing loss, particularly loss of speech discrimination, is suspicious for central/skull base pathology until proven otherwise.

■ Syndromes

Ramsay Hunt Syndrome (Herpes Zoster Oticus)

This syndrome is a varicella zoster infection that most commonly presents with a painful herpetic skin rash in the ear canal, pinna, or tympanic membrane, with associated hearing loss and facial nerve weakness. Vertigo can also occur.

Ototoxicity

Ototoxicity includes both hearing and balance toxicity due to an adverse effect of medical therapy. The most commonly implicated medications include aminoglycosides and platinum based chemotherapy.

- Risk factors: age (elderly), renal failure, loop diuretics, duration of medication, elevated serum levels of aminoglycosides

Vertigo

Vertigo is the hallucination of circling movement often accompanied by nausea, vomiting, sweating, and ataxia.

- The history and physical examination are the most important tools in making an accurate diagnosis. Specifics should include the onset, frequency, and duration of vertigo, as well as aggravating and relieving factors. Other otologic (e.g., hearing loss, tinnitus, aural pressure, ear discharge) and nonotologic (e.g., headache, nausea, facial weakness, double vision, voice or swallowing changes) symptoms are relevant and should be a standard part of the history. The underlying diagnosis can be categorized by the duration and frequency of the vertiginous episodes and are summarized in **Table 8.1**.

Benign Paroxysmal Positional Vertigo

Benign paroxysmal positional vertigo (BPPV) is by far the most common diagnosis in a patient with vertigo. BPPV is characterized by vertigo lasting seconds (less than a minute) often provoked by a rapid head movement, particularly neck extension or rotational head motion. It is thought that displaced otoliths floating inside the membranous labyrinth are the underlying pathology, causing position-induced asymmetric movements of the inner ear fluid. BPPV is more common with a history of previous ear infection, head injury, or Meniere's disease.

Meniere's Disease (Endolymphatic Hydrops)

Meniere's disease classically presents with episodic vertigo lasting minutes to hours, with accompanying tinnitus, sensorineural hearing loss, and, less commonly, aural pressure or fullness. Although episodic in nature with some hearing recovery between episodes, most patients will eventually have a permanent sensorineural hearing loss (moderate to severe) with natural disease progression.

Table 8.1 Vertigo: Common Diagnoses

Diagnosis	Duration	Head Movement	Other Otologic Symptoms	Hearing Loss	Treatment
Benign paroxysmal positional vertigo	Seconds	Provoked by head movement	No	No	Canalith repositioning or surgery (if recalcitrant)
Meniere's disease	Minutes to hours	Symptoms worse with head movement	Aural pressure; tinnitus—ipsilateral	Sensorineural hearing loss	Medical and surgical
Vestibular neuronitis	Hours to days	Symptoms worse with movement	None	None	Supportive
Labyrinthitis	Hours to days	Symptoms worse with head movement	Tinnitus	Sensorineural variable degree	Steroids, antibiotics if bacterial

Treatment is supportive, and as yet there is no broadly successful medical therapy for Meniere's disease. Currently, medical treatment includes betahistine and diuretics.

Ablative treatment using gentamicin instillation into the middle ear has been shown to successfully stop the vertiginous episodes by vestibular ablation due to the ototoxic characteristics of gentamycin. This is not without risk of permanent sensorineural hearing loss.

Vestibular Neuronitis

The etiology of vestibular neuronitis is unclear, and requires a clinical diagnosis of exclusion, with acute vertigo lasting hours to days without other otologic symptoms. Possible causes include viral, inflammatory, and vascular.

Labyrinthitis

Labyrinthitis is inflammation of the inner ear, including the cochlea and vestibular organs. Possible causes are viral, bacterial, and autoimmune disorders.

Acoustic/Vestibular Schwannoma

The common CPA tumor typically presents with a progressive gradual unilateral hearing loss (found in 85% of patients) and tinnitus (66%).[12] Imbalance symptoms rather than vertigo are more commonly reported and are present in 35 to 50% of patients.[12] If a sudden sensorineural hearing loss is the presenting complaint, about 1% of patients are found to have a vestibular schwannoma.[13,14] With increasing tumor size, signs and symptoms progress to include fifth nerve hypoesthesia and loss of corneal reflex. Large tumors can affect the lower cranial nerves, causing voice and swallowing dysfunction. With brainstem compression, hydrocephalus will result in headache and vision changes. Facial weakness is infrequent, and visual changes can be from lack of eye closure, hydrocephalus (blurring), or papilledema. Nystagmus, fast phase toward the ipsilateral side, is commonly present in larger tumors, and cerebellar signs may also occur.

- **Differential Diagnosis Vertigo (Common Causes)**
  - Vertebral-basilar insufficiency
  - Presyncope (often associated with hypertension treatment)
  - Medication adverse effects
  - Migraine
  - Hyperventilation

Vestibular Diagnostic Tests

Balance function testing is useful to assist in the diagnosis of many vestibular disorders, helping to distinguish between peripheral and central pathology and to quantify the degree of vestibular dysfunction. Vestibular and ocular motor systems are evaluated in the standard test battery.

Electronystagmogram (ENG)

The electronystagmogram (ENG) is based on the vestibular ocular reflex (VOR) and associated eye movements.

- Standard ENG (widely available) records the changes in eye position using surface electrodes to measure electrical potential between the cornea (+) and retina (−).
- Rotational head movement is normally accompanied by equal and opposite eye movements to maintain a stable retinal image mediated by the VOR.
- The test results are measured either as a surface electrical response output or using a video ENG system to record eye movements using a goggle camera and near-infrared light tracking system. Nystagmus is the main eye movement tracked and is described by direction and velocity (degree/s) from the slow phase of the eye movement.

Optokinetic Testing

Saccadic eye movements are quick movements used to track an object or move the target image to the fovea of the retina. Calibration of an ENG is done by asking patients to move their gaze between two test lights 10 degrees off center. The accuracy and symmetry of the eye movement is recorded.

Pursuit

The smooth pursuit system stabilizes images of moving objects on the fovea and is assessed by the subject tracking a moving light or pendulum.

Bithermal Caloric Tests

The lateral (horizontal) semicircular canal is stimulated by flushing the test ear canal with warm or cool water (7°C above and below normal body temperature) for 30 to 60 seconds. The temperature change stimulates internal fluid flow in the lateral (horizontal) semicircular canal. Surface electrodes record the corneoretinal electrical potential as the eyes move. Nystagmus is the normal physiological response using the mnemonic COWS (see Pearl) to indicate the appropriate direction of the fast phase of the nystagmus. Fixation suppression (patient is asked to look at a target) should occur during the caloric testing.

> **Pearl**
>
> User the mnemonic COWS: **C**old—**O**pposite; **W**arm—**S**ame.

- The velocity of the slow phase of the nystagmus is calculated and compared with that of the opposite ear. Less than a 20% difference is a normal, and 20% or greater represents a right- or left-sided weakness.
- Test cannot be performed with water if a tympanic membrane perforation is present.
- Results consistent with a peripheral disorder:
  - Unilateral caloric weakness (no other pathology on test)
  - Positional nystagmus
  - Direction fixed nystagmus
  - Bilateral or absent caloric weakness with history of labyrinthine disorder or ototoxicity
- Findings suggestive of a central disorder[15]:
  - Vertical nystagmus
  - Direction-changing nystagmus
  - Failure of fixation suppression during caloric testing
  - Abnormal saccadic or pursuit testing

Vestibular Evoked Myogenic Potentials

The vestibular evoked myogenic potential (VEMP) is an evoked electromyographic response test of the ipsilateral sternocleidomastoid muscle to a loud click stimulus presented to the ipsilateral ear. The VEMP test is used to assess the inferior vestibular nerve (afferent) and the spinocerebellar tract (efferent). This test is not yet routinely available.

■ Facial Nerve

The facial nerve is complex (see Chapter 3, page 83). It has motor, sensory, and general and specialized efferent/afferent nerve fibers for functional anatomy.

Assessment of Facial Paralysis

Acute facial paralysis (arising over hours or days) is a disabling condition, and most patients will seek emergency treatment. The most common cause of facial paralysis is Bell's palsy (> 50% of cases) followed by trauma (20% of cases). Neoplastic disease account for 5% of facial paralysis.

History

The history should address the facial weakness symptoms, the rate of onset, the duration, and the following associated symptoms:

- Otologic (ear pain, otorrhea or ear discharge, hearing loss, tinnitus, aural pressure, vertigo, or imbalance)
- Facial numbness (CN V)
- Hyperacusis (discomfort with loud noise exposure due to stapedial branch dysfunction)
- Dry eyes (reduced tearing)
- Past ear disorders or surgery

Pearl

Gradual onset (> 3 weeks) of facial weakness, multiple cranial nerve palsies, neck or facial mass, are suggestive of neoplastic etiology.

Physical Examination

The head and neck examination should include endoscopy to evaluate the anatomy of the nasopharynx (eustachian tube, posterior nasal space), palate movement, pharyngeal constrictor movement, and vocal cord movement.

- Otoscopy, assessment of CNs III to XII, neck and salivary gland palpation: Evaluate for mass lesions, asymmetry, muscle bulk of masseter and sternocleidomastoid

Neurologic Evaluation of Facial Nerve Motor Function

- Complete versus incomplete (paresis) using grading system (House-Brackmann grading system [Table 8.2])
- Assess main branches, motor function to upper, middle, and lower face for symmetry during rest and active movements
- Schirmer test (tear production assessment, ophthalmology referral)
- Sensory (Hitzelberger's sign)

Investigations

Laboratory Studies

- Complete blood cell count and erythrocyte sedimentation rate
- Serology (e.g., Lyme disease)
- Autoimmune (e.g., serum antinuclear antibody [ANA] and rheumatoid factor [RF])
- Cerebrospinal fluid assay

Table 8.2   House-Brackmann Facial Nerve Grading Classification[16]

Grade	Description
I	Normal function
II	Mild dysfunction: slight weakness on testing, can close eye, normal tone and symmetry at rest
III	Moderate gross dysfunction: at rest, normal tone and symmetry Synkinesis: not severe Movement: moderate weakness but active movement still observed Eye: can close with maximum effort
IV	Moderately severe: obvious weakness/asymmetry with movement At rest, normal tone and symmetry Eye closure incomplete
V	Severe: barely observed movement maximal effort Asymmetry at rest Eye closure incomplete
VI	Total paralysis: no movement, asymmetry at rest

Audiology

Pure-tone and speech discrimination testing.

Electrophysiological Tests

Electroneurography (ENoG), electromyography (EMG), nerve excitability test (NET).

Imaging

Computed tomography (CT) with contrast, magnetic resonance imaging (MRI) with gadolinium.

Differential Diagnosis

See **Table 8.3.**

Electrophysiologic Testing in Facial Paralysis

In patients with complete facial nerve paralysis, electrophysiological testing with EMG, ENoG, and NET can provide prognostic and diagnostic information, with certain limitations.

Pearl

Electrophysiological testing is not helpful in an incomplete paresis.

Table 8.3   Differential Diagnosis of Facial Paralysis

Diagnosis	Description
Idiopathic	• Bell's palsy (> 50%) • Melkersson-Rosenthal syndrome (recurrent familial facial palsy)
Infection	• Acute otitis media (serous or suppurative) • Chronic otitis media/cholesteatoma • Mastoiditis • Malignant otitis externa (skull base osteomyelitis) • Herpes zoster oticus (Ramsay Hunt syndrome) • Lyme disease (bilateral)
Trauma (> 20%)	• Penetrating trauma, face/temporal bone • Temporal bone fractures • Birth trauma • Iatrogenic injury (surgery of salivary gland, otologic, skull base) • Botox

Neoplasia	• Malignant
	  ○ Primary: salivary gland, melanoma, oral
	  ○ Metastatic: squamous cell (aerodigestive tract), melanoma, lymphoma, rhabdomyosarcoma, histiocytosis
	• Benign
	  ○ Glomus jugulare or tympanicum
	  ○ Facial neuroma
	  ○ Schwannoma of lower cranial nerves
	  ○ Meningioma

Congenital	• Möbius syndrome • Lower lip paralysis
Metabolic and systemic	• Autoimmune disorders (e.g., Wegener's granulomatosis, sarcoidosis) • Guillain-Barré syndrome

This testing is not useful in the first 3 days because wallerian degeneration has not yet occurred. The main limitation of EMG testing is that a severely neurapraxic but intact nerve cannot be distinguished from a complete degeneration in the acute phase. After 10 to 14 days, fibrillation potentials arise in the denervated muscles. If there are no voluntary motor units activated and fibrillation potentials are present on EMG testing, then complete nerve degeneration can be assumed to have occurred. An *incomplete* lesion has some motor units active and fibrillation potentials, whereas a *regenerating* nerve shows polyphasic motor unit potentials.[17]

- *Electromyography*: measurement of voluntary and evoked muscle unit responses.
- *Nerve excitability test*: threshold (in milliamperes, mA) to elicit barely visible muscle contraction on normal facial nerve compared to the side with facial weakness (< 3.5 mA difference yields a good prognosis).
- *Electroneurography*: quantitative test using high-level electrical current over main trunk of facial nerve for a compound action potential with surface electrodes to record depolarization of motor axons. Amplitude of the AP is proportional to the number of intact axons, and > 90% degeneration is consistent with a poor prognosis.

Sunderland Classification

The Sunderland classification categorizes nerve dysfunction as axonotmesis, neurapraxia, or neurotmesis[18] (**Table 8.4**).

Bell's Palsy

Bell's palsy is a diagnosis of exclusion of an acute facial paralysis of unknown etiology. The condition is usually temporary, and it affects 40 cases per 100,000 per year primarily in adults younger that age 45. The onset is rapid with few other symptoms, and it has a good prognosis. One third of patients will have an incomplete paresis, with more than 90% of those patients having a full recovery of facial nerve function.[19] The average length of time to recovery is 2 months, but it can take up to 6 months.

Table 8.4 Sunderland Classification of Nerve Dysfunction[18]

Classification	Description
Neurapraxia	• Nerve compression but intact and recovery expected • NET and ENoG Normal • EMG: no voluntary APs
Axonotmesis	• Wallerian (axonal) degeneration with intact endoneural sheaths • Test > 1 week • NET, and ENoG show complete degeneration • EMG no voluntary APs • > 10 to 14 days, fibrillation potentials become evident • Recovery expected
Neurotmesis	• Similar to axonotmesis plus loss of endoneural tubules • Electrophysiological test results similar to above but outcome unpredictable

Abbreviations: AP, action potentials; EMG, electromyography; ENoG, electroneurography; NET, nerve excitability test.

- Bell's palsy
  - One-third of patients with Bell's palsy have an incomplete paresis (> 90 % will have a complete recovery)
  - Two-thirds of Bell's palsy patients have a complete paralysis of which two-thirds will have a complete recovery

Signs and Symptoms

Signs and symptoms include eyebrow droop, paralysis of all the mimic muscles, stretching of the nasolacrimal duct, poor tear clearance (tearing), deficient conjunctival reflex, drooling, lack of food bolus clearance from inner cheek (buccinator paralysis), and hyperacusis (due to paralysis of the stapedius muscle). Lesions of the facial nerve can also cause loss of taste (in the anterior two thirds of the tongue).

Treatment

- Steroids: A meta-analysis demonstrated significant improvement in function with oral steroids (i.e., 1/mg/kg for 7 to 10 days) if started within 72 hours of onset.[20]
- Antivirals: An equivocal effect was found on the meta-analysis, but they are commonly given for 1 week.[21]

Pearl

- Protect eye/cornea: eyedrops, tape/patch at night, may require tarsorrhaphy.
- Prevent corneal abrasion/ulcer.

Ramsay Hunt Syndrome (Herpes Zoster Oticus)

This varicella-zoster infection can cause facial paralysis along with variable associated symptoms including hearing loss, tinnitus, and vertigo with a painful variable vesicular rash in the sensory distribution of CN V, VII, or X (neck, ear, tympanic membrane, or pharynx). Prognosis is more guarded than in Bell's palsy, and treatment should include antiviral therapy.

Melkersson-Rosenthal Syndrome

This syndrome is often familial and presents with a history of recurrent facial palsy and facial swelling with onset before age 20. Other symptoms include migraine and fissured tongue.

■ Swallowing, Voice, and Airway Considerations

- *Dysphagia* is defined as a difficulty with swallowing or an inability to swallow.

- *Dysphonia* is defined as an abnormally produced voice.
- *Dysarthria* is defined as defective articulation of speech.

The lower cranial nerves control aerodigestive tract function, including swallowing, voice/speech production, and airway protection. Larger skull base tumors can have a direct effect on the upper aerodigestive tract by direct mass effect causing dysphagia, change in voice quality, or airway obstruction.

- Partial nerve dysfunction may be subtle, and it requires a detailed history, physical examination, and special investigations. After surgical intervention, cranial nerve function is often worse with either transient or permanent neuropathy due to traction, transection, or heat injury during surgery.[22] The resulting neuropathy can vary from a mild reversible neurapraxia (conduction disruption), to a third-degree neurotmesis with loss of axon continuity and endoneural tube structure.[18] The pathology of the tumor will also influence nerve function depending on its predilection for invasion. For example, certain salivary gland tumors (adenoid cystic) are known to infiltrate the perineurium, whereas glomus jugulare tends to progressively invade the perineurium and then the endoneurium and to alter blood supply with larger tumor size.[23]
- Depending on tumor location, size, and pathology, specific cranial nerves are more likely affected. As tumor size increases, there is a higher incidence and degree of nerve dysfunction due to compression, loss of blood supply, or invasion.
- Although some patients have an isolated cranial neuropathy, many will have varying degrees of multiple nerve deficits. The effects of the neuropathies on aerodigestive tract function are logically based on their sensory and motor function[24,25] (**Table 8.5**).
- Multiple lower cranial neuropathies (see **Fig. 7.1** on page 181):
  - **Vernet's syndrome**: jugular foramen site; CNs IX, X, and XI affected
  - **Collet-Sicard syndrome** (intercondylar space syndrome): jugular foramen syndrome (dysfunction of CNs IX, X, and XI) with additional involvement of CN XII
  - **Villaret's syndrome**: Collet-Sicard and unilateral sympathetic involvement (Horner's syndrome)

■ Common Skull Base Tumors Associated with Cranial Nerve

Deficits Affecting Swallowing/Voice Function

- *Lateral skull base:* schwannoma, meningioma, epidermoid, paragangliomas (glomus jugulare, glomus tympanicum, glomus vagale), metastases to skull base

Table 8.5 Cranial Nerve Deficits: Effects on Swallowing, Voice, and Airway

Cranial Nerve	Swallowing	Voice	Airway
V Motor to temporalis, masseter, pterygoids, mylohyoid, tensor tympani, veli palatini Sensory: oral cavity, sinuses nose, palate, upper pharynx	Oral phase of swallowing ↓ Mastication ↓ Sensation Inappropriate bolus Nasal regurgitation	↓ Alteration oral cavity/oropharynx space ↓ Palate elevation Mild hypernasal voice quality	↓ Jaw movement Airway unlikely affected
VII Facial muscle	↓ Oral continence drooling	↓ Lips movement Articulation affected	N/A
IX Sensation pharynx palate	↓ Velopharyngeal closure Nasal regurgitation	Hypernasal voice	N/A
X Sensation: larynx Motor: palate/pharynx and larynx	Constrictor weakness Poor sensation, ↑ Aspiration ↓ Glottic closure	Pooling secretions ↓ Voice intensity Breathy weak "wet" voice	Bilateral: stridor, inability to abduct vocal folds Unilateral: ↓ Cough ↓ Subglottic air pressure ↓ Auto-PEEP ↓ Glottic closure
XII Motor: tongue	↓ Bolus formation and movement in oral phase ↓ Post-tongue base movement ↓ Pharyngeal clearance of bolus Reduced laryngeal elevation	↓ Articulation precision dysarthria	↑ Aspiration risk

Abbreviation: PEEP, positive end-expiratory pressure.

- *Anterior skull base:* nasopharyngeal carcinoma, schwannoma, meningioma, chordoma, sinus neoplasms (squamous cell carcinoma, salivary gland malignancies arising in a sinus), esthesioneuroblastoma, lymphoma, metastases

Normal Swallowing

Swallowing is divided into three phases:

1. *Oral phase* (duration variable but <5 seconds):
   a. Mastication of food, in conjunction with saliva, forms a bolus.
   b. The bolus is propelled posteriorly, and the soft palate elevates to prevent nasal regurgitation.
   c. The bolus is moved by the tongue posteriorly to enter the pharynx.
2. *Pharyngeal phase* (1–2 seconds):
   a. Transfer of the bolus to esophagus.
   b. Hyoid and larynx are elevated by strap muscles and tongue base.
   c. The vocal folds adduct, and the epiglottis is tipped posteriorly over the glottis.
   d. The tongue base moves posterior-inferior to propel the bolus
   e. The constrictor muscles (pharyngeal walls) sequentially contract to transit bolus into the upper esophageal sphincter.
   f. The upper esophageal sphincter opens for the bolus to pass into the upper esophagus.
3. *Esophageal phase*:
   a. Sequentially coordinated movement of bolus from superior to inferior.
   b. Relaxation of lower esophageal sphincter.

Normal Voice and Speech

Voice production is initiated by adduction (approximation) of the vocal folds (CN X, recurrent laryngeal nerve branch). During exhalation, aerodynamic forces cause oscillation or vibration of the surface cover of the vocal folds, which generates the sound source for speech. Both sensory and motor functions of the larynx are carried out by the vagus nerves (superior and recurrent laryngeal nerve branches).

- The vocal folds are normally adducted during swallowing and during normal coughing. During the cough reflex or during a voluntary cough, a rapid inhalation is followed by firm vocal fold adduction, raising subglottic air pressure. The release (abduction) of the vocal folds with rapid exhalation leads to a dramatic expulsion of air and secretions from below the vocal folds.
- Speech is an extremely complex coordinated task involving the motor and sensory control of not only the larynx but also the oral cavity (tongue, lips, and palate), pharynx, and hypopharynx. Depending on the shape of the vocal

tract (structures and space from just above the vocal folds up to the lips including the nasal cavity), the sound source is modified to generate various speech sounds.

Clinical Presentation: Dysphagia/Dysphonia

Alteration in aerodigestive tract function due to skull base pathology can vary from a mild change in voice to dramatic weight loss and aspiration pneumonia. The clinical history is critical in determining appropriate management. The onset, the swallowing problem or voice change, and the potential complications such as weight loss, shortness of breath, and choking are important aspects of the clinical presentation.

Partial nerve deficits are easily compensated in short-term voice tasks and, if present, are likely to worsen or become a complete paralysis postoperatively. Documenting the paresis preoperatively is helpful in planning postoperative decision making regarding swallowing function and likelihood of return in nerve function. **Table 8.6** lists the clinical symptoms. The presence of incomplete cranial nerve deficits may have subtle symptoms due to behavioral compensation, particularly in a slow-growing tumor such as a schwannoma or meningioma.

Table 8.6   Clinical Symptoms of Lower Cranial Nerve Palsy

Swallowing	Voice Speech	Airway

• Choking
• Change in diet
• Food stuck
• Time to onset of symptoms
  ○ < 2 seconds likely pharyngeal origin
• ≥ 2 seconds likely esophageal
  ○ Painful swallowing
  ○ Regurgitation of food
  ○ Throat clearing during eating
  ○ Coughing during eating
  ○ Drooling
  ○ Repeated pneumonia
	• Change in voice, e.g., weak, breathy, "wet" or gurgling (poor secretion clearance)
	• Nasal quality of voice
	• Difficulty with articulation, slurring, or tripping on words
		• Noisy breathing, e.g., stridor from bilateral CN X paralysis or larger tumor in airway
		• Shortness of breath
		• Weak cough
		• Nasal obstruction

- Aspiration is also under-recognized clinically and is associated with a four- to 13-fold increased risk of aspiration pneumonia.[26,27]
- The most problematic cranial neuropathy associated with dysphagia occurs in the vagus nerve, given its broad afferent and efferent connections within the larynx and pharynx. The presence of a unilateral vocal fold paralysis from a vagus neuropathy causes a 2.5 increased risk of aspiration over that in similar patients without a vocal fold paralysis.[28] The mortality rate from a hospital-acquired aspiration pneumonia is reported to be between 20% and 60%.[27]
- Dysphagia due to cranial nerve deficits can be quite complex. For example, a large lateral skull base CPA tumor with CNs V to XII affected will have multiple neuropathies contributing to the dysphagia. Lack of mastication and oral sensation (CN V) leads to poorly formed food boluses with reduced anterior tongue movement (CN XII) to manipulate bolus to the pharynx. The orbicularis oris muscle may be unable to keep the lips closed during the oral phase of swallowing (CN VII). The posterior tongue base (CN XII) lacks the ability to push the bolus posteriorly, and the pharyngeal phase is delayed with food residue in the valleculae. The constrictors (CN X) are weak on the same side with reduced pharyngeal propulsion of the bolus. The palate (CNs IX/X) cannot elevate and close the velopharyngeal space, and nasal regurgitation of food can occur.
- Laryngeal elevation to assist in glottic protection and opening the cricopharyngeus is reduced due to tongue and strap muscle weakness (CN XII). Even when the bolus arrives in the hypopharynx, the lower constrictors (CN X) cannot empty the pyriform fossa, and the cricopharyngeus (CN X) may not relax in order to permit bolus transition into the esophagus. All of the above leads to an increased risk of aspiration, and a poor cough (CN X) cannot clear the aspirated material before penetrating into the lower airway and lung.

Dysphonia

Dysphonia is most commonly associated with a vocal fold paralysis, which is typically a weak breathy voice with reduced loudness. The voice can also have a nasal quality if the palate does not close against the posterior pharyngeal wall at Passavant's ridge (a prominence on the posterior wall of the nasopharynx, caused by the contraction of the superior constrictor of the pharynx during swallowing).

Pearl

In rare cases, a large nasopharyngeal or clival mass can obstruct the posterior nasal space, causing a hyponasal voice and nasal obstruction symptoms.

Airway Obstruction

Airway obstruction at the level of the glottis can be observed with bilateral vocal fold paralysis.

The vocal folds cannot abduct (open), resulting in airway obstruction with stridor and shortness of breath. Airway management in these cases usually requires a tracheotomy. Other options include (micro)endoscopic approaches to increase the glottic opening with either a cordotomy or an arytenoidectomy. These procedures are not usually performed in the acute setting and often require subspecialty training in laryngology. Reinnervation of a bilateral vocal fold paralysis has rarely been done in a research setting.

The differential diagnosis for bilateral vocal fold paralysis includes postintubation laryngeal edema and glottic stenosis from prolonged intubation. Both conditions may require tracheotomy and assessment by an otolaryngologist. Tracheotomy is recommended in order to remove the endotracheal tube, and a nasogastric or oral gastric tube should also be replaced with a gastrostomy tube. Repeated nasoendoscopy is carried out to reevaluate the glottic function. If the airway obstruction does not improve, further surgical management with either endoscopic cordotomy or external approach laryngoplasty may be required to decannulate the patient.

■ Preoperative Evaluation

A *multidisciplinary approach* involving related specialists and health providers is advocated in order to provide the most comprehensive assessment and treatment options for patients with aerodigestive tract dysfunction or at risk of developing it.

Pearls

- It is recommended that patients be referred to an otolaryngologist head and neck surgeon for an examination of upper aerodigestive tract function including a detailed clinical examination and indirect endoscopy of the upper aerodigestive tract. Evaluation by a qualified speech-language pathologist with an oral mechanical exam and swallowing assessment (details below) is valuable in managing these patients with regard to both diagnosis and treatment.
- Patients should be counseled preoperatively about their risk of postoperative speech or swallowing difficulties. This can be done by a preoperative assessment of the tumor pathology, tumor location, and the patient's preoperative ability to compensate for deficits of cranial nerve function. If the risk of tracheostomy or percutaneous feeding tube is high, it should be discussed with the patient and be taken into consideration in the decisions regarding a specific surgical approach.

Imaging

Imaging with CT and MRI with contrast is routine, and a modified barium swallow (deglutition study; see below) may also be necessary.

Examination

A full head and neck examination is performed, as previously described. A full neurologic examination and cranial nerve assessment should also be done.

Cranial Nerves

CNs III, IV, VI: extra ocular eye movements, symmetry, and presence of nystagmus

CN V: open/close jaw to evaluate for trismus, strength, and symmetry

- Sensation V_1–V_3
- Corneal reflex

CN VII: symmetry at rest, and movement of facial muscles to evaluate upper and lower face, particularly eye closure

CN VIII: tuning fork assessment; Weber, Rinne, rapid evaluation of conductive/ sensorineural hearing loss

CN IX: palate elevation and symmetry, sensation of oral cavity, pharynx, gag reflex (with CN X)

CN XI: accessory nerve function: assess for symmetry, bulk, strength, and movement of sternocleidomastoid and trapezius muscle (e.g., head turn, shoulder shrug, raise arms overhead)

CN XII: anterior/posterior tongue bulk, fasciculation, movement and strength, symmetry

---

Examination Pearl

A slow-growing tumor such as a glomus jugulare may allow time for non–CN XI innervated muscles to compensate in shoulder muscle function, but close examination may disclose sternocleidomastoid and trapezius muscle wasting.

Neck

Examination includes the observation and palpation of masses, determining the location and size of masses, auscultation of masses, and assessment of lymphadenopathy.

CN XI: accessory nerve function: sternocleidomastoid and trapezius assessment for symmetry, bulk, strength, and movement (e.g., head turn, shoulder shrug, raise arms overhead)

A slowly growing tumor such as a glomus jugulare will allow time for compensatory non–CN XI innervated muscles to take over these functions, but close examination with the patient undressed will disclose the wasting.

Speech/Voice

Assess the patient's articulation, rate of speech, imprecision, and slurring.

- Voice weakness, breathy quality, poor cough, and a wet or gurgling quality to voice
- Rapid repetition of syllables /pa /ta/ ka/ or a similar task repeated four or five times to assess fatigability and dysdiadochokinesis of speech

Indirect Nasoendoscopy/laryngoscopy

Preoperative nasoendoscopy should be done on any patient with a lesion in the skull base along the tract of the vagus to evaluate the function of the larynx and pharynx.

- *Functional endoscopic evaluation of swallowing* (FEES) is a clinical assessment of swallowing conducted under endoscopic observation. It is a useful tool to evaluate dysphagia prior to resuming oral feeding; it is most often done by a speech-language pathologist or a otolaryngologist head and neck surgeon. A trial of various food and fluid consistencies is done, with observation of the swallowing by an endoscope and video monitor.
- Endoscopic evaluation of pharynx and larynx using flexible endoscope **(Fig. 8.1)**:
  - Observation during voice, respiratory, and swallowing tasks
    - Abduction and adduction of vocal folds noted bilaterally/symmetry
    - Glottic closure during voicing, swallowing (e.g., complete, incomplete, right/left sided glottis gap during adduction)
    - Rapid movements of vocal folds (dysdiadochokinesis)
    - Observation of pooling of secretions (pyriform fossa, valleculae) or aspiration
    - Swallowing tasks to evaluate constrictor function, tongue base movement, clearance, and pyriform and valleculae secretions (see FEES)
  - Utilized as medical record and as information for the patient as well as biofeedback for treatment

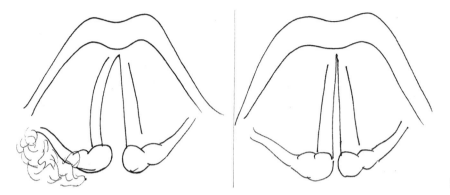

Fig. 8.1a,b **(a)** Unilateral vocal fold paralysis: incomplete glottic closure with a left vocal fold paralysis, a lateral position of the vocal fold with pooled secretions in the pyriform fossa. **(b)** Normal vocal fold position during adduction on endoscopy.

Special Investigations

Special testing may include audiology, speech pathology, and referral to other specialists.

- An audiogram should be performed routinely in any lateral skull base neoplasm, particularly when based near or at the internal auditory canal.
- Electronystagmogram (functional test vestibular function).
- Clinical swallowing assessment:
  - Bedside examination of swallowing
    - Bedside screening is highly correlated with FEES and fluoroscopic evaluation.
      - Clinical evaluation and screening tests can be done by speech pathologists or trained nurse practitioner.[29]
      - Different methodologies are described; one of the best-studied methods consists of a score from four clinical tests: a water swallow (50 mL), pharyngeal sensation, tongue movement, and voice change (91% sensitive, 93% negative predictive value).[29,30]
  - Functional endoscopic evaluation of swallowing (FEES)
    - Combination of clinical evaluation of swallowing during simultaneous endoscopic examination
    - Requires two trained clinicians, one to perform endoscopy and one to administer test bolus (more time and resource intensive than bedside clinical exam)

- Increases diagnostic sensitivity. Direct observation of pharyngeal and glottis tasks *during swallow:*
  - Observation of frank aspiration of secretions/test bolus
  - Coughing
  - Pooling of bolus material in vallecula or pyriform fossa
  - Incomplete movement of constrictor muscle (unilateral or bilateral) during swallowing
  - Dilated pyriform fossa (paresis)
  - Reduced laryngeal elevation
  - Reduced/absent posterior tongue movement
- Deglutition study
  - Fluoroscopic evaluation of swallow using different food consistencies
- Normal fluoroscopic swallow
  - Diagnostic and rehabilitative aspects to assessment
    - Recommendations to improve swallow function usually made when possible at the time of study by trained speech pathologist
  - Diagnosis of aspiration (may be "silent" without sensation, patient may not protect the airway)
- Manometry
  - Pharyngeal and upper esophageal dual-probe evaluation of intraluminal pressure during swallow
  - Determine coordination of swallow activity; muscle pressures at rest and during swallow
  - May help guide therapy, diagnosis, or surgical treatment (e.g., cricopharyngeus dysfunction)
  - Not routinely available in all hospitals

Treatment

Dysphagia

Treatment depends on the severity of the dysphagia and the patient's ability to manage secretions as well as the aspiration risk. Given the increased mortality in neurosurgical patients due to aspiration, early (within days or immediate) intervention to prevent aspiration pneumonia is strongly recommended in high-risk patients. Tumor location, preoperative swallowing, voice function, and the anticipated effects of surgical intervention should be considered in order to identify high-risk patients. For example, excision of large jugular foramen tumors (e.g., glomus jugulare) in patients who did not have preoperative compensation and are at high risk of aspiration should be managed aggressively *before* the onset of aspiration and other complications of the dysphagia. If it is judged in the immediate postoperative period (day 1 or 2) that there is a high likelihood of persistent cranial nerve injury, then a percutaneous gastric or jejunostomy feeding tube should be placed for nutrition and hydration.

- Mild dysphagia may only require a change in diet, with puréed food being tolerated in most cases.
- If a significant risk of florid aspiration is found on clinical, endoscopic, or imaging studies, patients may require nasogastric tube enteric feeds in the initial postoperative period.
- By 7 to 10 days, improvement in dysphagia can occur, with a reduction in postoperative inflammation and behavioral compensation. Clinical assessment with bedside screening evaluation is conducted by a trained nurse or a speech-language pathologist, who documents the symptoms of dysphagia or aspiration. If the patient fails the screening exam, endoscopic evaluation with FEES or a formal deglutition fluoroscopic study may be indicated.
- An oral mechanical exam is done during a bedside swallowing evaluation by a qualified speech-language pathologist and includes an assessment of labial closure (complete/incomplete), lingual range of motion, and facial symmetry. A poor functional exam result is associated with an increased risk of aspiration.

Pearl

If the patient is unable to swallow or if the aspiration risk remains high by 7 days postsurgery, a percutaneous gastric or jejunostomy feeding tube should be placed for nutrition and hydration. A gastric feeding tube is more comfortable, and removal of the nasogastric tube reduces edema in the hypopharynx as well as any gastroesophageal reflux (which is also an irritant).

Cranial nerve recovery could take up to 1 year, and central pathology can take longer to realize maximum functional improvement in swallowing and speech after neurosurgery.

Swallowing therapy with a speech-language pathologist is indicated and has been shown to help in resuming oral feeding in patients with a potential for behavioral compensation as well as neurologic recovery.

Voice

A paralyzed vocal fold is in a paramedian or more lateral position causing incomplete vocal fold closure during swallowing and contributes to aspiration. The presence of a vocal fold paralysis was found to have a 2.5 times higher change of aspiration on fluoroscopic evaluation.[28]

- The arytenoid tips anteroinferiorly with a lowering of vocal fold height, and the vocal fold will atrophy if paralysis persists. Voice quality can be very breathy and weak, with a poor cough.
- Some patients compensate well without intervention, but if they are floridly aspirating and cannot manage their secretions with multiple CN palsies, they may require surgical treatment to medialize their vocal fold, or in some cases a tracheotomy may be required (especially when patients are unable to clear pulmonary secretions).
- If a tracheotomy is required, often an enteral feeding tube is also necessary such as a percutaneous gastrostomy tube placed by an interventional radiologist or gastroenterologist.
- Treatment options for the dysphonia and less severe aspiration can be managed with temporary or permanent surgical intervention to medialize (reposition toward midline) the paralyzed vocal fold by injection augmentation or external medialization (thyroplasty).
- There are several types of materials that can be injected during a clinic procedure using endoscopic guidance transcutaneously or in the operating room under general anesthesia with a direct laryngoscopy[31] **(Table 8.7)**.

Options for Unilateral Vagal Paralysis

After skull base surgery, vagal paralysis is often persistent.[32] It is still present in 80% of cases at 1 year postsurgery, and patients with multiple cranial nerve deficits are far more likely to have more significant swallowing and voice symptoms requiring surgical rehabilitation.[22] Approximately 50% of patients with a vagal paralysis were found to experience aspiration, and half of them required a gastric tube for longer than 1 year.[22] There is some controversy about when to intervene.

- If a patient experiences significant aspiration usually accompanied by a weak and breathy voice, early intervention to medialize the paralyzed vocal fold can shorten the hospital stay and reduce the pneumonia risk.[33] There are now temporary materials that can be injected into a paralyzed vocal fold for either weeks or months, depending on the material used. This is ideal when it is anticipated that nerve function may recover. If vagal nerve recovery is not expected, then more permanent rehabilitative procedures can be performed to improve the swallowing and voice functions.
- Injection laryngoplasty, depending on material injected, can be temporary (weeks) or long term (9 to 18 months). Other procedures include medialization thyroplasty (neuroleptanalgesia, awake procedure) with insertion of a Silastic shim or Gore-Tex strip to alter the position of the paralyzed vocal fold toward the midline. This will permit improved closure against the normal vocal fold, higher subglottic air pressure to generate more effective cough,[34]

Table 8.7 Types of Injectable Products and Their Expected Duration of Effect

Material	Product	Source	Approval	Duration
Hyaluronic acid	Restylane	Streptococcus	FDA Off-label use in Canada	6–12 months
Gelatin	Radiesse Voice Gel®		FDA Health Canada	8–12 weeks
Collagen	Cymetra Cosmoplast Zyplast	Cadaveric skin Human fibroplasts Bovine	Off-label use	6–9 months 3–6 months 3–6 months
Synthetic polymer	Radiesse Voice® (calcium hydroxyapatite)	Synthetic spherical particles in sodium carboxymethylcellulose gel	FDA Health Canada approved	1–2 years

Abbreviation: FDA, Food and Drug Administration.

and reduced aspiration.[33] Some practitioners prefer to use an arytenoid adduction, which is a similar procedure, but the muscular process of the arytenoid is sutured such that the arytenoids rotate medially, and this provides an adducted position of the paralyzed vocal fold.[32,35] The goal is to surgically modify the position of the paralyzed vocal fold such that it rests in an adducted position and as close to midline as possible. This position permits the normal side to approximate to the paralyzed side during voicing and swallowing, which can dramatically improve the voice and, to varying degrees, ameliorate the choking and aspirating. The constrictor function is not improved at all with these procedures. Less commonly, a pharyngoplasty or plication of the dilated pyriform fossa is performed, along with laryngeal elevation by suspension of the hyoid bone to the mandible.[35]

- Other procedures to reduce nasal regurgitation are done occasionally, such as palatal adhesion to reduce hypernasality[36] or the fitting of an oral appliance with a palatal lift, which can be helpful in some patients.
- Cricopharyngeus or upper esophageal sphincter dysfunction can be addressed with a temporary measure (Botox injection) under local or general anesthesia. This is helpful when the deglutition study indicates that the cricopharyngeus is contributing to dysphagia and in a setting where nerve recovery is possible. Otherwise, the cricopharyngeus muscle can be excised endoscopically or externally.[36]

Pearls

The patients who are at risk of postoperative speech and voice complications are often predictable based on the tumor location, the preoperative voice and swallowing function, and the planned intervention.

- Aspiration is common in neurosurgical inpatients and often underdiagnosed.
- Aspiration pneumonia is a significant cause of morbidity and mortality and can be anticipated and to a large degree prevented by early intervention.
- A multidisciplinary approach to evaluate swallowing and voice function includes nursing, speech-language pathology, otolaryngology, respirology, and neurology.
- Bedside swallow assessment can be a useful screening tool, and further assessment using FEES or a video fluoroscopic swallowing study is often necessary to definitely evaluate swallowing function.
- Early and timely treatment for vocal fold paralysis can assist in reducing the risk of aspiration pneumonia and improving swallowing and the voice temporarily or permanently.
- Tracheotomy and a gastric or jejunostomy feeding tube may be necessary and often are required for the recovery period. In patients at high risk of aspiration, these procedures should be performed early before repeated bouts of aspiration pneumonia significantly debilitate the patient.
- Rehabilitative behavioral speech therapy for dysarthria and dysphagia is extremely helpful and should be offered to patients with those symptoms.

Tracheotomy Indications

- Airway obstruction: (1) supraglottic/laryngeal edema postintubation; (2) bilateral vocal fold paralysis; (3) large skull base tumor obstruction of the aerodigestive tract
- Pulmonary toilet: manage secretions/aspiration if severe
- Prolonged ventilator support requirement: (1) patient comfort; (2) reduce risk of glottis stenosis

■ References

Boldfaced references are of particular importance.

1. **Halmagyi GM, Cremer PD. Assessment and treatment of dizziness. J Neurol Neurosurg Psychiatry 2000;68:129–134**
2. Møller AR, Jannetta PJ. Evoked potentials from the inferior colliculus in man. Electroencephalogr Clin Neurophysiol 1982;53:612–620
3. Møller AR, Jannetta PJ. Interpretation of brainstem auditory evoked potentials: results from intracranial recordings in humans. Scand Audiol 1983;12:125–133
4. Møller AR, Jannetta PJ. Preservation of facial function during removal of acoustic neuromas. Use of monopolar constant-voltage stimulation and EMG. J Neurosurg 1984; 61:757–760
5. Møller AR, Jho HD. Responses from the brainstem at the entrance of the eighth nerve in human to contralateral stimulation. Hear Res 1988;37:47–52
6. Stockard JJ, Sharbrough FW, Tinker JA. Effects of hypothermia on the human brainstem auditory response. Ann Neurol 1978;3:368–370
7. Leggatt A. Electrophysiologic Audiotory Testing. Handbook of Clinical Neurology, Vol. 129: The Human Auditory System. 2015 Elsevier BV
8. Prass RL, Kinney SE, Lüders H. Transtragal, transtympanic electrode placement for intraoperative electrocochleographic monitoring. Otolaryngol Head Neck Surg 1987; 97:343–350
9. Silverstein H, Wazen J, Norrell H, Hyman SM. Retrolabyrinthine vestibular neurectomy with simultaneous monitoring of eighth nerve action potentials and electrocochleography. Am J Otol 1984;5:552–555
10. Krieg SM, Kempf L, Droese D, Rosahl SK, Meyer B, Lehmberg J. Superiority of tympanic ball electrodes over mastoid needle electrodes for intraoperative monitoring of hearing function. J Neurosurg 2014;120:1042–1047
11. Pou AM, Hirsch BE, Durrant JD, Gold SR, Kamerer DB. The efficacy of tympanic electrocochleography in the diagnosis of endolymphatic hydrops. Am J Otol 1996;17:607–611
12. Selesnick SH, Jackler RK, Pitts LW. The changing clinical presentation of acoustic tumors in the MRI era. Laryngoscope 1993;103(4 Pt 1):431–436
13. Higgs WA. Sudden deafness as the presenting symptom of acoustic neurinoma. Arch Otolaryngol 1973;98:73–76

14. Friedman RA, Kesser BW, Slattery WH III, Brackmann DE, Hitselberger WE. Hearing preservation in patients with vestibular schwannomas with sudden sensorineural hearing loss. Otolaryngol Head Neck Surg 2001;125:544–551

15. Kramer PD, Roberts DC, Shelhamer M, Zee DS. A versatile stereoscopic visual display system for vestibular and oculomotor research. J Vestib Res 1998;8:363–379

16. House JW, Brackmann DE. Facial nerve grading system. Otolaryngol Head Neck Surg 1985;93:146–147

17. Vrabec JT, Coker NJ. Acute paralysis of facial nerve. In: Bailey BJ, Johnson JT, Newlands SD, eds. Head and Neck Surgery–Otolaryngology, 4th ed. Philadelphia: Lippincott Williams & Wilkins; 2006:2139–2155

18. Sunderland S. A classification of peripheral nerve injuries producing loss of function. Brain 1951;74:491–516

19. Peitersen E. Bell's palsy: the spontaneous course of 2,500 peripheral facial nerve palsies of different etiologies. Acta Otolaryngol Suppl 2002;549:4–30

20. Salinas RA, Alvarez G, Daly F, Ferreira J. Corticosteroids for Bell's palsy (idiopathic facial paralysis). Cochrane Database Syst Rev 2010;3:CD001942

21. Quant EC, Jeste SS, Muni RH, Cape AV, Bhussar MK, Peleg AY. The benefits of steroids versus steroids plus antivirals for treatment of Bell's palsy: a meta-analysis. BMJ 2009;339:b3354

22. Oestreicher-Kedem Y, Agrawal S, Jackler RK, Damrose EJ. Surgical rehabilitation of voice and swallowing after jugular foramen surgery. Ann Otol Rhinol Laryngol 2010;119:192–198

23. Makek M, Franklin DJ, Zhao JC, Fisch U. Neural infiltration of glomus temporale tumors. Am J Otol 1990;11:1–5

24. Wilson-Pauwels L, Akeeson EJ, Stewart PA. Cranial Nerves: Anatomy and Clinical Comments. Hamilton, Ontario: Decker; 1998

25. Peterson KL, Fenn J. Treatment of dysphagia and dysphonia following skull base surgery. Otolaryngol Clin North Am 2005;38:809–817, xi xi.

26. Splaingard ML, Hutchins B, Sulton LD, Chaudhuri G. Aspiration in rehabilitation patients: videofluoroscopy vs bedside clinical assessment. Arch Phys Med Rehabil 1988;69:637–640

27. Smith Hammond CA, Goldstein LB. Cough and aspiration of food and liquids due to oral-pharyngeal dysphagia: ACCP evidence-based clinical practice guidelines. Chest 2006;129(1, Suppl):154S–168S

28. Leder SB, Suiter DM, Warner HL, Acton LM, Siegel MD. Safe initiation of oral diets in hospitalized patients based on passing a 3-ounce (90 cc) water swallow challenge protocol. QJM 2012;105:257–263

29. Martino R, Silver F, Teasell R, et al. The Toronto Bedside Swallowing Screening Test (TOR-BSST): development and validation of a dysphagia screening tool for patients with stroke. Stroke 2009;40:555–561

30. Bours GJ, Speyer R, Lemmens J, Limburg M, de Wit R. Bedside screening tests vs. videofluoroscopy or fibreoptic endoscopic evaluation of swallowing to detect dysphagia in patients with neurological disorders: systematic review. J Adv Nurs 2009;65:477–493

31. Sulica L, Rosen CA, Postma GN, et al. Current practice in injection augmentation of the vocal folds: indications, treatment principles, techniques, and complications. Laryngoscope 2010;120:319–325

32. Bielamowicz S, Gupta A, Sekhar LN. Early arytenoid adduction for vagal paralysis after skull base surgery. Laryngoscope 2000;110(3 Pt 1):346–351

33. Bhattacharyya N, Batirel H, Swanson SJ. Improved outcomes with early vocal fold medialization for vocal fold paralysis after thoracic surgery. Auris Nasus Larynx 2003; 30:71–75

34. Andersons JA. Voice Function After Thyroplasty in Unilateral Vocal Fold Paralysis. Toronto, ON, Canada: University of Toronto Press; 1999

35. Cheesman AD, Kelly AM. Rehabilitation after treatment for jugular foramen lesions. Skull Base 2009;19:99–108

36. Netterville JL, Jackson CG, Civantos F. Thyroplasty in the functional rehabilitation of neurotologic skull base surgery patients. Am J Otol 1993;14:460–464

■ Online Resources

An example of an Halmagyi Head Thrust Test: https://m.youtube.com/watch?v= CZXDNLLGG8k.

The Dix-Hallpike Position Test: http://www.youtube.com/watch?v=kEM9p4EX1jk.

Geotropic torsional nystagmus: http://www.youtube.com/watch?v=LUjPwbh9vOI.

An example of articulation, rate of speech during history, note imprecision, and slurring: http://www.youtube.com/watch?v=_7ZzmvavjQs&list=PLwPVTRO-4EcweD8 -AoclZrCII-Xz5CQZq&index=9.

An example of an endoscopy: http://www.youtube.com/embed/HYFrs80ZU-0?autoplay=1.

Examples of normal fluoroscopic swallow: http://www.youtube.com/embed/PwVreNr TKBw?autoplay=1 and http://www.youtube.com/embed/1sFNMk87558?autoplay=1.

9 Endocrinology

Skull-based endocrinology focuses on the management of pituitary/hypothalamic disruption by sellar and suprasellar lesions. There is a broad differential for lesions in the sellar and suprasellar areas (see Chapter 21, **Table 21.1** on page 498).

The mnemonic CAM-LIGHTS can be used to remember these lesions: **C**yst, **c**raniopharyngioma, **c**hordoma, **c**arcinoma, **A**denoma, **a**bscess, **a**rteriovenous fistulas, **M**eningioma, **m**etastasis, **L**ymphoma, **I**nfiltrative, **G**erm cell tumor, **H**ypophysitis, **H**istiocytosis X, **T**uberculosis, **S**arcoidosis.

- All lesions can present with symptoms and signs of mass effect: headache, decreased visual acuity, relative afferent pupillary defect, bitemporal hemianopsia, pale optic disk, diplopia, ptosis, and facial numbness.

■ Functional and Nonfunctional Pituitary Adenomas and Other Sellar Lesions

Prolactinoma

A lactotroph tumor of the anterior lobe of the pituitary produces prolactin, resulting in the clinical presentation of galactorrhea, infertility, and oligo- or amenorrhea in women.

- The majority of prolactinomas are larger in men than in women.[1]
- Men usually present later than women, and present with symptoms related to mass effect, such as headache and visual field defects.
- Men may also present with symptoms of hypogonadotropic hypogonadism, such as infertility, decreased libido, and erectile dysfunction. Men may also present with symptoms of hypopituitarism.[2]

Epidemiology

Prolactinoma accounts for approximately 40% of all pituitary tumors, with a prevalence variously noted to be 6 to 10 per 100,000 or 50 per 100,000.[3,4]

Pathophysiology

- Monoclonal expansion of a single cell that has likely undergone somatic mutation.
- Pituitary tumor transforming gene (PTTG) is overexpressed,[5] but it is expressed at higher levels in other pituitary tumors.[6]
- Familial and genetic considerations:
  - Multiple endocrine neoplasia-1 (MEN1): mutation in the *MEN1* gene, 40% of cases have a pituitary adenoma, most commonly a prolactinoma (other clinical manifestations include parathyroid adenomas, pancreatic islet cell/gastrointestinal adenomas)
  - Carney's complex: mutation in the *PRKAR1A* gene; presents with lentigines, myxomas, Schwann cell tumors, adrenal hyperplasia, and pituitary abnormalities (frequent hypersecretion of prolactin)
  - Familial isolated pituitary adenomas: 15% have mutations in the aryl hydrocarbon receptor-interacting protein *(AIP)* gene, 40% are prolactinomas[7]

Differential Diagnosis

Rule out other causes of elevated prolactin **(Table 9.1)**.

Table 9.1   Causes of Hyperprolactinemia[8, 9]

Physiological causes	Pregnancy, lactation, stress, coitus, sleep, exercise, mammary stimulation
Pathological sellar causes	Pituitary: prolactinoma, pituitary adenomas with mixed secretion of prolactin/growth hormone, surgery, trauma, hypophysitis Pituitary stalk damage: nonpituitary tumors (craniopharyngioma, germinoma, metastasis, meningioma), pituitary tumors other than prolactinoma, Rathke's cyst, granulomas, infiltrative lesions, cranial irradiation
Pharmacological causes	Antipsychotics especially neuroleptics, clomipramine, desipramine, amitriptyline, fluoxetine, metoclopramide, cimetidine, ranitidine, methyldopa, verapamil, labetalol, phenytoin, codeine, morphine, estrogens, protease inhibitors
Other	Primary hypothyroidism, chest wall injury, chronic renal failure, cirrhosis, epileptic seizures, polycystic ovarian syndrome, idiopathic hyperprolactinemia, macroprolactinemia, genetic

Diagnosis

- Measure prolactin level and request magnetic resonance imaging (MRI) of the sella.
- Levels generally correlate with tumor size; prolactin is usually > 200–250 μg/L (> 200–250 ng/mL) in macroprolactinomas.
- Rule out other causes of hyperprolactinemia **(Table 9.1)**.
- Macroprolactinemia:
  - Most prolactin is monomeric.
  - Macroprolactinemia occurs when there is a preponderance of a covalently bound polymeric form of inactive prolactin, which remains reactive to varying degrees in prolactin immunoassays.[10]
  - Normal biological activity; be suspicious when typical symptoms are absent.
  - Order a macroprolactin level when investigating asymptomatic hyperprolactinemia.
- Hook effect: assay artifact where a very high prolactin level saturates both the capture and signal antibodies, resulting in artifactually low prolactin results.[11,12] If the Hook effect is suspected, the assay should be repeated after a serial serum sample dilution.

Medical Treatment

- Dopamine agonists
  - Bromocriptine: Starting adult dose is 1.25 to 2.5 mg every night at bedtime, which can be increased by 2.5 mg as tolerated every 2 to 7 days until an optimal response is obtained. Maximum dose is 15 mg per day. Side effects include dizziness, headache, fatigue, nausea, and rhinitis.
  - Cabergoline: Starting adult dose is 0.5 mg weekly or 0.25 mg twice a week, which can be increased by 0.5 mg every 4 weeks until an optimal response is obtained. Maximum dose is 2 mg per week. Higher doses have been used off-label in studies. Side effects include headache, dizziness, and nausea.
  - Quinagolide: Starting adult dose is 0.025 mg per day for 3 days followed by 0.05 mg per day for 3 days, and then 0.075 mg per day. Further titration can be done at monthly intervals. The maximum dose is 0.9 mg per day. Side effects include dizziness, fatigue, headache, nausea, and vomiting.
  - Treat patients who are symptomatic to restore gonadal function, decrease prolactin levels, and decrease tumor size.[8]
  - First-line treatment is a dopamine agonist; cabergoline is more effective and better tolerated than bromocriptine.[13]
- In a placebo-controlled study, cabergoline in microprolactinomas, idiopathic hyperprolactinemia and empty sella resulted in normalization of prolactin in 95% of patients on 1 mg twice a week. Menses was restored in 82% of women with amenorrhea.[14]

- In a prospective study with macroprolactinomas, normal prolactin levels were achieved within 6 months in 81% of patients receiving cabergoline, and 92% had significant tumor shrinkage.[15]
- Visual fields normalized in 33% of patients and improved in 56% of patients in one series.[16]
- Results are similar to the impact of surgery on visual fields for giant non-functional tumors in another series[17]; of those who had visual field defects preoperatively, after surgery, 8.6% remained blind, 28% regained normal sight, and 67% had variable improvement.
- If the patient is symptomatic and does not achieve normalization of prolactin level or tumor shrinkage, increase the medical therapy to the maximum tolerated doses prior to considering surgery. Maximum dose for cabergoline is 2 mg/week. Higher doses have been used off-label in studies. Monitor with two-dimensional (2D) echocardiogram for valvular regurgitation if on high-dose cabergoline (> 2 mg a week).[8]
- A cerebrospinal fluid (CSF) leak can occur if a defect is revealed in the sellar floor after tumor shrinkage with a dopamine agonist.

Withdrawal of dopamine agonist therapy:

- Can consider withdrawal of therapy in patients who have been treated with a dopamine agonist for 2 years who no longer have an elevated prolactin and who have had significant tumor reduction as demonstrated on MRI.[8,18]
- Factors predicting remission:
  - Nadir prolactin level during treatment ≤ 5.4 µg/L (≤ 5.4 ng/mL) and nadir maximal tumor diameter ≤ 3.1 mm[19]
  - Size of tumor remnant prior to withdrawal of therapy: 18% increased recurrence risk for each millimeter[20]
  - Normalization of MRI and longer duration of treatment[21]
- Rates of recurrence after withdrawal[18,19,22–24]:
  - Idiopathic hyperprolactinemia 24–68%
  - Microadenomas 31–79%
  - Macroadenomas 36–93%
- Hyperprolactinemia is most likely to recur within the first year after withdrawal of dopamine agonists.[20,24]
- Follow prolactin every 3 months for 1 year, then annually; order an MRI if prolactin increases above the normal range.[8]
- Ongoing surveillance for increase in size of tumor is needed.

Other medical treatment options:

  - Can also consider an oral contraceptive pill in pre-menopausal women with amenorrhea and microprolactinoma.
  - In a small study, no significant change in size of microadenomas was found after 2 years on an oral contraceptive pill.[25]

Growth Hormone–Producing Tumor (Acromegaly)

Growth hormone–producing tumor is a somatotroph cell adenoma producing classic physical features of acromegaly (gigantism in children). It is characterized by:

- Enlargement of facial features (74%) and hands and feet in adults (86%)
- Other features[26,27] include cardiac disease (60%), excess perspiration (48%), arthralgia (46%), headache (40%), hypertension (39%), diabetes mellitus (38%), hypogonadism (38%), fatigue (26%), visual defect (26%), obstructive sleep apnea (13–50%), carpal tunnel syndrome (9%), colonic polyps (1.2% colonic cancer), multinodular goiter, benign prostatic hypertrophy, osteopenia, renal stones
  - There is early cardiovascular mortality if growth hormone (GH) excess is untreated (34% die due to cardiovascular disease).
  - Over 70% of tumors are macroadenomas at presentation.[27]

Epidemiology

The incidence is 3 cases/million persons/year; the prevalence is 60/million.[28]

Pathophysiology

Benign monoclonal: multiple genetic mutations have been associated with GH-producing adenomas, including Gs-α stimulating mutations, growth arrest and DNA damage-inducible (GADD) loss of function mutations, PTTG protein.[27]

Differential Diagnosis

- Rarely due to somatotroph hyperplasia, GH, or GH-releasing hormone (GHRH) production from an ectopic tumor. More primitive cell origin (mammosomatotroph) may co-secrete prolactin.
- Can have plurihormonal adenoma and GH-cell carcinoma.
- Genetic syndromes:
  - MEN1 (see above)
  - Familial isolated pituitary adenomas (FIPA): 30 to 50% have AIP aryl hydrocarbon–interacting protein gene (*AIP*) mutation[29]
  - McCune-Albright syndrome: somatotroph hyperplasia due to Gs-alpha mutation in GHRH receptor; patients also have café-au-lait lesions, osteodystrophy, and other endocrine hyperfunctioning states (e.g., premature menarche, hyperthyroidism, adrenal Cushing's)
  - Carney's syndrome (see above)

Table 9.2   Common conditions resulting in False-Positive and False Negative Testing in the Diagnosis of Acromegaly[31]

Conditions increasing IGF-1 levels
Pregnancy*
Thyrotoxicosis*
Glucocorticoids
Conditions decreasing IGF-1 levels
Estrogen therapy*
Hypothyroidism
Fasting*
Obesity
Poorly controlled diabetes*
Liver* and renal disease*

*Also causes increased and insuppressible GH levels.

Diagnosis

- Screening test: elevated insulin-like growth factor-1 (IGF-1).
- Confirm with 2-hour 75-g oral glucose suppression test; GH remains > 1 μg/L.[30]
- Consider causes of false positives and false negatives if lab testing does not correlate with clinical findings[31] **(Table 9.2)**.

Medical Treatment

- Consider medical therapy with a somatostatin analogue:
  - If patient is a poor surgical candidate due to high surgical risk from co-existing medical disorders.
  - If there is an invasive macroadenoma with no mass effect and low likelihood of surgical cure.[30]
  - If patient is not cured by surgery, patients are more likely to respond if the tumor is densely granulated in the histopathological examination.[32]
  - Preoperative treatment with a somatostatin analogue in macroadenomas may increase surgical remission rates[33–37]; however, further studies are needed, so pretreatment is not routinely recommended unless surgery is delayed.
- Other medical treatment options include dopamine agonists and growth hormone receptor antagonists (see **Table 9.3** for details about medical therapy for acromegaly).
- All patients should be screened for coexisting complications from acromegaly (with 2D echocardiogram, colonoscopy, hemoglobin A_{1c}, fasting glucose

Table 9.3   Medical Management of Acromegaly

Drug and Indication	Starting Adult Dose	Maximum Dose	Effectiveness	Side Effects	Cost*
SSA Octreotide LAR Lanreotide —Not surgically cured	20 mg IM every 4 weeks	40 mg IM every 4 weeks	↓ IGF-1 50–70% ↓ Tumor size in 30–50% of patients Improvement in LVH, BPH, sleep apnea	GI cramps, diarrhea (usually temporary) Gallstone "sludge" Hyperglycemia	20 mg/month = $25,000/year
Dopamine agonist – Cabergoline –Co-prolactin-secreting tumors –Patients with mild-moderate ↑ IGF-1 (25–50% above ULN) –In combination with SSA if partial response to SSA	1–2 mg po weekly in divided doses		↓ IGF-1 < 300 in 35% of patients	Nausea Dizziness Headache	2 mg/wk = $5,000/year
GH antagonist pegvisomant –Failure of surgery and other medical options	Load with 40 mg SC, then 10 mg SC daily, Check IGF-1 every 4-6 weeks, then increase then by 5 mg increments until IGF-1 normalized or at 30 mg daily	10–30 mg SC daily	Reduce-normalize IGF-1 levels in > 90% patients Does not suppress GH or tumor growth	↑ AST in 20% Check every month for 6 months, then every 6 months	20 mg/day = $80,000/year

Abbreviations: AST, aspartate aminotransferase; BPH, benign prostatic hypertrophy; GH, growth hormone; GI, gastrointestinal; IM, intramuscularly; LAR, long-acting release; LVH, left ventricular hypertrophy; SC, subcutaneous; SSA, somatostatin analogue; ULN, upper limits of normal.

* In North America, updated to 2014.

and lipids, prostate-specific antigen [PSA], bone mineral density [BMD], consider thyroid ultrasound, consider sleep study, plasma calcium level).

Adrenocorticotropic Hormone (ACTH)-Producing Tumor (Cushing's disease)

Cushing's disease is the result of a corticotroph adenoma overproducing ACTH. The classic features include the following[38]:

- Central weight gain (95%), supraclavicular and dorsal fat pads, moon facies (90%), thin skin (85%), menstrual irregularities (80%), hypertension (75%), psychosis and depression (75%), bruising (65%), proximal muscle weakness (60%), glucose intolerance (60%), osteopenia or fractures (50%), violaceous striae, acne, hirsutism, male-pattern alopecia, hypokalemia, increased thromboembolic events
- Early mortality if cortisol excess remains untreated

Epidemiology

The incidence of Cushing's disease is 1.2 to 1.7 cases/million/year.[39]

Pathophysiology

Pathophysiological findings include monoclonal expansion of corticotroph cells, usually microadenoma (80–85%), rarely hyperplasia, rarely familial (MEN1 is more typically a GH- or prolactin-producing tumor). Most tumors are densely granulated, basophilic, and often arise in the central part of the pituitary, due to the abundance of corticotrophs in that location.

Differential Diagnosis

- Exogenous steroids must be ruled out first.
- ACTH-dependent: pituitary adenoma or ectopic ACTH-producing tumor.
- ACTH-independent: adrenal adenoma, carcinoma, or hyperplasia.
- Pseudo-Cushing's: caused by depression, severe stress, chronic alcoholism, or central obesity.

Diagnosis in Three Steps[40]

1. Demonstrate abnormal excess from the hypothalamic-pituitary-adrenal (HPA) axis: at least two of the following should be abnormal:

- Lack of suppression of HPA axis by low-dose dexamethasone suppression test (DST)
  - 1 mg overnight DST: dexamethasone is taken between 11 PM and midnight, or
  - 2 day low-dose DST (0.5 mg every 6 hours for 48 hours)

  Either test is abnormal if the 8 AM cortisol is > 50 nmol/L after the last dose of dexamethasone.
- Overproduction of cortisol: elevated 24-hour urine for free cortisol (three- to fourfold elevation is very specific).
- Lack of diurnal variation of cortisol: elevated midnight salivary levels (cut point is assay-dependent).

Dexamethasone–corticotropin-releasing hormone (CRH) stimulation test can be done if the above results are inconclusive, especially if pseudo-Cushing's is suspected.

2. Measure ACTH to check for ACTH dependence (should be > 4 pmol/L in ACTH-dependent Cushing's).
3. With unsuppressed ACTH, decide if ACTH source is pituitary or ectopic (85–95% will be pituitary):
   - MRI sella: tumor size > 6 mm is suggestive of pituitary etiology[41,42] (also image the thorax/abdomen if ectopic source is suspected).
   - Inferior petrosal sinus sampling (IPSS) to confirm pituitary source of ACTH (stimulated by CRH or deamino-8-D-arginine vasopressin [DDAVP] 10 µg IV), sample blood from the left and right sinuses and central vein for plasma ACTH at baseline and 0, 2, 5, 10, and 15 minutes after CRH or DDAVP given.
     - In Cushing's disease, expect central/peripheral gradient ratio > 2:1 (with no CRH or DDAVP) and > 3:1 (stimulated with CRH or DDAVP).[42]
     - Lateralization with > 1.5:1 gradient between petrosal sinuses.
     - Conflicting studies:
       - More accurate lateralization with IPSS than with MRI (70% vs 49%, $p < 0.06$).[43]
       - When conventional MRI is negative or nondiagnostic, central venous sampling (CVS; cavernous and petrosal) is not as accurate in tumor localization as dynamic MRI (90% vs 52–65% with IPSS).[44]

The following testing is generally less helpful:

- High-dose DST (8 mg dexamethasone at midnight, followed by 8 AM plasma cortisol level) is less helpful because:
  - There is considerable overlap between the two populations (pituitary vs ectopic).[45]
  - There are different published cutoffs for the 8 AM plasma cortisol for the diagnosis of pituitary source (< 140 nmol/L, versus > 50% suppression, versus > 70% suppression from baseline 8 AM cortisol).

- Corticotropin-releasing hormone stimulation of ACTH and cortisol (ACTH should increase by > 50% 45 minutes after CRH in Cushing's disease).[46]
- Caveats for testing:
  - Pseudo-Cushing's: depression/alcoholism/severe stress/severe obesity.
  - False elevation in cortisol: increased cortisol-binding globulin (CBG) due to exogenous estrogen, pregnancy, hepatitis.
  - False-positive DST: drugs that alter dexamethasone metabolism such as phenobarbital, carbamazepine, and others.[40]
  - Incidental pituitary or adrenal masses can be "decoys" and not represent the actual ACTH-producing tumor.
  - Adrenal hyperplasia can be ACTH dependent or independent.

Medical Treatment

- Consider medical therapy if patient is a poor surgical candidate.
- Ketoconazole: A small retrospective study suggests that adequate presurgical treatment with ketoconazole or metyrapone in Cushing's disease may be associated with suppressed postoperative cortisol concentrations and an increased long-term remission rate[47]; however, further prospective studies are needed.
- Pasireotide somatostatin analogue (SSA) inhibits ACTH secretion via somatostatin type 5 receptor subset[48]; it normalizes urine free cortisol in 25% of patients. Side effect: hyperglycemia.

> It is critical to rule out hyperfunction due to overproduction of prolactin, growth hormone, or ACTH before surgery, as it can influence the choice of therapy, the preparation for surgery, and the need for hormonal coverage after surgery.

Nonfunctional Sellar Masses

Nonfunctional pituitary masses (adenomas and other pathologies) can present incidentally on imaging, with mass effect, hypopituitarism, or hyperprolactinemia due to stalk compression.

Pituitary Dysfunction in Extra-Adenoma Pathologies

These pathologies include cysts (e.g., Rathke's cleft cyst), craniopharyngiomas, parasellar tumors, and sellar metastases.

- Hypothalamic masses such as craniopharyngiomas are more likely to present with diabetes insipidus (DI), along with other tertiary hormone defects.

- Lymphocytic hypophysitis is more likely to present with headaches and secondary adrenal insufficiency.
- Presentations with CNs III, IV, V_1, V_2, and VI palsies are more likely secondary to pituitary apoplexy or other non-adenoma pathology (e.g., meningioma, lymphoma, or metastases).

> Hormonal hypofunction must be identified and treated preoperatively for all sellar and parasellar lesions (secretory or nonsecretory), especially hypocortisolism, hypothyroidism, and antidiuretic hormone (ADH) deficiency.

Aggressive Pituitary Adenomas

Aggressive pituitary adenomas are defined from a clinical perspective. They have an aggressive clinical behavior, recur early and frequently, and resist conventional treatment, including radiotherapy.[49]

- Approximately 25 to 55% of pituitary adenomas are invasive,[50-52] showing invasion of the surrounding structures, but the real percentage of aggressive pituitary adenomas is unknown.
- Suprasellar extension is not a criterion of invasiveness. Invasion refers to the bone erosion-invasion (Hardy grades III and IV; see Chapter 21, **Fig. 21.4**, on page 500), cavernous sinus invasion (Knosp grades 3 and 4; see **Fig. 21.5**, on page 501), or invasion of the sphenoid sinus (also shown in histopathology by the invasion of the sinus mucosa).
- Aggressive pituitary adenomas are nonmetastatic, but can share common histological features with pituitary carcinomas.[49]
- Typically they show atypical histological features, such as high mitotic activity, Ki-67 ≥ 3%, or extensive p53 immunopositivity.[53]
- Some histotypes of pituitary adenomas have been associated with a higher incidence of clinical aggressiveness. Some pituitary adenoma subtypes associated with clinical aggressiveness include:
  - Corticotroph tumors containing Crooke cells (cells that undergo massive accumulation of perinuclear cytokeratin in the presence of excess glucocorticoid); 60% of patients with Crooke cell tumors had recurrences at > 1 year follow-up (multiple recurrences in 24%). Average time to recurrence: 3.6 years.[54]
  - Silent corticotroph adenomas: tumors morphologically similar to ACTH-adenomas, but with no clinical or biochemical evidence of hormone excess.[55] Silent corticotroph adenomas, especially the subtype 3,[56] have been associated with clinical aggressiveness, although this correlation is controversial.[57]

○ Acidophil stem cell adenomas: rapidly growing plurihormonal adenoma, undifferentiated with focal immunopositivity to GH and prolactin (PRL).
• Patients affected by aggressive pituitary adenomas should undergo strict biochemical and radiological follow-up and multimodal treatment, including surgery, radiotherapy/radiosurgery, and/or chemotherapy (temozolomide).[49]

Nelson's Syndrome

• Aggressive corticotroph tumor growth after bilateral adrenalectomy for Cushing's disease presumably due to lack of feedback inhibition after adrenals are resected.
• Occurs after bilateral adrenalectomy in approximately 8 to 43% of patients[58]; 21% of patients in a recent systematic review.[59] There is a higher incidence among children.
• A small study suggests that stereotactic radiosurgery of pituitary tumors before bilateral adrenalectomy may decrease the incidence of Nelson's syndrome.[60]

Diagnosis

• Hyperpigmentation, mass effect from tumor.
• Check ACTH at 8 AM prior to steroid dose:
  ○ High ACTH levels (> 110 pmol/L) in addition to progressive elevation of ACTH on three occasions is diagnostic.[58]
• MRI of the sella (3 months postadrenalectomy, then every 6 months for 2 years, then yearly or if clinically indicated).[58]

Management of Nelson's Syndrome

• Surgery is first-line.
• Adjuvant radiotherapy: consider in patients with remnant tumor after transsphenoidal surgery.
• Stereotactic radiotherapy: data are limited and conflicting, with one study showing remission in 14%,[61] whereas another study showed no tumor regrowth at 7 years post–stereotactic radiosurgery.[62]
• Medical therapy (limited options):
  ○ Dopamine agonists: cabergoline can induce remission of Nelson's syndrome and tumor shrinkage.[63-65]
  ○ Selective somatostatin analogue: case report using pasireotide long-acting release (LAR) resulted in a significant decrease in ACTH level and reduction in tumor size.[66]
  ○ Temozolomide: alkylating agent may be effective, but more studies are needed.[67]

Pituitary Carcinoma

Epidemiology

Pituitary carcinoma accounts for 0.1% to 0.2% of pituitary tumors, defined as a pituitary tumor with craniospinal or systemic metastases.[68]

- Poor prognosis: 66% mortality in the first year of diagnosis.[69]
- Many pathological features overlap with atypical pituitary tumors.
- Prolactin-secreting pituitary carcinoma, corticotroph pituitary carcinomas, and growth hormone secreting carcinomas can occur.[70]
- There have been few reports of gonadotroph carcinomas, and thyroid-stimulating hormone (TSH)-secreting pituitary carcinomas are the most uncommon subtype.[71-73]
- Often, the clinical presentation is similar to that of adenomas, but pituitary carcinoma may be unresponsive to standard therapies and may recur quickly.
- 38.7% have systemic metastases, 45.2% craniospinal metastases, 16.1% have both.[74]
- Metastatic pituitary carcinoma from breast/lung primary accounts for 1% of all pituitary cancers.

Pathophysiology

Molecular mechanisms for progression from adenoma to carcinoma remain unclear.

- Molecular markers for an aggressive tumor: current markers have limitations
  - Ki-67 > 3% used to denote atypical pituitary tumor by World Health Organization (WHO) criteria,[53] but not all studies have demonstrated a difference in Ki-67 between pituitary carcinomas and other categories of adenomas.
  - p53 immunoreactivity correlates with pituitary tumor invasiveness.[75]

Treatment

- Surgery
- Radiation to prevent regrowth in partially resected tumors
- Medical therapy:
  - Control biochemical secretion: similar treatment to pituitary adenomas
  - Chemotherapy: data limited as there are no randomized studies
  - Most commonly reported agents used: cyclo-hexyl-chloroethyl-nitrosourea (CCNU; lomustine) and 5-fluorouracil until recently[70]
  - Current first-line therapy: temozolomide, with favorable response in 11 of 16 (69%) patients[76]

■ Special Situations

Pregnancy

In pregnancy, a normal pituitary increases by 30% in volume and 2.6 mm in height, due to hyperplasia of lactotrophs.[77]

- For intrasellar prolactinomas, usually stop dopamine agonist at conception.
- Risk of growth of prolactinoma in pregnant women:
  - ○ Microadenoma: 0 to 1.3%
  - ○ Macroadenoma: 10 to 25%; after surgery 3%[78]
- Macroprolactinomas that extend into the suprasellar region are treated with bromocriptine (or cabergoline) throughout pregnancy.[78]
- There are challenges to diagnose pituitary hyperfunction during pregnancy (prolactin, GH, or ACTH overproduction) due to normal physiological changes.
- New diagnoses of Cushing's are usually adrenal in origin in pregnancy.[79]
- It is challenging to assess for adrenal insufficiency (the morning cortisol in the third trimester rises to double the level—420 vs 980 nmol/L—in healthy women).
- For patients with hypofunction of the pituitary, the dose of L-thyroxine is typically increased by 30% in the first trimester, and the dose of hydrocortisone may need to increase slightly in the third trimester, to adjust for the normal physiological changes in each axis during pregnancy.
- One can try a dopamine agonist to reduce the size of normal lactotrophs and to reduce chiasmal compression when the combined mass of hyperplastic pituitary and tumor compromises the optic chiasm.
- Placental vasopressinase in third trimester can precipitate borderline diabetes insipidus.

Indications for Surgery

Surgical Indications for Mass Effect

- Visual compromise (decreased acuity or visual field defects), diplopia, headaches, or facial numbness in V_1 or V_2 distribution are indications for surgery.
- Prolactinomas usually respond to medical therapy with dopamine agonists even when there is significant mass effect.[80–82]
- Management of pituitary apoplexy is urgent surgery when there is visual compromise. Diplopia and headache may resolve spontaneously without surgical intervention.[83] See also Chapter 35, page 859.

Surgical Indications for Hyperfunction

Prolactinomas

- Medical treatment is first line (as above).
- Surgery is appropriate in symptomatic patients who cannot tolerate high doses of dopamine agonists or in those who do not respond to dopamine agonists.[8]

Acromegaly

- Surgery is the first-line therapy for all patients with surgically curable adenomas and for those with macroadenomas giving rise to mass effect.[30]
- Can consider surgery in those with macroadenomas without mass effect and a low likelihood of surgical cure to improve response to medical treatment.[30]

Cushing's Disease

- Surgery is first-line therapy for most patients, even in macroadenomas or invasive adenomas.[84]

Surgery and Pituitary Hypofunction

- Hypofunction may improve after surgery.
  - Improvement may be due to the restoration of normal hypothalamic-pituitary portal circulation and decrease in pituitary stalk compression.[85]
  - If there has been ischemic necrosis or destruction of the gland by tumor, then improvement in hormonal function is unlikely.
- 46 to 65% of patients had recovery of between one to three hormonal axes after surgery[17,86,87] **(Table 9.4)**.
- In one study of 234 patients,[87] 40% had preoperative hormonal deficit. Postoperatively, 22% had a new hormonal deficit (3–4% in other studies), and of those with preoperative hormonal deficit, 45 (48%) recovered from one to three deficiencies.
- A more recent meta-analysis found fewer than one third of patients with hormonal deficiencies recovered after transsphenoidal surgery.[88]

Preoperative Considerations

Baseline Tests for Hyper/Hypofunction

- Prolactin: need serial dilutions to rule out hook effect if it is a macroadenoma.
- TSH, free thyroxine (T_4)

Table 9.4   Percentage of Patients (of the Total) with Hormonal Deficiencies Pre- and Postoperatively

Study	↓ FSH + LH		↓ TSH		↓ ACTH	
	Preop	Postop	Preop	Postop	Preop	Postop
Marazuela et al[17]	70%	50%	23%	20%	20%	10%
Webb et al[87]	96%	30%	81%	34%	62%	38%

Abbreviations: ACTH, adrenocorticotropic hormone; FSH, follicle-stimulating hormone; LH, luteinizing hormone; TSH, thyroid-stimulating hormone.

- 8 AM cortisol, ACTH
  - Recall: False elevation in cortisol from increased cortisol-binding globulin due to estrogen (e.g., pregnancy, exogenous estrogen), hepatitis.
  - If suspect Cushing's disease, order a 24-hour urine for urinary free cortisol and/or 1 mg overnight DST and/or midnight salivary cortisol.
- Luteinizing hormone (LH), follicle-stimulating hormone (FSH), estradiol, or total and bioavailable testosterone.
- Growth hormone, IGF-1.
- Usual order of loss of function of pituitary hormones with a compressive lesion: GH > LH/FSH > TSH > ACTH > PRL (use the mnemonic *Go Look For The Adenoma Please*).

For patients with acromegaly or Cushing's disease: assess for metabolic decompensation (secondary diabetes mellitus, hypertension) and for cardiac dysfunction.

Who Gets Perioperative Glucocorticoid (GC) Coverage?

- No need for routine coverage for all patients, although some centers still cover all pituitary surgeries.
- Different centers have suggested different cutoffs for the use of basal (8 AM) cortisol to predict the need for intraoperative steroid coverage, and some centers do preoperative ACTH stimulation testing or insulin tolerance testing (ITT) (**Table 9.5**).

Recommendations for Glucocorticoid Coverage for Patients Not Already on It[94,99]

- If 8 AM preoperative basal cortisol > 220 nmol/L:
  - No perioperative GC coverage needed.

Table 9.5   Summary of Literature Examining Preoperative Basal Cortisol Levels Predicting Need for Perioperative Glucocorticoid (GC) Coverage

Preoperative Basal Cortisol Cutoff for No GC Coverage	Assessment Basis
> 400 nmol/L	ITT[89]
> 500 nmol/L	ITT[90]
> 215 nmol/L	ITT or metyrapone[91]
Normal stimulation: no coverage	ACTH stimulation[92]
> 450 nmol/L → no coverage 100–450 nmol/L → ITT to stratify < 100 nmol/L → coverage	ITT[23] or basal cortisol
> 500 nmol/L → no coverage 165–500 nmol/L → ITT to stratify < 165 nmol/L → coverage	ITT[93] or basal cortisol
≥ 224 nmol/L → no coverage < 223 nmol/L → coverage	Basal cortisol alone Intra- and postoperative observation[94]
> 350 nmol/L → no coverage 101–349 → ITT to stratify < 100 nmol/L → coverage	ITT[95] or basal cortisol
> 250 nmol/L → no coverage	Basal cortisol alone Intra- and postoperative observation[96]

Abbreviation: ITT, insulin tolerance testing.

- If 8 AM cortisol < 220 nmol/L:
  - Hydrocortisone 50 mg IV on call to the operating room, then every 8 hours on the day of surgery, followed by hydrocortisone per os 15 mg AM and 10 mg at 4 PM postoperative day 2 and 3, then baseline hydrocortisone dose.
  - Baseline hydrocortisone dose: In the past, a total dose of 20 to 30 mg daily baseline hydrocortisone was used; now, lower doses are used, e.g., hydrocortisone 10 mg per os in the morning and 5 mg daily at noon to 4 PM.[97]
- No GC coverage is needed for Cushing's disease patients, but need to watch closely for hypoadrenalism postoperatively if not covered (see below).
- These cutoff values do not apply to pregnant patients.

Postoperative Considerations

- Hormonal deficiencies:
  - The main concerns postoperatively in hospital are cortisol deficiency and water disturbances (diabetes insipidus, early and delayed hyponatremia).

- Cortisol deficiency:
  - There is a high risk if it was an extensive surgery or if there are multiple hormone deficiencies including a low prolactin level.
- Assessing for post-operative cortisol deficiency in patients not on perioperative glucocorticoid replacement:
  - Check 8 AM plasma cortisol daily on postoperative days 1 to 3 in addition to daily clinical assessments.
- Assessing for post-operative cortisol deficiency in patients requiring perioperative glucocorticoid replacement:
  - Check 8 AM plasma cortisol at least 24 hours after last dose of hydrocortisone (between days 3 and 5), to assess for recovery of HPA axis.[92]

Recommendations

There is controversy about the right postoperative approach to cortisol deficiency. It is reasonable to do the following[92,97–103] **(Table 9.6)**:

- Insulin tolerance testing (ITT) is the gold standard: 4 weeks after surgery (range of recommended timing of ITT from 5 to 8 days[99] to 1 to 3 months).[100]
- Can consider ACTH 250 μg stimulation test 4 months after surgery; the risk of secondary hypoadrenalism is very low (1.5%) when 30-minute post-ACTH cortisol is > 510 nmol/L.[101]
  - Note: patients on GC will need sick-day counseling.
  - Note: treatment of cortisol deficiency can unmask DI, because of the reversal of the reduced renal free water clearance seen with adrenal insufficiency.

Antidiuretic Hormone Deficiency

- Diabetes insipidus is common after transsphenoidal surgery (38.5% with isolated DI, usually on day 1 to 2; 21% with isolated hyponatremia, typically day 9; and 15.7% with combined DI and hyponatremia, with each component at the usual time).[102,103]

Table 9.6   Strategy for Postoperative Glucocorticoid Replacement (Does Not Apply to Pregnant Women)

Postoperative 8 AM cortisol (nmol/L)	Daily Glucocorticoid Replacement?	Insulin Tolerance Test?
< 100	Yes	No
100–250	Yes	Yes
251–399	No	Yes
≥ 400	No	No need

Differential diagnosis for polyuria:

- Postoperative mobilization of large volumes of crystalloid received intraoperatively
- Osmotic: glucose, mannitol, diuretics, urea (with total parenteral nutrition)
- Water-induced: psychogenic polydipsia versus central DI or nephrogenic DI

Central DI may present with one of the following clinical scenarios[104]:

- Usually transient (postoperative days 1 to 2)
- Permanent
- Triphasic (Low ADH due to axon shock resulting in DI, followed by elevated ADH due to release of preformed ADH, lasting 1–14 days, which may result in transient hyponatremia. Followed by low ADH after reserves are depleted which results in DI.)

Monitoring for Diabetes Insipidus

- Closely watch fluid balance (initially hourly ins and outs, running balance), twice daily serum and urine electrolytes and osmolality, urine specific gravity.

Treatment of Diabetes Insipidus

- Give DDAVP 1-2 μg IV/SC if all of the following criteria are met:
  - Urine output > 400 cc/hour × 2 hours (Note: patients with 200–400 cc/hour of urine output may have DI; however, this level of urine output can occur transiently when clearing intraoperative fluids, so one needs to interpret urine output based on the clinical scenario).
  - Urine specific gravity < 1.005.
  - Running total negative fluid balance.
  - Serum Na > 138 mmol/L (this will not rule out other causes of water diuresis, but ensures that the patient does not develop rapid hypernatremia while being investigated).
- If hypernatremic:
  - Will also need to replace free water losses by IV or per os.
  - Monitor water and Na content of oral and IV fluids, adjust as needed.
- If two or more doses of DDAVP are required postoperatively, then consider standing dose of DDAVP (e.g., DDAVP melt 60–120 μg sublingual every night; or intranasal DDAVP 10 μg every night).
  - Remind patient to drink only when thirsty and to adjust dose to allow breakthrough urination during day.
  - Reassess need for DDAVP in 2 weeks as outpatient (try holding the dose at night).

■ Assessing for Remission of a Hypersecretory Tumor After Surgery

Assessing for Remission of a Prolactinoma

The majority of patients with a prolactinoma are treated medically (see above).

- Prolactin levels lower than 10 µg/L on postoperative day 1 are predictive of remission in 100% of microadenomas and 93% of macroadenomas.[105]
- No patients with macroadenomas and prolactin levels between 10–20 µg/L on postoperative day 1 achieved remission.[105]

Recommendations

Order a prolactin test on postoperative day 1. A reading of < 10 µg/L indicates that the disease is in remission.

Assessing for Remission in Acromegaly

- Oral glucose suppression testing
  - One-week postoperative oral glucose tolerance test (OGTT) with GH nadir < 0.4 µg/L is highly predictive of cure.[106]
  - Most recent consensus guidelines suggest oral glucose suppression testing in a patient with a random growth hormone level > 1 µg /L. The nadir GH should be < 1 µg/L.[30]
- IGF-1 Levels:
  - Measure after 3 months as it may take a number of months to decline to the normal range.[106,107]

Recommendations

- At 1 week, order an oral glucose suppression test. A GH nadir < 0.4 µg/L indicates that the disease is under control.
- At 3 months, order a random GH level and IGF-1. If GH level is > 1 µg /L, order an oral glucose suppression test: the nadir GH should be less than 1 µg/L. IGF-1 levels should be within normal limits for age and sex.[30]

Assessing for Remission in Cushing's Disease

- No consensus for a definition of remission

Studies Assessing for Remission in Cushing's Disease with the Majority of Patients Receiving No Perioperative Steroids

- Postoperative cortisol levels were measured every 6 hours or 24 hours, then at 48 hours, and then at 10–12 days in one study.
  - In the cohort in which 80.6% of patients did not receive glucocorticoids, cortisol levels ≤ 96.6 nmol/L within 48 hours of surgery had a sensitivity of 73%, specificity of 100%, positive predictive value of 100%, and negative predictive value of 60%.[108] For cortisol levels drawn within 10 to 12 days of surgery, serum cortisol nadir less than or equal to157.3 nmol/L are associated with specificity and positive predictive value of 100%, sensitivity of 91%, and negative predictive value of 78% for disease remission.[108]
- Other studies have demonstrated varied levels of cortisol nadir for sustained remission.[109–113]

Recommendations

Predicting remission of Cushing's disease for patients on no GC coverage:

> Measure serum cortisol level every 6 hours for 48 hours postoperatively. Consider 8 AM cortisol postoperative day 10–12. In patients who have received no steroids, nadir cortisol level ≤ 157.3 nmol/L within 10 to 12 days has been found to be the best predictor of remission[108].
> Use a cutoff of ≤ 96.6 nmol/L for the early postoperative period (first 48 hours).

Studies Assessing for Remission in Cushing's Disease in Patients who have Received Perioperative Steroids

In patients who have received GCs:

- Postoperative cortisol levels > 24 hours after the last hydrocortisone dose:
  - Cortisol level of < 55.2 nmol/L during 48 hours postoperatively had a positive predictive value for remission of 100%.[114]
  - Other studies suggest that a postoperative cortisol level around 55.2 nmol/L predicts remission.[115,116]
- ACTH levels:
  - ACTH < 5 pg/mL 24 to 48 hours postoperatively was associated with a positive predictive value for remission of 100%.[114]

Recommendations

Predicting remission of Cushing's disease for patients on GC coverage:

Measure cortisol levels every 6 hours in the first 48 hours postoperatively. In patients who have received steroids, postoperative cortisol level < 55 nmol/L, during the first 48 hours postoperatively and 24 hours after the last dose of hydrocortisone, is predictive of remission.

Other Factors for Patients with Cushing's Disease

- For patients in remission, start daily hydrocortisone (20 mg in the morning and 10 mg 4 to 6 hours later). Taper over 6 months. Long-term follow-up is required.
- Be aware of factors that will increase cortisol-binding globulin (e.g., hepatitis or high estrogen states such as pregnancy) because the plasma cortisol level will be elevated, and may not truly reflect the free cortisol level.[113]
- Postoperative serum cortisol levels greater than 276 to 284 nmol/L are likely associated with the need for reoperation.[108,114]
- No single perioperative cortisol or ACTH cutoff value excludes all recurrences; therefore, these patients need long-term follow-up.[114]

Other Tests to Consider for Determining Remission

- ACTH levels[112,114]
- 1 mg DST
- 24-hour urine for free cortisol

Other Tests to Consider for Predicting Risk of Recurrence

- Cortisol and ACTH responses to ovine CRH: no cutoff values predicted recurrence.[116]
- Absolute increment in serum cortisol levels of > 193 nmol/L after desmopressin in the early postoperative period may help to identify those at risk for later recurrence.[118]

Follow-Up After Hospital Discharge

- Blood work 7 to 10 days postoperative:
  - Serum sodium, urine osmolality, free T_4[119] and 8 AM cortisol (if patient is on GC replacement, do these tests 24 hours after the last dose of hydrocortisone).
- Patient sees an endocrinologist 2 to 4 weeks after discharge; insulin tolerance test to be done 4 weeks after surgery if required.

Risk of Late Hyponatremia

- The syndrome of inappropriate secretion of ADH (SIADH) presents 0 to 28 days after surgery in 16% of patients (on average, postoperative day 4[120] to day 7.[119]
- Upon discharge, patients should be instructed to drink only when thirsty provided they have intact thirst regulation.
- Patients should be counseled on the symptoms of hyponatremia. If they develop headaches, malaise, nausea or lethargy, they should be instructed to seek emergent medical care.

For Patients Presenting with Hyponatremia

- Before SIADH is diagnosed, other causes of hyponatremia such as secondary adrenal insufficiency, secondary hypothyroidism and cerebral salt wasting should be ruled out.
- Treat with water restriction, with or without oral salt or 3% normal saline. The rate of correction will depend on the acuteness of the hyponatremia, and how symptomatic (correct hyponatremia faster if symptomatic, especially if the onset was acute).

Assessing for Other Pituitary Hormone Deficiencies

- *Free T_4*
  - Decrease in free T_4 by 50% 7 days postoperatively (its half-life) indicates there is little remaining thyrotroph function.
  - If free T_4 is below the normal range, start treatment with L-thyroxine. If free T_4 is in the bottom third of the normal range and the patient has symptoms of hypothyroidism, can consider treatment.
  - In secondary hypothyroidism, TSH may be low, normal, and even high (with inactive TSH), so it is not helpful to measure it.
  - Target free T_4 in the upper normal range.
  - Do not depend on TSH levels in patients with pituitary disease and suspected thyroid disturbances.
- *Sex hormones*
  - Men: LH, FSH, bioavailable testosterone checked at 1 to 2 months after surgery.
  - Premenopausal women: ask about menstrual cycle.
  - Postmenopausal women: FSH/LH are elevated normally; the ability of the pituitary to produce the expected high FSH and LH level can provide useful assessment of overall pituitary function.
- *Prolactin*
  - Hyperprolactinemia may indicate stalk compression/damage.
  - Very low level may be associated with panhypopituitarism.

- **Growth hormone**
  - Low IGF-1 and multiple hormone deficiencies or abnormal ITT (GH rises by less than 5 µg/L after plasma glucose falls to less than 2.2 mmol/L if GH deficient) diagnoses GH deficiency.

Patients at High Risk of Recurrence

- Patients with histopathological diagnosis of the tumors reported above.
- Nelson's syndrome.
- Ki-67 > 2.2% in one study predicted regrowth after surgery in nonfunctioning adenomas.[121] However, the value of the Ki-67/MIB1 labeling is controversial.[122]
- Aggressive pituitary tumors with massive invasion and rapid growth.[117]
- Pituitary carcinoma.

Patients need to be followed long-term for:

- Recurrence of hypersecretion if the underlying condition was a prolactinoma, Cushing's or acromegaly
- Pituitary hormone deficiency: monitor effectiveness of replacement hormones
- Recurrence of mass effect (serial MRIs, serial visual field and ophthalmologic assessments)
- Post-surgical tumor remnant
- Upon recurrence, one needs to consider repeat surgery, radiation or medical therapy where the latter is effective

Pituitary apoplexy

See Chapter 35.

■ References

Boldfaced references are of particular importance.
1. Delgrange E, Trouillas J, Maiter D, Donckier J, Tourniaire J. Sex-related difference in the growth of prolactinomas: a clinical and proliferation marker study. J Clin Endocrinol Metab 1997;82:2102–2107
2. Iglesias P, Bernal C, Villabona C, Castro JC, Arrieta F, Díez JJ. Prolactinomas in men: a multicentre and retrospective analysis of treatment outcome. Clin Endocrinol (Oxf) 2012;77:281–287
3. Daly AF, Rixhon M, Adam C, Dempegioti A, Tichomirowa MA, Beckers A. High prevalence of pituitary adenomas: a cross-sectional study in the province of Liege, Belgium. J Clin Endocrinol Metab 2006;91:4769–4775

4. Fernandez A, Karavitaki N, Wass JA. Prevalence of pituitary adenomas: a community-based, cross-sectional study in Banbury (Oxfordshire, UK). Clin Endocrinol (Oxf) 2010;72:377–382

5. Zhang X, Horwitz GA, Heaney AP, et al. Pituitary tumor transforming gene (PTTG) expression in pituitary adenomas. J Clin Endocrinol Metab 1999;84:761–767

6. Salehi F, Kovacs K, Scheithauer BW, et al. Immunohistochemical expression of pituitary tumor transforming gene (PTTG) in pituitary adenomas: a correlative study of tumor subtypes. Int J Surg Pathol 2010;18:5–13

7. Beckers A, Daly AF. The clinical, pathological, and genetic features of familial isolated pituitary adenomas. Eur J Endocrinol 2007;157:371–382

8. Melmed S, Casanueva FF, Hoffman AR, et al; Endocrine Society. Diagnosis and treatment of hyperprolactinemia: an Endocrine Society clinical practice guideline. J Clin Endocrinol Metab 2011;96:273–288

9. Glezer A, Bronstein MD. Approach to the patient with persistent hyperprolactinemia and negative sellar imaging. J Clin Endocrinol Metab 2012;97:2211–2216

10. Fahie-Wilson M, Smith TP. Determination of prolactin: the macroprolactin problem. Best Pract Res Clin Endocrinol Metab 2013;27:725–742

11. Comtois R, Robert F, Hardy J. Immunoradiometric assays may miss high prolactin levels. Ann Intern Med 1993;119:173

12. St-Jean E, Blain F, Comtois R. High prolactin levels may be missed by immunoradiometric assay in patients with macroprolactinomas. Clin Endocrinol (Oxf) 1996;44:305–309

13. Webster J, Piscitelli G, Polli A, Ferrari CI, Ismail I, Scanlon MF; Cabergoline Comparative Study Group. A comparison of cabergoline and bromocriptine in the treatment of hyperprolactinemic amenorrhea. N Engl J Med 1994;331:904–909

14. Webster J, Piscitelli G, Polli A, et al; European Multicentre Cabergoline Dose-finding Study Group. Dose-dependent suppression of serum prolactin by cabergoline in hyperprolactinaemia: a placebo controlled, double blind, multicentre study. Clin Endocrinol (Oxf) 1992;37:534–541

15. Colao A, Di Sarno A, Landi ML, et al. Macroprolactinoma shrinkage during cabergoline treatment is greater in naive patients than in patients pretreated with other dopamine agonists: a prospective study in 110 patients. J Clin Endocrinol Metab 2000;85:2247–2252

16. Shimon I, Benbassat C, Hadani M. Effectiveness of long-term cabergoline treatment for giant prolactinoma: study of 12 men. Eur J Endocrinol 2007;156:225–231

17. Marazuela M, Astigarraga B, Vicente A, et al. Recovery of visual and endocrine function following transsphenoidal surgery of large nonfunctioning pituitary adenomas. J Endocrinol Invest 1994;17:703–707

18. Dekkers OM, Lagro J, Burman P, Jørgensen JO, Romijn JA, Pereira AM. Recurrence of hyperprolactinemia after withdrawal of dopamine agonists: systematic review and meta-analysis. J Clin Endocrinol Metab 2010;95:43–51

19. Colao A, Di Sarno A, Guerra E, et al. Predictors of remission of hyperprolactinaemia after long-term withdrawal of cabergoline therapy. Clin Endocrinol (Oxf) 2007;67:426–433

20. Kharlip J, Salvatori R, Yenokyan G, Wand GS. Recurrence of hyperprolactinemia after withdrawal of long-term cabergoline therapy. J Clin Endocrinol Metab 2009;94:2428–2436

21. Huda MS, Athauda NB, Teh MM, Carroll PV, Powrie JK. Factors determining the remission of microprolactinomas after dopamine agonist withdrawal. Clin Endocrinol (Oxf) 2010;72:507–511

22. **Colao A, Di Sarno A, Cappabianca P, Di Somma C, Pivonello R, Lombardi G. Withdrawal of long-term cabergoline therapy for tumoral and nontumoral hyperprolactinemia. N Engl J Med 2003;349:2023–2033**

23. **Pereira O, Bevan JS. Preoperative assessment for pituitary surgery. Pituitary 2008;11:347–351**

24. Barber TM, Kenkre J, Garnett C, Scott RV, Byrne JV, Wass JA. Recurrence of hyperprolactinaemia following discontinuation of dopamine agonist therapy in patients with prolactinoma occurs commonly especially in macroprolactinoma. Clin Endocrinol (Oxf) 2011;75:819–824\

25. Testa G, Vegetti W, Motta T, et al. Two-year treatment with oral contraceptives in hyperprolactinemic patients. Contraception 1998;58:69–73

26. Mestron A, Webb SM, Astorga R, et al. Epidemiology, clinical characteristics, outcome, morbidity and mortality in acromegaly based on the Spanish Acromegaly Registry (Registro Espanol de Acromegalia, REA). Eur J Endocrinol 2004;151:439–446

27. **Melmed S. Medical progress: Acromegaly. N Engl J Med 2006;355:2558–2573**

28. Holdaway IM, Rajasoorya C. Epidemiology of acromegaly. Pituitary 1999;2:29–41

29. Chahal HS, Stals K, Unterländer M, et al. AIP mutation in pituitary adenomas in the 18th century and today. N Engl J Med 2011;364:43–50

30. Katznelson L, Laws ER Jr, Melmed S, et al. Acromegaly: an endocrine society clinical practice guideline. J Clin Endocrinol Metab 2014;99:3933–3951

31. **Kannan S, Kennedy L. Diagnosis of acromegaly: state of the art. Expert Opin Med Diagn 2013;7:443–453**

32. Bhayana S, Booth GL, Asa SL, Kovacs K, Ezzat S. The implication of somatotroph adenoma phenotype to somatostatin analog responsiveness in acromegaly. J Clin Endocrinol Metab 2005;90:6290–6295

33. Carlsen SM, Lund-Johansen M, Schreiner T, et al; Preoperative Octreotide Treatment of Acromegaly study group. Preoperative octreotide treatment in newly diagnosed acromegalic patients with macroadenomas increases cure short-term postoperative rates: a prospective, randomized trial. J Clin Endocrinol Metab 2008;93:2984–2990

34. Mao ZG, Zhu YH, Tang HL, et al. Preoperative lanreotide treatment in acromegalic patients with macroadenomas increases short-term postoperative cure rates: a prospective, randomised trial. Eur J Endocrinol 2010;162:661–666

35. Li ZQ, Quan Z, Tian HL, Cheng M. Preoperative lanreotide treatment improves outcome in patients with acromegaly resulting from invasive pituitary macroadenoma. J Int Med Res 2012;40:517–524

36. Pita-Gutierrez F, Pertega-Diaz S, Pita-Fernandez S, et al. Place of preoperative treatment of acromegaly with somatostatin analog on surgical outcome: a systematic review and meta-analysis. PLoS ONE 2013;8:e61523

37. Shen M, Shou X, Wang Y, et al. Effect of presurgical long-acting octreotide treatment in acromegaly patients with invasive pituitary macroadenomas: a prospective randomized study. Endocr J 2010;57:1035–1044

38. Newell-Price J, Bertagna X, Grossman AB, Nieman LK. Cushing's syndrome. Lancet 2006;367:1605–1617
39. Lindholm J, Juul S, Jørgensen JO, et al. Incidence and late prognosis of Cushing's syndrome: a population-based study. J Clin Endocrinol Metab 2001;86:117–123
40. Nieman LK, Biller BM, Findling JW, et al. The diagnosis of Cushing's syndrome: an Endocrine Society Clinical Practice Guideline. J Clin Endocrinol Metab 2008;93:1526–1540
41. Fielding JW, Raff H. CLINICAL REVIEW: Cushing's Syndrome: Important Issues in Diagnosis and Management. J Clin Endocrinol Metab 2006;91:3746–3753.
42. **Oldfield EH, Chrousos GP, Schulte HM, et al. Preoperative lateralization of ACTH-secreting pituitary microadenomas by bilateral and simultaneous inferior petrosal venous sinus sampling. N Engl J Med 1985;312:100–103**
43. **Booth GL, Redelmeier DA, Grosman H, Kovacs K, Smyth HS, Ezzat S. Improved diagnostic accuracy of inferior petrosal sinus sampling over imaging for localizing pituitary pathology in patients with Cushing's disease. J Clin Endocrinol Metab 1998;83:2291–2295**
44. Potts MB, Shah JK, Molinaro AM, et al. Cavernous and inferior petrosal sinus sampling and dynamic magnetic resonance imaging in the preoperative evaluation of Cushing's disease. J Neurooncol 2014;116:593–600
45. Aron DC, Raff H, Findling JW. Effectiveness versus efficacy: the limited value in clinical practice of high dose dexamethasone suppression testing in the differential diagnosis of adrenocorticotropin-dependent Cushing's syndrome. J Clin Endocrinol Metab 1997;82:1780–1785
46. Reimondo G, Paccotti P, Minetto M, et al. The corticotrophin-releasing hormone test is the most reliable noninvasive method to differentiate pituitary from ectopic ACTH secretion in Cushing's syndrome. Clin Endocrinol (Oxf) 2003;58:718–724
47. van den Bosch OF, Stades AM, Zelissen PM. Increased long-term remission after adequate medical cortisol suppression therapy as presurgical treatment in Cushing's disease. Clin Endocrinol (Oxf) 2014;80:184–190
48. McKeage K. Pasireotide: a review of its use in Cushing's disease. Drugs 2013;73:563–574
49. **Di Ieva A, Rotondo F, Syro LV, Cusimano MD, Kovacs K. Aggressive pituitary adenomas—diagnosis and emerging treatments. Nat Rev Endocrinol 2014;10:423–435**
50. Scheithauer BW, Kovacs KT, Laws ER Jr, Randall RV. Pathology of invasive pituitary tumors with special reference to functional classification. J Neurosurg 1986;65:733–744
51. **Thapar K, Kovacs K, Scheithauer BW, et al. Proliferative activity and invasiveness among pituitary adenomas and carcinomas: an analysis using the MIB-1 antibody. Neurosurgery 1996;38:99–106, discussion 106–107**
52. **Meij BP, Lopes MB, Ellegala DB, Alden TD, Laws ER Jr. The long-term significance of microscopic dural invasion in 354 patients with pituitary adenomas treated with transsphenoidal surgery. J Neurosurg 2002;96:195–208**
53. **DeLellis RA, Lloyd RV, Heitz PU, Eng C. World Health Organization Classification of Tumors: Tumors of Endocrine Organs. Geneva: WHO Press; 2004**

54. **George DH, Scheithauer BW, Kovacs K, et al. Crooke's cell adenoma of the pituitary: an aggressive variant of corticotroph adenoma. Am J Surg Pathol 2003;27: 1330–1336**

55. Scheithauer BW, Jaap AJ, Horvath E, et al. Clinically silent corticotroph tumors of the pituitary gland. Neurosurgery 2000;47:723–729, discussion 729–730

56. Kovacs K, Horvath E, Coire C, et al. Pituitary corticotroph hyperplasia preceding adenoma in a patient with Nelson's syndrome. Clin Neuropathol 2006;25:74–80

57. Jahangiri A, Wagner JR, Pekmezci M, et al. A comprehensive long-term retrospective analysis of silent corticotrophic adenomas vs hormone-negative adenomas. Neurosurgery 2013;73:8–17, discussion 17–18

58. Barber TM, Adams E, Ansorge O, Byrne JV, Karavitaki N, Wass JA. Nelson's syndrome. Eur J Endocrinol 2010;163:495–507

59. Ritzel K, Beuschlein F, Mickisch A, et al. Clinical review: outcome of bilateral adrenalectomy in Cushing's syndrome: a systematic review. J Clin Endocrinol Metab 2013; 98:3939–3948

60. Mehta GU, Sheehan JP, Vance ML. Effect of stereotactic radiosurgery before bilateral adrenalectomy for Cushing's disease on the incidence of Nelson's syndrome. J Neurosurg 2013;119:1493–1497

61. Jane JA Jr, Vance ML, Woodburn CJ, Laws ER Jr. Stereotactic radiosurgery for hypersecreting pituitary tumors: part of a multimodality approach. Neurosurg Focus 2003; 14:e12

62. Vik-Mo EO, Øksnes M, Pedersen PH, et al. Gamma knife stereotactic radiosurgery of Nelson syndrome. Eur J Endocrinol 2009;160:143–148

63. Pivonello R, Faggiano A, Di Salle F, Filippella M, Lombardi G, Colao A. Complete remission of Nelson's syndrome after 1-year treatment with cabergoline. J Endocrinol Invest 1999;22:860–865

64. Casulari LA, Naves LA, Mello PA, Pereira Neto A, Papadia C. Nelson's syndrome: complete remission with cabergoline but not with bromocriptine or cyproheptadine treatment. Horm Res 2004;62:300–305

65. Shraga-Slutzky I, Shimon I, Weinshtein R. Clinical and biochemical stabilization of Nelson's syndrome with long-term low-dose cabergoline treatment. Pituitary 2006;9: 151–154

66. Katznelson L. Sustained improvements in plasma ACTH and clinical status in a patient with Nelson's syndrome treated with pasireotide LAR, a multireceptor somatostatin analog. J Clin Endocrinol Metab 2013;98:1803–1807

67. Moyes VJ, Alusi G, Sabin HI, et al. Treatment of Nelson's syndrome with temozolomide. Eur J Endocrinol 2009;160:115–119

68. **Scheithauer BW, Kurtkaya-Yapicier O, Kovacs KT, Young WF Jr, Lloyd RV. Pituitary carcinoma: a clinicopathological review. Neurosurgery 2005;56:1066–1074, discussion 1066–1074**

69. Oh MC, Tihan T, Kunwar S, Blevins L, Aghi MK. Clinical management of pituitary carcinomas. Neurosurg Clin N Am 2012;23:595–606

70. Heaney AP. Clinical review: Pituitary carcinoma: difficult diagnosis and treatment. J Clin Endocrinol Metab 2011;96:3649–3660

71. Mixson AJ, Friedman TC, Katz DA, et al. Thyrotropin-secreting pituitary carcinoma. J Clin Endocrinol Metab 1993;76:529–533

72. McCutcheon IE, Pieper DR, Fuller GN, Benjamin RS, Friend KE, Gagel RF. Pituitary carcinoma containing gonadotropins: treatment by radical excision and cytotoxic chemotherapy: case report. Neurosurgery 2000;46:1233–1239, discussion 1239–1240

73. Roncaroli F, Nosé V, Scheithauer BW, et al. Gonadotropic pituitary carcinoma: HER-2/neu expression and gene amplification. Report of two cases. J Neurosurg 2003;99:402–408

74. Kaltsas GA, Grossman AB. Malignant pituitary tumours. Pituitary 1998;1:69–81

75. Thapar K, Scheithauer BW, Kovacs K, Pernicone PJ, Laws ER Jr. P53 Expression in Pituitary Adenomas and Carcinomas: Correlation with Invasiveness and Tumor Growth Fractions. Neurosurgery 1996;38:765–770; discussion 770–771

76. Ortiz LD, Syro LV, Scheithauer BW, et al. Temozolomide in aggressive pituitary adenomas and carcinomas. Clinics (Sao Paulo) 2012;67(Suppl 1):119–123

77. Gonzalez JG, Elizondo G, Saldivar D, Nanez H, Todd LE, Villarreal JZ. Pituitary glad growth during normal pregnancy: an in vivo study using magnetic resonance imaging. Am J Med 1988;85:217–220

78. Molitch ME. Medical management of prolactin-secreting pituitary adenomas. Pituitary 2002;5:55–65

79. Lindsay JR, Nieman LK. The hypothalamic-pituitary-adrenal axis in pregnancy: challenges in disease detection and treatment. Endocr Rev 2005;26:775–799

80. Verhelst J, Abs R, Maiter D, et al. Cabergoline in the treatment of hyperprolactinemia: a study in 455 patients. J Clin Endocrinol Metab 1999;84:2518–2522

81. Corsello SM, Ubertini G, Altomare M, et al. Giant prolactinomas in men: efficacy of cabergoline treatment. Clin Endocrinol (Oxf) 2003;58:662–670

82. Shimon I, Benbassat C, Hadani M. Effectiveness of long-term cabergoline treatment for giant prolactinoma: study of 12 men. Eur J Endocrinol 2007;156:225–231

83. Goguen JM. Pituitary apoplexy: Don't miss the diagnosis! Available at: http://endocrinologyrounds.ca/crus/endocdneng_1006.pdf. Accessed May 2014

84. Wagenmakers MA, Boogaarts HD, Roerink SH, et al. Endoscopic transsphenoidal pituitary surgery: a good and safe primary treatment option for Cushing's disease, even in case of macroadenomas or invasive adenomas. Eur J Endocrinol 2013;169:329–337

85. Arafah BM, Prunty D, Ybarra J, Hlavin ML, Selman WR. The dominant role of increased intrasellar pressure in the pathogenesis of hypopituitarism, hyperprolactinemia, and headaches in patients with pituitary adenomas. J Clin Endocrinol Metab 2000;85:1789–1793

86. Arafah BM. Reversible hypopituitarism in patients with large nonfunctioning pituitary adenomas. J Clin Endocrinol Metab 1986;62:1173–1179

87. Webb SM, Rigla M, Wägner A, Oliver B, Bartumeus F. Recovery of hypopituitarism after neurosurgical treatment of pituitary adenomas. J Clin Endocrinol Metab 1999;84:3696–3700

88. Murad MH, Fernández-Balsells MM, Barwise A, et al. Outcomes of surgical treatment for nonfunctioning pituitary adenomas: a systematic review and meta-analysis. Clin Endocrinol (Oxf) 2010;73:777–791

89. Pavord SR, Girach A, Price DE, Absalom SR, Falconer-Smith J, Howlett TA. A retrospective audit of the combined pituitary function test, using the insulin stress test, TRH and GnRH in a district laboratory. Clin Endocrinol (Oxf) 1992;36:135–139

90. Jones SL, Trainer PJ, Perry L, Wass JA, Bessser GM, Grossman A. An audit of the insulin tolerance test in adult subjects in an acute investigation unit over one year. Clin Endocrinol (Oxf) 1994;41:123–128

91. Hout WM, Arafah BM, Salazar R, Selman W. Evaluation of the hypothalamic-pituitary-adrenal axis immediately after pituitary adenomectomy: is perioperative steroid therapy necessary? J Clin Endocrinol Metab 1988;66:1208–1212

92. Inder WJ, Hunt PJ. Glucocorticoid replacement in pituitary surgery: guidelines for perioperative assessment and management. J Clin Endocrinol Metab 2002;87:2745–2750

93. Karaca Z, Tanriverdi F, Atmaca H, et al. Can basal cortisol measurement be an alternative to the insulin tolerance test in the assessment of the hypothalamic-pituitary-adrenal axis before and after pituitary surgery? Eur J Endocrinol 2010;163:377–382

94. Cozzi R, Lasio G, Cardia A, Felisati G, Montini M, Attanasio R. Perioperative cortisol can predict hypothalamus-pituitary-adrenal status in clinically non-functioning pituitary adenomas. J Endocrinol Invest 2009;32:460–464

95. Bhansali A, Dutta P, Bhat MH, Mukherjee KK, Rajput R, Bhadada S. Rational use of glucocorticoid during pituitary surgery—a pilot study. Indian J Med Res 2008;128:294–299

96. **De Tommasi C, Goguen J, Cusimano MD. Transsphenoidal surgery without steroid replacement in patients with morning serum cortisol below 9 μg/dl (250 Nmol/l). Acta Neurochir (Wien) 2012;154:1903–1915**

97. Behan LA, Rogers B, Hannon MJ, et al. Optimizing glucocorticoid replacement therapy in severely adrenocorticotropin-deficient hypopituitary male patients. Clin Endocrinol (Oxf) 2011;75:505–513

98. Auchus RJ, Shewbridge RK, Shepherd MD. Which patients benefit from provocative adrenal testing after transsphenoidal pituitary surgery? Clin Endocrinol (Oxf) 1997;46:21–27

99. Dökmetaş HS, Colak R, Keleştimur F, Selçuklu A, Unlühizarci K, Bayram F. A comparison between the 1-microg adrenocorticotropin (ACTH) test, the short ACTH (250 microg) test, and the insulin tolerance test in the assessment of hypothalamo-pituitary-adrenal axis immediately after pituitary surgery. J Clin Endocrinol Metab 2000;85:3713–3719

100. Agha A, Tomlinson JW, Clark PM, Holder G, Stewart PM. The long-term predictive accuracy of the short Synacthen (corticotropin) stimulation test for assessment of the hypothalamic-pituitary-adrenal axis. J Clin Endocrinol Metab 2006;91:43–47

101. Jayasena CN, Gadhvi KA, Gohel B, et al. Day 5 morning serum cortisol predicts hypothalamic-pituitary-adrenal function after transsphenoidal surgery for pituitary tumors. Clin Chem 2009;55:972–977

102. Seckl J, Dunger D. Postoperative diabetes insipidus. BMJ 1989;298:2–3

103. **Kristof RA, Rother M, Neuloh G, Klingmüller D. Incidence, clinical manifestations, and course of water and electrolyte metabolism disturbances following transsphenoidal pituitary adenoma surgery: a prospective observational study. J Neurosurg 2009;111:555–562**

104. Fisher C, Ingram WR. The effect of interruption of the supraoptico-hypophyseal tracts on the antidiuretic, pressor and oxytocic activity of the posterior lobe of the hypophysis. Endocrinology 1936;20:762–768

105. Amar AP, Couldwell WT, Chen JC, Weiss MH. Predictive value of serum prolactin levels measured immediately after transsphenoidal surgery. J Neurosurg 2002; 97:307–314

106. Feelders RA, Bidlingmaier M, Strasburger CJ, et al. Postoperative evaluation of patients with acromegaly: clinical significance and timing of oral glucose tolerance testing and measurement of (free) insulin-like growth factor I, acid-labile subunit, and growth hormone-binding protein levels. J Clin Endocrinol Metab 2005;90:6480–6489

107. Giustina A, Chanson P, Bronstein MD, et al; Acromegaly Consensus Group. A consensus on criteria for cure of acromegaly. J Clin Endocrinol Metab 2010;95: 3141–3148

108. Costenaro F, Rodrigues TC, Rollin GA, Ferreira NP, Czepielewski MA. Evaluation of Cushing's disease remission after transsphenoidal surgery based on early serum cortisol dynamics. Clin Endocrinol (Oxf) 2014;80:411–418

109. Simmons NE, Alden TD, Thorner MO, Laws ER Jr. Serum cortisol response to transsphenoidal surgery for Cushing disease. J Neurosurg 2001;95:1–8

110. Rollin GA, Ferreira NP, Junges M, Gross JL, Czepielewski MA. Dynamics of serum cortisol levels after transsphenoidal surgery in a cohort of patients with Cushing's disease. J Clin Endocrinol Metab 2004;89:1131–1139

111. Esposito F, Dusick JR, Cohan P, et al. Clinical review: early morning cortisol levels as a predictor of remission after transsphenoidal surgery for Cushing's disease. J Clin Endocrinol Metab 2006;91:7–13

112. Acebes JJ, Martino J, Masuet C, Montanya E, Soler J. Early post-operative ACTH and cortisol as predictors of remission in Cushing's disease. Acta Neurochir (Wien) 2007;149:471–477, discussion 477–479

113. AbdelMannan D, Selman WR, Arafah BM. Peri-operative management of Cushing's disease. Rev Endocr Metab Disord 2010;11:127–134

114. Hameed N, Yedinak CG, Brzana J, et al. Remission rate after transsphenoidal surgery in patients with pathologically confirmed Cushing's disease, the role of cortisol, ACTH assessment and immediate reoperation: a large single center experience. Pituitary 2013;16:452–458

115. Trainer PJ, Lawrie HS, Verhelst J, et al. Transsphenoidal resection in Cushing's disease: undetectable serum cortisol as the definition of successful treatment. Clin Endocrinol (Oxf) 1993;38:73–78

116. Lindsay JR, Oldfield EH, Stratakis CA, Nieman LK. The postoperative basal cortisol and CRH tests for prediction of long-term remission from Cushing's disease after transsphenoidal surgery. J Clin Endocrinol Metab 2011;96:2057–2064

117. Colao A, Grasso LF, Pivonello R, Lombardi G. Therapy of aggressive pituitary tumors. Expert Opin Pharmacother 2011;12:1561–1570

118. Romanholi DJ, Machado MC, Pereira CC, et al. Role for postoperative cortisol response to desmopressin in predicting the risk for recurrent Cushing's disease. Clin Endocrinol (Oxf) 2008;69:117–122

119. Ausiello JC, Bruce JN, Freda PU. Postoperative assessment of the patient after transsphenoidal pituitary surgery. Pituitary 2008;11:391–401

120. Jahangiri A, Wagner J, Tran MT, et al. Factors predicting postoperative hyponatremia and efficacy of hyponatremia management strategies after more than 1000 pituitary operations. J Neurosurg 2013;119:1478–1483

121. Šteňo A, Bocko J, Rychlý B, et al. Nonfunctioning pituitary adenomas: association of Ki-67 and HMGA-1 labeling indices with residual tumor growth. Acta Neurochir (Wien) 2014;156:451–461, discussion 461

122. Salehi F, Agur A, Scheithauer BW, Kovacs K, Lloyd RV, Cusimano M. Ki-67 in pituitary neoplasms: a review—part I. Neurosurgery 2009;65:429–437, discussion 437

10 Neuro-Ophthalmology

Of the manifold symptoms which may be produced by an intracranial growth, none are of greater interest and none of greater importance than the various disturbances on the part of the visual apparatus.

—Harvey Cushing, *Johns Hopkins Hospital Bulletin*, 1911

■ Introduction

This chapter reviews the aspects of the ophthalmic, visual field, pupil, motility, and optic nerve exam most relevant to the neurosurgeon. Some essential aspects of neuro-ophthalmology and corneal preservation are summarized below:

- By convention, confrontation fields are recorded from the patient's perspective, so that results from the neurologic exam can be compared with formal perimetry.
- Although bitemporal hemianopsia is the classic visual field defect in patients with chiasmal syndrome, many other field defects are possible.
- The relative afferent pupillary defect (RAPD) should not be confused with the efferent pupillary defect (blown pupil) of CN III palsy due to aneurysms
- When requesting an ophthalmology consult, always indicate whether the patient's pupils can be dilated or not.
- Papilledema should be excluded in all patients with cranial nerve (CN) VI palsy.
- Patients with combined CN VII palsy and corneal anesthesia usually require a tarsorrhaphy.
- A Tegaderm™ transparent dressing with lubricating ointment should be used rather than a cloth patch in patients with severe corneal exposure.

■ Visual Acuity

- The visual acuity of each eye should be tested separately, ideally both near and at distance, with the appropriate refractive correction in place. Use the palm of the hand rather than fingers to occlude the eye because patients can see through the interdigital spaces. If glasses are not available, make a small pinhole through a piece of paper. Patients older than 40 years of age may require reading glasses or bifocals when testing the near vision. If patients are in the supine position, and the near vision is being tested, raise the glasses so that the bifocal segment at the bottom of the glasses will be in the proper position.

- If patients are conscious but cannot verbalize, ask them to imitate fingers, or write down what they see. If patients do not appear conscious, document any aversion to bright light and the pupillary reaction to light.
- Visual acuity can be obtained with an eye chart or near card. Normal visual acuity is at least 20/20, 6/6, or logMAR 0.00. The minimum visual acuity required for driving in most jurisdictions is 20/40, 6/12, or logMAR 0.30.[1] Legal blindness can be defined as acuity in either eye less than 20/200, 6/60, or logMAR 1.00. If the patient cannot see the eye chart, then determine the maximum distance at which the examiner's fingers can be accurately counted. If the patient is unable to count fingers, test if the patient can perceive when your hand starts and stops moving. If hand motions cannot be detected, then test for light perception with a bright light. Ensure that the contralateral eye is well occluded with a tissue and/or the palm of the hand.
- The near and distance acuity measurements should correlate if the patient is using appropriate glasses. If the patient is unable to see the eye chart, but malingering is suspected, document the pupillary response and RAPD, and the optokinetic response. A positive optokinetic response usually indicates the vision potential is at least 20/400.
- All one-eyed patients should be instructed to use dress polycarbonate (shatter-proof lens) glasses during waking hours.

■ Color Vision

- Color vision loss is also known as dyschromatopsia. Color vision should be tested in each eye individually with the appropriate near correction. An asymmetric reading speed of the color plates may provide a clue to asymmetric optic nerve function. The most widely available test of color vision is the Ishihara color plates, but unfortunately 8% of the male population is red-green defective. Many color tests are available online and for smartphones.

■ Pupils

- Pupils should be tested in a dark room with the patient looking in the distance. Normal pupils should be round, equal in size, and constrict briskly to bright light. The size of the pupils in the light and the dark can be compared with a pupil gauge. If the pupillary reaction to light is normal, there is no need to test for the near reaction. Pupillary light-near dissociation occurs when the pupillary light reaction is poor, but the pupil reaction to near stimulus is better. An important cause of light-near dissociation in patients who present to the skull base surgeon is dorsal midbrain syndrome or Parinaud's syndrome.

- If the pupil is not round in the setting of facial trauma, gently elevate the lid to ensure that there is no globe rupture. An iris notch or tear in the iris sphincter with dilated pupil suggests traumatic mydriasis. Mimics of neurologically "blown" pupils include pharmacological dilation, angle closure glaucoma (misty cornea, mid-dilated pupil, elevated intraocular pressure, vomiting patient), sulcus intraocular lens after cataract surgery, and surgical iridectomy.

- Horner's syndrome is an oculosympathetic paresis, with ptosis, variable anhidrosis, and pupillary miosis (small pupil); it is more evident in the dark. The skull base surgeon may occasionally encounter Horner's syndrome in the setting of brainstem lesions, cavernous sinus lesions usually with CN VI involvement, skull base osteomyelitis, neuroblastoma, or after Swan-Ganz catheter insertion (see also Chapter 7, **Table 7.1**).

- Adie's tonic pupil is a parasympathetic defect at the ciliary ganglion. Early on, the Adie's pupil is mydriatic (enlarged pupil) and poorly reactive to light, with better reaction to a near stimulus. An isolated dilated pupil in a conscious patient with no extraocular muscle dysmotility or ptosis rarely, if ever, is associated with posterior communicating artery aneurysm.

- When light is shone in one eye of a normal subject, both pupils will constrict equally. The pupillary reaction in the illuminated eye is the direct response, and the reaction in the contralateral eye is the consensual response. The afferent pupil fibers hemidecussate in the chiasm, as do the pupillomotor fibers in the brainstem. This double hemidecussation enables equal pupillary innervation, and equal pupil size.

> **Examination Pearl**
>
> When a bright light is shone in one eye, there should be an initial brisk constriction of the pupil, with equal contralateral pupillary constriction, due to the consensual response.

- The swinging flashlight test compares the consensual pupillary light response of the two eyes. During the swinging flashlight test, if the pupil does not constrict, or frankly dilates when illuminated, an ipsilateral RAPD may be present. The RAPD is one of the most important objective signs in neuro-ophthalmology **(Fig. 10.1)**.

  ○ Although bilateral afferent pupillary defects can be seen, for example with bilateral optic neuritis, a RAPD cannot be bilateral. If a patient is suspected of having a relative afferent pupillary defect, there is often ipsilateral vision loss, visual field loss, and color vision loss. However, there are some important exceptions to consider. A midbrain lesion at the

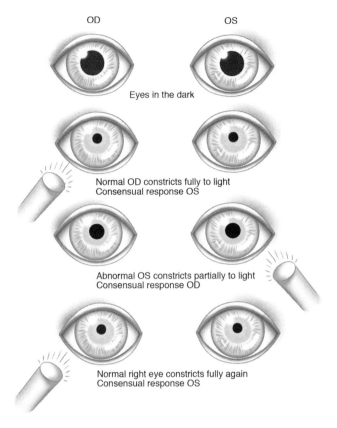

OD   OS

Eyes in the dark

Normal OD constricts fully to light
Consensual response OS

Abnormal OS constricts partially to light
Consensual response OD

Normal right eye constricts fully again
Consensual response OS

Fig. 10.1   Swinging flashlight test illustrating a left (OS) relative afferent pupillary defect (RAPD).

brachium of the superior colliculus can cause RAPD without acuity or field loss, because the geniculocalcarine fibers are not involved. Patients with unilateral optic neuritis may often have an ipsilateral RAPD, but retain 20/20 acuity. There may be decreased color perception, loss of contrast sensitivity, motion sensitivity, or visual field loss. Vision loss does not always correlate with an RAPD. A macular hole at the fovea of the retina may greatly decrease acuity, but because the amount of retina involved is small, there is no RAPD. A dense unilateral cataract may cause blindness, but should not cause an ipsilateral RAPD.

Examination Pearl

RAPD should not be confused with hippus, the rhythmic undulation in size of the pupil that is independent of illumination or accommodation, nor with the *efferent* pupillary defect (blown pupil) of CN III palsy due to aneurysm.

- When requesting an ophthalmology consult, clearly specify whether the pupils can be dilated. The nurse and ophthalmologist should document if and when dilating drops have been instilled in a neurosurgery patient. Dilating eyedrop bottles have a red top. The typical dilating drops used for examination are tropicamide, cyclopentolate, and phenylephrine.

■ Visual Fields

- Test the confrontation fields in each eye separately. Static objects are usually more difficult for the patient to discern than moving ones (statokinetic dissociation). Therefore, asking patients to count fingers in each quadrant may be more accurate than moving in targets from the periphery and waiting for a "yes-no" response to perceived movement.
- The Amsler grid tests the central 10 degrees of field and is especially useful for small homonymous occipital scotomas.
- Whenever possible, correlate perimetric findings with the visual acuity and the fundus examination. Visual field defects that respect the horizontal midline are nerve fiber bundle defects, with the exception of lesions above or below the calcarine fissure. Visual field defects respecting the vertical midline are due to chiasmal or retrochiasmal pathology, or rarely retinal lesions on either side of the fovea. Most chiasmal field defects are bitemporal hemianopsias (**Fig. 10.2a**). It is uncommon for neurosurgical lesions to cause nasal field defects respecting the vertical midline.[2] In the setting of binasal field loss, exclude optic nerve or retinal pathology, prior to considering intracranial lesions.
- The more posterior the visual pathway lesion, the closer the corresponding visual fibers from the two eyes, and the more congruent the homonymous hemianopsia. Complete homonymous field defects do not precisely localize the retrochiasmal pathology.
- Confrontation fields and Amsler grid testing are very useful, but formal perimetry can more accurately document and detect visual field loss. If patients are not cooperative for confrontation fields, they usually cannot perform formal perimetry either.
- Tangent screens are no longer used by most ophthalmologists. Goldmann perimetry (manual or kinetic perimetry) is not as readily available as automated/computerized (static) perimetry. The most common automated perimetry test used for neuro-ophthalmic diagnosis is a central 24-degree or central 30-degree threshold test, with test points about 6 degrees apart. The only neurologic field defects that a central 30-degree test may miss are small occipital scotomas and the temporal crescent of an anterior occipital lesion.
- In some countries the binocular Esterman field test is used as a screen to determine if the patient's visual field can meet a minimum standard for driving.

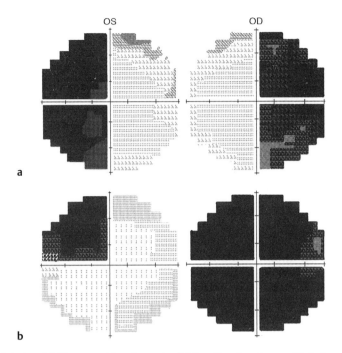

Fig. 10.2a,b **(a)** Bitemporal hemianopsia. **(b)** Junctional scotoma with lesion at the junction of the right optic nerve and chiasm.

An international symposium suggested a minimum peripheral vision standard for driving of 120 degrees of uninterrupted horizontal peripheral vision, with at least 40 degrees of vertical peripheral vision.[1]

■ Pituitary Tumors, Chiasmal Syndromes, and Medial Sphenoid Wing Meningioma

- Chiasmal lesions most commonly result in bitemporal hemianopsia. The bitemporal hemianopsia can be asymmetric, depending on the lateralization of the tumor. Monocular vision loss can result if a sellar mass compresses one optic nerve in a patient with a postfixed chiasm (See **Fig. 3.2c**, page 75). Junctional scotomas (monocular central scotoma with contralateral superotemporal field loss, Fig. **10.2b**) can occur when lesions compress the junction of the optic nerve and chiasm. Although the existence of Wilbrand's knee has been questioned, junctional scotomas are a well-documented clinical finding. A pituitary mass can cause incongruous homonymous hemianopsia (optic tract syndrome) in a patient with a prefixed chiasm (see Chapter 3, **Fig. 3.2b**).

- Pituitary lesions have to climb 10 mm above the sella before impinging on the chiasm. It is not uncommon for pituitary lesions to abut the chiasm on imaging, and yet perimetry appears normal.
- In general, pituitary tumors, growing from beneath the chiasm, cause bitemporal hemianopsia denser superiorly, whereas craniopharyngiomas compressing the chiasm from above cause bitemporal hemianopsia denser inferiorly, although this assumption is not always true.
- After chiasmal decompression surgery, visual recovery may be rapid and often occurs within 24 hours. If preoperative optical coherence tomography (OCT, see below) of pituitary adenoma shows that the average retinal nerve fiber layer is less than 75 μm, the prognosis for vision recovery may be less favorable.[3]
- Pituitary apoplexy, when symptomatic, is characterized by headache, visual acuity loss (unilateral or bilateral), visual field loss, and dysmotility. CN III palsy is more common than CN IV or VI palsy.[4]
- Tumors of the medial sphenoid wing can compress the optic nerve and present with early unilateral visual loss. Clinoidal meningiomas may also involve the cavernous sinus causing diplopia and facial numbness. Foster Kennedy syndrome (ipsilateral optic atrophy and contralateral papilledema) and painful ophthalmoplegia (Tolosa-Hunt syndrome) have been described with clinoidal meningioma (see also Chapter 7).

■ Anterior Segment Examination

- The normal cornea should be clear and glistening at all times. If there is any disruption of the corneal light reflex, a corneal epithelial defect should be suspected. A hand magnifier is a useful tool for bedside exams and can usually detect corneal foreign bodies, contact lenses, corneal abrasion, and Lisch nodules.
- In patients with CN VII palsy, it is essential to check corneal sensation. The combination of a CN VII palsy and corneal anesthesia often necessitates tarsorrhaphy prior to discharge from the hospital. Corneal sensation can be assessed by tangentially touching the cornea in different quadrants with a sterile filament (e.g., 6-0 silk suture). Alternatively, artificial tears can be instilled in either eye, and the amount of subjective sensation compared.
- If the direct ophthalmoscope is positioned about 50 cm from the eye, the red reflex can be examined. A central opacity in the red reflex may suggest a cataract. Posterior subcapsular cataracts in a young patient without history of diabetes mellitus or trauma may suggest neurofibromatosis type 2.
- Digital palpation through the closed eyelids can sometimes suggest markedly elevated intraocular pressure, but usually this is an inaccurate estimate. To better assess the intraocular pressure, a Perkins tonometer or Tono-Pen

can be borrowed from most emergency rooms, or from the ophthalmology operating room in the hospital. A vomiting patient complaining of a painful eye with a cloudy cornea and mid-dilated pupil suggests angle closure glaucoma.

■ Corneal Exposure

- In patients with corneal exposure, lubrication is essential. In ambulatory patients, lubricating drops can be used six times a day. If lubricating eyedrops are required more often than six times, preservative-free formulations can also be purchased over the counter. Lubricating ointment is a more effective moisturizer than drops, but it blurs the vision. For this reason many patients choose to use lubricating ointment only at bedtime.
- In patients with prolonged inability to protect their cornea, suggest using maximal lubrication, eye glasses, and humidifier, and consider suggesting tarsorrhaphy, punctal occlusion, Tegaderm™ transparent dressing[5]/moisture chambers, Lacrisert® moisture pellets, botulinum ptosis, external lid load weight (stuck on with double-sided tape), or gold weight implantation. Eyelid weights work by gravity. Therefore, if weighting down the upper lid, the patient must sleep with the head elevated.
- In a patient with poor eyelid closure, do not use a cloth eye patch. Cloth patches will abrade or desiccate the cornea. Instead, instill lubricating ointment and tape the eye closed or use a moisture chamber or intravenous plastic dressing (e.g., Tegaderm™) over the affected eye.

■ Fundus Examination

- *Papilledema* (nerve fiber layer edema) is bilateral optic disk edema from presumed increased intracranial pressure. Papilledema is caused by orthograde axoplasmic flow stasis at the optic nerve head. Patients with papilledema usually have retained central visual acuity, in contrast to the acuity loss in ischemic optic neuropathy and most cases of optic neuritis. The blood pressure should be checked in all patients with suspected papilledema, to exclude malignant hypertension. Usually diffuse fundus hemorrhages will accompany malignant hypertension, but these may be difficult to detect on direct ophthalmoscopy of patients with undilated pupils.
  - A modified Frisen scale can be used to clinically grade papilledema[6] (**Table 10.1**).
  - Optical coherence tomography (OCT) is akin to an optical ultrasound, and provides a more objective measure of the nerve fiber layer height, and the

Table 10.1   Modified Frisen Scale for Papilledema Grading[6]

Grade	Definition/Findings
0	Normal optic disk
I	Minimal papilledema: subtle C-shaped halo of disk edema with a normal temporal disk margin
II	Low-degree papilledema: circumferential halo of disk edema
III	Moderate papilledema: obscuration of one or more segments of the major blood vessels leaving the disk
IV	Marked papilledema: partial obscuration of a segment of major blood vessel on the disk
V	Severe papilledema: partial or total obscuration of all blood vessels on the disk

Note: for further information, go to http://content.lib.utah.edu/utils/getfile/collection/EHSL-Moran -Neuro-opth/id/140/filename/88.pdf.

progression of papilledema. In patients with papilledema and decreased retinal nerve fiber layer depth on OCT, it may be difficult to distinguish resolution of papilledema from atrophy of the nerve fiber layer. OCT analysis of the retinal nerve fiber layer and retinal ganglion cell layer in papilledema can be associated with misleading artifacts due to layer segmentation failures.[7]

o Despite OCT, distinguishing papilledema from pseudopapilledema may be difficult unless surface disk drusen or peripapillary nerve fibers can be identified. Further advances in OCT may enable axonal diameters to be accurately measured, thus facilitating a more definitive determination of subtle papilledema.

o OCT testing is most helpful when the measurements are normal. Structural measurements of the optic nerve in and of themselves may not be adequate for diagnosis. OCT measurements should be interpreted in light of severity and duration of vision loss, eye findings, perimetry, magnetic resonance imaging (MRI) scan, and prior OCT if available.

• Peripapillary retinochoroidal collaterals (often inappropriately called "optociliary shunt") may be seen with optic nerve sheath meningioma, optic nerve glioma, and chronic papilledema (**Fig. 10.3**). However, retinochoroidal collaterals are not specific for optic nerve tumors and are more commonly seen with central retinal vein occlusion.

• Nonarteritic ischemic optic neuropathy is a common age-related optic neuropathy, attributed to an ischemic spiral in an optic nerve that usually has a small cup/disk ratio. Bilateral sequential non-arteritic ischemic optic neuropathy more frequently causes the appearance of a unilateral swollen disk with contralateral disk pallor (**Fig. 10.4**), than does Foster Kennedy syndrome

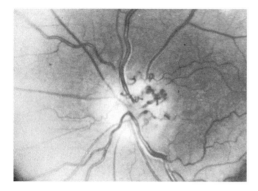

Fig. 10.3 Example of retinochoroidal collaterals.

(e.g., olfactory groove meningioma with ipsilateral optic atrophy and contralateral papilledema).

■ Orbit

- Enophthalmos may occur following orbital fracture, scirrhous metastatic carcinoma of the orbit (e.g., breast), and after ventriculoperitoneal shunting in childhood[8] (see also Chapter 20).
- Proptosis is a much more common presentation of orbital disease. An exophthalmometer can be used to measure proptosis, but globe protrusion can be easily estimated on overhead or malar view examination of the orbits. It is often useful to check for decreased orbital compliance (decreased retropulsion) by digital palpation through the closed eyelids. The globe is usually displaced opposite to the direction of the orbital tumor (displacement). Everting the eyelids may reveal fornix lesions.

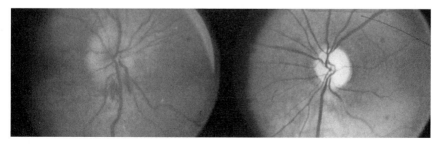

Fig. 10.4 Pseudo–Foster Kenney syndrome from bilateral sequential non-arteritic ischemic optic neuropathy, showing the appearance of a unilateral swollen disk with contralateral disk pallor.

- Spontaneous orbital pulsations may be seen with carotid cavernous fistulas, following removal of the orbital roof, and with sphenoid wing dysplasia (e.g., neurofibromatosis).
- The most common cause of unilateral or bilateral proptosis in an adult patient is thyroid-associated (Graves') orbitopathy. There is often lid retraction, conjunctival injection, and abnormal thyroid-stimulating hormone (TSH) blood test. The extraocular muscles may be enlarged characteristically with tendon sparing and preferential involvement of the inferior rectus and medial rectus muscles.
- High-flow carotid cavernous fistulas are rarely mistaken for Graves' disease due to their dramatic presentation and history of antecedent trauma. However, low-flow fistulas (dural arteriovenous fistulas [dAVFs]) usually seen in elderly hypertensive patients, may be mistaken for Graves' disease. The conjunctival injection of thyroid-associated orbitopathy is usually over the recti muscles. The conjunctival injection and episcleral venous dilation of a fistula extends 360 degrees around the eye and up to the limbus.
- The most common primary orbital malignancy in an adult is non-Hodgkin's lymphoma. On lid eversion, conjunctival "salmon patch" lesions may be seen in some cases. The orbit scan shows an infiltrative lesion that molds like putty with surrounding structures. The presentation of orbital lymphoma is usually indolent, and there is no orbital bone erosion.
- The differential diagnosis of well-circumscribed intraconal orbital tumors includes cavernous hemangioma, hemangiopericytoma/solitary fibrous tumor, schwannoma, neurofibroma, and fibrous histiocytoma.
- Fibrous dysplasia may be difficult to distinguish from meningioma. On imaging, meningioma may show a feathered bony surface, with a more homogeneous appearance, and with a dural tail and soft tissue changes. In contrast, fibrous dysplasia may be somewhat heterogeneous with smooth cortical boundaries. Rarely, fibrous dysplasia and meningioma may coexist. Prostate metastases to the orbital bone and occasionally metastatic breast cancer can mimic meningioma involving the orbital bones. The most common orbital metastases are lung cancer in men and breast cancer in women.
- Optic nerve sheath meningiomas are characterized by "tram track" appearance on axial imaging and "target sign" on coronal imaging. When sheath meningiomas cause vision loss or visual field loss, radiation therapy is recommended. Optic nerve gliomas characteristically show fusiform or globular enlargement of the optic nerve, and classically display sagittal kinking. Optic nerve gliomas in children are often associated with neurofibromatosis type 1 (NF1), and have much better prognosis than adult-onset malignant astrocytomas. The malignant astrocytomas of the optic nerve may present with the appearance of central retinal vein occlusion, and vision loss is usually severe and progressive.

- Orbital sarcoid can sometimes masquerade as optic nerve sheath meningioma or optic nerve glioma.[9]

■ Motility

- Extraocular motility and smooth pursuit eye movements can be examined by asking the patient to follow the examiner's finger or pen. The horizontal, vertical, and diagonal ocular rotations of the two eyes can be compared.

Monocular Diplopia

In monocular diplopia, the patient sees double even if one eye is occluded. Monocular diplopia should resolve when a patient looks through a pinhole. Causes of monocular diplopia include uncorrected astigmatism, dry eyes, cataract, and epiretinal membrane (wrinkling of the retina).

- Cerebral diplopia/polyopia attributed to cortical disease is uncommon, and cannot be eliminated even with pinhole occlusion.

Binocular Diplopia

Binocular diplopia is due to a misalignment of the visual axes from either nerve deficits or mechanical restriction. The diplopia should resolve if either eye is covered.

- Cranial nerve IV palsy is characterized by a head tilt to the shoulder opposite to the side of the palsy with vertical, diagonal, or torsional binocular diplopia. When the head is tilted toward the palsied eye, the affected eye may elevate markedly (Bielschowsky head tilt test). Checking the ocular alignment in different positions of gaze (three-step test) can help confirm a superior oblique palsy. With a right CN IV palsy, there is usually over-elevation of the right eye when the patient looks up and to the left, and less depression of the right eye when the patient looks down and to the left. Posttraumatic CN IV palsies are often bilateral. Dissection of the medial orbital periosteum as part of a surgical approach to the anterior cranial base,[10] and operations in the region of the tentorium can result in CN IV palsy.
- CN VI palsy results in esotropia, not exotropia. There is horizontal binocular diplopia more pronounced in the distance and on lateral gaze. In any patient with new-onset sixth nerve palsy, exclude papilledema and trigeminal nerve involvement.
- In cases of complete CN III palsy, there is a complete ptosis, and patients will not complain of diplopia unless they lift the ptotic eyelid. When patients

with oculomotor nerve palsy do notice diplopia, it is usually with diagonal separation. Compressive or posttraumatic oculomotor nerve palsies may result in later aberrant regeneration, such as lid-gaze synkinesis or pupil-gaze synkinesis. The most common lid-gaze synkinesis is elevation of the ptotic eyelid with attempted adduction, or infraduction of the palsied eye.

- Nerve palsies may be difficult to diagnose in the setting of orbital fractures because there may be periorbital swelling or mechanical entrapment of the extraocular muscles. If the patient fixates with the palsied eye due to contralateral amblyopia, the motility patterns may be confusing. Lesions at the orbital apex, cavernous sinus, or brainstem may result in multiple cranial nerve palsies. Myasthenia gravis can mimic almost any motility deficits.

- Ocular neuromyotonia is an uncommon cause of intermittent binocular diplopia, which can occur after parasellar external beam radiation and Gamma Knife radiosurgery.[11] Patients may report that their eyes are intermittently "stuck" in certain positions. A possible mechanism for neuromyotonia may be an injury that causes segmental demyelination, axonal hyperexcitability, and spasms of the extraocular muscles.

- Another uncommon cause of diplopia, seen in patients with complete bitemporal hemianopsia and phoria, is "hemifield slide." The loss of corresponding retinal areas between the two eyes from the bitemporal hemianopsia makes it difficult for the patient to fuse the two eyes together, and if there is an underlying phoria, objects may appear distorted along the vertical midline.

- The medical management of diplopia includes patching, tape occlusion of glasses, Fresnel prisms (stick-on prisms), and prisms ground into the spectacles. Sometimes spread of comitance over time will modestly improve the patient's alignment. Possible explanations for spread of comitance include a change in the elasticity (spasticity) of the extraocular muscles caused by the prolonged strabismus, and neural recalibration.

- Botulinum toxin injection in the antagonist of the palsied muscle can sometimes be of benefit. Strabismus surgery for paralytic strabismus can be performed 9 to 12 months later, if no substantial improvement in the ocular alignment is documented. The primary objective of strabismus surgery is to improve ocular alignment in the straight-ahead (primary) position. A secondary objective is to maximize the range of eye movement without binocular diplopia. Prisms are often combined with strabismus surgery.

- Complete CN III palsies are difficult to surgically rehabilitate because several extraocular muscles are involved. Frontalis sling ptosis repair of complete third nerve palsy may result in marked corneal drying, especially when Bell's phenomenon has been lost.

- CNs VI and IV palsies have a higher surgical success rate because only one muscle is involved. The remaining extraocular muscles can sometimes be transposed to provide vectorial force in the direction of the palsied muscle.

■ Nystagmus and Oscillatory Movements

- Nystagmus is an involuntary, repetitive eye movement. The ocular oscillations are initiated by slow eye movements that drive the eye away from the target.
- Bruns nystagmus is a form of nystagmus that occurs with eccentric gaze, in patients with large cerebellopontine angle (CPA) tumors (diameter > 3.5 cm) that compress the lateral brainstem.[12] There is a low-frequency, large-amplitude horizontal nystagmus when the patient looks toward the side of the lesion, attributed to defective gaze holding from compression of the cerebellar flocculus (neural integrator). When the patient looks away from the side of the lesion there is a high-frequency, small-amplitude nystagmus due to peripheral vestibular imbalance.
- Downbeat nystagmus occurs from lesions that compromise the vestibulo-cerebellum with defective vertical gaze holding. There is a slow upward drift of the eyes and corrective downward saccade. Structural lesions that cause downbeat nystagmus are often located at the cervical–medullary junction and include Chiari type I malformation, tumors at the foramen magnum, and platybasia.
- Convergence retraction nystagmoid movements sometimes occur with dorsal midbrain syndrome (Parinaud's syndrome). The eyes will bilaterally converge, and retract into the orbits with attempted upward saccades.
- Seesaw nystagmus, in which one eye rotates down and out while the other rotates up and in during a half cycle, with reversal in the next half cycle, is occasionally associated with parasellar tumors. It is thought that the chiasmal lesion impairs the subcortical pathway to the flocculus and inferior olivary nucleus.
- Patients with superior oblique myokymia may describe episodic tilting. The eye movements may be induced by looking down and in on the affected side. Rarely, midbrain astrocytoma can cause a movement disorder similar to superior oblique myokymia.
- *Spasmus nutans* usually occurs in the first year of life and is an intermittent, fine, shimmering eye movement that can be conjugate, disconjugate, disjunctive, or monocular. It is often accompanied by torticollis and head nodding. Most cases of spasmus nutans are benign and resolve with visual maturation. However, cases of chiasmal glioma and third ventricular tumor have been reported with spasmus nutans.

■ Radiation-Induced Optic Neuropathy

- Radiation-induced optic neuropathy (RION) can result in irreversible, severe vision loss months to years after radiation to the brain. Risk factors for RION include diabetes mellitus, older patients, and patients who have received prior chemotherapy. RION typically presents with acute, painless, and sometimes transient vision loss in one or both eyes, with peak onset at 1.5 years posttreatment. T1-weighted enhanced MRI may show marked enhancement of the optic nerves and chiasm.

- One study about fractionated stereotactic radiotherapy of benign anterior skull base tumors found that RION occurred in 10% of patients with skull base meningioma and 13% of patients with pituitary adenoma after treatment.[13]
- The long-term risk of RION in patients having single-fraction stereotactic radiosurgery (Gamma Knife) for benign skull base tumors is low (0–14%) if the dose to the anterior visual pathway is less than 12 Gy.[14,15]
- The treatment of RION is difficult. Systemic steroids, anticoagulants, and early hyperbaric oxygen have been suggested. The role of anti–vascular endothelial growth factor (VEGF) treatments such as bevacizumab requires further investigation.[16,17]
- The long-term effect of carbon-12 radiation for chordoma and chondrosarcoma remains the same, but electroretinogram and cortical potentials suggest a beneficial effect on visual pathways in the short term.[18]

■ Intraoperative Protection of the Eyes

- Many simple maneuvers can prevent ocular morbidity during skull base surgery. If the patient is positioned prone, ensure that there is no pressure on the globes. At the start of all surgical cases lubricate the corneas and tape the eyes shut. If the eyes are covered by a drape, use a sterile marking pen to diagram the eyes, to remind surgical assistants not to put pressure over the eyes. If operating on the orbit, the extraocular muscles can be identified, looped, and protected. If retrobulbar hemorrhage occurs during a neurosurgical operation, perform lateral canthotomy with cantholysis, and instil pressure-lowering eyedrops. If intraoperative facial nerve damage is suspected, a temporary or permanent tarsorrhaphy, with or without gold weight implantation, can be completed prior to the patient awakening.

■ References

Boldfaced references are of particular importance.

1. Colenbrander A, De Laey JJ. The International Council of Ophthalmology: vision requirements for driving safety with emphasis on individual assessment. February 2006. Available from: http://www.icoph.org/downloads/visionfordriving.pdf.
2. **Stacy RC, Jakobiec FA, Lessell S, Cestari DM. Monocular nasal hemianopia from atypical sphenoid wing meningioma. J Neuroophthalmol 2010;30:160–163**

3. Danesh-Meyer HV, Papchenko T, Savino PJ, Law A, Evans J, Gamble GD. In vivo retinal nerve fiber layer thickness measured by optical coherence tomography predicts visual recovery after surgery for parachiasmal tumors. Invest Ophthalmol Vis Sci 2008;49:1879–1885

4. Ranabir S, Baruah MP. Pituitary apoplexy. Indian J Endocrinol Metab 2011;15(Suppl 3):S188–S196

5. Airiani S, Braunstein RE, Kazim M, Schrier A, Auran JD, Srinivasan BD. Tegaderm transparent dressing (3M) for the treatment of chronic exposure keratopathy. Ophthal Plast Reconstr Surg 2003;19:75–76

6. Scott CJ, Kardon RH, Lee AG, Frisén L, Wall M. Diagnosis and grading of papilledema in patients with raised intracranial pressure using optical coherence tomography vs clinical expert assessment using a clinical staging scale. Arch Ophthalmol 2010;128:705–711

7. Kardon R. Optical coherence tomography in papilledema: what am I missing? J Neuroophthalmol 2014;34(Suppl):S10–S17

8. Bernardini FP, Rose GE, Cruz AA, Priolo E. Gross enophthalmos after cerebrospinal fluid shunting for childhood hydrocephalus: the "silent brain syndrome". Ophthal Plast Reconstr Surg 2009;25:434–436

9. Ing EB, Garrity JA, Cross SA, Ebersold MJ. Sarcoid masquerading as optic nerve sheath meningioma. Mayo Clin Proc 1997;72:38–43

10. Grabe HM, McKean EL, Eggenberger ER, Trobe JD. Persistent diplopia and superior oblique muscle dysfunction following dissection of the orbital periosteum in cranial base surgery. Br J Ophthalmol 2013;97:1330–1332

11. Much JW, Weber ED, Newman SA. Ocular neuromyotonia after gamma knife stereotactic radiation therapy. J Neuroophthalmol 2009;29:136–139

12. Lloyd SK, Baguley DM, Butler K, Donnelly N, Moffat DA. Bruns' nystagmus in patients with vestibular schwannoma. Otol Neurotol 2009;30:625–628

13. Astradsson A, Wiencke AK, Munck af Rosenschold P, et al. Visual outcome after fractionated stereotactic radiation therapy of benign anterior skull base tumors. J Neurooncol 2014;118:101–108

14. Leavitt JA, Stafford SL, Link MJ, Pollock BE. Long-term evaluation of radiation-induced optic neuropathy after single-fraction stereotactic radiosurgery. Int J Radiat Oncol Biol Phys 2013;87:524–527

15. Pollock BE, Link MJ, Leavitt JA, Stafford SL. Dose-volume analysis of radiation-induced optic neuropathy after single-fraction stereotactic radiosurgery. Neurosurgery 2014;75:456–460, discussion 460

16. Finger PT. Anti-VEGF bevacizumab (Avastin) for radiation optic neuropathy. Am J Ophthalmol 2007;143:335–338

17. Avery RA, Hwang EI, Jakacki RI, Packer RJ. Marked recovery of vision in children with optic pathway gliomas treated with bevacizumab. JAMA Ophthalmol 2014;132:111–114

18. Carozzo S, Schardt D, Narici L, Combs SE, Debus J, Sannita WG. Electrophysiological monitoring in patients with tumors of the skull base treated by carbon-12 radiation therapy. Int J Radiat Oncol Biol Phys 2013;85:978–983

11 Principles of Anesthesia in Skull Base Surgery

■ Basic Pathophysiological Consideration

Intracranial Pressure

Normal values of intracranial pressure (ICP) range from 3 to 15 mmHg (~ 5–20 cmH$_2$O). Two physiological mechanisms tend to limit the increase in ICP as the tumor increases in size:

- Displacement of intracranial blood volume by increasing venous outflow or reducing cerebral blood flow (CBF)
- Displacement of cerebrospinal fluid (CSF) from cranium to spinal subarachnoid space or by increasing CSF reabsorption

However, beyond a certain threshold, if intracranial contents continue to increase in volume, the ability to compensate is impaired and ICP increases steeply.[1–3]

Importance

Raised ICP is a common feature in skull base tumors that are:

- Large or cause significant edema and therefore create a large mass effect
- Obstruct CSF pathways and lead to obstructive hydrocephalus

Understanding this dynamic is critical for a safe anesthetic approach in skull base surgery. Symptoms and signs of raised ICP should be always identified during the preoperative patient evaluation (**Table 11.1**).

Carbon Dioxide

Carbon dioxide (CO$_2$) is the most potent cerebral vasodilator, and the manipulation of arterial carbon dioxide tension (partial pressure of carbon dioxide in arterial gas, Paco$_2$) results in modification of the CBF and the cerebral blood volume (CBV).

Table 11.1   Symptoms of Raised Intracranial Pressure (ICP) in Skull Base Tumors

Raised ICP related
- Headache (usually worse in the morning)
- Nausea and vomiting
- Papilledema
- Drowsiness/impairment of consciousness/somnolence
- Abnormal breathing pattern
- Hypertension + bradycardia
- Cushing's ulcer (esophageal, gastric, duodenal)

Other
- First-time seizure
- Difficulty with balance and coordination
- Dizziness
- Change in personality
- Weakness or loss of sensation in an arm or leg
- Facial pain, twitching, or paralysis
- Hearing loss
- Tinnitus (ringing in the ears)
- Double vision or vision loss
- Difficult in swallowing
- Speech difficulties
- Hoarseness

Importance

Hyperventilation induces hypocapnia, which decreases CBF, CBV, and ICP. The goal of a short-term temporary and therapeutic hyperventilation is generally to maintain partial pressure of carbon dioxide (Pco_2) in the range of 25 to 35 mmHg.[4,5] **Hyperventilation** is often used intraoperatively to produce brain relaxation, reduce ICP, and facilitate surgical exposure.

- There is no evidence that an aggressive hyperventilation ($Paco_2 < 25$ mmHg) offers an advantage over a more moderate hypocapnia, and it should be avoided because it has been shown to produce cerebral ischemia.[6]
- Following removal of the tumor, generally normocarbia (Pco_2 35–40 mmHg) is used to enable a return of normal cerebral circulation, to identify areas of poor hemostasis, and to enable normal brain to gradually reexpand into the surgical cavity.

Autoregulation

Autoregulation is the ability of the cerebral circulation to maintain a constant CBF by altering cerebrovascular resistance (CVR) despite variation in cerebral

Table 11.2   Other Factors Affecting Cerebral Blood Flow (CBF)

- Hematocrit
- Sympathetic tone
- β_1 stimulation: vasodilation
- α_2 stimulation: vasoconstriction
- Elevated central venous pressure
- Temperature
- Increased local metabolic activity (e.g., nitric oxide)
- High blood pressure

perfusion pressure (CPP). CBF is directly related to CPP and is remarkably stable over a wide range of mean arterial pressure (MAP). CPP is usually > 70 mmHg. However, autoregulation has limits that are usually cited as 60 and 150 mmHg.[7,8] Above and below these limits, CBF is passively dependent on MAP.

Importance

Both intracranial pathology (e.g., brain tumor, trauma, hypoxia, hypercapnia) and anesthetic agent (e.g., volatile agent in a dose-dependent way) may impair autoregulation and compromise CPP through effects on MAP or ICP. Other factors affecting CBF are presented in **Table 11.2**.

Hemodynamic Stability

Based on the physiological cerebral dynamics, an optimal blood pressure and heart rate management plays an important role in preventing major intraoperative and postoperative complications.

Importance

- The key goal is always to avoid severe variations in blood pressure, either high or low, during induction of anesthesia, at the time of intubation, during head-holder pins fixation, throughout the procedure, and at the time of extubation. **Hypotension** can lead to ischemia in areas of impaired autoregulation, whereas **hypertension** increases the risk for vasogenic edema and hemorrhage. The management of hypertension perioperatively always requires consideration of the effect of such treatment on intracranial dynamics and cardiovascular function. For example, in a patient with hypertension due to raised ICP for a tumor pressing on the brainstem, an acute normalization of blood pressure might cause worsening of a neurologic deficit.

- Heart rate and rhythm monitoring is critical during skull base surgery. Episodes of hypotension, hypertension, bradycardia, tachycardia, and extrasystoles can frequently occur during skull base surgery because of the proximity of the tumor to the brainstem (e.g., tachycardia, hypertension), fifth cranial nerve (e.g., tachycardia, hypertension, extrasystoles), tenth cranial nerve (e.g., bradycardia, hypotension), and the globe or orbital contents (trigeminal-vagal response with hypotension, bradycardia).

- Of particular note is the **trigeminocardiac reflex** (TCR) that can occur during procedures at the anterior, middle, and posterior skull base.[9] The TCR has been defined as a drop in MAP and heart rate of more than 20% compared with the baseline values before the stimulus and coinciding with the manipulation around the trigeminal nerve or the distribution of the trigeminal nerve branches.[10] Although TCR is rare (it has been reported to be in the range of 1.6 to 2.1%),[11] transient bradycardia, hypotension, or asystole can occur regardless of whether there is pressure on the brainstem during posterior fossa meningioma surgery.[12] Clear communication between the surgery and anesthesia teams is crucial if any of these signs occurs; tumor manipulation should be temporary stopped, and blood pressure or dysrhythmia treated if required, although they usually subside with interruption of the stimulus.

■ Preoperative Assessment

Given the complexity of most skull base surgeries, accurate and detailed preoperative assessment is crucial for effective and safe neuroanesthesia care. The clinical evaluation of patients with skull base tumors should be used to identify patients at greater risk of perioperative complications. Clear communication within the whole team in the operating room (e.g., surgeons, anesthetist, and nurses) and those outside the operating room (e.g., preoperative endocrinologists and the intensive care unit) is critical.

Symptoms Evaluation

Symptoms may vary according to the tumor location (e.g., meningioma, vestibular schwannoma, pituitary adenoma, chordoma), size, tumor growth rate, and involvement of adjacent structures, such as the brainstem, cranial nerves and arteries. Focal or global neurologic deficits should be clearly documented preoperatively and symptoms of raised ICP or seizures noted and accounted for by the anesthesia technique (**Table 11.1**).

Table 11.3   Skull Base Tumor: Symptoms Related to Pituitary's Hormones Level Changes

- Round face
- Disproportionate face, hands, and feet
- Tall stature
- Obesity
- Thin skin
- Joint pains
- Excess sweating
- Easy bruising
- Stretch marks
- Hypertension
- Hypokalemia, hypernatremia
- Diabetes mellitus

Hormones Secretion Assessment

Pituitary Tumors

Failure to recognize hypocortisolism, Cushing's disease, or acromegaly preoperatively can have serious consequences.

- **Acromegaly** can be associated with systemic hypertension, left ventricular hypertrophy, and diastolic dysfunction.[13] Growth hormone hypersecretion can cause potentially difficult airway management: enlarged and thickened tongue (macroglossia), hypertrophy of the laryngeal soft tissue, and epiglottis and prognathism with malocclusion. These patients also have marked bony and soft tissue hypertrophy, which can lead to excessive bleeding during surgery.
- **Cushing's disease** can be associated with hypertension, fluid retention, hyperglycemia, osteopenia, and obesity.[14] Pituitary adenomas in Cushing's disease may be quite small, and the surgical approach, particularly in the case of unoccluded intercavernous sinuses, may be associated with excessive bleeding[15] **(Table 11.3)**.
- All patients undergoing pituitary surgery are at risk of developing diabetes insipidus due to a perioperative antidiuretic hormone deficiency (see Chapter 9, page 239), but this is not usually encountered in the operating room.

Neurologic Assessment

A careful neurologic examination is of crucial importance, in particular to evaluate:

- The level of consciousness (i.e., is the patient alert and oriented, or somnolent and drowsy?)
- The presence or absence of baseline increased ICP **(Table 11.1)**

- Reactivity of the pupils
- Limb strength and movement
- Extent of neurologic deficits

In patients with clinically elevated ICP it may be necessary to prescribe an aggressive preoperative therapy with steroids and hyperosmolar agents to reduce edema; this therapy typically is started by the neurosurgeon.

Airway and Cardiorespiratory Assessment

Assessment of the airway and cardiorespiratory system is important in planning a smooth anesthesia induction and emergence, avoiding any maneuver that raises ICP or causes airway irritability, bronchospasm, laryngospasm, or cardiovascular instability.

Critical for airway management is the prospective assessment of whether or not the patient's airway potentially poses difficulties.[16] In particular, the anesthesiologist needs to be experienced with alternative methods of intubation (e.g., tracheotomy, submental orotracheal intubation) that have been described in the literature for transfacial or transmaxillary approaches to the cranial base (e.g., chondrosarcomas), when neither nasal nor orotracheal intubation is indicated for limiting the exposure of the cranial base.[17,18]

Blood Work

Preoperative blood work should include an assessment of preoperative hemoglobin, international normalized ratio (INR), glucose, CO_2, and, if necessary, hormonal values such as 8 AM cortisol, free thyroxine (T_4), growth hormone, and insulin-like growth factor-1 (IGF-1: somatomedin C).

Diagnostic Imaging

Diagnostic brain imaging should be assessed to identify the type of tumor; its location and vascularity; the evidence of mass effect, midline shift, hydrocephalus, or edema; and the amount of space around the basal cisterns and posterior fossa.

■ Intraoperative Management

General Problems

Intracranial Pressure Management

In the operating room, raised ICP may be controlled by the use of any of the following[19,20]:

- Head-up position
- Free venous drainage
- Hyperventilation
- Anesthesia agent (e.g., reduce volatile anesthetic, change to intravenous anesthetic)
- Hyperosmolar agents (e.g., mannitol/hypertonic saline)
- Drainage of CSF
- Avoidance of the development of ischemic or hemorrhagic brain by continuous retraction or vascular injury

Fluid Management

Fluid optimization is crucial in neuroanesthesia. Patients undergoing skull base surgery frequently present with coexisting endocrine and electrolytes disorders (e.g., diabetes insipidus, Cushing's disease, fluid retention), and in these patients the choice of fluid is determined by the nature of the disorder involved.

- There is no specific evidence to support the optimal use of crystalloids over colloids in terms of patient outcome.[21]
- Maintenance of normal osmolarity or mild hyperosmolarity of plasma is desirable, avoiding hypo-osmolar and dextrose-containing solution. Normal saline (0.9% NaCl) commonly is the fluid of choice because it is slightly hyperosmolar (308 mOsm) and is thought to attenuate formation of brain edema.[22]
- Fluid management strategies need to be individualized and directed by an understanding of the underlying pathophysiological mechanisms. These patients often experience rapid changes in intravascular volume caused by positioning, administration of diuretics, bleeding, or marked cerebral edema. For many years, a restrictive fluid management in neuroanesthesia has been the treatment of choice.[23] Recent evidence has changed this approach completely.[24]
- The goals for a rational fluid administration should be to maintain an adequate cardiac output and electrolytes balance; to replace urinary output, blood loss, and insensible loss; and to avoid excessive fluid resuscitation.[25]

Seizure Prevention

Patients with skull base tumors often present first with headache and seizure, primarily due to increased ICP by the growing tumor. Seizure activity is associated with increased neuronal activity, increased CBF and CBV, and consequently increased ICP.[26]

- **Seizure prophylaxis** is not typically considered as part of the anesthesia plan; the anesthesiologist needs to be aware of whether the patient has re-

ceived (or needs to receive prophylactically) antiseizure medications perioperatively to prevent potential cerebral injuries.

* **Anticonvulsant agents** such as phenytoin may decrease the duration of action of non-depolarizing muscle relaxant.[27,28]

Steroid Supplementation

Steroids can be used to replace physiological levels lost due to interruption of
the hypothalamic-pituitary axis (e.g., craniopharyngioma or pituitary macroadenoma) or as a means of reducing cerebral edema.

* For replacement, **hydrocortisone** 25 or 50 mg IV is often used perioperatively (see also Chapter 9).
* For peritumoral edema, to reduce swelling (not the size of the tumor in itself), to decrease ICP, and to improve associated neurologic deficit, **dexamethasone** 2 to 10 mg IV is considered most often.[29,30]

Hyperosmolar Agents

Osmotic agents are commonly used intraoperatively to reduce ICP, improve
cerebral perfusion, and facilitate surgical exposure before opening of the dura
or as needed.

* There is little evidence to support the use of one specific agent (e.g., mannitol vs hypertonic saline).[31]
* When using **mannitol** (0.25 to 1 g/kg, 15 to 20 minutes before opening of the
dura mater), the anesthesiologist needs to consider the osmotic-mediated
diuresis that can result in important intravascular volume-depletion, hypotension, and imbalance of electrolytes such as sodium and potassium.
* The use of **hypertonic saline** (3 mL/kg; the optimal dose is not known[32]) is
effective in reducing ICP without the disadvantage of subsequent osmotic
diuresis. However, plasma osmolarity, sodium concentration, and renal function need to be carefully monitored during administration.[33]
* Both mannitol and hypertonic saline should be used carefully in a patient
with a history of congestive heart failure because they induce a transient
increase in intravascular volume.
* The use of **furosemide** (0.2 to 0.5 mg/kg) is not supported by the evidence
and is at the discretion of the anesthetist.[34]

Glucose Control

Both hyperglycemia and hypoglycemia should be avoided because they have
been demonstrated to have adverse metabolic and cerebral ischemic effects.[35]

- There is no definitive evidence to support a very "tight" glucose control in critically ill patients,[36] and whether it improves outcome in elective craniotomy is yet to be proven.
- A perioperative continuous insulin infusion protocol might be justifiable only in selected cases assessed by an endocrinologist preoperatively in those skull base tumors (e.g., some pituitary tumors) that are associated with diabetes, or in patients with insulin-dependent diabetes.

Pain Control

Pain control postcraniotomy remains challenging and controversial, as there are no large-scale trials determining effective treatments and side effects.[37] In transsphenoidal approaches, postoperative pain is usually moderate, and it can be controlled with modest doses of opioids and acetaminophen.

- A **multimodal analgesia** approach has been proposed in order to reduce opioids' side effects and achieve an effective pain control.[38]
- Measures to decrease postoperative pain include scalp nerves block, and incision line and pin-site infiltration with bupivacaine or ropivacaine.[39,40]
- Typically modest intravenous doses of **morphine** (10–15 mg) or **hydromorphone** (1–2 mg) are safe without a significant increase of their adverse effects or delayed emergence from anesthesia.
- Acetaminophen can be used safely in addition to opioids.
- The use of nonsteroidal anti-inflammatory drugs remains controversial because they may contribute to bleeding or postoperative renal failure.[41]

Nausea and Emesis Prevention

Women and any patient undergoing infratentorial surgery are at particularly high risk for postoperative nausea and vomiting.[42]

- **Prophylactic antiemetics,** including ondansetron (4 mg) and steroids (dexamethasone 10 mg), are often administered intraoperatively to reduce the undesirable effects of vomiting.[43]
- Although there is no convincing evidence in favor of one antiemetic agent over another, it might be wise to avoid, if possible, the use of antihistamines (e.g., dimenhydrinate), which can cause drowsiness, or antidopaminergics (e.g., droperidol), which can cause extrapyramidal symptoms.
- Blood in the stomach after transsphenoidal surgery is common and can be associated with significant postoperative nausea and vomiting.[44] The use of throat packing that is placed into the oropharynx and attached onto the external surface of the patient and appropriately labeled can prevent this postoperative complication to a large degree.

Temperature Control

Measuring body temperature is now the standard-of-care during prolonged general anesthesia as the anesthesia-induced impairment of normal thermoregulatory control has been largely described.[45] Prospective randomized trials demonstrated in a variety of patient populations that even mild hypothermia might have a negative effect on immune function, coagulation, the cardiovascular system, and recovery behavior.[46]

- Skull base procedures might require prolonged surgical time and mild hypothermia may occur spontaneously.
- Endocrine disturbances can be associated with pituitary tumors and can cause temperature regulation abnormalities that are more common postoperatively.
- Brain temperature is typically 0.5°C lower than the commonly measured tympanic and esophageal temperature, but little is known about its effect during general anesthesia and craniotomy.
- Utilizing an IV fluid warming system and a forced air-warming device is helpful in minimizing heat loss in the intraoperative phase.
- The main goal is to avoid a drop in body temperature to below 36°C in the perioperative phase and the possible subsequent negative effects.
- Hyperthermia or fever is relatively rare during general anesthesia. However, acute hyperthermia has been reported as a potential complication following stereotactic radiosurgery for a large pituitary tumor.[47]

Antibiotic Prophylaxis

Antibiotic prophylaxis in craniotomy is effective in preventing surgical-site infections even in low-risk patients.[48]

- For cranial base surgery, a broad-spectrum coverage of gram-positive and gram-negative organisms for at least 48 hours is recommended.[49]

Monitoring

Standard monitors, including temperature monitoring and urine output, are generally appropriate, with the addition of a large-bore venous access and an arterial line to monitor blood pressure or drawn blood sample intraoperatively. A central venous access is rarely indicated, but should be considered if required by the patient's medical status or if the potential risk of air embolism is high.

Special Requirements

- **Cranial nerve electromyograms (EMGs):** desirable during resection of tumors involving the cranial nerves (see Chapter 3, page 89).

- **Armored EMG electrode embedded endotracheal tube**: desirable for lesions that potentially place the lower cranial nerves at risk. It is used to monitor the recurrent laryngeal nerve, a branch of the vagus nerve.[50] It is imperative that the neuroanesthesiologist be experienced in the optimal placement of this specific endotracheal tube to guarantee the correct intraoperative nerve monitoring. Somatosensory and brainstem evoked potentials have never been shown to be of benefit in improving outcomes in randomized controlled trials, although some centers use them routinely.
- **Lumbar subarachnoid catheter:** desirable for selected cases in which there is no risk of transtentorial or transforaminal herniation. Usually inserted after anesthesia induction, it can be useful to drain CSF intraoperatively and minimize brain retraction. In cases of expected CSF leakage (e.g., extended transsphenoidal approach with planned breach of the arachnoid cisterns), lumbar drainage is used to reduce the risk of postoperative CSF leak and meningitis.

Surgical Positioning

The correct position of the patient and the patient's head is crucial to facilitate an optimal exposure of the lesion while ensuring that the position is physically safe for the patient.

- Patients with skull base tumors can be placed in the supine, semilateral, lateral, prone, or sitting/semisitting position, with the head elevated.[51]
- The anesthetist often has poor access to the patient's face and airway during the procedure, so special care must be taken in securing the patient's airway, intravenous lines, and arterial line at the beginning of the procedure.
- Increased ICP, venous congestion with edema, or bleeding and airway compromise are generally the most frequent intraoperative problems that can occur as a result of incorrect patient positioning.
- Skull base surgery can be complex, and **rhabdomyolysis** can occur postoperatively due to a prolonged position. This has been reported as a highly under-recognized complication in neurosurgery that can occur particularly in patients in the lateral position, more frequent in obese patients, and it can lead to lactic acidosis and renal failure.[52,53]
- Other important **postoperative complications** related to patient positioning are peripheral neuropathies due to nerve compression, skin breakdown, and corneal abrasion. If the patient is expected to have a high likelihood of corneal exposure (e.g., from a facial nerve palsy) postoperatively, a temporary tarsorrhaphy with instilled lubrication of the cornea can prevent early postoperative corneal ulceration (see also Chapter 10, page 268).

Lateral Position

There are several methods for placing the patient into the lateral position:

- An axillary roll is positioned under the upper part of the chest to prevent pressure on and injury to axillary structures. This is a commonly used method.
- The dependent arm is allowed to rest on a well-padded arm-board placed superior to the top of the bed. This, too, is a commonly used method.
- In both of the above approaches, supports are placed along the patient's abdomen and back, paddings are positioned between and under the legs, and the patient is well strapped and taped into position.
- Two modifications of the lateral position are often used for skull base surgery, and particular attention must be paid to avoid kinking/obstruction of the endotracheal tube as well as obstruction of the venous outflow due to compression of the jugular vein:
  - **Park-bench position** (e.g., vestibular schwannoma): The trunk is rotated 15 degrees from the lateral position into the semiprone position, and the head is flexed and then rotated toward the floor.
  - **Semiprone position** (e.g. cerebellopontine angle [CPA] tumors): The head is turned down.

Prone Position

The head is typically fixed in a Sugita®, Mayfield®, or other similar head clamp in neutral position; it has to be positioned carefully to maximize venous outflow and avoid kinking of the endotracheal tube. Two bolsters usually support the chest of the patient, with the goal of avoiding or minimizing pressure on the chest, abdomen, male genitals, and breasts. Paddings are used for arms and knees; ankles are elevated to allow toes to hang freely.

- The prone position is most often used for the suboccipital midline approach and is associated with a higher risk of complications than other positions.[54] When turning the patient from the supine to the prone position, care should be taken to assess the patient for hemodynamic and respiratory changes, particularly in patients with increased ICP or mass effect on the brainstem or cerebellum.
- Although the **cardiovascular responses** to turning the patient prone have not been fully understood, data suggest that the left-ventricular ejection fraction and cardiac index may decrease, potentially causing hemodynamic instability.[55] Thus, in turning the patient to the prone position, it is important for the anesthesiologist to have a plan for disconnecting and reconnecting the monitor in an organized manner to avoid excessive "window" monitoring and to intervene promptly if necessary.
- **Prolonged prone positioning and excessive fluid administration** can sometimes be associated with venous congestion and facial edema, but more rarely with swelling of the tongue, soft palate, pharynx, and arytenoid.[56–58]

After a prolonged procedure, the presence of upper airway swelling should be ascertained when deciding whether to extubate the patient in the operating room. Although no test has been proven to have high sensitivity and specificity in recognizing postoperative upper airway edema, the cuff leak test,[59] visual inspection of the airway[60] (e.g., laryngoscopy, bronchoscopy), and spirometry[50] (e.g., flow-volume loops on the anesthetic machine) are the most common tests used to assess the risk for extubation.

- Although a rare occurrence, **retinal ischemia and blindness** have been reported, particularly in a prolonged procedure with significant hypotension and associated blood loss.[61] The risk of **air embolism** is lower in the prone or lateral positions than in the sitting position.[51]

Sitting Position

The sitting position has been used for surgery of posterior fossa tumors. It can provide an optimal surgical exposure by lowering ICP; it also promotes gravity drainage of blood and CSF. However, positioning of the patient should proceed slowly to avoid an episode of hypotension due to a decreased venous return.

- **Specific complications** related to this position include hemodynamic instability (e.g., hypotension), venous air embolism **(Table 11.4)**,[62] quadriplegia, pneumocephalus, and compressive peripheral neuropathy.[63]
- It has been suggested that absolute contraindications for this position are patients with a ventriculoatrial shunt, pulmonary hypertension, a patent foramen ovale, and symptomatic cerebral ischemia.[64]

Anesthesia Induction and Maintenance

There is no definitive evidence to suggest that one specific induction technique is the most effective. Similarly, there is no evidence to suggest that one agent is superior to another for maintenance of anesthesia in neurosurgery[34] or specifically in skull base surgery.

- The goals of anesthesia during induction include maintenance of CPP, hemodynamic stability, and airway control, as well as prevention of secondary brain injury **(Table 11.5)**.
- It is critical to guarantee a **smooth and rapid induction,** avoiding large changes in blood pressure, episodes of coughing or straining during a highly stimulating maneuver such as laryngoscopy, intubation, head pinning, and patient positioning. Usually these goals can be achieved using propofol or thiopental as induction agents, whereas etomidate and ketamine can be used occasionally only in hemodynamically unstable patients. These agents are supplemented with opioid (e.g., fentanyl and/or remifentanil), intravenous

Table 11.4   Venous Air Embolism During Skull Base Surgery

Clinical etiology
1. The head is above the level of the heart
2. Air entry through exposed venous vasculature

Clinical diagnosis
1. Cardiac dysrhythmias
2. Blood pressure fluctuation
3. Low end-tidal CO_2
4. Elevated central venous pressure readings
5. Asynchrony with the ventilator in previously adequate control ventilation
6. Surgeon may notice tiny air bubbles in the exposed field

Devices for detection available during surgery
1. Transesophageal echocardiography: high sensitivity, invasive; expertise required
2. Precordial Doppler: high sensitivity, not invasive, limitation in obese patients
3. Transcranial Doppler: high sensitivity, not invasive; expertise required
4. Esophageal stethoscope: low sensitivity, not invasive

Treatment
1. Notify the surgeon
2. Flood surgical site
3. Give oxygen 100%
4. Stop N_2O if part of the anesthesia technique
5. Lower operative site
6. Aspiration though a central venous access
7. Compression of the jugular veins
8. Cardiopulmonary support (fluid, pressors, inotropes)

lidocaine. and a muscle relaxant with different effect on CBF and the cerebral metabolic rate of oxygen ($CMRO_2$).[65]

- In patients with a large posterior fossa tumor, extensive movements of the head and neck should be avoided as medullary or spinal cord compression can occur with these maneuvers.
- **Maintenance of anesthesia** can be achieved with intravenous or inhalation agents, and the choice is largely at the discretion of the anesthetist based on experience and ability to achieve a smooth and rapid emergence at the end of the surgery.[34] Generally, the choice of short-acting agents such as remifentanil or desflurane may offer some advantage in elderly patients who are at risk for a delayed emergence from anesthesia.
- It is critical to guarantee a **stationary surgical field** throughout the procedure, particularly during a fully endoscopic endonasal approach. Being that the head is fixed in the Sugita, Mayfield, or other similar frames, any patient movement carries the risk of increased ICP, possible cervical spine injury, or

Table 11.5   Prevention of Secondary Brain Injury: Provide the Six N's

Avoid hypoxia:	Normoxia
Avoid hypercarbia:	Normocarbia
Avoid hypotension:	Normotension
Avoid hyper/hypovolemia:	Normovolemia
Avoid hyper/hypoglycemia:	Normoglycemia
Avoid hyperthermia:	Normothermia

direct intracranial injury by the use of the surgical instruments. It is important to remember that endoscopic surgery for base skull tumor can be highly stimulating (e.g., direct basal dura or trigeminal nerve irritation), and an **appropriate depth of anesthesia** must be accomplished to enable sensitive cranial nerve monitoring, avoid patient movement, and guarantee a good surgical visualization. Maintaining a low-normal range of blood pressure throughout the surgery can be helpful in improving operative conditions and in controlling bleeding due to surgical dissection and manipulation of highly vascularized structures, such as the turbinate.

- In cases in which **cranial nerve monitoring** is required intraoperatively (e.g., cranial nerve [CN] VII during CPA tumors surgery), a muscle relaxant should wear off after induction, and the patient should remain off muscle relaxants for the dissection of the cranial nerves such as the facial nerve. In addition, an intravenous anesthetic agent should be preferred, considering that inhalation agents suppress somatosensory evoked potential responses in a dose-dependent manner and are only minimally influenced by total intravenous anesthesia. Usually a combination of a low-level inhalation agent, propofol infusion, and a short-acting opioid such as remifentanil can permit good neurophysiological monitoring, providing a stable and secure level of anesthesia.

- Although it is controversial, **Valsalva maneuvers** reaching an intrathoracic pressure of 30 to 40 cmH$_2$O, are sometimes requested by the surgeon before the closure, in order to check for bleeding and CSF leak in the surgical cavity.[66,67]

Anesthesia Emergence

A smooth emergence from anesthesia without coughing, straining, and asynchrony with the ventilator is crucial to avoid arterial hypertension, bleeding in the surgical bed, brain edema, or dislodgment of the graft where used. Close and constant discussion between the anesthetist and the surgeons is also important when reaching the end of the surgery.

Step 1

It is wise to keep the patient under deep anesthesia until the closure has been completed, the anesthesiologist again has access to the head, and the head clamp has been removed.

Step 2

It is important to ascertain the presence of edema and airway swelling.[68] The use of pharyngeal packs intraoperatively is common for endoscopic procedures but might cause swelling of the tongue postoperatively.[69]

Such situations might compromise airway patency after extubation, and if necessary a cuff leak test, a fiberoptic exam of the airway, or a direct laryngoscopy to assess airway swelling should be considered. The decision to delay the extubation to allow the edema to resolve may be a prudent option in some cases. In other cases, keeping the patient intubated for no specific reason can also place the patient at significant risk of complications associated with prolonged intubation (e.g., nosocomial pneumonia, tracheostomy).

Step 3

Although the patient is still under deep anesthesia and still intubated, adequate **spontaneous ventilation should be maintained**, the cuff of the tube gently deflated, and, if the breathing remains regular, the patient can be extubated without any further stimulation. An oral airway can be positioned if needed, until the patient is more awake.

Step 4

After extubation, the goal is to keep the patient comfortable so that a postoperative neurologic evaluation can be performed.

Immediate Complications

- In rare cases of intraoperative trauma to cranial nerves or respiratory centers, postoperative airway control and ventilator support may be required.
- **Delayed emergence** is not infrequent after prolonged skull base tumor resection, and potential causes such as seizure, intracranial hematoma, pneumocephalus, hypothermia, and metabolic acidosis should be investigated.
- **Hemorrhagic complications** during and after an endoscopic endonasal approach of skull base tumors are rare but can be life-threatening due to potential lesions of the sphenopalatine arteries or internal carotid artery.[70] More frequently, immediate postoperative bleeding can be usually controlled with packing, and it is wise to assess the presence of blood in the upper airway

before extubation. An oropharyngeal pack as described earlier can be very effective in preventing aspiration of blood into the airway as well.

- Having a **good blood pressure stability** is crucial in the immediate postoperative period because hypertension may contribute to the development of postoperative edema and hematoma.[71] This complication can be very serious in particular after skull base surgery. The neurologic status of the patient can suddenly deteriorate and the patient can develop bradycardia, hypertension, and irregular or absent respiration (Cushing's triad) secondary to brainstem or cerebellum infarction or compression, and require a rapid re-intubation. Discussion with the surgeons will help the anesthetist to assess the risk of postoperative bleeding and deterioration from all these causes.

■ References

Boldfaced references are of particular importance.

1. Miller JD, Garibi J, Pickard JD. A clinical study of intracranial volume pressure relationships. Br J Surg 1973;60:316
2. Smith M. Monitoring intracranial pressure in traumatic brain injury. Anesth Analg 2008;106:240–248
3. Mokri B. The Monro-Kellie hypothesis: applications in CSF volume depletion. Neurology 2001;56:1746–1748
4. Gelb AW, Craen RA, Rao GS, et al. Does hyperventilation improve operating condition during supratentorial craniotomy? A multicenter randomized crossover trial. Anesth Analg 2008;106:585–594
5. Marsh ML, Marshall LF, Shapiro HM. Neurosurgical intensive care. Anesthesiology 1977;47:149–163
6. **Brain-Trauma Foundation: Joint Section on Neurotrauma and Critical Care. Hyperventilation. J Neurotrauma 2000;17:513–520**
7. Paulson OB, Strandgaard S, Edvinsson L. Cerebral autoregulation. Cerebrovasc Brain Metab Rev 1990;2:161–192
8. Lucas SJ, Tzeng YC, Galvin SD, Thomas KN, Ogoh S, Ainslie PN. Influence of changes in blood pressure on cerebral perfusion and oxygenation. Hypertension 2010;55:698–705
9. **Koerbel A, Gharabaghi A, Samii A, et al. Trigeminocardiac reflex during skull base surgery: mechanism and management. Acta Neurochir (Wien) 2005;147:727–732, discussion 732–733**
10. **Schaller B, Probst R, Strebel S, Gratzl O. Trigeminocardiac reflex during surgery in the cerebellopontine angle. J Neurosurg 1999;90:215–220**
11. Etezadi F, Orandi AA, Orandi AH, et al. Trigeminocardiac reflex in neurosurgical practice: An observational prospective study. Surg Neurol Int 2013;4:116
12. Usami K, Kamada K, Kunii N, Tsujihara H, Yamada Y, Saito N. Transient asystole during surgery for posterior fossa meningioma caused by activation of the trigeminocardiac reflex: three case reports. Neurol Med Chir (Tokyo) 2010;50:339–342

13. **Colao A, Ferone D, Marzullo P, Lombardi G. Systemic complications of acromegaly: epidemiology, pathogenesis, and management. Endocr Rev 2004;25(1):102–152**

14. Chabre O. [Cushing syndrome: Physiopathology, etiology and principles of therapy]. Presse Med 2014;43(4 Pt 1):376–392

15. Lake MG, Krook LS, Cruz SV. Pituitary adenomas: an overview. Am Fam Physician 2013;88:319–327

16. Apfelbaum JL, Hagberg CA, Caplan RA, et al; American Society of Anesthesiologists Task Force on Management of the Difficult Airway. Practice guidelines for management of the difficult airway: an updated report by the American Society of Anesthesiologists Task Force on Management of the Difficult Airway. Anesthesiology 2013; 118:251–270

17. Biglioli F, Mortini P, Goisis M, Bardazzi A, Boari N. Submental orotracheal intubation: an alternative to tracheotomy in transfacial cranial base surgery. Skull Base 2003;13: 189–195

18. **Sekhar LN. Surgery of the Cranial Base Tumors. New York: Raven Press; 1993**

19. Wolfe TJ, Torbey MT. Management of intracranial pressure. Curr Neurol Neurosci Rep 2009;9:477–485

20. Lang SS, Kofke WA, Stiefel MF. Monitoring and intraoperative management of elevated intracranial pressure and decompressive craniectomy. Anesthesiol Clin 2012; 30:289–310

21. Bulger EM, May S, Brasel KJ, et al; ROC Investigators. Out-of-hospital hypertonic resuscitation following severe traumatic brain injury: a randomized controlled trial. JAMA 2010;304:1455–1464

22. Tommasino C, Moore S, Todd MM. Cerebral effects of isovolemic hemodilution with crystalloid or colloid solutions. Crit Care Med 1988;16:862–868

23. Shenkin HA, Bezier HS, Bouzarth WF. Restricted fluid intake. Rational management of the neurosurgical patient. J Neurosurg 1976;45:432–436

24. Oppitz PP, Stefani MA. Acute normovolemic hemodilution is safe in neurosurgery. World Neurosurg 2013;79:719–724

25. Tommasino C. Fluids and the neurosurgical patient. Anesthesiol Clin North America 2002;20:329–346, vi vi.

26. Meldrum BCA. Metabolic consequences of seizures. In: Siegel GJ, Agranoff BW, Albers RW, et al, ed. Basic Neurochemistry: Molecular, Cellular and Medical Aspects. Philadelphia: Lippincott-Raven; 1999

27. Ornstein E, Matteo RS, Schwartz AE, Silverberg PA, Young WL, Diaz J. The effect of phenytoin on the magnitude and duration of neuromuscular block following atracurium or vecuronium. Anesthesiology 1987;67:191–196

28. Alloul K, Whalley DG, Shutway F, Ebrahim Z, Varin F. Pharmacokinetic origin of carbamazepine-induced resistance to vecuronium neuromuscular blockade in anesthetized patients. Anesthesiology 1996;84:330–339

29. **Ryken TC, McDermott M, Robinson PD, et al. The role of steroids in the management of brain metastases: a systematic review and evidence-based clinical practice guideline. J Neurooncol 2010;96:103–114**

30. Galicich JH, French LA, Melby JC. Use of dexamethasone in treatment of cerebral edema associated with brain tumors. J Lancet 1961;81:46–53

31. Fink ME. Osmotherapy for intracranial hypertension: mannitol versus hypertonic saline. Continuum (Minneap Minn) 2012;18:640–654
32. Mortazavi MM, Romeo AK, Deep A, et al. Hypertonic saline for treating raised intracranial pressure: literature review with meta-analysis. J Neurosurg 2012;116:210–221
33. **Strandvik GF. Hypertonic saline in critical care: a review of the literature and guidelines for use in hypotensive states and raised intracranial pressure. Anaesthesia 2009;64:990–1003**
34. **Todd MM. Outcomes after neuroanesthesia and neurosurgery: what makes a difference. Anesthesiol Clin 2012;30:399–408**
35. Gisselsson L, Smith ML, Siesjö BK. Hyperglycemia and focal brain ischemia. J Cereb Blood Flow Metab 1999;19:288–297
36. Kavanagh BP, McCowen KC. Clinical practice. Glycemic control in the ICU. N Engl J Med 2010;363:2540–2546
37. de Gray LC, Matta BF. Acute and chronic pain following craniotomy: a review. Anaesthesia 2005;60:693–704
38. Leslie K, Williams DL. Postoperative pain, nausea and vomiting in neurosurgical patients. Curr Opin Anaesthesiol 2005;18:461–465
39. **Bala I, Gupta B, Bhardwaj N, Ghai B, Khosla VK. Effect of scalp block on postoperative pain relief in craniotomy patients. Anaesth Intensive Care 2006;34:224–227**
40. **Garavaglia MM, Das S, Cusimano MD, et al. Anesthetic approach to high-risk patients and prolonged awake craniotomy using dexmedetomidine and scalp block. J Neurosurg Anesthesiol 2014;26:226–233**
41. Kelly KP, Janssens MC, Ross J, Horn EH. Controversy of non-steroidal anti-inflammatory drugs and intracranial surgery: et ne nos inducas in tentationem [and lead us not into temptation]? Br J Anaesth 2011;107:302–305
42. Audibert G, Vial V. [Postoperative nausea and vomiting after neurosurgery (infratentorial and supratentorial surgery)]. Ann Fr Anesth Reanim 2004;23:422–427
43. Gan TJ, Meyer T, Apfel CC, et al; Department of Anesthesiology, Duke University Medical Center. Consensus guidelines for managing postoperative nausea and vomiting. Anesth Analg 2003;97:62–71 table of contents.
44. Neufeld SM, Newburn-Cook CV. What are the risk factors for nausea and vomiting after neurosurgery? A systematic review. Can J Neurosci Nurs 2008;30:23–34
45. Sessler DI. Temperature monitoring and perioperative thermoregulation. Anesthesiology 2008;109:318–338
46. Pannen BH. [Normothermia and hypothermia from an anaesthesiological viewpoint]. Anaesthesist 2007;56:940–944
47. Kalapurakal JA, Silverman CL, Akhtar N, et al. Acute hyperthermia following stereotactic radiosurgery for pituitary adenoma. Br J Radiol 1999;72:1218–1221
48. **Korinek AM, Golmard JL, Elcheick A, et al. Risk factors for neurosurgical site infections after craniotomy: a critical reappraisal of antibiotic prophylaxis on 4,578 patients. Br J Neurosurg 2005;19:155–162**
49. Carrau RL, Snyderman C, Janecka IP, Sekhar L, Sen C, D'Amico F. Antibiotic prophylaxis in cranial base surgery. Head Neck 1991;13:311–317

50. Modrykamien AM, Gudavalli R, McCarthy K, Liu X, Stoller JK. Detection of upper airway obstruction with spirometry results and the flow-volume loop: a comparison of quantitative and visual inspection criteria. Respir Care 2009;54:474–479

51. Ruskin K, Rosenbaum SH, Rampil IJ. Fundamentals of Neuroanesthesia: A Physiologic Approach to Clinical Practice. Oxford: Oxford University Press; 2013

52. **De Tommasi C, Cusimano MD. Rhabdomyolysis after neurosurgery: a review and a framework for prevention. Neurosurg Rev 2013;36:195–202, discussion 203**

53. **Garavaglia M, Mak T, Cusimano MD, et al. Body mass index as a risk factor for increased serum lactate during craniotomy. Minerva Anestesiol 2013;79:1132–1139**

54. Rozet I, Vavilala MS. Risks and benefits of patient positioning during neurosurgical care. Anesthesiol Clin 2007;25:631–653, x

55. Toyota S, Amaki Y. Hemodynamic evaluation of the prone position by transesophageal echocardiography. J Clin Anesth 1998;10:32–35

56. Edgcombe H, Carter K, Yarrow S. Anaesthesia in the prone position. Br J Anaesth 2008;100:165–183

57. El Hassani Y, Narata AP, Pereira VM, Schaller C. A reminder for a very rare entity: massive tongue swelling after posterior fossa surgery. J Neurol Surg A Cent Eur Neurosurg 2012;73:171–174

58. Lam AM, Vavilala MS. Macroglossia: compartment syndrome of the tongue? Anesthesiology 2000;92:1832–1835

59. Ochoa ME, Marín MdelC, Frutos-Vivar F, et al. Cuff-leak test for the diagnosis of upper airway obstruction in adults: a systematic review and meta-analysis. Intensive Care Med 2009;35:1171–1179

60. Bentsianov BL, Parhiscar A, Azer M, Har-El G. The role of fiberoptic nasopharyngoscopy in the management of the acute airway in angioneurotic edema. Laryngoscope 2000;110:2016–2019

61. Ho VT, Newman NJ, Song S, Ksiazek S, Roth S. Ischemic optic neuropathy following spine surgery. J Neurosurg Anesthesiol 2005;17:38–44

62. Mirski MA, Lele AV, Fitzsimmons L, Toung TJ. Diagnosis and treatment of vascular air embolism. Anesthesiology 2007;106:164–177

63. Standefer M, Bay JW, Trusso R. The sitting position in neurosurgery: a retrospective analysis of 488 cases. Neurosurgery 1984;14:649–658

64. Porter JM, Pidgeon C, Cunningham AJ. The sitting position in neurosurgery: a critical appraisal. Br J Anaesth 1999;82:117–128

65. **Miller RD. Effects of anesthetics on cerebral blood flow and cerebral metabolic rate. In: *Miller's Anesthesia*, 7th ed. New York: Elsevier; 2007**

66. **Prabhakar H, Bithal PK, Suri A, Rath GP, Dash HH. Intracranial pressure changes during Valsalva manoeuvre in patients undergoing a neuroendoscopic procedure. Minim Invasive Neurosurg 2007;50:98–101**

67. **Wendling W, Sadel S, Jimenez D, Rosenwasser R, Buchheit W. Cardiovascular and cerebrovascular effects of the applied Valsalva manoeuvre in anaesthetized neurosurgical patients. Eur J Anaesthesiol 1994;11:81–87**

68. Figueredo-Gaspari E, Fredes-Kubrak R, Canosa-Ruiz L. [Macroglossia after surgery of the posterior fossa]. Rev Esp Anestesiol Reanim 1997;44:157–158

69. Kawaguchi M, Sakamoto T, Ohnishi H, Karasawa J. Pharyngeal packs can cause massive swelling of the tongue after neurosurgical procedures. Anesthesiology 1995;83: 434–435

70. Raymond J, Hardy J, Czepko R, Roy D. Arterial injuries in transsphenoidal surgery for pituitary adenoma; the role of angiography and endovascular treatment. AJNR Am J Neuroradiol 1997;18:655–665

71. Basali A, Mascha EJ, Kalfas I, Schubert A. Relation between perioperative hypertension and intracranial hemorrhage after craniotomy. Anesthesiology 2000;93:48–54

12 Endovascular Interventions for Skull Base Lesions

The management of skull base lesions has undergone evolution in the last two decades thanks to advances in endovascular techniques to either help manage these lesions before or after open surgery, or as an alternative approach to an open procedure.

- Interventional neuroradiology (INR) is a branch of interventional radiology that encompasses image-guided procedures involving the head, neck, and spine.

The primary applications of endovascular techniques in the management of skull base lesions are embolization of lesions (e.g., skull base tumors and fistulas), balloon test occlusion, vessel sacrifice, and inferior petrosal sinus sampling.

■ Embolization of Skull Base Lesions

Embolization is a procedure to obliterate the vascular supply to a lesion. Since the first treatment of a posttraumatic carotid cavernous fistula in the 1930s, by placing a long muscle fragment marked with a clip in the internal carotid artery (Brooks's[1] technique), a number of studies on embolization have explored the value of presurgical tumor embolization, its cost-efficiency, and its ability to decrease surgical blood loss and to reduce operative and recovery time.[2-9]

General Principles

A thorough understanding of the vascular anatomy is mandatory in all endovascular procedures. Awareness of normal anatomy of the blood vessels, as well as of the anatomic variants, the collateral pathways, and anastomoses between the extracranial and intracranial vessels, is important to ensure safe and successful treatment.[10,11] Knowledge of the anastomoses, such as among the internal carotid artery (ICA), vertebral artery (VA), and external carotid artery (ECA) branches, as well as the arterial supply to the cranial nerves, is essential for neurointerventional procedures.

Embolic agents

In 1970, Charles Dotter's group reported the first use of occlusive embolic particles to treat arterial bleeding.[3] An autologous blood clot was delivered endovascularly via superselective catheter injection in order to control acute upper gastrointestinal bleeding. Since then, a plethora of occlusive, prothrombotic materials have been used in the endovascular treatment of arterial bleeding (including fascial strips and silk threads, which have now been replaced in clinical use by more modern products).

- The new generation of embolic agents can be classified as permanent or temporary (enabling recanalization over time).[12] Embolic agents can also be classified according to their physical properties: mechanical devices, particles, and liquid **(Table 12.1)**.

Mechanical Devices

- Balloon: Inflatable balloons are used for the obliteration of large vessels, such as the carotid and vertebral arteries.[13-16]
  - Detachable balloons (Balt, Goldballoons, Balt Extrusion, Montmorency, France) are not currently Food and Drug Administration (FDA) approved, but are available in most countries, as of August 2014.
  - Care must be used when employing detachable balloons in the cerebral circulation, as they have the potential risk of spontaneously deflating over time or rupturing once deployed, and then embolizing into the distal arterial circulation.
- Coil: There are several types of coils **(Table 12.1)**. The most commonly used coils, the detachable coils, enable accurate positioning before permanent deployment.
  - Although widely available, coils are not usually the preferred tool in the embolization process. They enable a more proximal occlusion of the blood supply and are better for large vessel occlusion. But for tumors, coils block access for future embolization through the same vessel, which makes it not necessarily the best option.

Particles

Gelfoam is one of the most commonly used particles.

- Gelfoam is used in either powder form (40 to 60 μm) or in solid form as strips. The strips are cut down to a size of a few millimeters and then are injected under pressure into the target vessel, often referred to as "torpedoes."
- The ability of Gelfoam to expand with hydration is one of its key advantages.
- Used in most embolization after the use of Gelfoam, it offers temporary proximal arterial control, which enables the option of future access.

Table 12.1 Embolic Agents

Agent	Type	Examples	Cost	Permanent (P) or Temporary (T)
Liquid agents	• Cyanoacrylates	• N-butyl-cyanoacrylate (n-BCA) Trufill → (Codman Neurovascular, Raynham, MA)	$$	P
	• Precipitated polymers	• Onyx → (ev3, Irvine, CA)	$$$$	P
	• Sclerosing agents	• Absolute ethanol	$	P
Particles	• Gelatin foam (Gelfoam, Upjohn, Kalamazoo, MI)	• Sponge • Powder	$	T
	• Polyvinyl alcohol (PVA) foam	• Contour → emboli (Boston scientific, Natick, MA) • PVA foam embolization particles (Cook Medical, Bloomington, IN)	$$	P
	• Spherical emboli	• Spherical contour SE™ (Boston Scientific, Natick, MA) • Bead Block™ (Terumo Medical, Somerset, NJ) • Embospheres → (Biosphere Medical, Rockland, MA)	$$	P
	• Silk suture	• 3-0 or 5-0 suture	$	P
Mechanical devices	• Coils	• Bare platinum coils (detachable) • Bioactive coils: polyglycolic-polylactic acid (fibered detachable) • Hydrogel incorporated coils (expanded detachable) • Berenstein coils (pushable)	$$–$$$	P
	• Detachable balloons	• BaltGoldballoons (Balt Extrusion, Montmorency, France)	$$$	P

Polyvinyl alcohol (PVA) comes in a variety of sizes (45–150 to 1,000–1,180 μm).

- Cerebral angiography might not demonstrate all the small arterious micro-anastomoses, especially for vessels ranging from 50 to 80 μm in size.[17] Knowledge of the local microanatomy is important in choosing the appropriate-sized PVA particles. With the use of Gelfoam or PVA, the vessel can recanalize over time (faster with the Gelfoam than with PVA). Thus, these materials are often used in the presurgical embolization of lesions, when definitive surgical treatment is planned within 24 to 72 hours.[18]

Liquids

Cyanoacrylates (also called "glue") and precipitated polymers are the most common liquid embolic agents used. Glue has classically been considered an effective and permanent agent for the occlusion of vascular lesions.[19]

INR Pitfalls

The durability and permanence of glue has been called into question.[20] Further complicating the use of glue in embolization procedures is the fact that glue is technically challenging to deliver into the cerebral circulation, and its use requires experience because polymerization of glue starts on contact with anions in the blood.[21] Although this is somewhat altered by formulation with Ethiodol, it still poses a technical challenge. Rapid polymerization in a microcatheter can also cause glue to adhere to the microcatheter prior to its removal, with the risk of catheter breakage. Furthermore, a lesion treated with glue will often become less pliable and stiffer, making a subsequent surgical excision more difficult.[22]

- *Precipitated polymers.* Onyx (ev3, Irvine, CA), a precipitated polymer (also known as nonadhesive liquid embolic agents), is a newer embolic agent that has become an alternative to glue.
  - Advantages of Onyx: It is nonadhesive, and although physically occupying spaces within the vasculature, it does not adhere to the vessel walls. This enables longer injections than with glue, and the ability to control the rate of embolization. Onyx can be deployed more slowly than glue, and often entails a more controlled delivery. For instance, injection of Onyx can be stopped, an angiogram injection performed, and then a decision regarding more embolization can be made. This can all be done with significantly less risk of embedding the catheter in a vessel than with the use of glue.[21]
  - Disadvantages of Onyx: the need to flush the catheter in vivo with dimethyl sulfoxide (DMSO), which is potentially toxic to the endothelium,

painful in awake patients, and requires a DMSO-compatible catheter. Onyx also produces a rather pungent smell of garlic on the patient's breath.

Indications for and Goals of Embolization

- Indications[7,22–27]
  - Prior to surgery (head and neck surgeries)
  - Adjuvant therapy (stabilize or reduce inoperable tumors, epistaxis)
  - Dural arteriovenous fistula
  - Relief of symptoms (pain) in palliative situation
  - Recurrent nonsurgical lesions
- Goals[7,22–27]
  - Devascularize lesion
  - Occlude surgically inaccessible blood supply
  - Sacrifice large vessels (endovascular approach enables prior testing before occlusion)
  - Facilitate surgical access (e.g., allowing decrease blood loss at skin incision)

Complications of Embolization

- Neurologic
  - Vessel injury with dissection or rupture, which may cause subarachnoid, subdural, or intracerebral hemorrhage
    - Frequency: The N-Butyl-Cyanoacrylate (n-BCA) Trial Investigators Study found an average vessel perforation rate of 1.9% in glue (flow-directed microcatheter) versus 5.8% in PVA.[28]
  - Thromboembolic events
    - 9% symptomatic.[29]
    - Other studies found lower risk, which varies with the embolic agents and lesions treated; 1.9% thromboembolic events and 3.8 to 5.8% stroke.[28]
  - Trapped microcatheter
    - Frequency: 7.4% for n-BCA versus 0% for PVA.[28] As for Onyx, the percent varies but can be as low as 2.5% and as high as 8.5%.[22,30]
  - Cranial nerve injury
  - Specific complications related to vascular lesion embolization:
    - Rupture, hemorrhage (with or without intraparenchymal hematoma), venous drainage obstruction.
    - In arteriovenous malformation (AVM) treatment, 14% treatment-related neurologic deficit rate, a 2% persistent disabling deficit rate, and 1% mortality.[31]
    - In carotid-cavernous fistula (CCF), worsening of symptoms is possible but usually transient (it occurs as the cavernous sinus thromboses).

- Specific complications related to tumor embolization:
  - Most common: fever and localized pain[25]
  - Intratumoral hemorrhage
  - Swelling (generally responds to corticosteroids)
  - Scalp infarction
- Nonneurologic[32]
  - Allergic reactions
  - Groin complications (infection, hematoma, pseudoaneurysm, arterial occlusion) in 0.2%, with a 0.5% risk of hematoma requiring surgery or transfusion
  - Renal failure 0.2%
  - Deep venous thrombosis (DVT) or pulmonary embolization when treating arteriovenous malformations from venous shunting[18]

Embolization of Tumors

The most common skull base–related embolized tumors are paragangliomas (glomus tumors), meningiomas, and angiofibromas.[26,27,33] Less common are metastases, esthesioneuroblastomas, schwannomas, chordomas, and hemangiopericytomas.[27]

- **Timing:** Tumor embolization is usually performed 24 to 72 hours prior to surgery, although this a matter of debate. This timing is believed to enable maximal thrombosis of the vessels prior to recanalization.[4–6,27] In meningioma, delaying surgery up to 7 to 9 days has been reported; it enables tumor softening and minimizes blood loss.[34,35] This has not been routinely observed in all series, with the risk of confusing the grade and even overgrading due to findings of necrosis and enlarged nuclei, as found in embolized meningiomas.[36]

Meningiomas

Although meningiomas are common, preoperative embolization is rarely done for convexity lesions whose blood supply can be easily taken at resection. Skull base tumors such as clival meningiomas have a deep blood supply (usually off the ICA) that is difficult to access; endovascular access to the feeding pedicle (usually the meningohypophyseal trunk) is often difficult, and embolic material can reflux into the ICA.[37]

- *Olfactory groove meningiomas,* which are commonly supplied by the anterior ethmoidal artery, cannot be embolized due to the risk of inadvertent introduction of embolic material into the ophthalmic artery via anastomotic connections.[38]
- *Cavernous and parasellar meningiomas* receive blood supply from the meningohypophyseal trunk and the inferolateral trunk; these vessels can be difficult

to embolize and require surgeons with extensive experience.[39,40] ICA-supplied skull base meningiomas have been embolized with a good outcome.[41]

- A retrospective analysis of 470 treated meningiomas found an average of 27% embolized skull base location meningiomas, including olfactory groove, planum sphenoidale/tuberculum, sphenoid wing, and cerebello-pontine angle.[42]
- Some requirements for preoperative embolization have been elaborated[42]:
  - Tumors size above 3 cm in diameter and with 50% of feeders from accessible ECA branches.
  - Imaging-confirmed deep supply or hypervascularity of the lesion.
  - Eloquent locations.
  - Significant calcified meningiomas are not generally embolized.
- Regarding the outcome after embolization, complete tumor devascularization has been described as beneficial in many studies.[37,43]
- Regarding the choice of embolic agents, PVA is most commonly used. Glue is the best known agent, and it offers good result. It enables occlusion of feeders and intratumoral vessels, which prevent intratumoral bleeding.[44] Onyx has been reported in few cases and no definitive conclusions may be drawn yet.[45]

Paragangliomas

Paragangliomas are highly vascular, and embolization is frequently performed prior to surgery.[46–49]

- In some cases, paragangliomas may secrete vasoactive substances. Release of vasoactive mediators can occur during angiography and lead to a hypertensive crisis.
- Direct percutaneous puncture of the tumor can be performed when arterial feeders are too small to navigate from a peripheral access point (such as from femoral or radial access) or when the transarterial approach carries a high risk.[26,50,51]
- Facial nerve palsy has been reported after embolization of paragangliomas. Although some reports show less injury after embolization, this is not a consistent finding.[52,53]
- Decreased extent of the procedure and less blood loss have been observed after embolization.[48,53,54] Blood loss dropped from 599 to 263 mL with embolization, and simple excision was achieved in 97% versus 82% with an estimated mean devascularization of 76%.[54]

Angiofibromas

Juvenile angiofibromas (JAFs) are rare lesions, accounting for 0.05% of all head and neck neoplasms.[55] Although benign, JAFs can be locally invasive into the nasopharynx, and even intracranial extension is possible. They often arise in the sphenopalatine fossa.[23] The precise origin can be difficult to determine, as they present commonly with considerable size. It is commonly agreed that the posterior choanal tissue is the origin of the JAF.

Angiography is essential prior to surgery for two reasons:

- To obtain detailed vessels architecture:
  - Assess the vascularization of JAFs for surgical planning, delineate normal and pathological anastomosis, and assess retinal supply.[56]
  - Correlations have been made between the size of the JAF and its blood supply. In general, ECA branches and the target vessels for presurgical embolization are often branches of the internal maxillary artery (IMAX) such as the sphenopalatine artery, accessory meningeal artery, and superior pharyngeal artery.
  - In the Andrews classification, stage III and IV JAFs have tumor invading the infratemporal fossa, orbit, and extending intracranially, and have supply from ICA branches, anterior and posterior ethmoidal arteries, the inferolateral trunk, meningohypophyseal trunk (MHT), and other vessels.[57]
- To provide treatment of embolization followed by complete surgical removal[6]:
  - Embolization is often unsafe.[6,23,55,57,58]
  - In some instances, direct percutaneous puncture can be an option, when the ICA is the main vascular supply.[59,60]
  - Careful angiographic images should be obtained and thoroughly inspected prior to embolization to assess dangerous anastomosis; occasionally, the use of temporary balloon occlusion of the proximal blood supply from the ICA or VA may be an adjunctive safety measure.[61]
  - Intraoperative blood loss ranges from 915 to 3,000 mL versus 450 mL with embolization.[56]

Embolization of Vascular Lesions

Vascular lesions of the skull base region encompass a variety of types, including CCF, dural arteriovenous fistula (dAVF), and AVM. Other vascular lesions, which are mostly low-flow lesions, include capillary, capillarovenous, venous, or lymphatic malformations.[25–27,62,63]

Carotid Cavernous Fistula

Carotid cavernous fistula can be classified using the Barrow classification[64]:

- Type A: direct (high flow) between the carotid artery and the cavernous sinus (CS) (spontaneous intracavernous aneurysm rupture or traumatic)
- Indirect (low flow) dural shunt (spontaneous)
  - Type B: shunt between ICA branches and the CS

- ○ Type C: shunt between ECA branches and the CS
- ○ Type D: shunt between both ECA and ICA branches and the CS

Treatment

Urgent treatment is usually required in direct CCFs, as they are high flow and often present with vision loss, high intraocular pressure, and even venous reflux into the cortical veins.[65]

- Endovascular repair has become the preferred strategy for CCF treatment; specifically, the transarterial approach is usually employed for direct CCFs and transarterial/transvenous approaches for indirect CCFs.
- Detachable balloons, coils, PVA, liquid embolic agents, and stents have all been used in the treatment of CCFs, with the goal of closing the fistula while preserving flow within the ICA.[66–71]
- For indirect CCFs, the favored approach is transvenous embolization, starting from the femoral or jugular veins. Indirect CCFs have also been treated via direct canalization of the ophthalmic vein. The goal is to access the cavernous sinus and then pack the appropriate part with coil to shut down the shunting.[72–76] CCFs supplied by the ICA branches are particularly thought to be more safely treated with transvenous embolization.[77]
- Transarterial embolization is possible for accessible feeders, especially those from the ECA. Once again, coils, PVA, or liquid embolic agents can also be used.
- Up to a 98% rate of successful occlusion of direct CCF has been achieved in countries where the detachable balloon method is available. In institutions where series included balloon and other devices, the rate was between 88 and 94%.[71,78] The largest series on indirect CCF reported a 90% success rate using the transvenous approach.[78,79]

Dural Arteriovenous Fistula

As classified by Borden et al or Cognard et al (see **Table 25.5**, page 695), a dAVF is a shunt between extracranial (and meningeal) arteries and the dural venous sinus, dural veins, or cortical veins. Although some institutions consider open surgery as the best treatment, the advancements in endovascular treatment, with new devices, embolic agents, and catheters, have made it a valid and proven option for dAVF.

Goal

The goal, which correlates with the surgical disconnection, is the obliteration of the fistulous connection. The vein is the known recruiting source, and obliteration has to include either both sides or at least the venous side.

- Complete obliteration will result in cure.[80–82] Incomplete embolization enables new arterial supply to form and necessitates a second endovascular attempt or a new approach, such as open surgery. If neurosurgical excision is advocated, the initial embolization provides partial devascularization and decreased bleeding, which can be significant and rapid in dAVF (including just incising the scalp).[83]
- Approaches to dAVF embolization can be divided into transarterial or transvenous, or both.
  - **Transarterial:** usually favored for small dAVFs or those with venous occlusion or stenosis, where the access is restricted. A common initial strategy is to shut down the small feeders, which increase the flow in the main arterial supply. This increases the chance for the embolic agent (glue or Onyx) to penetrate the venous side, the ultimate end point. This strategy can also be used as an initial step, before the transvenous approach.
  - **Transvenous:** usually selected for large, complex dAVFs with a nonfunctional and isolated dural sinus. Access with a microcatheter followed by occlusion of the disease segment with coil is commonly performed.

Of note, when femoral transarterial or transvenous treatment is impossible or unsuccessful, options include direct access either by direct puncture (carotid), cutdown to expose vessels (superior ophthalmic vein to access cavernous sinus), or even through a bur hole position on the known cortical drainage vein.[84–86]

- Some factors have been shown to improve the cure rate:
  - Treatment through meningeal arterial supply offers a higher success rate than using the superficial temporal or occipital arteries to penetrate via the transosseous branches of the skull, which are millimetric and tortuous.[87]
  - High-flow dAVFs are better treated by using a balloon to occlude the flow, or by embolization using a coil.[88]
  - As described above, occlude the smaller supply to increase the flow in the main feeder.
- Success rates depend on the type of embolic agent used—glue versus Onyx:
  - Cyanoacrylate (glue). More studies are available considering this agent, as it has been available for a long time. On initial transarterial approach, cure was achieved in only 30% versus 81% for a transvenous approach. In one study, a combined approach offered a 54% cure rate. Delayed thrombosis of a residual shunt has been described, with a follow-up angiogram showing complete occlusion in 88% of patients with residual flow at the end of the initial procedure.[89,90] In a study involving 170 patients, cure was achieved in 60% and 69% of patient without and with cortical venous drainage, respectively. At follow-up, these numbers increase to 85% and 89%, with overall clinical improvement in 93%. These numbers seem more accurate with larger groups being included compared with case series,

with an initial cure rate of 63 to 100%.[91–94] For those that do not occlude with surgery or embolization, Gamma Knife radiosurgery is an option.
○ Onyx: Available studies showed an immediate cure rate ranging from 62 to 95%.[30,95–98] At follow-up angiogram, the cure rate has even reached 100%.[95,96]

■ Occlusion Test

Provocative testing is performed in an attempt to predict if a clinical deficit will appear following a vessel occlusion or sacrifice.

Balloon Test Occlusion

Balloon test occlusion (BTO) of the ICA is a relatively common endovascular procedure to assess cerebrovascular reserve.

- Balloon test occlusion incorporates multiple methods of clinical and radiographic evaluation. It requires:
  ○ A detailed clinical exam before, during, and after the occlusion
  ○ Timed angiographic imaging
  ○ Cerebral blood flow imaging

Temporary occlusion of a vessel is a well-accepted evaluation prior to surgery in which arterial sacrifice or prolonged temporary occlusion is considered.[99] The following factors must be taken into consideration[22]:

- Whenever possible, the vessel must be temporarily occluded at the level that would simulate the proposed sacrifice.
- Neurologic testing should evaluate the possible consequences of the proposed vascular occlusion.

Technique

There are several techniques for performing a BTO. One of the most common techniques is as follows:

- A neurologic exam is completed prior to the test. Two or more days before the test a baseline single photon emission computed tomography (SPECT) study is performed to assess cerebral perfusion as a control.
- Bilateral femoral arterial access is achieved (one side will be used during inflation for repeat angiography) with the patient awake.
- The patient is heparinized to an activated clotting time (ACT) goal of above 300; at this level, clot formation decreases.

- An initial diagnostic cerebral angiogram is performed (ICA and dominant VA usually), with the occasional use of cross-compression (manual compression of the contralateral carotid during the injection) to demonstrate the anterior communicating artery. The Allcock maneuver assesses the posterior communicating artery while the VA is injected and the ipsilateral carotid is compressed.
- After inflation of the balloon and confirmation of proper occlusion with contrast stagnation, the angiogram is repeated in the contralateral ICA and dominant VA. The neurologic assessment should be reviewed with the patient prior to the procedure and the inflation, and the patient is examined continuously during occlusion.
- Twenty-five minutes postocclusion, the radiotracer is administered intravenously and at the 30-minute mark the balloon is deflated and significant backflow is performed to minimize the risk of thrombus embolization; for extra safety an aspiration can be performed through the catheter.
- The heparin is reversed, the sheaths are withdrawn, and hemostasis is achieved by manual compression.

If at any moment, the patient's clinical status changes, the procedure is aborted and this is considered a failed BTO. On the angiographic study, an important component is the timing of the venous delay:

- The appearance of the first cortical vein on the injected side is the beginning of the venous phase. Images are reviewed, and one of the considerations for vessel sacrifice acceptance is when the delay between the appearance of the first cortical vein on the injected side and the contralateral and occluded hemisphere is no longer than 2 seconds.[100,101]

There are number of adjunctive tests that can be performed to improve either the clinical or imaging aspect:

- Neurologic function. These tests either assess neurologic function or are used to increase the accuracy of the evaluation.
  - Hypotension challenge[102–108]
  - Neuropsychological testing[109–111]
  - Electroencephalography (EEG)[112–115]
  - Somatosensory evoked potentials (SSEP)[116–119]
- Cerebral blood flow
  - Angiography[100,120,121]
  - Stump pressure[101,122–126]
  - Transcranial Doppler (TCD)[127–129]
  - Xenon imaging[107]
  - Xenon computed tomography (CT)[99,122,130,131]
  - CT perfusion (CTP)[132–135]
  - Positron emission tomography (PET)[115,136–139]

- Single-photon emission computed tomography (SPECT)[119,123,126,140–143]
- Magnetic resonance perfusion and *blood oxygenation level dependent* (BOLD) magnetic resonance imaging (MRI)[144,145]
- Computer simulation[146,147]

Complications

Many of the complications seen during BTOs are common to all interventional procedures. In the case of BTO, some studies show a higher rate of thrombo-embolic stroke, but these earlier reports had a low number of patients.[148] In high-volume centers, an overall 4 to 7% risk has been reported, with a 1.6% rate of asymptomatic complications, including dissection, pseudoaneurysm, and embolus, and a 1.6% rate of symptomatic (neurological deficit), of which 0.4% were permanent.[99]

It is not uncommon for patients to have discomfort or experience a vasovagal reaction when the balloon is inflated. However, this should be only transient, and appropriate rescue medications such as epinephrine and glycopyrrolate should always be available.

Risk

The main issue regarding a BTO is mostly its reliability. It is well known that this test is not perfect. That is, one can never be completely certain that the patient's passing the BTO will mean that the patient will not experience any neurologic sequela of the planned vessel sacrifice. Discuss with the patient the reliability and risks of this technique in detail!

Two major reviews have addressed this issue. In one review of 254 patients, in which the ICA was sacrificed without a test occlusion, an average stroke rate of 26% and mortality rate of 12% were found.[22] The second review included 262 patients who passed the BTO, and it found a 13% stroke rate and 3% mortality.[120] Although this statistically significant difference supports the utility of the BTO, it also favors the use of one of the adjunctive tests listed in **Table 12.1.**

Venous Test Occlusion

Venous test occlusion (VTO) is not as widely performed as BTO.

Indications

- Occlusion of a venous structure is anticipated.
- There is concern as to the occlusions effect on the venous drainage. As is often seen in venous thrombosis causing infarction, symptoms can be delayed,

as it is the venous stasis that can precipitate a venous infarct. This event can occur even if the patient had passed the VTO clinically during the procedure.

To try to avoid provoking the same feared consequence one is hoping to prevent, that is, venous infarction after vessel sacrifice, multiple approaches are used. The following three components, taken together, are needed to assess if the patient passes or fails a VTO:

- Clinical status of the patient.
- Measuring the venous pressure proximal to the site of occlusion and ensuring it does not rise above a certain level. Studies have shown that an increase of less than 10 mmHg confirms a safe occlusion while concomitantly providing data on the potential effects of the occlusion.[149,150]
- The assessment of collateral flow and venous congestion.

Vessel Occlusion Option

There are multiple ways to sacrifice a vessel, either via endovascular techniques or directly during open surgery. Briefly, vessel occlusion can be achieved from the INR standpoint with a detachable balloon, coil, or both.

■ Venous Sampling

The selective venous sampling of the inferior petrosal sinuses can provide essential information in the workup of a cushingoid state, which was first reported in 1977.[151,152]

Indications

The indications for venous sampling are as follows, along with a contra-indication[22,151–155]:

- Adrenocorticotropic hormone (ACTH)-dependent Cushing's syndrome
- Differentiation of pituitary versus ectopic ACTH source
- Lateralization of the source of higher ACTH production in the event of negative or equivocal MRI of the pituitary
- Discrepancy among clinical, imaging, and biochemical tests
- Persistent or recurrent Cushing's syndrome after pituitary surgery: a relative indication that may be difficult to assess due to the disturbed venous flows that may occur post–pituitary surgery
- Contraindication: not reliable for growth hormone sampling for acromegaly[156,157]

- Indication beyond the scope of this chapter: locating a parathyroid adenoma, in recurrent hyperparathyroidism after surgery[158–161]

Technique for Inferior Petrosal Sinus Sampling (IPSS)

- The patient is given a local anaesthetic for the groin punctures and mild sedation whenever required (2 mg IV midazolam and 25 mg IV fentanyl).
- A 6-French (F) sheath is inserted in the right femoral vein and a 5F sheath is inserted in the left femoral vein. The larger 6F sheath is used for peripheral sampling. The patient is heparinized afterward to an ACT of 300.
- A 5F Envoy (Codman Neurovascular, Raynham, MA) catheter is placed over a guidewire under roadmap guidance in the bilateral jugular veins.
- A microcatheter is introduced with a micro-guidewire. The inferior petrosal sinuses are accessed bilaterally.
- Once both microcatheters are positioned in the inferior petrosal sinuses (IPSs), the blood in the sinuses is sampled.
- The technique requires a surgical staff of three—one for each site (peripheral, left, and right IPS). One or two baseline samples are taken, followed by injection of corticotropin-releasing hormone (CRH) or more widely available desmopressin repeated sampling is obtained at 0, 1, 3, 5, 10, and 15 minutes. As a matter of practice, all samples are very carefully labeled and are transported to the lab. The catheters and sheaths are removed, and hemostasis is achieved by manual compression.

Special Features

Cavernous sinus and jugular venous sampling is also possible. Most authorities would argue that cavernous sinus sampling is technically more challenging, and in most studies it has an accuracy similar to that of IPSS.[162,163] On the other hand, jugular venous sampling is usually used if the endovascular specialist is inexperienced. The specificity of the jugular venous sampling in one study was 100% and the sensitivity was 83%, which would suggest that patients with negative or equivocal results be referred to a more experienced center for proper IPSS.[164]

Results and Reliability

A ratio of central (IPSS) ACTH level to peripheral (sheath) ACTH level is calculated. An ACTH gradient of ≥ 2.0 before CRH administration, or ≥ 3.0 after CRH, is diagnostic of a pituitary source of ACTH. Using these ratios, the IPSS has a sensitivity of 95% and specificity of 100% before CRH, and specificity and sensitivity of 100% after CRH.[165]

If the ratio varies from one side to the other between the withdrawal times, always suspect a labeling error. It is easy to make a mistake with this high number of samples collected, so careful attention should be paid.

Prepare all the sample vials before commencing the procedure, and a non-surgeon staff member should be responsible for labeling and collection.

Complications

Venous sampling is a safe procedure, with a complication rate as low as 0.001% with an experienced operator; in inexperienced hands it is slightly higher—usually below 1%.[166] There have been case reports of transient or permanent neurologic deficits associated with IPSS. These complications often involve the brainstem and related cranial nerves (CNs). Of note, often CN VI and VII are affected. As well, rare instances of brainstem edema, brainstem infarct, and reversible encephalopathy syndrome have been reported.[166–172] Venous hypertension or thrombosis, in deep cerebral veins, are the likely pathophysiological explanation proposed for these adverse events.[166,173] The use of a smaller microcatheter may in fact facilitate access to these small veins and potentially occlude them.[173]

- Subarachnoid haemorrhage has also been reported.[167,174]
- As for dissection on the arterial side, venous damage and cases of deep venous thrombosis and death from pulmonary embolism have been reported as well.[175]

■ Endovascular Approach for Traumatic and Iatrogenic Lesions

Traumatic Lesions

Head trauma is quite common and can produce a variety of injuries. Vascular injury (e.g., aneurysm, fistula, transected artery, dissection) as immediate or delayed sequelae of penetrating skull injuries or fractures of the skull base are quite challenging to manage.[176]

- Up to 1.1% of trauma is associated with a blunt carotid or vertebral injury.[177]
- An associated mortality rate of 23 to 31% and permanent severe neurologic deficit rate of 48 to 58% are reported.[177,178]
- A grading scale has been elaborated to described injury to the carotid artery[179]:
  o Grade I: irregular wall or < 25% lumen stenosis
  o Grade II: dissection, raised flap, intraluminal clot, or intramural hematoma with ≥ 25% lumen stenosis

- ○ Grade III: pseudoaneurysm
- ○ Grade IV: occlusion
- ○ Grade V: transection with active extravasation

The feasibility of a successful endovascular repair of a traumatically induced skull base vascular injury depends on the nature of the vessel injury. Traumatic aneurysms/pseudoaneurysms that occur in the context of trauma to the skull base are usually of the dissecting type that might require treatment with the use of vascular stenting and even coil placement. The use of covered stents (polytetrafluoroethylene [PTFE]-covered JoStent, JoMed, Helsingborg, Sweden) has been proposed and used in petrous and cavernous ICA pseudoaneurysms after head injury and skull base fractures.[176] In other scenarios, venous or arterial vessel sacrifice is the only option (example: a knife attack into the jugular vein requires sacrificing the vein prior to removing the weapon).

Iatrogenic Lesions

Vessel injury is a possible complication in all the skull base approaches.

- **Iatrogenic lesions in transsphenoidal surgery (TSS):**
  - ○ Injury from the ICA is one of the most severe complications in TSS.[180,181] There is a 1% risk of arterial injuries during or after TSS with a morbidity and mortality of 24% and 14%, respectively.[180] Endoscopic approaches are widely used, and many reports confirm a decreased overall complication rate when compared with the microsurgical route.[182–184] Other authors feel that the risk of vessel injury in endoscopic procedures could be slightly higher with this laterally oriented approach.[185] If proper packing and hemodynamic control cannot be obtained when such a complication occurs, then endovascular management can be considered, such as coiling or vessel occlusion. If the patient cannot tolerate the BTO, a stent-graft can be used with low risk.[180]
  - ○ Another reported complication following pituitary surgery is vasospasm. Endovascular surgery, either by injection of intra-arterial medication or mechanical angioplasty, has always been a treatment considered for vasospasm when medical management failed.[186]

Intra-Arterial Injection of Chemotherapy

Intra-arterial injection of chemotherapy might be a consideration in the treatment of head and neck tumors. It has been described as an option in patient care. Either used alone or in combination with radiotherapy, it is an evolving and emerging INR procedure. Every neurosurgeon and ear, nose, and throat (ENT) surgeon should keep this in mind when reviewing treatment options.[26,63,187]

■ References

Boldfaced references are of particular importance.

1. Brooks B. The treatment of traumatic arterio-venous fistula. South Med J 1930;23: 100–106

2. Rutka J, Muller PJ, Chui M. Preoperative Gelfoam embolization of supratentorial meningiomas. Can J Surg 1985;28:441–443

3. Teasdale E, Patterson J, McLellan D, Macpherson P. Subselective preoperative embolization for meningiomas. A radiological and pathological assessment. J Neurosurg 1984;60:506–511

4. Dean BL, Flom RA, Wallace RC, et al. Efficacy of endovascular treatment of meningiomas: evaluation with matched samples. AJNR Am J Neuroradiol 1994;15:1675–1680

5. Macpherson P. The value of pre-operative embolisation of meningioma estimated subjectively and objectively. Neuroradiology 1991;33:334–337

6. Moulin G, Chagnaud C, Gras R, et al. Juvenile nasopharyngeal angiofibroma: comparison of blood loss during removal in embolized group versus nonembolized group. Cardiovasc Intervent Radiol 1995;18:158–161

7. **Macht S, Turowski B. [Neuroradiologic diagnostic and interventional procedures for diseases of the skull base]. HNO 2011;59:340–349**

8. **Mine B, Delpierre I, Hassid S, De Witte O, Lubicz B. The role of interventional neuroradiology in the management of skull base tumours and related surgical complications. B-ENT 2011;7(Suppl 17):61–66**

9. **Péreza RA, Espinosa-García H, Alcalá-Cerra G, de la Rosa Manjarréz G, Gómez FO, Barrios AR. [Embolization of skull-base hypervascular tumors: description of a series of cases and proposal of a therapeutic algorithm]. Bol Asoc Med P R 2013; 105:20–27**

10. Oh MS, Kim MH, Chu MK, Yu KH, Kim KH, Lee BC. Polyarteritis nodosa presenting with bilateral cavernous internal carotid artery aneurysms. Neurology 2008;70:405

11. Sharma S, Kumar S, Mishra NK, Gaikwad SB. Cerebral miliary micro aneurysms in polyarteritis nodosa: report of two cases. Neurol India 2010;58:457–459

12. Stehbens WE. Atypical cerebral aneurysms. Med J Aust 1965;1:765–766

13. Topaloglu R, Kazik M, Saatci I, Kalyoncu M, Cil BE, Akalan N. An unusual presentation of classic polyarteritis nodosa in a child. Pediatr Nephrol 2005;20:1011–1015

14. Toyoda K, Tsutsumi K, Hirao T, et al. Ruptured intracranial aneurysms in pediatric polyarteritis nodosa: case report. Neurol Med Chir (Tokyo) 2012;52:928–932

15. Uemura J, Inoue T, Aoki J, Saji N, Shibazaki K, Kimura K. [A case of polyarteritis nodosa with giant intracranial aneurysm]. Rinsho Shinkeigaku 2013;53:452–457

16. Thompson B, Burns A. Subarachnoid hemorrhages in vasculitis. Am J Kidney Dis 2003;42:582–585

17. Geibprasert S, Pongpech S, Armstrong D, Krings T. Dangerous extracranial-intracranial anastomoses and supply to the cranial nerves: vessels the neurointerventionalist needs to know. AJNR Am J Neuroradiol 2009;30:1459–1468

18. Repa I, Moradian GP, Dehner LP, et al. Mortalities associated with use of a commercial suspension of polyvinyl alcohol. Radiology 1989;170:395–399

19. Wikholm G. Occlusion of cerebral arteriovenous malformations with N-butyl cyanoacrylate is permanent. AJNR Am J Neuroradiol 1995;16:479–482

20. Rao VR, Mandalam KR, Gupta AK, Kumar S, Joseph S. Dissolution of isobutyl 2-cyano-acrylate on long-term follow-up. AJNR Am J Neuroradiol 1989;10:135–141

21. Vaidya S, Tozer KR, Chen J. An overview of embolic agents. Semin Intervent Radiol 2008;25:204–215

22. **Harrigan MR, Deveikis JP. Handbook of Cerebrovascular Disease and Neurointerventional Technique. Dordrecht, the Netherlands: Humana Press; 2013.**

23. **Byrne JV. Tutorials in Endovascular Neurosurgery and Interventional Neuroradiology. Berlin: Springer; 2012:361.**

24. Broomfield S, Bruce I, Birzgalis A, Herwadkar A. The expanding role of interventional radiology in head and neck surgery. J R Soc Med 2009;102:228–234

25. **American Society of Interventional and Therapeutic Neuroradiology. Head, neck, and brain tumor embolization. AJNR Am J Neuroradiol 2001;22(8, Suppl):S14–S15**

26. **Gandhi D, Gemmete JJ, Ansari SA, Gujar SK, Mukherji SK. Interventional neuroradiology of the head and neck. AJNR Am J Neuroradiol 2008;29:1806–1815**

27. Jindal G, Gemmete J, Gandhi D. Interventional neuroradiology applications in oto-laryngology, head and neck surgery. Otolaryngol Clin North Am 2012;45:1423–1449

28. n-BCA Trail Investigators. N-butyl cyanoacrylate embolization of cerebral arteriove-nous malformations: results of a prospective, randomized, multi-center trial. AJNR Am J Neuroradiol 2002;23:748–755

29. Qureshi AI, Luft AR, Sharma M, Guterman LR, Hopkins LN. Prevention and treatment of thromboembolic and ischemic complications associated with endovascular proce-dures: Part II—Clinical aspects and recommendations. Neurosurgery 2000;46:1360–1375, discussion 1375–1376

30. Lv X, Jiang C, Zhang J, Li Y, Wu Z. Complications related to percutaneous transarterial embolization of intracranial dural arteriovenous fistulas in 40 patients. AJNR Am J Neuroradiol 2009;30:462–468

31. Hartmann A, Pile-Spellman J, Stapf C, et al. Risk of endovascular treatment of brain arteriovenous malformations. Stroke 2002;33:1816–1820

32. Citron SJ, Wallace RC, Lewis CA, et al; Society of Interventional Radiology; American Society of Interventional and Therapeutic Neuroradiology; American Society of Neu-roradiology. Quality improvement guidelines for adult diagnostic neuroangiography. Cooperative study between ASITN, ASNR, and SIR. J Vasc Interv Radiol 2003;14(9 Pt 2):S257–S262

33. Shahinian HK. Endoscopic Skull Base Surgery. Totowa, NJ: Humana; 2008:193

34. **Chun JY, McDermott MW, Lamborn KR, Wilson CB, Higashida R, Berger MS. De-layed surgical resection reduces intraoperative blood loss for embolized menin-giomas. Neurosurgery 2002;50:1231–1235, discussion 1235–1237**

35. Nania A, Granata F, Vinci S, et al. Necrosis score, surgical time, and transfused blood volume in patients treated with preoperative embolization of intracranial meningio-mas. Analysis of a single-centre experience and a review of literature. Clin Neurora-diol 2014;24:29–36

36. Barresi V, Branca G, Granata F, Alafaci C, Caffo M, Tuccari G. Embolized meningiomas: risk of overgrading and neo-angiogenesis. J Neurooncol 2013;113:207–219

37. **Bendszus M, Rao G, Burger R, et al. Is there a benefit of preoperative meningioma embolization? Neurosurgery 2000;47:1306–1311, discussion 1311–1312**

38. White DV, Sincoff EH, Abdulrauf SI. Anterior ethmoidal artery: microsurgical anatomy and technical considerations. Neurosurgery 2005;56(2, Suppl):406–410, discussion 406–410

39. Robinson DH, Song JK, Eskridge JM. Embolization of meningohypophyseal and infero-lateral branches of the cavernous internal carotid artery. AJNR Am J Neuroradiol 1999;20:1061–1067

40. Peltier J, Fichten A, Havet E, Foulon P, Page C, Le Gars D. Microsurgical anatomy of the medial tentorial artery of Bernasconi-Cassinari. Surg Radiol Anat 2010;32:919–925

41. Waldron JS, Sughrue ME, Hetts SW, et al. Embolization of skull base meningiomas and feeding vessels arising from the internal carotid circulation. Neurosurgery 2011;68:162–169, discussion 169

42. Raper DM, Starke RM, Henderson F Jr, et al. Preoperative embolization of intracranial meningiomas: efficacy, technical considerations, and complications. AJNR Am J Neuroradiol 2014;35:1798–1804

43. Singla A, Deshaies EM, Melnyk V, et al. Controversies in the role of preoperative embolization in meningioma management. Neurosurg Focus 2013;35:E17

44. Kominami S, Watanabe A, Suzuki M, Mizunari T, Kobayashi S, Teramoto A. Preoperative embolization of meningiomas with N-butyl cyanoacrylate. Interv Neuroradiol 2012;18:133–139

45. Shi ZS, Feng L, Jiang XB, Huang Q, Yang Z, Huang ZS. Therapeutic embolization of meningiomas with Onyx for delayed surgical resection. Surg Neurol 2008;70:478–481

46. Murphy TP, Brackmann DE. Effects of preoperative embolization on glomus jugulare tumors. Laryngoscope 1989;99:1244–1247

47. White JB, Link MJ, Cloft HJ. Endovascular embolization of paragangliomas: a safe adjuvant to treatment. J Vasc Interv Neurol 2008;1:37–41

48. Naik SM, Shenoy AM, Nanjundappa, et al. Paragangliomas of the carotid body: current management protocols and review of literature. Indian J Surg Oncol 2013;4:305–312

49. Tikkakoski T, Luotonen J, Leinonen S, et al. Preoperative embolization in the management of neck paragangliomas. Laryngoscope 1997;107:821–826

50. Quadros RS, Gallas S, Delcourt C, Dehoux E, Scherperel B, Pierot L. Preoperative embolization of a cervicodorsal paraganglioma by direct percutaneous injection of Onyx and endovascular delivery of particles. AJNR Am J Neuroradiol 2006;27:1907–1909

51. Shahinian HK, Kabil MS, Jarrahy R, Thill MP. Endoscopic Skull Base Surgery. New York: Humana Press; 2010:1013–1193

52. Marangos N, Schumacher M. Facial palsy after glomus jugulare tumour embolization. J Laryngol Otol 1999;113:268–270

53. Chan JY, Li RJ, Gourin CG. Short-term outcomes and cost of care of treatment of head and neck paragangliomas. Laryngoscope 2013;123:1645–1651

54. Power AH, Bower TC, Kasperbauer J, et al. Impact of preoperative embolization on outcomes of carotid body tumor resections. J Vasc Surg 2012;56:979–989

55. Yi Z, Fang Z, Lin G, et al. Nasopharyngeal angiofibroma: a concise classification system and appropriate treatment options. Am J Otolaryngol 2013;34:133–141

56. Ballah D, Rabinowitz D, Vossough A, et al. Preoperative angiography and external carotid artery embolization of juvenile nasopharyngeal angiofibromas in a tertiary referral paediatric centre. Clin Radiol 2013;68:1097–1106

57. Andrews JC, Fisch U, Valavanis A, Aeppli U, Makek MS. The surgical management of extensive nasopharyngeal angiofibromas with the infratemporal fossa approach. Laryngoscope 1989;99:429–437

58. Chan KH, Gao D, Fernandez PG, Kingdom TT, Kumpe DA. Juvenile nasopharyngeal angiofibroma: vascular determinates for operative complications and tumor recurrence. Laryngoscope 2014;124:672–677

59. Casasco A, Herbreteau D, Houdart E, et al. Devascularization of craniofacial tumors by percutaneous tumor puncture. AJNR Am J Neuroradiol 1994;15:1233–1239

60. Tranbahuy P, Borsik M, Herman P, Wassef M, Casasco A. Direct intratumoral embolization of juvenile angiofibroma. Am J Otolaryngol 1994;15:429–435

61. **Casasco A, Houdart E, Biondi A, et al. Major complications of percutaneous embolization of skull-base tumors. AJNR Am J Neuroradiol 1999;20:179–181**

62. Flint PW, Cummings CW. Cummings Otolaryngology–Head & Neck Surgery, 5th ed. Philadelphia: Mosby/Elsevier; 2010

63. **Valavanis A, Christoforidis G. Applications of interventional neuroradiology in the head and neck. Semin Roentgenol 2000;35:72–83**

64. **Barrow DL, Spector RH, Braun IF, Landman JA, Tindall SC, Tindall GT. Classification and treatment of spontaneous carotid-cavernous sinus fistulas. J Neurosurg 1985;62:248–256**

65. Halbach VV, Hieshima GB, Higashida RT, Reicher M. Carotid cavernous fistulae: indications for urgent treatment. AJR Am J Roentgenol 1987;149:587–593

66. Li J, Lan ZG, Xie XD, You C, He M. Traumatic carotid-cavernous fistulas treated with covered stents: experience of 12 cases. World Neurosurg 2010;73:514–519

67. Tiewei Q, Ali A, Shaolei G, et al. Carotid cavernous fistulas treated by endovascular covered stent grafts with follow-up results. Br J Neurosurg 2010;24:435–440

68. **Morón FE, Klucznik RP, Mawad ME, Strother CM. Endovascular treatment of high-flow carotid cavernous fistulas by stent-assisted coil placement. AJNR Am J Neuroradiol 2005;26:1399–1404**

69. Madan A, Mujic A, Daniels K, Hunn A, Liddell J, Rosenfeld JV. Traumatic carotid artery-cavernous sinus fistula treated with a covered stent. Report of two cases. J Neurosurg 2006;104:969–973

70. Luo CB, Teng MM, Chang FC, Chang CY. Transarterial balloon-assisted n-butyl-2-cyanoacrylate embolization of direct carotid cavernous fistulas. AJNR Am J Neuroradiol 2006;27:1535–1540

71. Wang W, Li YD, Li MH, et al. Endovascular treatment of post-traumatic direct carotid-cavernous fistulas: a single-center experience. J Clin Neurosci 2011;18:24–28

72. Goldberg RA, Goldey SH, Duckwiler G, Vinuela F. Management of cavernous sinus-dural fistulas. Indications and techniques for primary embolization via the superior ophthalmic vein. Arch Ophthalmol 1996;114:707–714

73. Biondi A, Milea D, Cognard C, Ricciardi GK, Bonneville F, van Effenterre R. Cavernous sinus dural fistulae treated by transvenous approach through the facial vein: report of seven cases and review of the literature. AJNR Am J Neuroradiol 2003;24:1240–1246

74. Benndorf G, Bender A, Lehmann R, Lanksch W. Transvenous occlusion of dural cavern-ous sinus fistulas through the thrombosed inferior petrosal sinus: report of four cases and review of the literature. Surg Neurol 2000;54:42–54

75. Halbach VV, Higashida RT, Hieshima GB, Hardin CW, Pribram H. Transvenous emboli-zation of dural fistulas involving the cavernous sinus. AJNR Am J Neuroradiol 1989; 10:377–383

76. Halbach VV, Higashida RT, Hieshima GB, Hardin CW, Yang PJ. Transvenous embolization of direct carotid cavernous fistulas. AJNR Am J Neuroradiol 1988;9:741–747

77. **Halbach VV, Higashida RT, Hieshima GB, Hardin CW. Embolization of branches arising from the cavernous portion of the internal carotid artery. AJNR Am J Neu-roradiol 1989;10:143–150**

78. **Ducruet AF, Albuquerque FC, Crowley RW, McDougall CG. The evolution of endo-vascular treatment of carotid cavernous fistulas: a single-center experience. World Neurosurg 2013;80:538–548**

79. Meyers PM, Halbach VV, Dowd CF, et al. Dural carotid cavernous fistula: definitive endovascular management and long-term follow-up. Am J Ophthalmol 2002;134: 85–92

80. De Keukeleire K, Vanlangenhove P, Kalala Okito JP, Hallaert G, Van Roost D, Defreyne L. Transarterial embolization with ONYX for treatment of intracranial non-cavernous dural arteriovenous fistula with or without cortical venous reflux. J Neurointerv Surg 2011;3:224–228

81. Luo CB, Chang FC, Mu-Huo Teng M, et al. Transarterial Onyx embolization of intracra-nial dural arteriovenous fistulas: a single center experience. J Chin Med Assoc 2014; 77:184–189

82. Rangel-Castilla L, Barber SM, Klucznik R, Diaz O. Mid and long term outcomes of dural arteriovenous fistula endovascular management with Onyx. Experience of a single tertiary center. J Neurointerv Surg. 2014;6:607–613

83. Greenberg MS, Greenberg MS. Handbook of Neurosurgery, 7th ed. Tampa, FL: Green-berg Graphics/Thieme; 2010

84. Liu A, Liu J, Qian Z, et al. Onyx embolization of cavernous sinus dural arteriovenous fistulas via direct transorbital puncture under the guidance of three-dimensional re-constructed skull image (reports of six cases). Acta Neurochir (Wien) 2014;156:897–900

85. Kim MJ, Shin YS, Ihn YK, et al. Transvenous embolization of cavernous and paracav-ernous dural arteriovenous fistula through the facial vein: report of 12 cases. Neuro-intervention 2013;8:15–22

86. Vanlandingham M, Fox B, Hoit D, Elijovich L, Arthur AS. Endovascular treatment of intra-cranial dural arteriovenous fistulas. Neurosurgery 2014;74(Suppl 1):S42–S49

87. Jung C, Kwon BJ, Kwon OK, et al. Intraosseous cranial dural arteriovenous fistula treated with transvenous embolization. AJNR Am J Neuroradiol 2009;30:1173–1177

88. Andreou A, Ioannidis I, Nasis N. Transarterial balloon-assisted glue embolization of high-flow arteriovenous fistulas. Neuroradiology 2008;50:267–272

89. Kirsch M, Liebig T, Kühne D, Henkes H. Endovascular management of dural arteriove-nous fistulas of the transverse and sigmoid sinus in 150 patients. Neuroradiology 2009;51:477–483

90. Fok KF, Agid R, Souza MP, terBrugge KG. Thrombosis of aggressive dural arteriovenous fistula after incomplete embolization. Neuroradiology 2004;46:1016–1021

91. Agid R, Terbrugge K, Rodesch G, Andersson T, Söderman M. Management strategies for anterior cranial fossa (ethmoidal) dural arteriovenous fistulas with an emphasis on endovascular treatment. J Neurosurg 2009;110:79–84

92. Guedin P, Gaillard S, Boulin A, et al. Therapeutic management of intracranial dural arteriovenous shunts with leptomeningeal venous drainage: report of 53 consecutive patients with emphasis on transarterial embolization with acrylic glue. J Neurosurg 2010;112:603–610

93. Kiyosue H, Hori Y, Okahara M, et al. Treatment of intracranial dural arteriovenous fistulas: current strategies based on location and hemodynamics, and alternative techniques of transcatheter embolization. Radiographics 2004;24:1637–1653

94. Tomak PR, Cloft HJ, Kaga A, Cawley CM, Dion J, Barrow DL. Evolution of the management of tentorial dural arteriovenous malformations. Neurosurgery 2003; 52:750–760, discussion 760–762

95. Abud TG, Nguyen A, Saint-Maurice JP, et al. The use of Onyx in different types of intracranial dural arteriovenous fistula. AJNR Am J Neuroradiol 2011;32: 2185–2191

96. Cognard C, Januel AC, Silva NA Jr, Tall P. Endovascular treatment of intracranial dural arteriovenous fistulas with cortical venous drainage: new management using Onyx. AJNR Am J Neuroradiol 2008;29:235–241

97. Hu YC, Newman CB, Dashti SR, Albuquerque FC, McDougall CG. Cranial dural arteriovenous fistula: transarterial Onyx embolization experience and technical nuances. J Neurointerv Surg 2011;3:5–13

98. Chandra RV, Leslie-Mazwi TM, Mehta BP, et al. Transarterial Onyx embolization of cranial dural arteriovenous fistulas: long-term follow-up. AJNR Am J Neuroradiol 2014;35:1793–1797

99. Mathis JM, Barr JD, Jungreis CA, et al. Temporary balloon test occlusion of the internal carotid artery: experience in 500 cases. AJNR Am J Neuroradiol 1995;16:749–754

100. Abud DG, Spelle L, Piotin M, Mounayer C, Vanzin JR, Moret J. Venous phase timing during balloon test occlusion as a criterion for permanent internal carotid artery sacrifice. AJNR Am J Neuroradiol 2005;26:2602–2609

101. Wang AY, Chen CC, Lai HY, Lee ST. Balloon test occlusion of the internal carotid artery with stump pressure ratio and venous phase delay technique. J Stroke Cerebrovasc Dis 2013;22:e533–e540

102. Devagupthapu SR, Khatri R, Qureshi AI. Balloon test occlusion with hypotensive challenge using a novel agent Fenoldopam: a first experience. J Neurosurg Anesthesiol 2011;23:270–271

103. Standard SC, Ahuja A, Guterman LR, et al. Balloon test occlusion of the internal carotid artery with hypotensive challenge. AJNR Am J Neuroradiol 1995;16:1453–1458

104. Wong GK, Poon WS, Chun Ho Yu S. Balloon test occlusion with hypotensive challenge for main trunk occlusion of internal carotid artery aneurysms and pseudoaneurysms. Br J Neurosurg 2010;24:648–652

105. McIvor NP, Willinsky RA, TerBrugge KG, Rutka JA, Freeman JL. Validity of test occlusion studies prior to internal carotid artery sacrifice. Head Neck 1994;16:11–16

106. Dare AO, Gibbons KJ, Gillihan MD, Guterman LR, Loree TR, Hicks WL Jr. Hypotensive endovascular test occlusion of the carotid artery in head and neck cancer. Neurosurg Focus 2003;14:e5

107. Marshall RS, Lazar RM, Young WL, et al. Clinical utility of quantitative cerebral blood flow measurements during internal carotid artery test occlusions. Neurosurgery 2002;50:996–1004, discussion 1004–1005

108. Dare AO, Chaloupka JC, Putman CM, Fayad PB, Awad IA. Failure of the hypotensive provocative test during temporary balloon test occlusion of the internal carotid artery to predict delayed hemodynamic ischemia after therapeutic carotid occlusion. Surg Neurol 1998;50:147–155, discussion 155–156

109. Marshall RS, Lazar RM, Pile-Spellman J, et al. Recovery of brain function during induced cerebral hypoperfusion. Brain 2001;124(Pt 6):1208–1217

110. Lazar RM, Marshall RS, Pile-Spellman J, et al. Continuous time estimation as a behavioural index of human cerebral ischaemia during temporary occlusion of the internal carotid artery. J Neurol Neurosurg Psychiatry 1996;60:559–563

111. Marshall RS, Lazar RM, Mohr JP, et al. Higher cerebral function and hemispheric blood flow during awake carotid artery balloon test occlusions. J Neurol Neurosurg Psychiatry 1999;66:734–738

112. Morioka T, Matsushima T, Fujii K, Fukui M, Hasuo K, Hisashi K. Balloon test occlusion of the internal carotid artery with monitoring of compressed spectral arrays (CSAs) of electroencephalogram. Acta Neurochir (Wien) 1989;101:29–34

113. Cloughesy TF, Nuwer MR, Hoch D, Vinuela F, Duckwiler G, Martin N. Monitoring carotid test occlusions with continuous EEG and clinical examination. J Clin Neurophysiol 1993;10:363–369

114. Herkes GK, Morgan M, Grinnell V, et al. EEG monitoring during angiographic balloon test carotid occlusion: experience in sixteen cases. Clin Exp Neurol 1993;30:98–103

115. Murphy KJ, Payne T, Jamadar DA, Beydoun A, Frey KA, Brunberg JA. Correlation of continuous EEG monitoring with [O-l5]H2O positron emission tomography determination of cerebral blood flow during balloon test occlusion of the internal carotid artery. Experience in 34 cases. Interv Neuroradiol 1998;4:51–55

116. Kuroda S, Yonekawa Y, Kawano T, et al. [SEP monitoring during balloon occlusion test or operation for vertebro-basilar aneurysms]. No Shinkei Geka 1991;19:343–348

117. Schellhammer F, Heindel W, Haupt WF, Landwehr P, Lackner K. Somatosensory evoked potentials: a simple neurophysiological monitoring technique in supra-aortal balloon test occlusions. Eur Radiol 1998;8:1586–1589

118. Su CC, Watanabe T, Yoshimoto T, Ogawa A, Ichige A. Proximal clipping of dissecting intracranial vertebral aneurysm—effect of balloon Matas test with neurophysiological monitoring. Case report. Acta Neurochir (Wien) 1990;104:59–63

119. Kaminogo M, Ochi M, Onizuka M, Takahata H, Shibata S. An additional monitoring of regional cerebral oxygen saturation to HMPAO SPECT study during balloon test occlusion. Stroke 1999;30:407–413

120. van Rooij WJ, Sluzewski M, Slob MJ, Rinkel GJ. Predictive value of angiographic testing for tolerance to therapeutic occlusion of the carotid artery. AJNR Am J Neuroradiol 2005;26:175–178

121. Sorteberg A, Bakke SJ, Boysen M, Sorteberg W. **Angiographic balloon test occlusion and therapeutic sacrifice of major arteries to the brain. Neurosurgery 2008;63:651–660, 660–661**

122. Barker DW, Jungreis CA, Horton JA, Pentheny S, Lemley T. Balloon test occlusion of the internal carotid artery: change in stump pressure over 15 minutes and its correlation with xenon CT cerebral blood flow. AJNR Am J Neuroradiol 1993;14:587–590

123. Kato K, Tomura N, Takahashi S, et al. Balloon occlusion test of the internal carotid artery: correlation with stump pressure and 99mTc-HMPAO SPECT. Acta Radiol 2006; 47:1073–1078

124. Kurata A, Miyasaka Y, Tanaka C, Ohmomo T, Yada K, Kan S. Stump pressure as a guide to the safety of permanent occlusion of the internal carotid artery. Acta Neurochir (Wien) 1996;138:549–554

125. Morishima H, Kurata A, Miyasaka Y, Fujii K, Kan S. Efficacy of the stump pressure ratio as a guide to the safety of permanent occlusion of the internal carotid artery. Neurol Res 1998;20:732–736

126. Tomura N, Omachi K, Takahashi S, et al. Comparison of technetium Tc 99m hexamethylpropyleneamine oxime single-photon emission tomograph with stump pressure during the balloon occlusion test of the internal carotid artery. AJNR Am J Neuroradiol 2005;26:1937–1942

127. Galego O, Nunes C, Morais R, Sargento-Freitas J, Sales F, Machado E. Monitoring balloon test occlusion of the internal carotid artery with transcranial Doppler. A case report and literature review. Neuroradiol J 2014;27:115–119

128. Bhattacharjee AK, Tamaki N, Wada T, Hara Y, Ehara K. Transcranial Doppler findings during balloon test occlusion of the internal carotid artery. J Neuroimaging 1999; 9:155–159

129. Eckert B, Thie A, Carvajal M, Groden C, Zeumer H. Predicting hemodynamic ischemia by transcranial Doppler monitoring during therapeutic balloon occlusion of the internal carotid artery. AJNR Am J Neuroradiol 1998;19:577–582

130. Erba SM, Horton JA, Latchaw RE, et al. Balloon test occlusion of the internal carotid artery with stable xenon/CT cerebral blood flow imaging. AJNR Am J Neuroradiol 1988;9:533–538

131. Linskey ME, Jungreis CA, Yonas H, et al. Stroke risk after abrupt internal carotid artery sacrifice: accuracy of preoperative assessment with balloon test occlusion and stable xenon-enhanced CT. AJNR Am J Neuroradiol 1994;15:829–843

132. Ebara M, Murayama Y, Saguchi T, et al. Balloon test occlusion with perfusion CT imaging utilizing intraarterial contrast injection. Interv Neuroradiol 2006;12(Suppl 1): 241–245

133. Jain R, Hoeffner EG, Deveikis JP, Harrigan MR, Thompson BG, Mukherji SK. Carotid perfusion CT with balloon occlusion and acetazolamide challenge test: feasibility. Radiology 2004;231:906–913

134. Lorberboym M, Pandit N, Machac J, et al. Brain perfusion imaging during preoperative temporary balloon occlusion of the internal carotid artery. J Nucl Med 1996; 37:415–419

135. Okudaira Y, Arai H, Sato K. Cerebral blood flow alteration by acetazolamide during carotid balloon occlusion: parameters reflecting cerebral perfusion pressure in the acetazolamide test. Stroke 1996;27:617–621

136. Brunberg JA, Frey KA, Horton JA, Deveikis JP, Ross DA, Koeppe RA. [15O]H2O positron emission tomography determination of cerebral blood flow during balloon test occlusion of the internal carotid artery. AJNR Am J Neuroradiol 1994;15:725–732

137. Katano H, Nagai H, Mase M, Banno T. Measurement of regional cerebral blood flow with H2(15)O positron emission tomography during Matas test. Report of three cases. Acta Neurochir (Wien) 1995;135:70–77

138. Kawai N, Kawanishi M, Shindou A, et al. Cerebral blood flow and metabolism measurement using positron emission tomography before and during internal carotid artery test occlusions: feasibility of rapid quantitative measurement of CBF and OEF/CMRO . Interv Neuroradiol 2012;18:264–274

139. Murphy KJ, Deveikisz JP, Brunberg JA, Jamadar DA, Frey KA. [O-15]H2O positron emission tomography determination of cerebral blood flow reserve after intravenous acetazolamide during balloon test occlusion of the internal carotid artery. Interv Neuroradiol 1998;4:57–62

140. Monsein LH, Jeffery PJ, van Heerden BB, et al. Assessing adequacy of collateral circulation during balloon test occlusion of the internal carotid artery with 99mTc-HMPAO SPECT. AJNR Am J Neuroradiol 1991;12:1045–1051

141. Peterman SB, Taylor A Jr, Hoffman JC Jr. Improved detection of cerebral hypoperfusion with internal carotid balloon test occlusion and 99mTc-HMPAO cerebral perfusion SPECT imaging. AJNR Am J Neuroradiol 1991;12:1035–1041

142. Ryu YH, Chung TS, Lee JD, et al. HMPAO SPECT to assess neurologic deficits during balloon test occlusion. J Nucl Med 1996;37:551–554

143. Moody EB, Dawson RC III, Sandler MP. 99mTc-HMPAO SPECT imaging in interventional neuroradiology: validation of balloon test occlusion. AJNR Am J Neuroradiol 1991;12:1043–1044

144. Michel E, Liu H, Remley KB, et al. Perfusion MR neuroimaging in patients undergoing balloon test occlusion of the internal carotid artery. AJNR Am J Neuroradiol 2001;22:1590–1596

145. Ma J, Mehrkens JH, Holtmannspoetter M, et al. Perfusion MRI before and after acetazolamide administration for assessment of cerebrovascular reserve capacity in patients with symptomatic internal carotid artery (ICA) occlusion: comparison with 99mTc-ECD SPECT. Neuroradiology 2007;49:317–326

146. Charbel FT, Zhao M, Amin-Hanjani S, Hoffman W, Du X, Clark ME. A patient-specific computer model to predict outcomes of the balloon occlusion test. J Neurosurg 2004;101:977–988

147. Kailasnath P, Dickey PS, Gahbauer H, Nunes J, Beckman C, Chaloupka JC. Intracarotid pressure measurements in the evaluation of a computer model of the cerebral circulation. Surg Neurol 1998;50:257–263

148. Simonson TM, Ryals TJ, Yuh WT, Farrar GP, Rezai K, Hoffman HT. MR imaging and HMPAO scintigraphy in conjunction with balloon test occlusion: value in predicting sequelae after permanent carotid occlusion. AJR Am J Roentgenol 1992;159:1063–1068

149. Spetzler RF, Daspit CP, Pappas CT. The combined supra- and infratentorial approach for lesions of the petrous and clival regions: experience with 46 cases. J Neurosurg 1992;76:588–599

150. Schmid-Elsaesser R, Steiger HJ, Yousry T, Seelos KC, Reulen HJ. Radical resection of meningiomas and arteriovenous fistulas involving critical dural sinus segments: ex-

perience with intraoperative sinus pressure monitoring and elective sinus reconstruction in 10 patients. Neurosurgery 1997;41:1005–1016, discussion 1016–1018

151. Kharb S, Gundgurthi A, Pandit A, et al. Inferior petrosal sinus sampling: final solution to a riddle called "Cushing's syndrome." Med J Armed Forces India 2013;69: 74–77

152. Corrigan DF, Schaaf M, Whaley RA, Czerwinski CL, Earll JM. Selective venous sampling to differentiate ectopic ACTH secretion from pituitary Cushing's syndrome. N Engl J Med 1977;296:861–862

153. Bonelli FS, Huston J III, Carpenter PC, Erickson D, Young WF Jr, Meyer FB. Adrenocorticotropic hormone-dependent Cushing's syndrome: sensitivity and specificity of inferior petrosal sinus sampling. AJNR Am J Neuroradiol 2000;21:690–696

154. Deipolyi A, Karaosmanoğlu A, Habito C, et al. The role of bilateral inferior petrosal sinus sampling in the diagnostic evaluation of Cushing syndrome. Diagn Interv Radiol 2012;18:132–138

155. Deipolyi AR, Hirsch JA, Oklu R. Bilateral inferior petrosal sinus sampling with desmopressin. J Neurointerv Surg 2013;5:487–488

156. Crock PA, Gilford EJ, Henderson JK, et al. Inferior petrosal sinus sampling in acromegaly. Aust N Z J Med 1989;19:244–247

157. Doppman JL, Miller DL, Patronas NJ, et al. The diagnosis of acromegaly: value of inferior petrosal sinus sampling. AJR Am J Roentgenol 1990;154:1075–1077

158. Miller DL, Doppman JL, Krudy AG, et al. Localization of parathyroid adenomas in patients who have undergone surgery. Part II. Invasive procedures. Radiology 1987; 162(1 Pt 1):138–141

159. Miller DL, Chang R, Doppman JL, Norton JA. Localization of parathyroid adenomas: superselective arterial DSA versus superselective conventional angiography. Radiology 1989;170(3 Pt 2):1003–1006

160. Chaffanjon PC, Voirin D, Vasdev A, Chabre O, Kenyon NM, Brichon PY. Selective venous sampling in recurrent and persistent hyperparathyroidism: indication, technique, and results. World J Surg 2004;28:958–961

161. Jones JJ, Brunaud L, Dowd CF, Duh QY, Morita E, Clark OH. Accuracy of selective venous sampling for intact parathyroid hormone in difficult patients with recurrent or persistent hyperparathyroidism. Surgery 2002;132:944–950, discussion 950–951

162. Graham KE, Samuels MH, Nesbit GM, et al. Cavernous sinus sampling is highly accurate in distinguishing Cushing's disease from the ectopic adrenocorticotropin syndrome and in predicting intrapituitary tumor location. J Clin Endocrinol Metab 1999;84:1602–1610

163. Oliverio PJ, Monsein LH, Wand GS, Debrun GM. Bilateral simultaneous cavernous sinus sampling using corticotropin-releasing hormone in the evaluation of Cushing disease. AJNR Am J Neuroradiol 1996;17:1669–1674

164. Ilias I, Chang R, Pacak K, et al. Jugular venous sampling: an alternative to petrosal sinus sampling for the diagnostic evaluation of adrenocorticotropic hormone-dependent Cushing's syndrome. J Clin Endocrinol Metab 2004;89:3795–3800

165. Oldfield EH, Doppman JL, Nieman LK, et al. Petrosal sinus sampling with and without corticotropin-releasing hormone for the differential diagnosis of Cushing's syndrome. N Engl J Med 1991;325:897–905

166. Doppman JL. There is no simple answer to a rare complication of inferior petrosal sinus sampling. AJNR Am J Neuroradiol 1999;20:191–192

167. Miller DL, Doppman JL, Peterman SB, Nieman LK, Oldfield EH, Chang R. Neurologic complications of petrosal sinus sampling. Radiology 1992;185:143–147

168. Hinchey J, Chaves C, Appignani B, et al. A reversible posterior leukoencephalopathy syndrome. N Engl J Med 1996;334:494–500

169. Lefournier V, Gatta B, Martinie M, et al. One transient neurological complication (sixth nerve palsy) in 166 consecutive inferior petrosal sinus samplings for the etiological diagnosis of Cushing's syndrome. J Clin Endocrinol Metab 1999;84:3401–3402

170. Kitaguchi H, Tomimoto H, Miki Y, et al. A brainstem variant of reversible posterior leukoencephalopathy syndrome. Neuroradiology 2005;47:652–656

171. Seyer H, Honegger J, Schott W, et al. Raymond's syndrome following petrosal sinus sampling. Acta Neurochir (Wien) 1994;131:157–159

172. Sturrock ND, Jeffcoate WJ. A neurological complication of inferior petrosal sinus sampling during investigation for Cushing's disease: a case report. J Neurol Neurosurg Psychiatry 1997;62:527–528

173. Gandhi CD, Meyer SA, Patel AB, Johnson DM, Post KD. Neurologic complications of inferior petrosal sinus sampling. AJNR Am J Neuroradiol 2008;29:760–765

174. Bonelli FS, Huston J III, Meyer FB, Carpenter PC. Venous subarachnoid hemorrhage after inferior petrosal sinus sampling for adrenocorticotropic hormone. AJNR Am J Neuroradiol 1999;20:306–307

175. Blevins LS Jr, Clark RV, Owens DS. Thromboembolic complications after inferior petrosal sinus sampling in patients with Cushing's syndrome. Endocr Pract 1998;4:365–367

176. Redekop G, Marotta T, Weill A. Treatment of traumatic aneurysms and arteriovenous fistulas of the skull base by using endovascular stents. J Neurosurg 2001;95:412–419

177. Kerwin AJ, Bynoe RP, Murray J, et al. Liberalized screening for blunt carotid and vertebral artery injuries is justified. J Trauma 2001;51:308–314

178. Biffl WL, Moore EE, Ryu RK, et al. The unrecognized epidemic of blunt carotid arterial injuries: early diagnosis improves neurologic outcome. Ann Surg 1998;228:462–470

179. Biffl WL, Moore EE, Offner PJ, Burch JM. Blunt carotid and vertebral arterial injuries. World J Surg 2001;25:1036–1043

180. Raymond J, Hardy J, Czepko R, Roy D. Arterial injuries in transsphenoidal surgery for pituitary adenoma; the role of angiography and endovascular treatment. AJNR Am J Neuroradiol 1997;18:655–665

181. Kocer N, Kizilkilic O, Albayram S, Adaletli I, Kantarci F, Islak C. Treatment of iatrogenic internal carotid artery laceration and carotid cavernous fistula with endovascular stent-graft placement. AJNR Am J Neuroradiol 2002;23:442–446

182. Cappabianca P, Alfieri A, Colao A, et al. Endoscopic endonasal transsphenoidal surgery in recurrent and residual pituitary adenomas: technical note. Minim Invasive Neurosurg 2000;43:38–43

183. Cappabianca P, Cavallo LM, Colao A, de Divitiis E. Surgical complications associated with the endoscopic endonasal transsphenoidal approach for pituitary adenomas. J Neurosurg 2002;97:293–298

184. Cappabianca P, Cavallo LM, Colao A, et al. Endoscopic endonasal transsphenoidal approach: outcome analysis of 100 consecutive procedures. Minim Invasive Neurosurg 2002;45:193–200
185. Ciric I, Rosenblatt S, Zhao JC. Transsphenoidal microsurgery. Neurosurgery 2002;51:161–169
186. Mansouri A, Fallah A, Cusimano MD, Das S. Vasospasm post pituitary surgery: systematic review and 3 case presentations. Can J Neurol Sci 2012;39:767–773
187. Kerber CW, Wong WH, Howell SB, Hanchett K, Robbins KT. An organ-preserving selective arterial chemotherapy strategy for head and neck cancer. AJNR Am J Neuroradiol 1998;19:935–941

13 Hi-Tech Tools in Skull Base Surgery

■ 3D Endoscopy

- Endoscopes are part of the armamentarium of skull base surgeons, in both pure endoscopic and microsurgical endoscope-assisted approaches.[1,2]
- The lack of three-dimensionality of the two-dimensional (2D) endoscope has been compensated by the introduction of the three-dimensional (3D) endoscope systems,[3–5] with large applications in transsphenoidal surgery.[6,7]
  - Advantages: 3D deepness of the surgical field, faster training curve for nonexperts.
  - Disadvantages: dizziness, fatigue, eyestrain,[3,8] cost, excessive magnification in some cases. The models that do not offer high definition lack fine differentiation of the colors of different structures.

■ Image-Guided and Robotic Skull Base Surgery

Neuronavigation technology has great advantages in skull base surgery, by fusing computed tomography (CT) and magnetic resonance imaging (MRI) and yielding real-time multiplanar images and 3D reconstructions for orientation during the approaches.

- Image guidance systems are optically based or work by means of electromagnetic tracking devices.
- Intraoperative CT and MRI offer real-time updates of the surgical results. Intraoperative MRI suites require dedicated instruments, such as nonferromagnetic surgical instrumentation, and they are still in limited use because of their very high costs.
- Ultrasound-based navigation systems enable intraoperative navigation and visualization of different structures at lower costs than with intraopera-

tive CT/MRI, with applications in open skull base surgery as well as in endoscopy.[9–11]

- Intraoperative navigation systems can be integrated with virtual endoscopy in endonasal transsphenoidal surgery, providing additional anatomic information and improving surgical orientation, especially in the presence of anatomic variants.[12,13]
- Robotic surgery, such as the da Vinci® surgical system (Intuitive Surgical Inc., Sunnyvale, CA) or the neuroArm® (University of Calgary, Canada),[14] which is an MR-compatible image-guided robot, enables free-hand surgery for multiple purposes, facilitating a precise, bimanual, tremor-free surgical dissection under microscopic 3D visualization. In the otolaryngology–head and neck surgery field, robotic surgery is used above all for transoral robotic surgery procedures,[15–18] with some limited case reports in skull base surgery by means of extended approaches (e.g., incision of soft palate and resection of hard palate). Its adoption and application in skull base surgery is currently limited by the size of the robotic arms and the instruments.
- Modifications of the Da Vinci robotic arms and concentric tube robotic instruments with needle-sized tentacle-like arms are currently under investigation for their use in robotic transnasal skull base surgery.[19]

■ Ultrasonic Surgical Aspirator

The available ultrasonic surgical aspirators include the Cavitron ultrasonic aspirator (CUSA; Valleylab, Boulder, CO), the Sonopet ultrasonic aspirator (Stryker, Kalamazoo, MI), and the Sonastar ultrasonic aspirator (Braun, Aesculap, Center Valley, PA). These tools use different technologies, and the interested reader should refer to the technical information provided by the manufacturers.

- A titanium tip oscillates at a frequency of 23 to 25 kHz (ultrasound), disintegrating tissue and, at the same time, aspirating it through a central channel.[20]
- The level of irrigation, suction, and vibration can be set on the control counsel; a foot switch is used to activate the device.
- Different settings and several tip variations can be used for different kinds of tissues, including bone. By using low level of irrigation, the heat generated allows the aspirator to be used for cutting and/or coagulating.[21]
- Standard CUSA displacement: 10 to 350 µm.[22]
- The manipulation of the hand piece provides "tactile feedback," which is useful when treating difficult tumors, such as skull base meningiomas and schwannomas.[21]

- Specific microprobes and modified hand-pieces enable the use of ultrasonic aspiration in transsphenoidal surgery,[23-26] facilitating the resection of the clinoid processes, clivus, odontoid process, and crista galli via the endonasal route.[27]
- Ultrasonic aspirators have been shown to provide safe, quick, and effective devascularization of dura mater attached to the brain in cases of reoperation,[28] confirming its potential use in skull base surgery as well.
- Ultrasonic bone aspirators are safe, quick, and effective tools in orbital surgery,[29,30] turbinoplasty,[31] skull base osteoma,[32] and facial nerve decompression.[33]
- Advantages: ultrasonic aspirators are very useful for debulking tumors and for partial hemostasis, as in the central debulking of vestibular schwannomas without damaging the capsule.
- Disadvantages: Ultrasonic aspirators are expensive tools. The disposable tip is also a disadvantage in that it adds to the cost.

The normal saline irrigating solution of the CUSA may be replaced by H_2O_2 (3%), offering an uninterrupted delivery of peroxide to the tumor at the same time as the ultrasonic aspiration is being done, potentially reducing blood loss in vascular tumors.[34,35]

■ Water-Jet Dissection

Water-jet dissection has been shown to be useful for resection of brain tumors, with preservation of vessels and cranial nerves,[36] although it has not been standardized for use in skull base surgery.

- The pulsed laser-induced liquid jet (LILJ) is a hybrid technique in which the photoacoustic energy of the laser is used to provide high-flow kinetic energy in the water jet.[3,4]
- An LILJ consists of a bayonet-shaped catheter incorporating a jet generator surrounded by a suction tube, with the jet energy source provided by a pulsed holmium:yttrium-aluminum-garnet (Ho:YAG) laser system. The laser pulse forms a large vapor bubble in the water flow and provides an expansion of the confined vapor bubbles, causing a high-velocity pulsed liquid jet (velocity ~ 20 m/s).
- The temperature of the water jet remains below 37°C (41°C is the temperature reported to cause neuronal damage[37,38]).
- An LILJ has been shown to provide precise dissection of skull base tumors (pituitary adenomas, meningiomas, craniopharyngiomas), with the great advantage of sparing perforators around tumors and preserving visual function.[39,40]

■ Laser

Used since the 1960s, lasers have wide application for surgical removal of intracranial tumors. It is also used in skull base surgery and endoscopic transsphenoidal approaches.

- The laser wavelength is absorbed by water. The laser is used to vaporize and coagulate small vessels.
- Lasers can be conveyed through a flexible optical fiber (diameter ~ 1 mm) and can be set at different powers, exposure times, and in pulsed or continuous wave.
- The neodymium (Nd):YAG laser has a wavelength of 1,060 to 1,340 nm. It is widely used in neurosurgery,[41,42] although it has deep penetration and entails the risk of tissue injury.[43,44]
- The CO_2 laser has also been used in neurosurgery[45], with the same limits of thermal dispersion in the tissue.[46] The problem of thermal dispersion is less relevant in endonasal surgery, and CO_2 laser can be used for pedicled nasoseptal flap tailoring.[47]
- The thulium laser, initially used for third ventriculostomy, has a more limited penetration and diffusion, in comparison with the other kinds of lasers, and higher cut precision.[48]
- The thulium laser is used in meningioma surgery for debulking, shrinking, and coagulating the tumor as well as its basal implant.[49–51]
- Lasers can be used under continuous irrigation to reduce the thermal damage on the peritumoral structures.
- In comparison to the CUSA, the thulium laser adds to the debulking/shrinkage of the tumor as well as the coagulation of the tissue and small vessels, avoiding the use of the ultrasonic aspirator with a bipolar.

> **Surgical Anatomy Pearl**
>
> Cranial nerves and vessels around the tissue should be protected with cottonoids.

■ Cryosurgery

A cryoprobe is used for simple, rapid freezing of vascular lesions. The freezing cryoprobe achieves adhesion to any tissue surfaces and may be used as a tumor retractor after its frozen tip and the tumor surface are firm enough to allow tumor removal without further dissections.[52] Popularized in the 1960s and 1970s for brain lesions and arteriovenous malformations, the technique is still used in skull base surgery, especially for orbital vascular tumors.

■ Excimer Laser-Assisted Nonocclusive Anastomosis

Excimer laser-assisted nonocclusive anastomosis (ELANA) is used in vascular neurosurgery or for the management of complex skull base tumors involving sacrifice of the main arteries, when high-flow bypass may be required.

- The ELANA technique uses an excimer laser/catheter system for performing an extracranial-to-intracranial or intracranial-to-intracranial bypass using a large-caliber conduit without occlusion of the recipient artery.

Technique

An anastomotic ring is attached to a recipient artery with sutures. A laser suction catheter is then passed down the lumen of the open donor vessel, placing it against the sidewall of the recipient artery. The activation of the laser enables a precise arteriotomy, separating the arteriotomy flap from the recipient, and avoiding its migration into the lumen of the recipient by suction. After removal of the catheter from the donor vessel with the small flap attached, the proximal donor lumen can be sewn end-to-end.[53-55]

■ References

Boldfaced references are of particular importance.

1. **Perneczky A, Fries G. Endoscope-assisted brain surgery: part 1—evolution, basic concept, and current technique. Neurosurgery 1998;42:219–224, discussion 224–225**
2. **Di Ieva A, Tam M, Tschabitscher M, Cusimano MD. A journey into the technical evolution of neuroendoscopy. World Neurosurg 2014;82:777–789**
3. Barkhoudarian G, Del Carmen Becerra Romero A, Laws ER. Evaluation of the 3-dimensional endoscope in transsphenoidal surgery. Neurosurgery 2013;73(1, Suppl Operative):ons74–ons78, discussion ons78–ons79
4. Becker H, Melzer A, Schurr MO, Buess G. 3-D video techniques in endoscopic surgery. Endosc Surg Allied Technol 1993;1:40–46
5. Singh A, Saraiya R. Three-dimensional endoscopy in sinus surgery. Curr Opin Otolaryngol Head Neck Surg 2013;21:3–10
6. **Bolzoni Villaret A, Battaglia P, Tschabitscher M, et al. A 3-dimensional transnasal endoscopic journey through the paranasal sinuses and adjacent skull base: a practical and surgery-oriented perspective. Neurosurgery 2014;10(Suppl 1):116–120, discussion 120**
7. **Tabaee A, Anand VK, Fraser JF, Brown SM, Singh A, Schwartz TH. Three-dimensional endoscopic pituitary surgery. Neurosurgery 2009;64(5, Suppl 2):288–293, discussion 294–295**

8. Brown SM, Tabaee A, Singh A, Schwartz TH, Anand VK. Three-dimensional endoscopic sinus surgery: feasibility and technical aspects. Otolaryngol Head Neck Surg 2008; 138:400–402

9. Rygh OM, Cappelen J, Selbekk T, Lindseth F, Hernes TA, Unsgaard G. Endoscopy guided by an intraoperative 3D ultrasound-based neuronavigation system. Minim Invasive Neurosurg 2006;49:1–9

10. Strowitzki M, Kiefer M, Steudel WI. A new method of ultrasonic guidance of neuro-endoscopic procedures. Technical note. J Neurosurg 2002;96:628–632

11. McGrath BM, Maloney WJ, Wolfsberger S, et al. Carotid artery visualization during anterior skull base surgery: a novel protocol for neuronavigation. Pituitary 2010; 13:215–222

12. Schulze F, Bühler K, Neubauer A, Kanitsar A, Holton L, Wolfsberger S. Intra-operative virtual endoscopy for image guided endonasal transsphenoidal pituitary surgery. Int J CARS 2010;5:143–154

13. Wolfsberger S, Neubauer A, Bühler K, et al. Advanced virtual endoscopy for endoscopic transsphenoidal pituitary surgery. Neurosurgery 2006;59:1001–1009, discussion 1009–1010

14. Sutherland GR, Lama S, Gan LS, Wolfsberger S, Zareinia K. Merging machines with microsurgery: clinical experience with neuroArm. J Neurosurg 2013;118:521–529

15. McLeod IK, Mair EA, Melder PC. Potential applications of the da Vinci minimally invasive surgical robotic system in otolaryngology. Ear Nose Throat J 2005;84:483–487

16. O'Malley BW Jr, Weinstein GS, Snyder W, Hockstein NG. Transoral robotic surgery (TORS) for base of tongue neoplasms. Laryngoscope 2006;116:1465–1472

17. Van Abel KM, Moore EJ. The rise of transoral robotic surgery in the head and neck: emerging applications. Expert Rev Anticancer Ther 2012;12:373–380

18. Austin GK, McKinney KA, Ebert CS Jr, Zanation AM. Image-guided robotic skull base surgery. J Neurol Surg B Skull Base 2014;75:231–235

19. Gilbert H, Hendrick R, Remirez A, Webster R III. A robot for transnasal surgery featuring needle-sized tentacle-like arms. Expert Rev Med Devices 2014;11:5–7

20. Reinhardt HF, Gratzl O. [Ultrasonic resection of brain tumors]. Ultraschall Med 1984; 5:260–264

21. Brock M, Ingwersen I, Roggendorf W. Ultrasonic aspiration in neurosurgery. Neurosurg Rev 1984;7:173–177

22. Desinger K, Liebold K, Helfmann J, Stein T, Müller G. A new system for a combined laser and ultrasound application in neurosurgery. Neurol Res 1999;21:84–88

23. Baddour HM, Lupa MD, Patel ZM. Comparing use of the Sonopet(®) ultrasonic bone aspirator to traditional instrumentation during the endoscopic transsphenoidal approach in pituitary tumor resection. Int Forum Allergy Rhinol 2013;3:588–591

24. Cappabianca P, Cavallo LM, Esposito I, Barakat M, Esposito F. Bone removal with a new ultrasonic bone curette during endoscopic endonasal approach to the sellar-suprasellar area: technical note. Neurosurgery 2010;66(3, Suppl Operative):E118, discussion E118

25. Oertel J, Krauss JK, Gaab MR. Ultrasonic aspiration in neuroendoscopy: first results with a new tool. J Neurosurg 2008;109:908–911

26. Yamasaki T, Moritake K, Nagai H, Uemura T, Shingu T, Matsumoto Y. A new, miniature ultrasonic surgical aspirator with a handpiece designed for transsphenoidal surgery. Technical note. J Neurosurg 2003;99:177–179

27. Rastelli MM Jr, Pinheiro-Neto CD, Fernandez-Miranda JC, Wang EW, Snyderman CH, Gardner PA. Application of ultrasonic bone curette in endoscopic endonasal skull base surgery: technical note. J Neurol Surg B Skull Base 2014;75:90–95

28. Galarza M, Sood S, Pomata HB. Use of ultrasonic aspiration for dural opening in cranial reoperations: technical note. Neurosurgery 2005;57(1, Suppl):E216, discussion E216

29. Cho RI, Choe CH, Elner VM. Ultrasonic bone removal versus high-speed burring for lateral orbital decompression: comparison of surgical outcomes for the treatment of thyroid eye disease. Ophthal Plast Reconstr Surg 2010;26:83–87

30. Sivak-Callcott JA, Linberg JV, Patel S. Ultrasonic bone removal with the Sonopet Omni: a new instrument for orbital and lacrimal surgery. Arch Ophthalmol 2005;123:1595–1597

31. Greywoode JD, Van Abel K, Pribitkin EA. Ultrasonic bone aspirator turbinoplasty: a novel approach for management of inferior turbinate hypertrophy. Laryngoscope 2010;120(Suppl 4):S239

32. Pagella F, Giourgos G, Matti E, Colombo A, Carena P. Removal of a fronto-ethmoidal osteoma using the Sonopet Omni ultrasonic bone curette: first impressions. Laryngoscope 2008;118:307–309

33. Samy RN, Krishnamoorthy K, Pensak ML. Use of a novel ultrasonic surgical system for decompression of the facial nerve. Laryngoscope 2007;117:872–875

34. Lichtenbaum R, de Souza AA, Jafar JJ. Intratumoral hydrogen peroxide injection during meningioma resection. Neurosurgery 2006;59(4, Suppl 2):ONS470–ONS473, discussion ONS473

35. Ammirati M, Lamki TT, Pillai P, Powers C. Intra-tumoral ultrasonic aspirator delivery of H2O2—a novel approach to resecting highly vascularized intracranial tumors. Technical note and case report. Clin Neurol Neurosurg 2013;115:1891–1893

36. Piek J, Oertel J, Gaab MR. Waterjet dissection in neurosurgical procedures: clinical results in 35 patients. J Neurosurg 2002;96:690–696

37. Hirano T, Nakagawa A, Uenohara H, et al. Pulsed liquid jet dissector using holmium:YAG laser—a novel neurosurgical device for brain incision without impairing vessels. Acta Neurochir (Wien) 2003;145:401–406, discussion 406

38. Matsumi N, Matsumoto K, Mishima N, et al. Thermal damage threshold of brain tissue—histological study of heated normal monkey brains. Neurol Med Chir (Tokyo) 1994;34:209–215

39. Ogawa Y, Nakagawa A, Washio T, Arafune T, Tominaga T. Tissue dissection before direct manipulation to the pathology with pulsed laser-induced liquid jet system in skull base surgery—preservation of fine vessels and maintained optic nerve function. Acta Neurochir (Wien) 2013;155:1879–1886

40. Ogawa Y, Nakagawa A, Takayama K, Tominaga T. Pulsed laser-induced liquid jet for skull base tumor removal with vascular preservation through the transsphenoidal approach: a clinical investigation. Acta Neurochir (Wien) 2011;153:823–830

41. Beck OJ. Use of the Nd-YAG laser in neurosurgery. Neurosurg Rev 1984;7:151–157

42. Beck OJ, Frank F. The use of the Nd-YAG laser in neurosurgery. Lasers Surg Med 1985; 5:345–356

43. Yamagami T, Handa H, Takeuchi J, et al. Extent of thermal penetration of Nd-YAG laser—histological considerations. Neurosurg Rev 1984;7:165–170

44. Jain KK. Complications of use of the neodymium: yttrium-aluminum-garnet laser in neurosurgery. Neurosurgery 1985;16:759–762

45. Killory BD, Chang SW, Wait SD, Spetzler RF. Use of flexible hollow-core CO2 laser in microsurgical resection of CNS lesions: early surgical experience. Neurosurgery 2010;66:1187–1192

46. Ryan RW, Wolf T, Spetzler RF, Coons SW, Fink Y, Preul MC. Application of a flexible CO(2) laser fiber for neurosurgery: laser-tissue interactions. J Neurosurg 2010; 112:434–443

47. Nation JJ, Shkoukani M, Guthikonda M, Folbe AJ. A novel technique for pedicled naso-septal flap takedown in revision skull base surgery. J Neurol Surg B Skull Base 2013;74:225–227

48. Xia SJ. Two-micron (thulium) laser resection of the prostate-tangerine technique: a new method for BPH treatment. Asian J Androl 2009;11:277–281

49. Passacantilli E, Anichini G, Delfinis CP, Lenzi J, Santoro A. Use of 2-μm continuous-wave thulium laser for surgical removal of a tentorial meningioma: case report. Photomed Laser Surg 2011;29:437–440

50. Passacantilli E, Antonelli M, D'Amico A, et al. Neurosurgical applications of the 2-μm thulium laser: histological evaluation of meningiomas in comparison to bipolar forceps and an ultrasonic aspirator. Photomed Laser Surg 2012;30:286–292

51. Passacantilli E, Anichini G, Lapadula G, Salvati M, Lenzi J, Santoro A. Assessment of the utility of the 2-μ thulium laser in surgical removal of intracranial meningiomas. Lasers Surg Med 2013;45:148–154

52. Endo S, Nishijima M, Takaku A. Cryosurgical retraction in the removal of intracranial vascular tumors—technical note. Neurol Med Chir (Tokyo) 1993;33:44–45

53. Tulleken CA, Verdaasdonk RM, Berendsen W, Mali WP. Use of the excimer laser in high-flow bypass surgery of the brain. J Neurosurg 1993;78:477–480

54. Tulleken CA, Verdaasdonk RM. First clinical experience with Excimer assisted high flow bypass surgery of the brain. Acta Neurochir (Wien) 1995;134:66–70

55. van Doormaal TP, Klijn CJ, van Doormaal PT, et al. High-flow extracranial-to-intracranial excimer laser-assisted nonocclusive anastomosis bypass for symptomatic carotid artery occlusion. Neurosurgery 2011;68:1687–1694, discussion 1694

II Skull Base Surgery

14 Transcranial Approaches to the Skull Base

■ 14.1 Presurgical Considerations Regarding the Approach

When deciding on a surgical approach to the skull base, the surgeon must consider the lesion, the patient, his or her own preferences and expertise, as well as the surgical team and the environment in which the team operates. The surgeon must gauge the abilities of the surgical team (e.g., is the planned surgery within the team's capabilities and training?), and must assess the equipment and resources available (e.g., is neuronavigation available?). Undertaking approaches with which the surgeons and the surgical team have little or no experience is irresponsible, unfair to the patient, and could lead to avoidable complications.

* The lesion and its effects on the patient must be carefully considered. Asymptomatic lesions rarely need a surgical approach on a first assessment, unless the working diagnosis suggests a poor prognosis if left untreated. Asymptomatic patients who have lesions that have been shown to be growing, particularly in eloquent areas with impending neurologic deficit, should have appropriate counseling regarding the natural history of the disease and the pros and cons of surgery. Symptomatic patients should be assessed for a correlation between the symptoms and the lesion. Those patients in whom the lesion and symptoms cannot be deemed related should undergo a similarly focused discussion with their surgeons regarding the benefits and risks of surgery in a frank and honest fashion. In many of these circumstances, observation of the patient with serial imaging may be the most prudent approach.

Patients who have lesions that correlate well with their symptoms (e.g., the patient with a large pituitary adenoma and a bitemporal visual field defect) should be considered candidates for surgery after medical assessment and an assessment of the likelihood of being helped by a surgical approach. Patients who are unlikely to be helped by surgery (e.g., the patient with a small cavernous sinus meningioma and ophthalmoparesis) should be managed by alternative techniques such as radiosurgery (see Chapter 30).

Considerations of the patient's age, physiological status, and comorbidities should be carefully weighed before recommending surgery. Whether surgery will hold a reasonable likelihood of benefit depends on the symptom–anatomy correlation and the degree to which effects on critical structures can be reversed, or at the very least critical function can be preserved and damage minimized.

- Once it is decided that a patient will benefit from surgery, the surgeon and the team must determine the goals of surgery (e.g., tissue diagnosis, debulking, resection, decompression), the most appropriate approach, and the methods to achieve this approach. The approach must be determined by considering the eloquence of the surgical corridor and the degree to which the corridor will provide sufficient access to achieve the goals of surgery. For example, if the goal of surgery is to achieve a gross total resection but the approach selected would only provide a subtotal resection or biopsy, then either the goal or the approach should be reconsidered. The goal must align with the proposed surgical approach. The goal and the surgical plan should be discussed with the patient and the family.
- Determining the surgical approach is based in part on an evaluation of the size, texture, vascularity, and firmness of the lesion; the degree of extension to cranial nerves, vessels, and brain structures; the degree of brain edema and shift of structures; the intracranial pressure and hydrocephalus; and the number of "compartments" (e.g., a cranial fossa, a paranasal sinus, a particular bone, an extracranial space) in which the lesion resides. Whether the

Example 1: A 40-year-old, otherwise healthy, patient with no prior surgery presented with a large sellar and suprasellar mass with visual compromise and normal prolactin levels. A lesion in a large sella turcica would be best treated via an approach through the sphenoid sinus using appropriate local tissues for repair.

Example 2: A 60-year-old patient presented with an extensive basal frontal lesion with marked frontal lobe edema, and extension through the dura, arachnoid, pia mater, and skull base into the ethmoid and sphenoid bones. The patient will likely need an approach that provides wide access to each compartment and the ability to reconstruct the neuro-aerodigestive tract barriers, ideally with vascularized tissue, as well as management of intracranial and CSF pressures. This might mean a subfrontal approach with orbitocranial osteotomy and pericranial flap reconstruction. A failure to consider these issues in a comprehensive manner when planning whether and how to approach a particular patient with a particular lesion is doomed to fail.

lesion is intradural or extradural must be determined. Also, the degree to which vascularized or nonvascularized tissues are necessary to repair a particular corridor, once lesion management has been completed, must be assessed. The surgeon must ensure that a reconstruction can be performed before embarking on access.

■ Intraoperative, Preincisional Considerations

The surgical plan should clearly describe the surgical approach and the imaging to be used. The plan should be reviewed by all members of the team. A comprehensive, standardized, specialty-specific checklist should be developed in a meeting of all surgical, anesthesia, and nursing team members. The following issues should be discussed: surgical goals, patient positioning, antibiotic and seizure prophylaxis, blood and fluid treatment plans, deep vein thrombosis prophylaxis, anesthesia and monitoring techniques, the availability and functioning of surgical equipment, management of intracranial pressure and cerebrospinal (CSF), tissue reconstruction, and the postoperative discharge plan.

- **Cerebrospinal fluid diversion**. Patients at risk of CSF leak or in need of brain relaxation (or both) should be considered for CSF diversion. CSF diversion can be done via a lumbar drain (LD) or an external ventricular drain (EVD). Lumbar drains are considered for those patients in whom the basal CSF cisterns will be accessed late in the procedure and in whom brain relaxation will facilitate the access, but not place the patient at undue risk of herniation. Those patients with large tumors that cause significant mass effect or shift of structures from one compartment to another should be considered for EVD rather than LD if CSF drainage is thought to be of use and if access to the basal cisterns will occur late in the procedure. Patients undergoing procedures that involve wide opening of the basal cisterns and opening of the barriers of the neuro-aerodigestive tract will require CSF diversion in the intensive care unit for several days postoperatively. Those who are at low or no risk of postoperative CSF leak can have their drains removed and the site stitched before they leave the operating room.

■ Intrasurgery Performance

Optimum performance of the team requires constant communication among all members. Any unexpected findings or change in plans of any of the discussed preincisional issues should be discussed immediately. Staff changes during the procedure should be communicated, and proper continuity of care ensured by standardized means of communications such as checklists. A thorough explanation of the intraoperative events and findings should be clearly documented in the patient record and communicated to the staff who will be managing the patient postoperatively, such as the intensive care unit staff.

■ Specific Approaches

The open approaches selected should facilitate (1) viewing the lesion with maximal safe access, (2) treating the lesion (e.g., excision), (3) avoiding complications with critical structures, and (4) providing the best ability to reconstruct. Every surgical plan should avoid complications by having a thorough plan for (1) access, (2) treatment, and (3) reconstruction. Views, surgical approaches, and techniques can be thought of, or classified, in a number of different ways. The type of skin incision does not define a surgical approach. Rather, the incision is created *after* a consideration of the following issues, to define the sort of access through the skull. The accomplished skull base surgeon will consider each issue with every patient:

1. Whether the relation to the skull base is (a) from below upward, or "subbasal"(e.g., transsphenoidal); (b) from above downward or "suprabasal" (e.g., pterional); or (c) by traversing the skull base (e.g., transcranial), or "transbasal."
2. Whether the lesion is viewed from (a) anterior, (b) anterolateral, (c) lateral, (d) posterolateral, or (e) posterior.
3. Whether the bones transgressed are (a) frontal, (b) temporal, (c) occipital, (d) sphenoid, (e) ethmoid, (f) maxillary, or (g) a combination of bones (e.g., frontal-temporal, transsphenoidal-ethmoidal). This conceptualization can be further subdivided according to the components of the particular bone transgressed (e.g., translabyrinthine, transcochlear, or transcondylar).
4. Whether the approach is primarily for the central midline or non-midline structures or both (see Chapter 2, **Fig. 2.3b**, page 12).
5. Whether the approach is primarily extradural, intradural, interdural, or transdural.
6. The relations with specific brain structures such as a lobe of the brain (e.g., subfrontal lobe or paracerebellar).
7. The natural brain pathways to the skull base or the positions to which the skull base lesion may extend (e.g., through fissures such as the frontal interhemispheric fissure, the sylvian fissure, or the posterior interhemispheric fissure).
8. Whether the resection of the lesion will occur as a whole (en-bloc) or progressively (piecemeal).

■ 14.2 Anterior Approaches

These approaches are classified according to whether they approach the lesion at the skull base from below (i.e., subbasal), from above (suprabasal), or directly parallel to or through the base (transbasal)[1,2] **(Fig. 14.1)**. The suprabasal and transbasal approaches generally go through the frontal bone, and the subbasal ones extend through the nasal cavity, ethmoid bones, sphenoid bone, and occasionally the maxilla. These approaches can be used for lesions from the frontal sinus to C2 and even further along the cervical spine. However, their widest extent is in the anterior and central skull base. Those anterior subbasal (subcranial) approaches are generally limited laterally by the optic nerves or medial orbital walls and internal carotid arteries (ICAs), whereas the suprabasal or transbasal ones are not.[3]

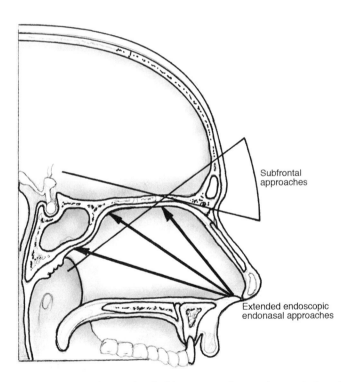

Fig. 14.1   Anterior approaches to the skull base. According to the surgical angle and the potential transgression of the bone, the approaches can be subbasal, suprabasal, or transbasal (see text). The figure also shows the possible surgical angles of the endonasal approaches.

Should the Lesion Be Approached from Above or Below the Skull Base?

In deciding whether to approach a midline lesion from above or below, in addition to considering the optic nerves and ICAs, the slope and particular anatomy of the anterior cranial fossa floor in relation to the position of the lesion should also be considered. This is particularly true for lesions, such as meningiomas, that are in the region of the planum sphenoidale. Intradural lesions along the planum in patients who have a steeply sloping planum are difficult to access from a purely anterior subfrontal approach unless the planum is drilled. These patients may be better served by an extended transsphenoidal approach as long as there is no encasement or extension of the tumor around the ICAs or anterior cerebral arteries (ACAs). If there is encasement, an anterior-lateral approach may be better.

- For the anterior approaches mentioned above, the degree to which one might have to use brain retraction is also a deciding factor. In this respect, one needs to consider the degree to which the lesion extends away from the floor. Although it may seem paradoxical, the higher the lesion extends up from the skull base, the more one might consider a more basally oriented approach. For example, for a large frontal fossa lesion that extends upward significantly, one may choose to perform an orbitocranial osteotomy in addition to a frontal craniotomy in order to avoid frontal lobe injury from brain retraction, if the relaxation provided by CSF drainage is insufficient. The less it extends away from the skull base, the more likely that simple measures such as an LD and a simple craniotomy will be sufficient.
- The subcranial approaches generally avoid brain retraction but are limited in their intracranial extent laterally without significantly more dissection. They also demand a high degree of experience and ability to reconstruct.
- Because the subbasal anterior approaches tend to be limited by the position of the lesion in relation to the ICAs, lesions that significantly extend laterally may be better approached suprabasally.

Should a Lumbar Drain Be Placed?

Access that interrupts the neuro-aerodigestive tract barriers to CSF must be reconstructed to prevent meningitis. If CSF leak is not a risk, then a vascularized repair is less critical, although one should always be prepared for a CSF leak. If the CSF barriers are penetrated, placement of CSF diversion is strongly recommended before accessing the lesion. If the lesion is large, but not so large as to place the patient at risk of herniation of brain, then an LD is often helpful.

Bilateral or Unilateral Approach?

This decision is largely defined by the lesion and its relation to critical structures like the ICAs. In general, the more the lesion extends across the midline and extends beyond the contralateral ICA, the more likely the surgeon would want to be able to access the contralateral ICA for control in the event of an ICA injury. Furthermore, if one is taking a purely interhemispheric approach and requiring access to purely midline structures such as the interhemispheric fissure, the more likely one would want a bilateral but more limited lateral approach.

Suprabasal Approaches: Subfrontal Approach

Indications

This approach is indicated for any lesion, intradural or extradural, of the anterior cranial fossa, including the frontal sinus, unilateral or bilateral, such as a tumor, aneurysm, or traumatic CSF leak. See subsection "Should the Lesion Be Approached from Above or Below the Skull Base", above.

Position

The patient is placed in a supine, semi-reclining position, with the head higher than the heart. The head is in neutral position, not turned for midline or paramidline lesions. For more laterally placed craniotomies to access lesions on both sides of the ICA or optic nerves, the head can be turned 15 to 30 degrees. The vertex is extended to allow the frontal lobes to relax by gravity. If fascia lata or fat is required for a repair, it should be prepared at this time and included in the sterile field.

Navigation

The position of the lesion and the frontal sinus should be projected and marked onto the scalp. The bony opening should be planned first and then the optimal incision planned afterward. In centers without frameless stereotaxy, this can also be accomplished by reference to surface landmarks and preoperative imaging correlation.

Incision

The incision can be unilateral or bilateral depending on whether the bony approach is unilateral or bilateral, how close to the midline the bony exposure is planned, and cosmetic considerations. For "mini" approaches, the incision can be placed above, in, or below the eyebrow. Local anesthetic with adrenaline for all incisions is recommended unless contraindicated (e.g., prior radiation, extensive scar, infection, allergy, hypertension, vascular concerns). The standard unilateral incision is a reverse question-mark shape starting in a crease close to the tragus and continuing to the midline of the hairline. For those cases where an orbitocranial osteotomy is fashioned, the incision can be taken lower and repaired with a fine subcuticular stitch. Careful hemostasis of the scalp should be maintained at all times by the eventual use of scalp clips (e.g., Raney clips) or hemostats.

- For patients requiring a bifrontal approach, a bony opening at the midline or, for cosmetic reasons (to avoid incisions near the forehead), a coronal incision is used. This generally extends from helix to helix, or if more basal exposure or temporal exposure is required, from the tragus or even lower. Although a number of variations exist on the coronal exposure (e.g., zigzag, sinusoidal) **(Fig. 14.2)**, the one that is in the same position as the coronal suture or parallel to it is the one that is most often used in neurosurgery. This variation maximizes the length of any pericranial/periosteal vascularized flap and yields very good cosmesis. The length of a pericranial flap should be estimated on the preoperative imaging, and the position of the coronal incision should be planned with this length in mind.

❖ Scalp Flap: Surgical Approach

Always try to preserve all the layers of the scalp and the superficial temporal artery and vein in the opening. These are all vascularized layers that can be important to the health of the scalp in the event of radiation, or be used if vascularized tissue is required.

- ◈ If the preoperative plan includes opening the frontal sinus and performing a vascularized periosteal flap reconstruction, then it is easiest to leave the periosteal layer on the bone when elevating the scalp and to raise it in a second layer based on the supraorbital artery and nerve along the orbital rim. If there is a low likelihood of requiring a periosteal flap, it is best to elevate it together with the other layers of the scalp and leave it attached. If the flap is needed at the end of the procedure, it can be easily dissected with care using a No. 15 scalpel or with fine nontraumatic scissors. Care should be taken to leave the galea aponeurotica in place, especially on the first surgery.
- ◈ The region of the frontalis branch of the facial nerve and the temporal fat pad should be managed carefully to avoid postoperative frontalis nerve palsy (see Chapter 2, **Fig. 2.19**, page 63). In coronal scalp incisions, this region should be managed the same way on both sides. In a unilateral approach, elevate the superficial fat pad and get to the deep fat pad and ele-

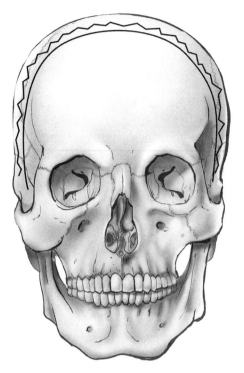

Fig. 14.2 Examples of coronal incisions in the anterior bifrontal approaches.

vate both with the scalp. In a unilateral or bilateral approach, carry the scalp at least as far as the orbital rim. If an orbitocranial osteotomy is planned with exposure near or across the midline, the nasal frontal suture is exposed in the midline. If a more lateral exposure is required, the zygomatic bone to the orbitofacial foramen is exposed.

- In the event that the supraorbital nerve is contained within a foramen, it usually can be extended into a notch with the use of an osteotome directed away from the globe. The supraorbital artery and vein should be preserved whenever possible with the nerve. If the distance between the superior orbital rim and the supraorbital foramen is more than 5 mm, often it is best to just sacrifice the nerve rather than create a large defect. The dissection is carried onto the superior orbital roof at this point, particularly if a transbasal approach with an orbitocranial osteotomy is planned. The orbital contents are protected with cottonoids, and the dissection proceeds with communication with the anesthesia team in the event of a trigeminal-vagal response due to the manipulation of orbital contents. The scalp is either stitched carefully or held in place with rubber bands connected to the stitches or by carefully placed hooks. The scalp is kept moist throughout the remainder of the procedure.

Craniotomy

Prior to craniotomy, the brain should be relaxed by means of an LD, hyperventilation, osmotic diuretics, or combinations of these maneuvers. The decision regarding the extent of the craniotomy has been described above. If a bilateral exposure is planned, control of the superior sagittal sinus (SSS) is crucial. It is quite safe to place one or more bur holes directly over the sinus using a perforator with an automatic stop function that halts the perforator once it is through bone as long as the perforator is held perfectly perpendicular to the bone. Carefully strip the SSS from the bone prior to elevation of the bone flap. Place one or multiple bur holes elsewhere. Bone dust can be preserved and placed into antibiotic solution for the remainder of the surgery and, if required, can be used in the reconstruction. If control of the SSS is not required, then place a bur hole high up on the frontal bone adjacent to the SSS to avoid any deformity of the forehead.

◈◈ Variation: At least one bur hole is placed in the "keyhole" after some elevation of the temporalis muscle, even in purely frontal craniotomies. Four bur holes can be done, combined with the cranioplastic "bridge technique" that leaves small bridges of bone between the bur holes. When the craniotomy is replaced, the bone rests on these bridges, providing a perfect contour of the skull and biomechanical stability that usually obviates the need for expensive miniplates in simple craniotomies.[4]

◈ If a bifrontal craniotomy is required, the same set of holes are placed on the contralateral side. The craniotome is taken straight across the base of the frontal bone through the frontal sinus bilaterally. The basal cut should be taken as low on the frontal fossa as possible to provide skull base access without the need for frontal lobe retraction. In the event of a deep midline internal crest on the frontal bone, a bridge is left in the midline and then it is "cracked" in the same fashion as the other bridges.

Frontal Sinus Exenteration

If only a tiny hole has been created in the frontal sinus, it can be repaired safely with bone wax. If it is a larger opening, strip and remove the frontal sinus mucosa carefully. Use a fine high-speed drill to remove any remaining fragments of mucosa. The sinus can be de-functioned after complete exenteration with fat packing and plugging of the frontal-nasal duct.

• There is no controlled or randomized evidence for removal of the posterior wall of the frontal sinus, so-called cranialization of the sinus. Apart from the case of trauma with comminuted fractures of the posterior wall of the frontal sinus (see Chapter 34, page 846), it seems that there is no role for cranialization in the contemporary management of skull base lesions.

Dural Management

Apply tack-up stitches to the edges of the dura. If the lesion is extradural, transbasal, or has extensive vascular supply arising extradurally (e.g., meningioma), or an orbital osteotomy is planned, the extradural space is now developed. After appropriate brain relaxation, use a dural or periosteal dissector to carefully elevate the anterior skull base dura. If needed, the ethmoidal and other penetrating arteries can be bipolared and divided. If a midline exposure is sought, the midline is dissected and a decision regarding the olfactory nerves ought to have been made preoperatively and discussed with the patient. Preservation of one set of olfactory nerves is desirable but must be predetermined based on the goals of the surgery. If the nerves are divided, the dura should be over-sewn immediately. If the midline is required, the SSS is suture ligatured carefully, with one suture ligature above and one below the planned position of the transection of the SSS, which ought to be as low to the skull base as possible. Dural access to the base can be achieved by cutting along the base, with a flap created along the base or along the SSS (near the foramen cecum) if the hemispheric fissure is the main corridor of access.

Wherever possible, all bridging veins should be preserved.

Lesion Management

Lesion management is discussed in the chapters that address each type of lesion. Some key points:

- Normal anatomic structures will be fixed in their origin from the brain and exit from the skull base; for example, the trigeminal nerve will always exit the pons on its midpoint and lateral aspect regardless of what the tumor has done to the pons. Its branches will always exit at the superior orbital fissure (SOF) (V_1), foramen rotundum (V_2), and foramen ovale (V_3). So whenever tumors or other lesions distort the anatomy, try to find the normal structure where one would expect to find it entering or exiting the space of interest.
- Preserve the arachnoid. Because blood vessels and nerves run in the subarachnoid space, preserving the arachnoid and always keeping the normal arachnoid with the patient will generally preserve the critical vessels, nerves, and brain.

Reconstruction: Dura Mater

Close the dura primarily. If the dura cannot be repaired, a duraplasty can be performed using autologous tissue such as the fascia lata or temporalis fascia. If other tissues are available, try not to use the pericranium for dural reconstruction, so as not to compromise the integrity of the scalp. A variety of commercially available dural substitutes can also be used. Some forms of these products may not be acceptable to the patient because of cultural or religious reasons, so the source of such products should be discussed preoperatively with the patient. The dural closure can be reinforced with fibrin glue, although no randomized controlled evidence supports this practice.

Reconstruction: Pericranial Flap (Fig. 14.3)

If there has been a broad opening of the CSF pathways and the neuro-aerodigestive pathways are opened, vascularized tissue coverage is the goal. The preserved periosteal flap is the one most used for this purpose. If it is absent and the scalp is in satisfactory condition, a galea flap or vascularized free flap such as a radial forearm flap based on the superficial temporal can also be used.

In bringing the periosteal flap down, care should be taken to be certain that the flap is not kinked over the base of the craniotomy opening. If the flap has to take a sinuous course up over a large bridge of bone at the base and the flap is at risk of necrosis, it may be best to remove the orbital bar so as to provide a flat and straight path for the vascularized flap. The flap should not be under tension and should be long enough to reach to the deepest part of the opening. The flap can be placed directly against the dura, or against a fat graft adjacent to the dura. If possible, the flap should be sutured to the dura at several spots so that it does not move in the closure. If there is a wide opening into the nasal

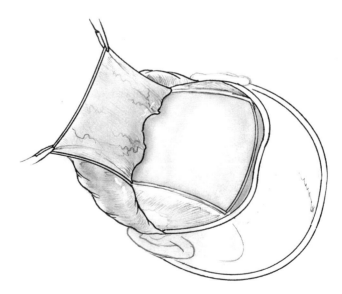

Fig. 14.3 Harvesting of the pericranial flap in the coronal approach.

cavity, it is also possible to place a fat graft and fibrin glue external to the peri-cranial flap. In the setting of a good flap, repair of the bone defect in the anterior skull base is not always necessary (see also Chapter 27, page 711).

Reconstruction: Bone and Soft Tissues

Care should be taken to ensure that any bony defects of the forehead that are visible are repaired with inert materials. If the frontal sinus has been opened, and even if repaired, cements such as methyl methacrylate are contraindicated because of the high risk of infection. In this instance, inert titanium mesh or plates can be used. In the absence of these options, bone dust and sutures can be utilized. A subgaleal drain can be used with or without a cranial wrap dressing.

Transbasal Approaches: Uni- or Bilateral Orbital-Cranial Subfrontal Transbasal, Nasofrontal Transbasal

There are a number of modifications of the transbasal approach.[5,6] The simplest involve drilling through the ethmoid and/or sphenoid planum in order to access the paranasal sinus regions. The more complex approaches incorporate an osteotomy that basically extends the approach to a transbasal point of view. The osteotomies can include only the orbit, the frontal-nasal complex, and the orbit, or the bilateral orbital roofs and the nasofrontal complex. The osteotomy(ies) can be combined with a drilling through the ethmoids and/or the sphenoid, in order to access the nasal cavity, the clivus, or down to C2.

◈◈ Variation: The approach may be limited to the midline, and done with a basal removal of the medial orbital and nasofrontal complex for malignant disease of the nasofrontal ethmoidal complex.[1,2,7] This osteotomy can be extended unilaterally or bilaterally to the orbital roof and rim, in order to widen the working spaces.

◈◈ In the event that the osteotomies are performed, the pericranial flap reconstruction should be brought in under (inferior) to the osteotomy and the osteotomized piece should be drilled slightly to widen the space for the flap so as not to strangulate it by using a flap that is too tight fitting.

◈ Orbital and orbito-nasofrontal osteotomies are replaced with the aid of titanium miniplates or, if these plates are unavailable, with heavy suture.

Complications

Complications can be classified as follows: (1) related to the approach (e.g., frontalis palsy, supraorbital numbness, alopecia along the incision, SSS injury, hemorrhage, anosmia, periorbital swelling, ptosis, diplopia); (2) related to the treatment of the lesion (e.g., neural injury such as cranial nerve or pituitary stalk, venous/arterial/perforator infarction, brain contusion, seizures); (3) related to the reconstruction (e.g., cosmetic deformities, CSF leak, meningitis); or (4) systemic (e.g., deep vein thrombosis, pneumonia).

Suprabasal Interhemispheric Approach to the Anterior Skull Base

Indications

This approach is suggested for the treatment of anterior skull base lesions, such as olfactory groove meningiomas, craniopharyngiomas, and dural arteriovenous fistulas[8,9] (see Chapter 19, **Fig. 19.2**, page 461).

Position

The patient is placed in the supine position, with the head fixed in a head clamp in the neutral position with the nose straight up, slightly elevated from the level of the heart, and with the face horizontal (parallel to the floor) or slightly extended.

❖ Surgical Approach

- ◈ Place at least two bur holes perfectly perpendicular on the SSS or on each side of it. Carefully dissect the SSS.
- ◈ Make a frontal bone flap between the coronal suture and the frontal sinus according to the size of the lesion. If the lesion is perfectly midline, then the approach can be performed on each side, or, for a right-handed surgeon, more to the right side.
- ◈ Using the microscope, perform interhemispheric dissection along the falx. Stay in the subarachnoid space and avoid going subpial. Identify and pre-

Surgical Anatomy Pearl

Spare all cortical veins in the dural opening. Be careful about those that enter the sinus in the top of the anterior third of the SSS. The dura can be opened with the base at the SSS or the base at the frontal skull base. A wider opening in the dura is worthwhile to avoid dividing the bridging veins and to enable working around these veins.

serve the anterior cerebral arteries. Reach the appropriate location along the anterior skull base and the pathology to be treated. Lateral retraction of one of the frontal lobes may be required, but avoid bifrontal retraction at all times.

Anterior Approaches to the Skull Base from Below

Transsphenoidal Approach

The sphenoid bone is the key to the skull base, and so it is no surprise that the transsphenoidal sinus (TSS) approaches have the most versatility in approaching lesions of the skull base. A number of variations exist in the TSS approaches, but the basic premise to unlock the sphenoid sinus and its adjacent neighbors remains constant. Access to the sphenoid sinus requires the establishment of a sufficient corridor in which to access and maneuver instruments at the skull base. This requires displacement or removal of part or all of the turbinates of the nasal cavity. The microscopic approaches generally displace and compress them using specula for the nasal cavity and displacement of the septum, whereas the endoscopic approaches tend to remove part or all of the middle and inferior turbinate depending on the area required for access. Although the microscope offers unparalleled stereoscopic vision, the endoscopic offers unparalleled panoramic vision and the ability to observe far beyond the midline. The initial access and mode of visualization differ, but ultimately, for midline structures, the techniques used at the tumor level are similar.

For a description of the endoscopic approaches, both standard and extended, see Chapter 16.

Sublabial Transsphenoidal Approach

This approach offers a wider exposure to the sphenoid in the event of small nostrils, such as occurs in young children.

Position of the Head

Use of head fixation is optional. Most surgeons maintain a neutral head position, although some prefer the head laterally flexed toward the surgeon by about 10 degrees or with mild extension (no more than 10 to 15 degrees) and some with rotation by approximately 10 to 20 degrees. Maintaining the anatomic neutral position minimizes the chances for surgeon disorientation. In pituitary surgery, avoid hyperextension of the head, as it leads to an approach that is too anterior, reaching the planum sphenoidale instead of the sella turcica.

❖ Surgical Approach

◈ Apply topical adrenaline with or without local anesthetic or a nasal agent such as xylometazoline, for nasal mucosa vasoconstriction.

◈ Administer local anesthetic along the floor and the nasal septum in order to assist in the elevation of the flap of mucosal tissue from the sublabial position.

◈ After preparation and elevation of the upper lip, infiltrate local anesthetic with diluted 1:100,000 or 1:200,000 adrenaline, and in a few minutes make a sublabial incision, and elevate the mucosa and periosteum with a dissector to expose the anterior nasal spine and inferior and lateral parts of the piriform aperture, creating one large pocket or two pockets (**Fig. 14.4**).

◈ Elevate the mucosa from the floor of the nasal cavity. Occasionally the spine can be drilled or removed with a small rongeur, but not more than 2 to 3 mm of bone.

◈ Elevate the mucosa in the anteroposterior direction with a superior and inferior dissection along the septum, reaching the vomer bone, more posteriorly.

◈ Separate the mucosa from the perpendicular plate and dissect it from the septal cartilage (columella) on both sides.

◈ Detach the columella from the vomer bone and perpendicular plate.

◈ Insert a nasal speculum and open the blades to straddle the perpendicular plate and expose the sphenoid bone rostrum, and remove it (with rongeurs).

◈ Identify the sphenoid ostia and enlarge them as required, to gain access into the sphenoid sinus.

◈ Strip the sphenoid sinus mucosa and remove the intrasinus septa.

◈ Based on the location of the pathology, drill or remove the bone of the sellar floor for access to the pituitary, the tuberculum sellae for access to more superoanterior lesions, and the clivus for posterior fossa approaches.

Surgical Anatomy Pearl

Check the anatomy of the sphenoid sinus septa carefully in the computed tomography (CT) scan before the approach.

Surgical Anatomy Pearl

Carefully localize the intrasphenoidal sinus anatomy: the planum sphenoidale superiorly, the sellar floor in the middle with cavernous sinuses and parasellar ICAs laterally, and the clivus inferiorly with paraclival ICAs laterally (see Chapter 2, **Fig. 2.15**, page 54). The most caudal extension of the clivus resection enables visualization and access to the atlas and to the tip of the odontoid process.

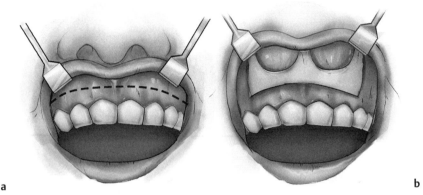

a   b

Fig. 14.4a,b   Sublabial transsphenoidal approach. **(a)** Sublabial incision. **(b)** Exposure of the anterior nasal spine and inferior piriform aperture. (Adapted from Day JD, Koos WT, Matula C, Lang J. Color Atlas of Microneurosurgical Approaches. Stuttgart, New York: Thieme; 1997.)

Transnasal Interseptal Approach

❖ Surgical Approach

The preparation of the nasal cavity and mucosa is similar to that in the sublabial approach.

◈ Enlarge the nostril and protect the nasal wing with an elevator or by using a nasal speculum **(Fig. 14.5a)**.

◈ Make a transfixion incision at the muco-squamosal junction just inside the nose along the septum.

◈ Elevate the mucosa and perichondrium from the septal cartilage **(Fig. 14.5b)**.

◈ Separate the mucosa from the septum on both sides.

◈ Perform luxation of the cartilaginous septum, detaching its posterior attachment on the perpendicular lamina of the ethmoid.

◈ Introduce a self-retaining speculum between the two septal mucosa layers, open the valves, and reach the floor of the sphenoid sinus.

Surgical Anatomy Pearls

Use the right length of speculum to reach the sinus; excessive opening of the speculum may cause skull base fractures **(Fig. 14.5c,d)**.

The position of the speculum in relation to the sphenoid sinus might eventually be checked by a lateral intraoperative X-ray.

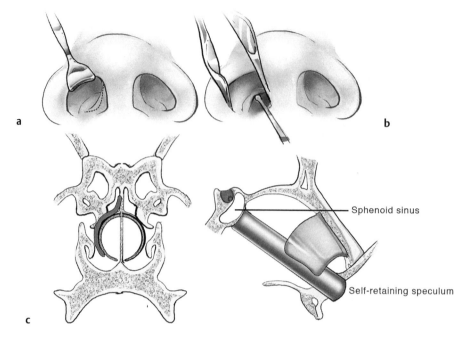

a

b

Sphenoid sinus

Self-retaining speculum

c

d

Fig. 14.5a–d Transnasal interseptal approach. (See text for a description of the panels.) (Adapted from Day JD, Koos WT, Matula C, Lang J. Color Atlas of Microneurosurgical Approaches. Stuttgart, New York: Thieme; 1997.)

◈ Open the floor of the sphenoid sinus, connecting the two sphenoid ostia, or drill off the front wall of the sphenoid.

◈ Access the sphenoid sinus, strip the mucosa out, and remove the septa, for correct identification of the landmarks.

Disadvantages of Microscopic Transsphenoidal Approaches

Disadvantages include long and narrow corridors, limited by the nasal structures, and limited exposure to the midline, particularly when visualized by microscope.

■ 14.3 Anterolateral Approaches

These approaches generally avoid the frontal sinus (depending upon the sinus lateral extension) and may or may not involve removal of the temporal squamous

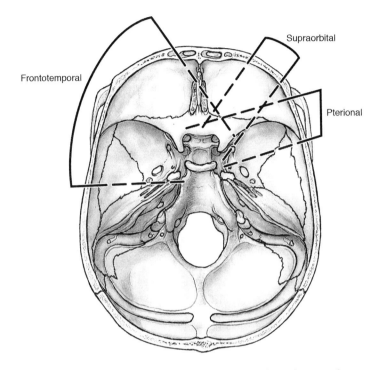

Fig. 14.6 Schematic representation of the angles of potential visualization of some antero-lateral approaches (pterional, supraorbital, extended frontotemporal).

bone in addition to the frontal bone. The frontotemporal craniotomy is the most common of these with variations such as the pterional, osteoplastic, fronto-temporal orbitocranial, and the orbitozygomatic approach. Like the anterior approaches, these approaches can be classified as suprabasal, transbasal, and subbasal based on the views they provide. They can also be classified as intra-dural, interdural, or extradural. **Fig. 14.6** shows a schematic representation of the angles of potential visualization of some anterolateral approaches.

Frontotemporal Craniotomy

This is a unilateral approach that is very useful for lesions of the regions of the anterior and middle fossa floor. It cannot easily access the frontal pole and anterior or superior interhemispheric fissure, and it provides less direct visu-alization of the contralateral ICA. Although it provides a limited pericranial flap, it can provide a temporalis muscle flap for reconstruction. Much of what was described for the anterior suprabasal approaches applies to the frontotemporal craniotomy.

Position

The patient is placed in the supine, semi-reclining position, with the head higher than the heart. Often a shoulder roll is placed to minimize strain on the neck. The head is often turned 15 to 45 degrees, depending on the pathology. The vertex is extended to allow the frontal lobes to relax by gravity.

Navigation

See above (page 337).

Incision

The standard unilateral incision is a reverse question-mark shape starting in a crease close to the tragus and coming to the midline of the hairline (**Fig. 14.7**). For those cases where an orbitocranial osteotomy is fashioned, the incision can be taken lower and repaired with a fine subcuticular stitch. For relatively small lesions in the posterior aspect of the middle fossa floor or tentorial incisura (e.g., basilar aneurysm), occasionally a straight incision or an inverted U-shaped incision centered just in front of the ear will suffice.

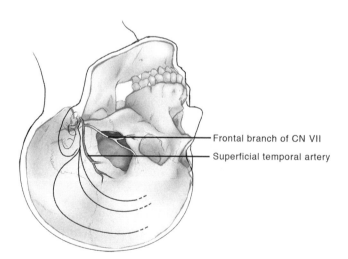

Frontal branch of CN VII
Superficial temporal artery

Fig. 14.7 Anterolateral approaches, surgical position. Based on the surgical plan, different incisions can be used. Note the position of the superficial temporal artery and the frontal branch of the facial nerve. The *dotted lines* show the eventual incision on the forehead, which, whenever necessary, should be sutured with subcuticular stitches at the end of the procedure.

Scalp Flap

As stated above, always try to preserve all the layers of the scalp and the superficial temporal artery and vein in the opening. These are all vascularized layers that can be important to the health of the scalp in the event of radiation, or can be used if vascularized tissue is required. Because these approaches rarely utilize a pericranial flap reconstruction, the pericranium is usually left attached with the other layers of the scalp. The scalp dissection is carried onto the superior orbital roof at this point, particularly if a transbasal approach with an orbitocranial osteotomy is planned. It is of paramount importance to understand the anatomy of the soft tissues in the pterional region (see **Fig. 2.19**, page 63).

- If a free bone flap is planned, then the temporalis muscle is elevated after the interfascial dissection as described above. The temporalis is mobilized most commonly from inferior to superior and either it can be completely disconnected at the superior temporal line (STL) or a small cuff of muscle can be left at the STL.
- If an osteoplastic flap is planned, the temporalis muscle is left attached to the bone and the bone flap turned. This technique is not possible if a transbasal orbitocranial or orbitozygomatic approach is planned.

> **Surgical Anatomy Pitfall**
>
> The temporalis muscle should not be denervated by any cuts across its belly in order to avoid postoperative atrophy.[10]

Craniotomy

Prior to craniotomy, the dura should be relaxed by means of an LD, hyperventilation, osmotic diuretics, or combinations of these maneuvers. One or more bur holes can be used for the approach, with at least one placed in the "keyhole." In the pterional technique, the bone of the pterion, the lateral sphenoid ridge, and the ridges of the orbital roof are drilled off. In the orbitocranial and orbitozygomatic approaches, this bone is removed en bloc and then replaced at the end of the procedure, usually providing less of a bone defect postoperatively.

Middle Fossa Floor

If access to the middle fossa floor is required, an extradural dissection is carried out along the floor. If this is extensive, this is usually combined with an orbitozygomatic (OZ) or a zygomatic arch osteotomy. The dissection is carried in an anterior to a posterior direction from the lesser sphenoid wing to the greater sphenoid wing to identify the foramen rotundum and foramen spinosum. The middle meningeal artery is carefully identified, bipolared, and divided. Any vascular supply to lesions can also be taken in this step. The foramen ovale and arcuate eminence can then be identi-fied. If more dissection is required, the greater superficial petrosal nerve, which runs parallel and often on top of the petrous ICA, is identified and dissected using magnification allowing access to the horizontal petrous ICA segment.

> **Surgical Anatomy Pearl**
>
> The petrous ICA has no bony covering in 30 to 40% of cases, and if there is any bone, it is often a millimeter or thinner.

- In the transbasal exposures or those requiring access to the infratemporal fossa, the middle fossa floor will be removed by high-speed drill under magnification.

Dural Management

Tack-up stitches are routinely applied to the edges of the dura.

In extradural lesions, stitches are placed in the inferior temporal dura and allowed to hang on hemostats. For intradural lesions, the dura is opened in a C-shaped fashion along the sylvian fissure and tacked up.

- The decision of whether to open the sylvian fissure depends on the lesion and its relation to the arachnoid. Carefully study this fissure and consider the location on the preoperative imaging. It is often not necessary to open the dura for lesions of the lateral cavernous sinus wall or for lesions such as tri-geminal schwannomas, which are truly interdural or only in Meckel's cave and not in the subdural space. In these sorts of cases, an interdural approach is much preferred. For all aneurysms, that sit in the subarachnoid space, the fissure is opened. For lesions in the subdural space, such as meningiomas, the arachnoid is preserved along with the vessels of the sylvian fissure, if possible.

Lesion Management

Lesion management is discussed in the chapters addressing each lesion.

A few points:

- Identify the middle meningeal artery early at the foramen spinosum, bipolar it well, and clearly cut it. If necessary, pack the foramen spinosum with he-mostatic material such as methyl-cellulose (e.g., Surgicel).
- Identify the foramen rotundum and ovale and preserve the nerves within them.
- Preserve all veins. Try more dissection and altering the approach before sac-rificing a vein. Often with effort, they can be preserved, though it takes more time. Never take the vein of Labbé, especially if it is dominant.

- Be careful in dissection of the middle fossa floor near the geniculate ganglion. Use the microscope and dissect the length of the greater superficial petrosal nerve (GSPN). If you cannot avoid stretching it, it may be better to divide it than risk facial nerve palsy.

Reconstruction: Pericranial Flap

If there has been a broad opening of the CSF pathways and the neuro-aerodigestive pathways are opened, vascularized tissue coverage is the goal. The sphenoid sinus is most commonly invaded or opened between the foramen ovale and foramen rotundum. If so, a strip of the temporalis muscle can be transferred in the extradural position to repair any defect after the dura has been secured.

- The flap should not be under tension and should be long enough to reach to the deepest part of the opening. The flap can be placed directly against the dura, and fat graft followed by fibrin glue can be placed into the sphenoid. If possible, the flap should be sutured to the dura at several spots so that it does not move in the closure.

Reconstruction: Bone and Soft Tissues

Care should be taken to ensure that any bony defects of the forehead that are visible are repaired with inert materials as described above. Defects in the sphenoid wing or lateral orbit can be replaced with bone cements or titanium mesh if the frontal sinus has not been breached.

Frontotemporal-Orbitozygomatic Approach

The frontotemporal-orbitozygomatic (FTOZ) approach, considered the workhorse of skull base surgery, is a modification of the frontotemporal craniotomy.[11] By means of the extension of the frontotemporal craniotomy with an orbitocranial (OC) or orbitozygomatic (OZ) osteotomy, a larger surgical corridor allows wider and shallower access and more ability to access deeper and higher structures with less retraction[12] (**Fig. 14.8**).

This approach allows the surgeon a wider view of basal structures. The addition of the OC or OZ osteotomies increases the view angles by 75% in the subfrontal approach, 46% in the pterional approach, and 86% in the subtemporal approach.[13] The OZ approach significantly enlarges the angles of maneuvering when compared with the pterional approach (about 37 degrees vs 27 degrees, respectively). The approach with maxillary extension offers a further, but less significant, widening of exposure in comparison with the OZ alone.[12]

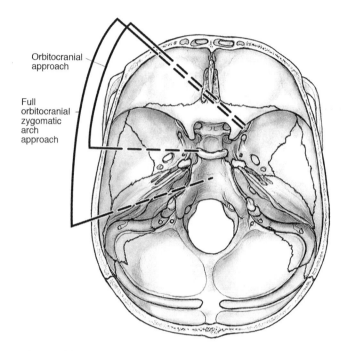

Orbitocranial
approach

Full
orbitocranial
zygomatic
arch
approach

Fig. 14.8 Schema of the working area and angle of potential visualization provided in the orbitocranial and orbitozygomatic approaches.

Indications

This approach provides basal exposure of the anterior and middle fossa structures such as the cavernous sinus, as well as extradural access to the infratemporal fossa and paranasal sinuses.[14]

- The OC approach provides wider access to lesions placed anterior to the oculomotor trigone, whereas the extension to include the zygomatic arch provides wider access to those locations that are posterior to the oculomotor trigone such as the basilar artery apex and the interpeduncular region.[14-17] Both the OC and the OZ provide access to the regions as described, regardless of pathology (e.g., aneurysms, craniopharyngiomas, pituitary macroadenomas, chordomas). By minimizing retraction, venous injury and contusion risks are minimized.
- ◈◈ A variant of the FTOZ approach involving the forced opening of the patient's mouth has been described for widening the surgical corridor toward the infratemporal space. It can be used for treatment of pathologies both with splanchno- and neurocranial involvement. The forced opening of the mouth keeps the coronoid process of the mandible lower and away from

the operating field, providing unobstructed access to the pterygoid and pterygopalatine fossae, and the lateral wall of the maxillary, sphenoid, and ethmoid sinuses, without using a transfacial approach.[18]

For Frontotemporal Craniotomy with Orbitozygomatic Osteotomy

Position

Patient positioning depends on the location of the lesion; more anterior and central lesions require less head rotation than laterally placed and posterior lesions. For a lesion in the anterior clinoid process (ACP) region, the patient is placed in the supine position with the head fixed and elevated 20 degrees, slightly hyperextended and rotated contralaterally approximately 10 to 30 degrees, with the zygomatic bone positioned parallel to the floor. As stated above, preoperative lumbar drainage might be inserted; a small amount of CSF can be gradually drained before or during surgical maneuvers.

❖ Surgical Approach

◈ The incision is made as indicated above. Once the orbital rim is approached, inform the anesthetist because dissection of the periorbita may cause a vasovagal response.

◈ Dissect the periosteum along the zygomaticofrontal suture and then closely follow the bone right into the orbit while carefully elevating the periorbita. Always stay right on the bone.

Surgical Anatomy Pearls

◈ Avoid use of the monopolar cautery for mobilization of the temporal muscle, instead introduce an elevator in the inferior margin of the posterior incision and elevate the deep fascia from posterior to anterior and from the zygomatic arch to the superior temporal line. This maneuver preserves the innervation and vascularization of the temporal muscle, avoiding postoperative muscle atrophy, cosmetic defects, and swallowing dysfunction.

◈ A meticulous skeletonization of the zygomatic arch from soft tissue makes the osteotomy easier. Free the inferior margin of the arch from the attachment of the masseteric fascia.

◈ Perform a bone flap by using one to four bur holes. Connect the holes using a craniotome.

◈◈ Variation: You may consider the "bridge technique" for the craniotomy: leave cuts between the bur holes incomplete except for small 2-mm bridges of bone that are cracked free when the bone flap is elevated (see above, page 340).

◈   Dissect the periorbita until reaching the superior and inferior orbital fissures, about 2.5 cm deep. Insert the tip of the dissector (Penfield No. 4, for example) in the fissures. Cottonoids are placed to protect the periorbita during the dissection. When introduced in the inferior orbital fissure (IOF), the tip of the dissector can be seen in the temporal fossa.

◈   When the periorbita has been dissected and the zygomatic bone has been fully exposed, incise the temporalis muscle on its posterior margin, and elevate and mobilize it as indicated above.

Orbitozygomatic Osteotomy: Variations

• The OZ approach can be full or partial (the zygomatic arch remains intact and only the orbit is opened[14]).

• Orbitozygomatic craniotomies can be performed in one-, two-, or three-piece flaps.[19] In general, the one-piece orbitozygomatic approach enables the frontotemporosphenoidal craniotomy to be elevated along with the orbitozygomatic osteotomy, whereas the two-piece orbitozygomatic approach elevates the frontotemporosphenoidal bone flap first and then the orbitozygomatic part is separated afterward.[20]

• The cuts of the OZ osteotomy are generally performed by using a reciprocating saw, but the use of the same footplate for the craniotomy has been advocated as a safe and quick approach.[21] Reciprocating saws generally leave much smaller gaps in the bone cuts than do craniotomies with footplates.

> **Surgical Pearl**
>
> During osteotomy, self-retaining retractors may be used, not to retract the brain but for protecting the dura.

One-Piece FTOZ Approach

This approach is recommended for access to high-positioned basilar artery aneurysms or to the temporal fossa[22,23] (**Fig. 14.9**).

Advantage

This approach provides maximal exposure with minimal bone loss.[24]

Disadvantages

The visualization of important structures is more limited than with the multi-piece osteotomies, and the whole flap may be lost in the event of postoperative

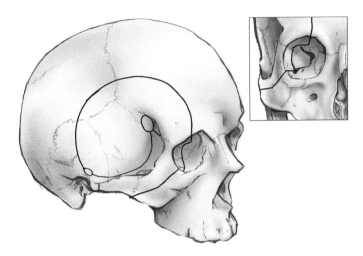

Fig. 14.9   One-piece frontotemporal-orbitozygomatic (FTOZ) approach.

bone flap infection. There are three types of one-piece OZ approach, based on the volume of anatomic exposure required as well as the location of the lesion[25] **(Fig. 14.10)**.

1. Total: for exposure of the anterior and middle cranial fossa **(Fig. 14.10a)**
2. Temporal: for exposure of the middle cranial fossa and interpeduncular region through the transsylvian route **(Fig. 14.10b)**
3. Frontal: for exposure of the anterior cranial fossa **(Fig. 14.10c)**

❖ **Surgical Approach: Six bony cuts are required for the one-piece FTOZ**

◈ First cut: from the MacCarty bur hole (which is the keyhole exposing the anterior cranial base superiorly and the orbit inferiorly) at the frontosphenoidal suture 7 mm superior and 5 mm posterior to the frontozygomatic suture[26] **(Fig. 14.9)**; use the craniotome footplate, cutting along the curvilinear line of the standard frontotemporal craniotomy.[27] Whenever possible, the most medial part of the cutting should be positioned lateral to the frontal sinus, to avoid entering it. If the sinus is entered, it has to be repaired. The frontal sinus may be exenterated and packed, and the epicranium from the frontal region may be turned over the sinus, and eventually sutured at the dura, in order to avoid communication between the intracranial cavity and the sinus itself, potentially causing infections, CSF leaks, muceles, or pneumocephalus.[28] Small holes can be plugged with bone wax.

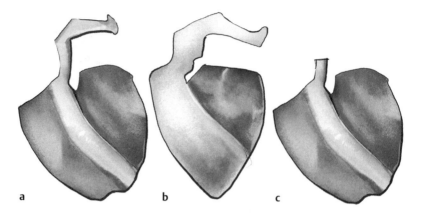

Fig. 14.10a–c One-piece FTOZ approach: variants. (See text for a description of the panels). (Adapted from Aziz KM, Froelich SC, Cohen PL, Sanan A, Keller JT, van Loveren HR. The one-piece orbitozygomatic approach: the MacCarty burr hole and the inferior orbital fissure as keys to technique and application. Acta Neurochir (Wien) 2002;144:15–24.)

◈ Second cut: in the lateral wall of the orbit, from the keyhole to the IOF. Protect the periorbita with a dissector or a retractor.

◈ Third cut: across the body of the zygoma, from the lateral orbital edge to the anterolateral edge of the IOF.

◈ Fourth cut: across the posterior end of the zygomatic root of the temporal bone.

◈ Fifth cut: extends the first cut through the supraorbital ridge.

◈ Sixth cut: across the orbital roof to the MacCarty keyhole.

> **Pearl**
>
> Advise the anesthesist that the orbital contents will be manipulated since a vasovagal response may occur with this maneuver.

The cuts do not necessarily reach one another. Small amounts of leftover bone can be gently cracked by means of a small osteotome.

Two-Piece FTOZ Approach

This approach is recommended, as it is the simplest. It is also recommended for pathologies involving the orbital rim or roof, such as sphenoid wing meningiomas with hyperostosis.[23]

Advantages

The two-piece OZ approach has been quantitatively shown to enable more extensive orbital roof removal and to facilitate visualization of the basal frontal lobe, with a lower incidence of enophthalmos and a better cosmetic outcome.[29] In cases of bone flap infection, the orbit is rarely affected and can be preserved.

❖ Surgical Approach

The two-piece FTOZ approach involves five separate sequential bone cuts to free the orbit and zygomatic arch[14,30] **(Fig. 14.11)**:

◈ First cut: through the medial orbital rim and roof (made just lateral to the supraorbital notch and extends directly posteriorly, approximately 2.5 cm from the inner table of the skull). A cut more medial to the supraorbital notch may be required, depending on the size and localization of the pathology (cribriform plate, sphenoid region).

◈ Second cut: through the roof and lateral wall of the orbit from the posterior end of the first cut, extending in a medial to lateral direction along the posterior orbital roof to the most lateral extent of the SOF, just anterior to it. Carry the cut down to the lateral orbit, approximately halfway to the IOF.

◈ Third cut: extends to the IOF (made in an inferior to superoposterior direction to come close to the second cut).

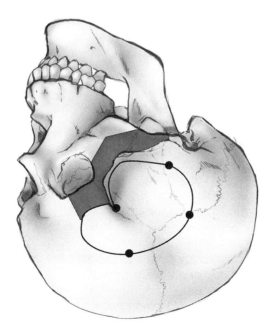

Fig. 14.11 Two-piece FTOZ approach.

◈ Fourth cut: part 1, from the inferior orbital fissure through the anterior aspect of the zygomatic bone above the zygomaticofacial foramen.

◈ Fourth cut: part 2, through the posterior aspect of the zygomatic bone. The two steps together create a V-shaped cut, for an easy reconstruction at the end.

Surgical Pearl
The periorbita must be carefully protected (second surgeon putting a retractor into the orbit, for example).

◈ Fifth cut: through the root of the zygomatic process of the temporal bone. Mobilize the temporalis muscle anteriorly. The cut can be made perpendicularly to the process, or in an oblique fashion, beginning at the inferior and posterior edge of the arch and advancing posteriorly and superiorly; this latter way facilitates repositioning of the bone for reconstruction and avoids injury to the temporomandibular joint.

◈ Last step: A 5- to 6 mm-osteotome is used to remove the orbitozygomatic bone en bloc.

Three-Piece FTOZ Approach

This approach is recommended for anterior or middle fossa approaches.[20]

Advantage

This approach preserves the masseter fascia.

Disadvantage

It requires more careful reconstruction.

❖ Surgical Approach

◈ Two cuts are used for the section of the zygomatic arch:
 1. First cut: vertical section of the posterior part of the arch, immediately anterior to the temporomandibular joint (TMJ)
 2. Second cut: anterior cut, posterior to the union of the zygomatic arch and the zygoma

◈ Mobilize the arch inferiorly along with the masseter muscle.

◈ Perform a craniotomy (one or more bur holes).

◈ The orbital removal cuts resemble the steps summarized in the two-piece approach: an orbital rim cut laterally to the frontal medial edge of the craniotomy. Extend the cut backward over the orbital roof for approximately 1 cm before the SOF, and then change direction and cut toward the IOF into the lateral orbital wall. Cut the orbital rim from the union between the zygomatic arch and the zygoma to the IOF.

◈ At the end of the OZ osteotomy, further extradural dissection can then be performed, removing further bone, whenever required, as in the temporopolar approach, where bone removal at the anterior and middle skull base is furthered, to reach the sphenocavernous and petroclival regions.[31]

Further Modifications of the OZ Approach

- **Modified osteoplastic orbitozygomatic craniotomy** without removing of the zygoma in which the orbital rim component extends from lateral to the supraorbital foramen/notch to the frontozygomatic suture.[23]
- **Extension of the one-piece FTOZ approach to the glenoid fossa**: in this approach, an en-bloc resection of the glenoid fossa and root of the zygomatic arch and an FTOZ osteotomy are utilized to increase the exposure to the region medial to the TMJ, to the posterior part of the temporal fossa, and to the vertical segment of the petrous ICA, and facilitate the reconstruction of the TMJ.[32] Be careful not to injure the ICA when doing the medial cut for the glenoid as the ICA runs close to this region.

◈ Following the zygomatic osteotomy, the temporal craniotomy may be extended toward the root of the zygoma, and an osteotomy of the ascending ramus of the mandible below the capsule is performed.

◈ After the TMJ transection, the skull base bone can be drilled to reach the ICA. The eustachian tube may be transected.

- **One-piece pedunculated FTOZ craniotomy**: The creation of a subperiosteal tunnel beneath the temporal muscle enables hinging the one-piece bone flap on the temporal muscle, reducing the risk of atrophy of the temporal muscle and improving the cosmetic results.[33]

Surgical Anatomy Pearl
Avoid injury to the internal maxillary artery.

- **One-and-a-half fronto-orbital approach**: coronal incision, frontotemporal craniotomy with extension of the frontal craniotomy over the midline, and an OZ osteotomy[34] (**Fig. 14.12**).

Reconstruction

For good cosmetic and functional results, the restoration of the bony defect is required.[35]

To reconstruct the OZ osteotomy, place three titanium miniplates: (1) medially

Surgical Pearl
For a good bone repositioning with optimal cosmetic results, it is advisable to position the miniplates before the bone cuts.

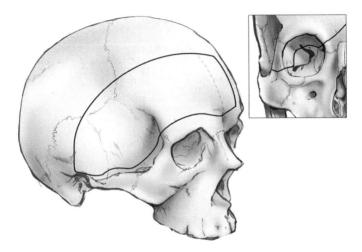

Fig. 14.12 One-and-half fronto-orbital craniotomy. *Inset:* The eventual orbitotomy extension in the approach. (Adapted from Sekhar LN, Fessler RG. Atlas of Neurosurgical Techniques. New York: Thieme; 2006.)

across the first cut, (2) at the zygomatic bone cuts, and (3) at the zygomatic root.

◈ The bone flap can be repositioned as described above for the other craniotomies (plates or buttons with or without synthetic bone cements, or nonabsorbable sutures (e.g., silk) in cases using the bridge technique.

◈ Eventual defects in the keyhole or at the level of the pterion, frontal, or temporal bones can be filled with cement bone (Norian® [Synthes, West Chester, PA], Monument® [Synthes], methyl methacrylate, calcium phosphate) or, alternatively, covered with titanium mesh or bone dust from the saw with a suture carried across the bur hole.

◈ The temporalis muscle is repositioned in its anatomic position and secured with nonabsorbable sutures through mini-holes in the bone, to the pericranium or the eventual cuff of fascia and muscle, if left at the beginning of the muscle dissection.

◈ The interfascial dissection should be repaired; suture the dissected leaflet to the galea.

◈ Suture the scalp in two layers.

Postoperative Care

It is mandatory to keep the conjunctiva and cornea well lubricated and moist to prevent edema and scarring, above all in cases in which the periorbita is injured during the dissection and periorbital fat herniates. Ice packs or cold compresses can reduce symptomatic pain. Ptosis may occur for several weeks or months but almost always improves over time.

- Patients should exercise their jaw by opening it and moving it from side to side to minimize TMJ pain and "a frozen jaw."[14]

> **Pearl**
>
> Ophthalmologic follow-up is recommended.

Complications

Overall, postoperative complications related to the OZ approach occur in up to a maximum of 21.3% of cases; cranial nerve palsy occurs in up to 9.3% of cases,[19] but most are related to the management of the lesion rather than to the osteotomy itself.

Complications related to the OZ approach can be summarized as follows[19,21,35]:

- Damage to orbital contents: ocular movement palsy (2.4%), optic nerve injury, blindness, enophthalmos, pulsating exophthalmos, ptosis
- CSF leakage, pseudomeningocele
- Poor cosmetic outcome: transient frontalis muscle paresis and temporalis wasting, with sinking of the muscle; almost 80% of patients are satisfied with the cosmetic outcome[19]
- TMJ-chewing problems

"Mini"–Anterolateral Approaches

These approaches consist of small frontal or frontotemporal craniotomies performed through an incision above, through, or below the eyebrow, centered on the pterional region.

- **Lateral supraorbital approach.** This approach has been shown to be valid alternative that is less invasive and much faster than the classic pterional approach for the treatment of aneurysms and anterior/middle cranial base lesions,[36] as well as for intradural anterior clinoidectomy.[37] The approach is a modified pterional approach, but, in comparison, it is more anterior and subfrontal, less invasive, and faster (in some cases it requires less than 10 minutes) (**Fig. 14.13**). Described essentially for treatment of aneurysms, including basilar artery aneurysms, if they are located superiorly to the posterior clinoid process.[36]

Advantages

This approach is quick and minimally invasive, and entails less cosmetic deformity than the pterional or eyebrow approach (the latter is not well accepted

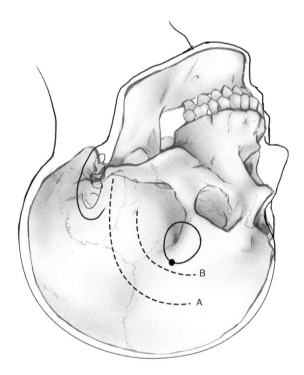

Fig. 14.13 Lateral supraorbital approach: incision line and craniotomy. Note the different incision lines of the pterional approach *(line A)* versus the lateral supraorbital approach *(line B)*.

cosmetically in patients with thin or light eye brows). Also, there is less postoperative temporal muscle atrophy and no postoperative chewing deficits.

Disadvantages

When larger and more temporal exposures are needed, this approach is not indicated. Moreover, the essential key point of this approach is having brain relaxation (pharmacologically, by means of the elevation of the head or by means of CSF subtraction).[38] In the case of a swollen brain, this approach might be contraindicated.

Moreover, some cases of cotton granulomas have been described, caused by cottons accidentally left in the surgical cavity, due to the small size of the surgical field or the use of cottonoids without strings.

❖ Surgical Approach

◈ The positioning of the patient is similar to that in the pterional approach.

◈ The skin incision is curvilinear but shorter than in the pterional approach, without reaching the ear.

◈ Dislocate the skin–galea muscle flap in one single layer anteriorly, retracting it by means of hooks, to visualize the superior orbital rim and the anterior zygomatic arch.

◈ Make a single bur hole, just posterior to the insertion line of the temporal muscle.

◈ The footplate craniotome is used to cut a bone flap sized approximately 3 × 3 × 4 cm.

◈ Drill the lateral sphenoid ridge.

◈ Open the dura in a curvilinear fashion.

Surgical Anatomy Pearl
The sylvian fissure lies on the temporal edge of the craniotomy.

◈ Closure: Fix the bone flap back with two rivet-type cranial clamps, miniplates, or heavy suture fixation.

• **Supraorbital keyhole craniotomy.** This approach uses a single bur hole and a small craniotomy to treat frontal to supra- and parasellar region lesions with less invasiveness that in other approaches.[39] This craniotomy can be used for microsurgical techniques, or endoscopic techniques, or combined techniques (endoscope-assisted microscopic approaches; see Chapter 17).

❖ Surgical Approach

◈ Make a skin incision within the eyebrow or slightly superior to it, possibly in a wrinkle, lateral to the supraorbital incisura (**Fig. 14.14**).

◈ Dissect the subcutaneous tissue in a frontal direction, cutting the frontal muscle with a monopolar cautery, until the frontal bone is reached.

◈ Make a gentle retraction of the inferior margin of the frontal muscle and of the orbicular muscle downward, in order to avoid periorbital ecchymosis/hematoma.

◈ Mobilize the temporal muscle laterally, exposing the temporal line.

◈ Drill a single bur hole posteriorly and inferiorly to the temporal line, in the keyhole, eventually enlarging it with punches.

◈ Cut a basal straight line with the craniotome from the hole to the medial direction, avoiding the frontal sinus whenever possible.

◈ Cut a C-shaped line from the bur hole to the medial border of the previous cut, creating the bone flap.

◈ Drill the inner edge of the bone above the orbital rim, protecting the dura with a retractor, in order to enlarge the surgical angle.

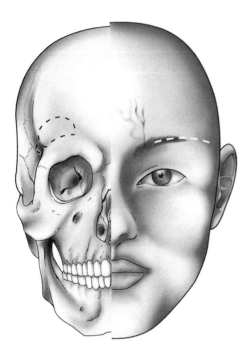

Fig. 14.14 Supraorbital keyhole craniotomy: eyebrow incision and position of the bur hole and craniotomy. Note the position of the supraorbital foramen and its contents.

◈ Open the dura in a curved fashion, with the base parallel to the supraorbital rim, or proceed with an extradural dissection to the anterior skull base, depending on the pathology.

Reconstruction

The small bone flap can be fixed with miniplates or, better, with a titanium rivet-type skull clamp (e.g., CranioFix®, Aesculap, Center Valley, PA) and eventually with bone cement to fill the gap, in order to completely cover the bur hole.

◈ After suturing the subcutaneous layers, skin can be sutured intracutaneously, with good cosmetic results and a high reported rate of patient satisfaction.[40]

Optic Canal Decompression and Anterior Clinoidectomy (Fig. 14.15)

Optic nerve decompression (OND) and anterior clinoidectomy (AC) may be used alone or as a component of more extensive operations that require access to these areas or decompression of the optic nerve. For this reason, a close inspection of the preoperative imaging is required; special attention should be paid to the location of the posterior ethmoid air cells, as these can extend into the ACP and are almost always present medial to the optic canal. AC exposes the paraophthalmic segment (or clinoidal segment) of the ICA, and thus provides access to the region and proximal control of the ICA. The approaches to each area can be performed extradurally or intradurally, depending on the lesion as well as on the experience and preference of the surgeon. For example, a meningioma of the anterior clinoid region with hyperostosis of the ACP can be devascularized extradurally, and the AC can provide space required for access. Identifying the entrance to the optic canal and opening the falciform ligament is useful for the OND, and this is frequently performed intradurally.

Extradurally, the posterior orbit is exposed and drilled via an anterolateral approach (see above). The base of the ACP is identified and its center is drilled with copious irrigation (as with all drilling), leaving a thin "eggshell" of bone on the 360-degree external walls of the ACP. Once the walls are sufficiently thin, they are reflected inward toward the center of the decompression. Drilling may be started with a small diamond matchstick shaped drill bit or a small round one (3 mm or less).

The intradural exposure requires that the dura over the ACP be opened and reflected anteriorly toward the posterior orbit and then the ACP drilled as above.

For the OND, the falciform ligament is cut and then a flap of dura over the ACP and the posterior orbit is reflected and the optic nerve canal drilled at an approximately 30-degree angle that is matched to the angle provided on the preoperative imaging. The imaging demonstrates the position of the ethmoid air cells. Drilling parallel to the walls of the optic canal will provide a 180-degree decompression. If the posterior ethmoid air cell is intentionally or unintentionally opened in a small area, it should be repaired with fat and fibrin glue. If required, the optic strut can be accessed by continuing to drill laterally, releasing both the optic nerve and the ICA.

Anterior Petrosal Approach[41] (Fig. 14.16)

- A relatively confined middle fossa transpetrosal lateral and anterolateral approach to the apex of the petrous bone and the tentorial incisura, the anterior superior posterior fossa space and cerebral peduncle, and the top of the anterolateral pons.
- The craniotomy and extradural approach are performed as previously described.
- This approach can be performed via a pterional, frontotemporal craniotomy alone or combined with an orbitozygomatic or zygomatic osteotomy.

❖ **Surgical Approach**

◈ Elevate the dura along the petrous ridge, exposing the middle fossa foramina and dividing the middle meningeal artery. Posteriorly, expose the arcuate eminence.

◈ Continue to dissect the dura in an anteromedial fashion, and uncover the GSPN.

◈ A self-retaining retractor may be used for holding the temporal dura away from the skull base, particularly as one advances more medially.

◈ Identify the following petrosectomy landmarks delimiting the area of bone, which has to be drilled to access the clivus, cerebellopontine angle (CPA), and posterior fossa: (1) intersection of the GSPN with the trigeminal nerve, (2) porus trigeminus, (3) intersection of the arcuate eminence with the petrous ridge, and (4) intersection of the lines projected along the axes of the GSPN and the arcuate eminence.

◈ Drill the bone window between the GSPN anteriorly and V_3 medially.

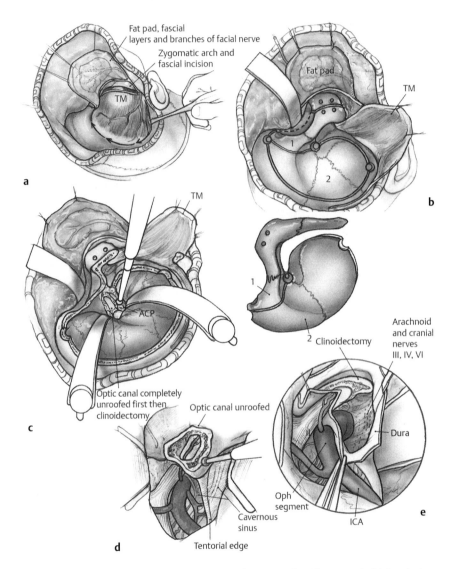

Fig. 14.15a–e Optic nerve decompression and anterior clinoidectomy. **(a,b)** Surgical approach of an FTOZ for **(c)** anterior clinoid process (ACP) drilling and **(d)** unroofing of the optic canal. **(e)** Extradural clinoidectomy with exposure of the carotid dural rings and cavernous sinus. ICA, internal carotid artery; TM, temporalis muscle; Oph, ophthalmic. (From Alvernia JE, Guclu B, Sindou M. Cavernous Sinus Meningiomas. In: Nader R. et al. (Eds). Neurosurgery Tricks of the Trade. New York: Thieme; 2014:155.)

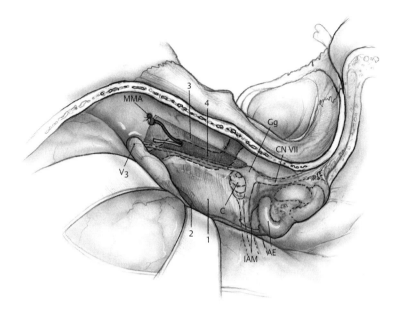

Fig. 14.16   Anterior petrosectomy: Kawase approach via extradural skull base dissection of the middle fossa. 1, Kawase triangle; 2, trigeminal impression; 3, Glasscock triangle; 4, petrous carotid; AE, arcuate eminence overlying the anterior semicircular canal; C, cochlea; Gg, geniculate ganglion; IAM, internal auditory meatus; MMA, middle meningeal artery; V_3, mandibular nerve. (From Baai AA, Agazzi S, van Loveren H. Combined Anterior and Posterior Petrosectomy. In: Nader R. et al. (Eds). Neurosurgery Tricks of the Trade. New York: Thieme; 2014:34.)

◈ If the ICA is involved or requires proximal control, this can be achieved by uncovering the genu of the intrapetrous ICA in the posterolateral (Glasscock's) triangle (see Chapter 2, **Table 2.4**, page 20).

◈ Drill further into the anterior apex of the petrous bone posterior and medial to the ICA and the cochlea, which is covered by the otic capsule. The tensor tympani muscle and eustachian tube run parallel to the ICA and should be avoided.

◈ Expose the dura of the posterior fossa, using as an upper landmark the superior petrosal sinus, which can then be ligated (generally medially, at the porus trigeminus).

◈ If the lesion is intradural, one can then turn to the intradural space and cut the tentorium medially, lifting the medial margin with a stitch or right-angled hook.

◈ Open the dura to access the basilar artery, anterior inferior cerebellar artery (AICA), or cranial nerves (CNs) V and VI.

■ 14.4 Lateral and Transtemporal Approaches

Lateral approaches to the skull base may involve traversing primarily the temporal bone (containing the ear, facial nerve, sigmoid sinus, jugular bulb, and petrous ICA). These approaches can incorporate surrounding articulating bones (parietal, occipital, sphenoid, and zygomatic bones).

See an overview of the lateral, posterolateral, and posterior approaches to the skull base in **Fig. 14.17**. Review temporal bone anatomy in Chapter 2, **Fig. 2.7**, page 23.

Indications for Lateral Surgical Approaches

- Neoplastic disease[42–44]
  - ○ Benign tumors (schwannomas, meningiomas, epidermoid tumors, cholesterol granulomas, lipomas, paragangliomas/glomus tumors, neurofibromas)

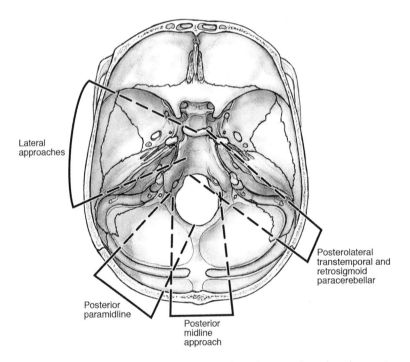

Fig. 14.17 Potential angles of visualization in the lateral, posterolateral, and posterior approaches to the skull base.

- ○ Primary malignant tumors (chordomas, squamous cell carcinoma, basal cell carcinoma, adenocarcinoma, adenoid cystic carcinoma, sarcoma)
- ○ Metastatic malignant tumors (melanoma, carcinoma)
- Trauma (penetrating and crush injury to the temporal bone)
- Hearing implant surgery
  - ○ Cochlear implantation.
  - ○ Auditory brainstem implantation or auditory midbrain implantation.
  - ○ Preoperative histology/biopsy: usually required for suspicious lesions suggestive of a malignancy, obtained by tissue sampling through the ear canal or incisional biopsy. Fine needle aspiration may be performed on cervical lymph nodes, or deeply seated skull base tumors using CT guidance. Usually not required for characteristic benign lesions based on imaging.

Intraoperative Considerations and Monitoring

- Image guidance equipment: registration with preoperative CT or magnetic resonance imaging (MRI), with fiducial markers in more complex cases
- Cranial nerve monitoring (see also Chapter 3, page 89)
  - ○ Real-time electromyography (EMG) can be selectively applied to the motor supply of CNs V, VII, X, XI, and XII (masseter, facial musculature, vocal cords, sternocleidomastoid muscle, and tongue) through bipolar needle electrodes.
  - ○ Electrocochleography (ECochG) may be helpful in hearing preservation for very small tumors, whereas somatosensory evoked potentials are generally not necessary.
  - ○ Electrically evoked auditory brainstem responses (EABR) in the case of auditory brainstem implantation.

■ Types of Lateral Approaches

See also the transpetrous approaches schema in **Fig. 14.18**.

Translabyrinthine Approach

Indication

This approach is used for CPA tumors (most commonly vestibular schwannoma), vestibular neurectomy, and temporal bone fractures.[45]

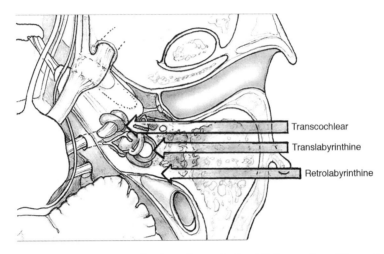

Fig. 14.18   Transpetrous approaches (see Chapter 2, **Fig. 2.7,** for a review of the anatomy).

Advantages

This approach entails minimal or no cerebellar retraction with excellent exposure of the internal auditory canal and the facial nerve. It provides a wide surgical field, especially in a well-pneumatized mastoid.[46]

Disadvantages

Hearing and vestibular function are sacrificed. Extensive bone removal is required. The exposure may be limited in a bone with an anterior sigmoid sinus and a high-riding jugular bulb. There is a risk of a CSF leak from unobliterated air cells.

Positioning

The patient is placed in the supine or lateral position with a three- or four-pin head frame. A wide postauricular scalp shave and antiseptic skin prep are performed. Preoperative antibiotics are prescribed. Navigation setup and registration are performed.

Neuromonitoring

If monitoring is available, the facial nerve is monitored (along with the trigeminal and vagal nerves if the tumor is large enough to warrant it).

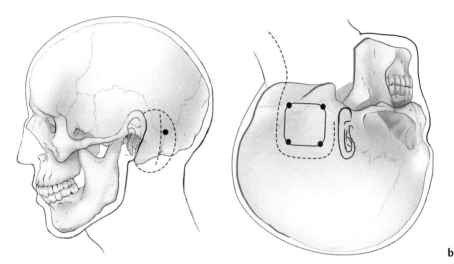

a   b

Fig. 14.19a,b Postauricular incisions for translabyrinthine or retrosigmoid approaches: variations. The *dashed lines* show possible skin incisions. **(a)** A single bur hole in the region of the asterion can be performed for a circular craniotomy. **(b)** Multiple bur holes, eventually extending the craniotomy toward the foramen magnum by means of a craniectomy.

Skin Incision

A postauricular C-shaped incision is made from the mastoid tip to the supra-pinna area and 1 cm more medial and posterior than the most medial aspect of the tumor, posteriorly to the pinna attachment **(Fig. 14.19)**.

❖ Surgical Approach (Fig. 14.20):

◈ Soft tissue dissection. Reflect the skin flap anteriorly and the mastoid periosteal flap inferiorly; elevate the inferior attachment of the temporalis muscle.

◈ Mastoidectomy. Skeletonize and decompress the tegmen mastoideum, sigmoid sinus, and posterior fossa dura, and expose the endolymphatic sac. Make the posterior canal wall thinner, open the antrum, and expose fully the bony labyrinthine of the semicircular canals. Self-retaining retractors may be placed but are not always required.

◈ Labyrinthectomy. Remove all three semicircular canals and expose the vestibule. The superior petrosal sinus is identified to mark the uppermost limit of the posterior fossa exposure.

◈ Identification of the jugular bulb. Dissect the retrofacial air cell followed by creation of a trough inferior to the vestibule that defines the lower edge

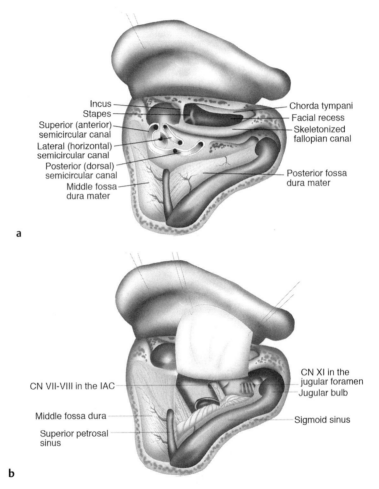

Fig. 14.20a,b **(a)** Right-sided translabyrinthine approach, with **(b)** visualization of the cerebellopontine angle (CPA) nerves after dura opening. IAC, internal auditory canal.

of the internal auditory canal. Drill down toward the jugular bulb (often through bone marrow) to establish the lowest limit of this exposure. Identify the cochlear aqueduct by moving forward and medial to the retrofacial tract.

◈ Internal auditory canal (IAC). Once the inferior limit of the IAC is identified, remove circumferentially the bone (posterior 180 degrees) around it, by creating a trough between the vestibule and the posterior fossa dura, connecting to the trough just above the jugular bulb. Slowly lean forward with the drill to reveal a color transition from yellow to pink, to safely locate the dura of the IAC without injury to its contents.

Surgical Anatomy Pearl

Particular care is needed in uncovering the anterior-superior aspect of the IAC where the facial nerve is most vulnerable. Small bone fragments over the IAC are removed to provide at least a 180-degree exposure. Fully uncover the dura of the posterior fossa by removing the bone at the porus acusticus.

Surgical Anatomy Pearl

The facial nerve location relative to the IAC and the tumor capsule is identified in the anterior superior position in the IAC and can be confirmed with a neurostimulator. Roots of the lower cranial nerves and the trigeminal nerve are identified to serve as lower and upper landmarks of the approach.

◈ Dural opening and tumor removal (see also Chapter 22). Incise the posterior fossa dura and achieve full exposure of the CPA. CSF is released to provide decompression.

◈ If required, bipolar the posterior tumor capsule and enter the tumor to initiate tumor debulking using sharp and blunt dissections facilitated with bipolar coagulation. The tumor capsule is gradually collapsed to permit further exposure of neurovascular structures. The ultrasonic aspirator can be helpful for internal debulking.

◈ The identification of the roots of CNs VII and VIII permit further medial-to-lateral tumor reduction until most (80%) of the CPA component is removed.

◈ Final stage of tumor removal and facial nerve dissection: Attention is turned toward the IAC, whereby the dura is opened. The facial nerve is identified via stimulation. Cut the vestibular nerve, dissect carefully the tumor from the facial nerve.

◈ Debulk the tumor within the IAC to facilitate a lateral-to-medial dissection. The facial nerve is followed under direct vision toward the porus and into the CPA. Once the course of the nerve is established, achieve a more aggressive debulking to reduce the tension and traction along the nerve leading to gradual and complete tumor removal.

Surgical Anatomy Pearl

At the brainstem, identify the flocculus and choroid plexus as landmarks. The facial nerve is superior to the ponto-medullary junction.

◈ Temporal bone resection cavity obliteration. An abdominal fat graft may be used for obliteration of the dead space. Some surgeons like to add a dural graft to delineate a dural border; bone wax to obliterate mastoid air cells, including the antrum; and fibrin glue placement between the fat. A titanium mesh or miniplate may be placed as a remnant of the mastoid cortex for cosmesis. Stitch the musculoperiosteal flap together to cover the area of the temporal bone drilling, forming a two-layer skin closure.

◈ Dressing. A head bandage is placed with very gentle or no pressure. Eventually, a closed suction drain is placed for abdominal or lateral thigh fat or a fascia donor site (not always required).

Modified Translabyrinthine (TL) Approaches

❖ Surgical Approach

◈◈ **Transotic approach**. In this modification, a slightly larger area of posterior fossa exposure can be achieved, including a circumferential exposure of the IAC.[47,48] The advantage of a modest increase in exposure must be weighed against the extra surgical time and a slightly worse cosmetic appearance due to soft tissue retraction into a larger surgical defect. There are three distinct differences from a standard TL approach:

1. The postauricular incision is extended to transect the external acoustic canal (EAC) to ensure that the canal can be oversewn to create a blind sac closure. The medial ear canal, its skin lining, the tympanic membrane, and the ossicles (incus and malleus) are removed.

2. An extended radical mastoidectomy (subtotal petrosectomy) is performed along with removal of the cochlea and medial temporal bone posterior to the petrous carotid artery. The eustachian tube opening can now be directly obliterated with soft tissues and wax.

3. At the completion of this approach, the fallopian canal is suspended while the IAC is skeletonized close to 360 degrees circumferentially.

◈◈ **Transcochlear approach**. This modification is the most aggressive in terms of medial temporal bone exposure with the intent of accessing the anterior aspect of the petrous apex and the petroclival junction through the temporal bone[49,50] (**Fig. 14.18**). The limiting factors to accessing these anterior regions in a lateral approach are the presence of the cochlea and the fallopian canal. In the transcochlear approach, a full transotic approach is completed. The fallopian canal is uncovered from the stylomastoid foramen to the IAC to allow a full decompression and transposition of the facial nerve posteriorly. To do so, the labyrinthine segment (the narrowest segment) and the geniculate ganglion will have to be decompressed with great care and the GSPN cut. The entire intrapetrous facial nerve can now be transposed posteriorly and protected with cottonoids; once completed, tumors at the petroclival junction and the petrous apex can now be accessed.

• This technique requires advanced knowledge and experience in temporal bone surgery as well as a clear justification for its use; the added exposure must be weighed against the likelihood of significant facial nerve injury and longer duration of surgery, particularly when dealing with benign disease. It can be considered as an option of facial nerve reconstruction in the event of a segmental facial nerve transection in a translabyrinthine or transotic approach. It creates length from the intra-petrous facial nerve, sufficient to permit a primary anastomosis to the proximal stump of the facial nerve, avoiding an interpositional graft. The more common approach to this scenario is to use the greater auricular or a sural nerve graft instead (see Chapter 28).

◈◈ **Presigmoid/Retrolabyrinthine Transpetrosal Approach ± Labyrinthec-tomy**. Petroclival lesions such as meningiomas, chondrosarcomas, and CN V and VI schwannomas can be accessed by this approach.[51] The retrolabyrin-thine component of this approach, which can preserve hearing, can be used to assess tumors of the CPA, vestibular neurectomy, and endolymphatic sac tumors.[52] In this approach, the same skin incision and mastoidectomy are performed to expose the sigmoid sinus, lateral semicircular canal, and teg-men mastoideum. The facial nerve is identified in its descending segment, and the retrofacial air cell tract is cleared. However, the semicircular canals are skeletonized to identify the posterior semicircular canal and superior semicircular canal. The bone posterior to the sigmoid sinus is removed to facilitate decompression of the sinus. The bone covering the dura over the posterior fossa and middle cranial fossa is then skeletonized and removed, or a wide craniotomy is performed to expose the posterior and middle cra-nial fossa and to preserve bone flaps. Care is taken to avoid injury to the superior petrosal sinus. The endolymphatic sac and duct are divided. Dura is then removed over the Trautmann's triangle, the area bounded by the sigmoid sinus, bony labyrinth, and superior petrosal sinus. The superior petrosal sinus is ligated medially. The tentorium is then divided perpen-dicular to the superior petrosal sinus and then parallel to the transverse sinus.[53] The vein of Labbé is protected.[54] Further anterior exposure may be achieved by performing a labyrinthectomy (partial or complete) to expose the IAC. However, this is at the expense of hearing loss.

Infratemporal Fossa Approach

Review the topographic anatomy of the temporal bone and infratemporal re-gion in Chapter 2.

Indications for Surgery

The indications need to be balanced against the risks of surgery, especially facial nerve and lower cranial nerve injury. Nonsurgical options, including observa-tion and chemoradiotherapy, should be considered. Radiotherapy has largely supplanted surgery in this area, especially for benign tumors. There are three types of approaches[44,55]:

- **Type A**
  - Tumors of the jugular foramen (Fisch class C and D glomus tumors), cholesteatoma of the ICA and petrous apex, schwannomas of CNs IX to XII, and skull base lesions such as carotid artery aneurysms, glomus vagale tumors, and choristomas
- **Type B**
  - Petrous apex lesions (such as mucosal cysts, dermoid and epidermoid cysts) and lesions of the clivus (including chordomas and chondrosarcomas)
- **Type C**
  - Juvenile nasopharyngeal angiofibroma (class III and IV), nasopharyngeal carcinoma, infratemporal fossa tumors involving the peritubal space and parasellar regions

Overview of Exposure (Fig. 14.21)

- **Type A:** from the sigmoid sinus to the mandibular fossa and petrous apex

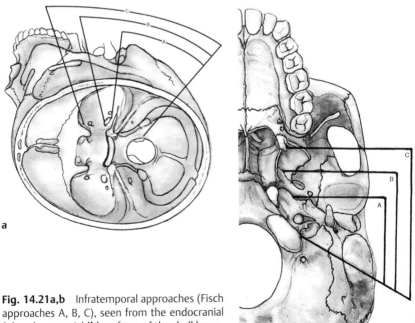

a

b

Fig. 14.21a,b Infratemporal approaches (Fisch approaches A, B, C), seen from the endocranial **(a)** and exocranial **(b)** surfaces of the skull base.

- **Type B:** from the sigmoid sinus to the petrous apex, including the foramen ovale and the horizontal segment of the ICA
- **Type C:** from the sigmoid sinus to the cavernous sinus including the foramen rotundum and foramen lacerum

❖ Surgical Step Highlights for Each Approach

- **Type A**
- ◈ Make a cervicotemporal wide postauricular skin incision. Transect the external auditory canal, remove the external canal skin, and remove the tympanic membrane. Perform blind sac closure. The facial nerve is exposed in the parotid. The great vessels and lower cranial nerves (X, XI, XII) are exposed in the neck.
- ◈ Perform a subtotal petrosectomy including removal of retrolabyrinthine, retrofacial, hypotympanic, and supralabyrinthine air cells.
- ◈ Decompress and translocate anteriorly the facial nerve in its tympanic (horizontal) and mastoid (vertical) segments.
- ◈ Obliterate the eustachian tube and displace the mandible anteriorly.
- ◈ Dissect and expose the jugular bulb, involving the following steps:
  - Ligation of the sigmoid sinus superior to the emissary vein and tumor, and ligation of the inferior jugular vein inferior to the tumor
  - Opening of the jugular bulb and the use of a Yankauer sucker to allow visualization during heavy bleeding
  - Obliteration of the posterior venous drainage pathways (condylar veins) and anterior venous drainage pathways through two or three openings of the inferior petrosal sinus
- ◈ Obliterate the middle ear cleft with fat and the temporalis muscle flap.

- **Type B**

It includes all of the above steps described for type A plus the following:

- ◈ Identify the facial nerve in its main trunk and frontal branch. The facial nerve is then protected with retractors.
- ◈ Cut and reflect anteriorly the zygomatic arch together with the temporalis muscle.
- ◈ Make a subtotal petrosectomy as in type A, and expose the condylar fossa, mandibular condyle, intratemporal carotid artery, middle meningeal artery, and mandibular nerve.
- ◈ Cut the condyle of the mandible and displace it inferiorly. There is further drilling away of the skull base from the condylar fossa and anteriorly toward the foramen ovale through the eustachian tube. This can continue to the petrous apex and clivus. The cavity is then obliterated with fat and temporalis muscle.

- **Type C**

It includes all of the above steps described for type A and B plus the following:

◈ Following completion of the subtotal petrosectomy as in types A and B, divide the middle meningeal artery and section the mandibular branch of the trigeminal nerve. Displace the mandibular condyle inferiorly and drill away the pterygoid process and surrounding bone of the skull.

◈ Section the maxillary branch of the trigeminal nerve and then expose the ICA from the carotid foramen to the foramen lacerum and the cavernous sinus. This includes drilling toward the horizontal portion of the carotid into the cavernous sinus.

◈ Expose the infratemporal fossa, pterygopalatine fossa, parasellar region, and nasopharynx, and remove the tumor.

◈ Rewire the zygomatic arch into place and fill the cavity with temporalis, fat graft, or local muscle flaps.

Middle Cranial Fossa (MCF) Approach

Indication

This approach is indicated for small vestibular or facial schwannomas (with an IAC component and no CPA tumor and with residual hearing), repair of selected meningoencephaloceles and CSF leaks due to tegmen defects, repair of superior semicircular canal dehiscence, and facial nerve decompression.

Advantages

Hearing preservation is more likely, and wide access is provided to the middle cranial fossa.[56]

Disadvantages

This approach provides a limited view of the medial IAC and can be associated with a higher rate of facial palsy since the facial nerve is located superior to the acoustic and inferior vestibular nerves and often displaced superiorly. Temporal lobe retraction is difficult.

Internal Auditory Canal Exposure

Surgical Approach

◈ Center the bone flap using the external auditory canal and the incisura as landmarks. The dimensions of the flap depend on the surgical indication and disease. Inferior bony extension of the bone flap should extend to the

Surgical Anatomy Pearl

The following techniques aid in the identification of the IAC medial to the superior SCC and the facial hiatus:

- Blue line the superior semicircular canal. The IAC is 60 degrees to the superior SCC.[57]
- Identify the GSPN and follow this to the geniculate ganglion (Gg). From the Gg, trace the course of the labyrinthine segment of CN VII to the IAC.[58]
- Bisect the superior SCC and the GSPN and start uncovering the bone over the IAC from medial to lateral.[59]

middle fossa floor marked by the root of the zygoma. If wider exposure is required, the flap can be extended anteriorly and posteriorly to improve exposure along the floor of the middle cranial fossa.

◈ Use a lumbar drain to relax the temporal lobe. Dexamethasone and mannitol may also be used.

◈ Perform a progressive extradural dissection and decompression along the floor of the middle cranial fossa to identify bony landmarks (**Fig. 14.16**); natural dehiscence in the tegmen and sometimes by opening into the middle ear space could ensure accurate identification of the superior semicircular canal (SCC) and the facial hiatus in bones that are more flat and amorphous.

◈ If required, place a self-retaining retractor once the brain is sufficiently slack.

Lateral Skull Base Surgery–Related Complications

Specific postoperative complications include the following:

- Hemorrhage
  - Most likely within the immediate postoperative period.
  - Either arterial or venous, most commonly from vessels that may not have been cauterized.
  - If significant, may produce a fall in Glasgow Coma Scale (GCS) score and require emergency craniotomy for evacuation of hematoma.
  - Extradural hematoma risk of 0.2% has been reported in patients treated with the middle fossa approach.[44]
- CSF leak
  - Presents with wound leak, rhinorrhea, or otorrhea.
  - Wounds typically leak from the lower edge due to dependency and may be require skin-reinforcing sutures and pressure bandage.
  - Rhinorrhea or otorrhea may be due to inadequate obliteration of mastoid air cells of the aditus ad antrum.

- o Treatment is head elevation and lumbar drain insertion.
- o Operative treatment requires waxing of the middle fossa floor or blind sac closure of the external auditory canal; removal of the ear canal skin, tympanic membrane, incus, and malleus; and obliteration of the eustachian tube (with muscle and bone wax).
- Facial nerve injury
  - o The rate of injury is higher with larger tumors due to stretching and thinning of the nerve over the tumor.
  - o Facial transposition when performed in infratemporal fossa approaches carries a much higher rate of paresis. In type A, at best 80% of patients recover to House-Brackmann (H-B) grade II but if the epineurium is removed for tumor infiltration, then at best 70% recover to H-B grade III. In the type B approach, due to stretching of the nerve at the main trunk in the parotid, there is at least a 3% risk of upper face temporary facial weakness. In the type C approach, there is at least a 2% risk of permanent weakness of the frontal branch of the facial nerve.[44]
  - o Preservation of the nerve may necessitate subtotal tumor excision especially in the portion adherent to the nerve. The residual tumor requires surveillance postoperatively with serial MRI scanning.
  - o Inadequate eye closure requires meticulous eye care, including lubricating drops, ointment, the use of taping, an eye shield, or temporary tarsorrhaphy. Temporary tarsorrhaphy can be performed as a first step in operations in which there is a significant risk of postoperative facial nerve paresis.
  - o Consider intraoperative nerve grafting if the nerve is sacrificed or postoperative facial reanimation if recovery is unlikely or has not occurred.
- Cerebellar injury
  - o Minimized by eliminating or significantly reducing cerebellar retraction.
  - o Patients present with ataxia, dysmetria, and dysdiadochokinesis (ipsilateral).
  - o May be due to infarction, hemorrhage, or edema; visible on CT or MRI scan.
  - o Retraction may also result in injury to the flocculus and cerebellar peduncle or CN VI, resulting in diplopia.
  - o Usually managed expectantly unless there is evidence of raised intracranial pressure or hemorrhage.
- Dural venous sinus thrombosis
  - o Most commonly occurring in the sigmoid sinus and transverse sinus.
  - o May be due to sigmoid sinus compression or injury.
  - o Consider thrombophilia screen in at-risk individuals.
  - o Can rarely cause venous infarction of adjacent cerebellar hemisphere, causing cerebellar ataxia, ipsilateral dysmetria, and dysdiadochokinesis.
  - o Given the risk of pulmonary embolism, consider anticoagulation and discussion with a hematologist to balance the risks of postoperative bleeding and embolism.

- Other cranial nerve injuries
  - Resection of V_2 and V_3 in the infratemporal fossa approaches results in facial and tongue anesthesia.
  - Injury to the jugular bulb may result in CN IX and X paresis or paralysis, which in turn may result in dysphagia and dysphonia. They require immediate management by nasogastric tube and early percutaneous

---

Lateral Skull Base Approaches to Hearing Implant Surgery

There exists a rapidly expanding variety of options to treat conductive hearing loss, mixed hearing loss, and sensorineural hearing loss.[60]

- Types of implants:
  - Bone conducting implant: Bonebridge® (MED-EL, Innsbruck, Austria)
  - Cochlear implant (CI)
  - Auditory brainstem implant (ABI)
- Otologic highlights:
  - Bonebridge®
    - A recess for the bone conducting floating mass transducer (BC-FMT) measuring 15.8 mm wide by 8.7 mm deep is typically drilled out in the mastoid bowl at the sinodural angle before being screwed into position using two titanium screws provided with the implant.
    - Usually requires decompression of the middle fossa or posterior fossa dura and may involve dural venous sinus decompression.
    - The receiver stimulator is placed posterior superior under temporalis muscle and fascia.
  - Cochlear implantation
    - Involves insertion of the electrode into the cochlea via cochleostomy or round window.
    - Access to the middle ear from a postauricular approach involves drilling a mastoidectomy; identifying the sigmoid sinus, tegmen mastoideum, lateral semicircular canal, and antrum; and skeletonizing the posterior canal walls.
    - The facial recess (between the chorda tympani nerve, facial nerve and incus buttress) is opened and widened to expose the round window (RW) niche. This is drilled away to expose the RW membrane. The membrane is opened and the electrode is inserted slowly and through the RW. The remaining electrode is coiled into the mastoid cavity.
  - Auditory brainstem implantation
    - Sugita head-frame, Leila retractors, and ABR audiometry setup.
    - Retrosigmoid craniotomy, exposure, and opening of dura.
    - Gradual decompression of cerebellum to expose the CPA and drain CSF.
    - Identification of the root exit zone of CNs VII, VIII, and IX as well as the choroid plexus to determine the foramen of Luschka (the entrance to the lateral recess of the fourth ventricle).
    - A silicone test electrode is inserted into the lateral recess where the cochlear nucleus is located, and electrically EABRs are measured to confirm a functional neural pathway and the correct location.
    - The implant paddle is then inserted and the position is fine tuned using EABR.

gastrostomy as well as possible tracheostomy to avoid the high risk of aspiration pneumonia.

- Hearing loss
  - ○ Complete sensorineural hearing loss is expected following the translabyrinthine approaches including its modifications.
  - ○ Hearing preservation following middle cranial fossa surgery is variable but has been reported in a recent large series study.[56] According to the American Academy of Otolaryngology–Head and Neck Surgery, 65% of patients with class A hearing (signifying pure-tone average, PTA, hearing level ≤30 decibels, and word recognition score (WRS) ≥70%) preoperatively may have preserved the same class of hearing at 5 years. The rate is 67% in patients with class B hearing (PTA hearing level >30. ≤50 decibels, WRS ≥50%).
  - ○ Maximal conductive hearing loss occurs following the infratemporal fossa approaches due to removal of the lateral ossicular chain.

■ 14.5 Posterolateral Approaches

The orientation of the skull base in this region shifts 90 degrees from a horizontal to an oblique vertical position and is associated with a progression from the middle to the posterior fossa space. The anterior, anterolateral, and lateral approaches access the skull base from its horizontal orientation, as opposed to the posterior and posterolateral approaches that approach it from its vertical orientation. Those approaches that transgress the tentorium access both the horizontal and vertical orientation. From the posterolateral superficial to deep direction, including the transverse sinus and the associated entrance of the vein of Labbé, guard the entrance to the tentorium. The veins of the tentorial incisura (e.g., straight sinus) guard the exit of the tentorium medially. The sigmoid sinus and the superior petrosal sinus define the access from a lateral direction. Working anteriorly, one enters through the temporal bone (e.g., translabyrinthine approach); working posteriorly, one enters through the paracerebellar space and the posterior fossa (e.g., retrosigmoid paracerebellar approach, RSPCA).

Decision-Making Points

- When considering whether to perform a particular approach, review the variety of issues raised above, particularly with respect to the anatomy of the lesion, its effect on the brain, and the experience of the surgeon and the team. In particular, look for such factors as distortion of the fourth ventricle, hydrocephalus, herniation downward or upward, and widening of the CSF pathways created by extra-axial lesions or arachnoid cysts along the corridor of access. Take advantage of naturally created corridors whenever they are available.

- Lesions purely posterior to the IAC are simply approached via a RSPCA.
- Lesions between the IAC and the entrance to Meckel's cave can be approached via a RSPCA or one of the transtemporal approaches (or with a combination).
- Lesions purely medial to the entrance to Meckel's cave require either an anterior extended transsphenoidal transclival approach or transbasal approach (see above), extensive transtemporal approach such as a transcochlear or total petrosectomy approach if more extensive, or an anterolateral transpetrousapex approach (Kawase approach, **Fig. 14.16**), if the lesions are limited in extent and superiorly placed. If the lesion is extending along the clivus to its inferior third, then an inferior access (RSPCA) is applied. If there is a limited corridor (< 1 cm) developed by a purely anteriorly placed clival lesion, a transcondylar approach may be required.
- Use CSF drainage to your advantage. Draining the cisterna magna almost always relaxes the cerebellum and if repeated several times, will provide access to the paracerebellar space.
- Angle the microscope to the available space rather than retract the cerebellum.
- Rotating the patient from side to side allows the cerebellum to move under the effects of gravity and opens corridors of access, especially in the RSPCA.
- With the patient placed in the lateral or park-bench position, tilting the bed away from the surgeon provides more access to the petrous face and associated structures, whereas tilting it toward the surgeon facilitates visualization of the brainstem.

Retrosigmoid Paracerebellar Approach

This is the most versatile of the approaches of the posterior fossa and can be enlarged depending on the size and/or extension of the lesion. For example, for a microvascular decompression of the trigeminal nerve, the bony opening would be smaller than for an extensive schwannoma extending from the tentorium to the jugular foramen or below. A suprajugular extension of the approach, by drilling between the acoustic meatus and the jugular foramen, medially to the endolymphatic depression, may allow removal of tumors extending into the upper part of the jugular foramen without a more extensive skull base approach.[61]

Indications

This approach is indicated most commonly for CPA tumors (with mostly cisternal component or residual hearing), lateral cerebellar, petrous face or lateral clival lesions up to Meckel's cave, auditory brainstem implantation, vestibular neurectomy, and microvascular decompression.

Position

Planning the position of the head is critical to allow the cerebellum to drop away with gravity. Once that is defined, determine the positioning of the body. The body is positioned and snugly secured prior to the positioning of the head. Once the patient is positioned, perform a test by tilting the bed to ensure that the patient and endotracheal tube and all lines are stable and safe.

- Sitting position. This position requires an appropriate head clamping system and microscope setup. The surgeon will require armrests. The advantage is that CSF and blood are allowed to drain downward from the surgical site.[51] Many anesthetists object because of the concern about air embolism. Brain retraction may be required.
- Lateral position and its variants. Most centers have experience with the lateral positions. Depending on the body habitus of the patient and the length of the neck, access to the space between the shoulder and the head may be variable. If extremely narrow, this may be an argument for a transtemporal approach.
  - In the vast majority of cases, sufficient space is available or can be created. The ipsilateral shoulder should be allowed to fall forward and away from the surgeon (so-called park-bench position) or taped inferiorly to open the space and enable maneuverability of the surgeon and microscope. The vertex can be tilted down toward the floor to open the space between the ipsilateral shoulder and the ear.
  - Pressure on the brachial plexus and axillary artery should be avoided by placing extra soft padding on the chest wall (incorrectly often called an axillary roll), or by allowing the dependent arm to rest slightly below the level of the bed on a well-padded arm board by having the patient overhang the top end of the bed by a length equivalent to slightly more the width of the arm.
  - The patient's body should be well secured to allow rolling of the bed from side to side as well as to allow the cerebellum to fall away by gravity and provide visualization of the brainstem (toward surgeon) or the petrous face (away from surgeon).
  - Tilting the operating table from side to side (the tilt test) before draping the patient to ensure there is no movement is good practice.
- Supine position, with the head turned 90 degrees.

Navigation

Given the lack of surface landmarks posteriorly, many navigation systems operate better if surface fiducials are added to the patient's head prior to the frameless stereotactic imaging scan. Before marking the skin, the surgeon should identify

Surgical Anatomy Pearl

Removing enough mastoid is critical to avoid cerebellar retraction in these cases. Insufficient mastoid removal is the most common reason for needing cerebellar retraction.

the surface landmarks, specifically the superior nuchal line (SNL). The surgeon should carefully run the flat pad of his or her distal index finger parallel with the SNL from the occipital muscles upward. There is almost always a palpable groove at the SNL (see also Chapter 2, **Fig. 2.16**). Note that the surface landmark for the foramen magnum is the tip of the mastoid process.

> **Surgical Pearl**
>
> The surgeon should first plane the bone opening required to access the lesion and then fashion the best incision that will allow access to the lesion itself and reconstruction of normal barriers like dura, bone and skin.

- In planning the approach, an inline view that takes the surgeon in line with the petrous face will minimize brain retraction and show how much of the mastoid should be removed.
- After a shave, mark out the lesion, the pertinent anatomy (e.g., sinuses), and then the required bone opening. Only after all of the above mark the skin incision.

Incision

A variety of incisions are possible (**Fig. 14.19**). The simplest, a straight oblique line parallel to the hairline, centered two-thirds laterally to the midline along the SNL will access many smaller lesions at the petrotentorial junction.

❖ Modified Approach

◈◈ For wider exposure, the linear incision can be extended to a sigmoid (S-shaped) incision coming over the mastoid and under the ear, if required, at the top end and toward the midline at the inferior end, if required (**Fig. 14.22a**). There is rarely any need to take the inferior aspect of the incision below the tip of the mastoid, and doing so only risks injuring the C2 nerve root, the occipital muscles, and potentially the vertebral artery.

◈◈ For larger lesions, a C-shaped incision based on the ear is also used, especially when combined with any drilling of the temporal bone.

◈◈ For lesions far lateral or traversing the tentorium, an inverted U-shaped incision mobilizes the thick occipital muscles out of the exposure and can be very helpful. It also keeps a well-vascularized flap present if radiation might be required later.

Craniotomy

Exposure of the venous sinuses ensures sufficient lateral and superior exposure. If there is herniation of the cerebellar tonsils, decompress the foramen magnum. The first bur hole can be done over the angle between the transverse and

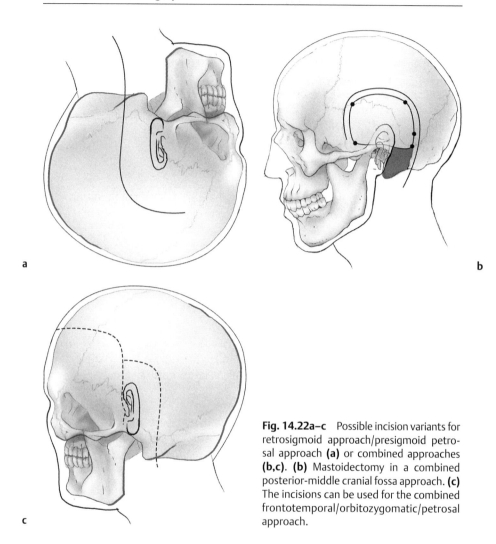

Fig. 14.22a–c Possible incision variants for retrosigmoid approach/presigmoid petrosal approach **(a)** or combined approaches **(b,c)**. **(b)** Mastoidectomy in a combined posterior-middle cranial fossa approach. **(c)** The incisions can be used for the combined frontotemporal/orbitozygomatic/petrosal approach.

sigmoid sinuses (see asterion on **Fig. 2.17a** in Chapter 2). Place one or several bur holes, but be careful in the lateral cut not to damage the mastoid emissary vein, which varies in size from tiny to huge (look for it on the preoperative imaging). Perform rongeuring or drilling of the bone using a high-speed drill (with dural protection using a spatula) until the sigmoid sinus is seen or until the exposure is sufficiently lateral to avoid placing a brain retractor.

Dural Incision

The cerebellum can herniate when the dura of the posterior fossa is incised. To avoid this, routinely make a small transverse incision parallel to the foramen

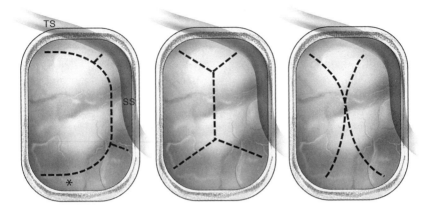

Fig. 14.23 Retrosigmoid dural incisions, variations (right side). The asterisk in the first option shows where the incision cut should begin, in order to open the cisterns for cerebrospinal fluid (CSF) release. TS, transverse sinus; SS, sigmoid sinus.

magnum at the inferior aspect of the dural exposure (leaving enough dura to suture at the closure!) **(Fig. 14.23)**. Then, under magnification, use a small brain spatula to expose the cisterna magna and open it under direct vision. Allow the CSF to drain for a few minutes and repeat as often as is required to achieve brain relaxation. This incision can then be extended into a C-shaped opening that parallels the sigmoid and transverse sinuses. The dural flap created is left spread out on the cerebellum, thus keeping it moist. The lateral component is stitched up to the muscle with appropriate relaxation cuts. This opening has the advantage of staying moist and being closable most of the time.

◈◈ The alternatives, including cruciate and X-shaped incisions, provide access as well, but often desiccate and require a dural graft for closure.

Intradural Steps

The tentorium is first inspected for any bridging veins, which are carefully taken down if this area requires exposure. Follow the tentorial petrous junction down and then the petrous bone face to the IAC and, if required, to the jugular foramen.

> **Surgical Pearl**
>
> Continual readjustment of the microscope avoids the need to retract the cerebellum in most cases.

Reconstruction

The RSPCA is a simple procedure for closure. Care should be taken to gently reapproximate the muscles and then to close the fascia in layers. If the mastoid has been opened, the air cells must be carefully waxed when opened and during closure of the incision.

Internal Auditory Canal Exposure[51]

Exposure of the IAC is required when a tumor extends into it; drilling of the posterior wall of the IAC begins after significant debulking is achieved within the CPA. Although the IAC may be approached from either the medial (cerebellar) or the lateral (petrous) direction, the lateral approach is safer and easier. The degree of bony removal is dependent on the lateral extension of the tumor and the relative position of the posterior SCC, the most likely portion of the inner ear to be at risk. Ideally, a 180-degree posterior decompression of the IAC is achieved. There are no consistent landmarks for the posterior SCC that limit the medial exposure of the fundus; measurements taken from the posterior lip of the porus acusticus on MRI or CT images and intraoperative navigation will help define the safety margin during the drill-out. Exposed air cells must be obliterated with bone wax. Diamond burs are used to uncover the dura of the IAC prior to opening and tumor exposure. A clear determination of the location of the facial nerve at the level of the fundus facilitates early identification and tracking of the nerve from a medial to lateral direction. A 30- or 45-degree endoscope may be used to facilitate exposure of the most lateral aspect of the IAC to achieve complete tumor removal (see Chapter 17).

Posterior Petrosal Transtentorial Approach: Posterior and Middle Fossa Approach

This approach combines the middle cranial fossa approach with the posterior fossa approaches, such as the transmastoid, translabyrinthine or, rarely nowadays, transcochlear approaches, for the management of complex multicompartment tumors (e.g., giant petroclival meningiomas).

❖ Surgical Approach

◈ Make the incision in a C-shaped curvilinear fashion around the ear, with the posterior part terminating at least 1 cm more medial than the posteromedial aspect of the lesion and below the mastoid tip, with the anterior part curving around the ear toward the tragus (**Fig. 14.22b**).

◈◈ An alternative skin incision is a combination of two incisions, a reverse question-mark incision starting at the tragus (see above for the frontal temporal craniotomy), with a curvilinear extension so as to create a three-pronged incision, providing access to the middle fossa and posterior fossa (**Fig. 14.22c**).

◈ Two scalp flaps are used, one anteriorly reflected for the temporal dissection and middle cranial fossa craniotomy, the other one posterior, with the sternocleidomastoid and splenius capitis muscles, which can be detached and retracted posteriorly or inferiorly (preserving their innervation and vascularization).

◈ Perform a retrolabyrinthine mastoidectomy that exposes the middle and posterior fossa dura and the full length of the superior petrosal sinus and sigmoid sinus (see transtemporal approaches).

◈ One large or two smaller flaps can be turned after exposure and dissection of the transverse sinus off the inner aspect of the bone flap. For this purpose, the exposure can be done during the mastoidectomy, or three perpendicularly placed bur holes can be placed directly onto the transverse sinus, which are then stripped from the undersurface of the bone.

◈◈ Variation: Perform the mastoidectomy at this stage, although it is advisable to do it before the craniotomy to avoid venous injury.

◈ Cut the middle fossa dura parallel to the middle fossa floor and then anterior to the sigmoid sinus.

◈ Suture, ligate, and divide the superior petrosal vein and then cut the tentorium.

◈◈ Translabyrinthine and even transcochlear extensions can be added to the simple retrolabyrinthine mastoidectomy as required.

■ 14.6 Posterior Approaches

Midline Occipital Approach (Fig. 14.24)

This approach is used above all others for posterior fossa midline lesions. It can also be used for supracerebellar infratentorial lesions (e.g., pineal tumors and lesions around the posterior deep venous complex), for Chiari malformation treatment, and for other entities.

Disadvantages

This approach may require downward cerebellar retraction and sacrifice of cerebellar bridging veins to the tentorium, as well as the precentral cerebellar vein. Occipitocervical extension, can be used to access the craniovertebral juncture (CVJ), foramen magnum, vertebral arteries, and other entities.

Positions: Prone/Concorde, sitting or in lateral decubitus.

❖ Occipitocervical Exposure: Surgical Approach

◈ Midline skin incision: The length and extent are defined by the size and location of the tumor.

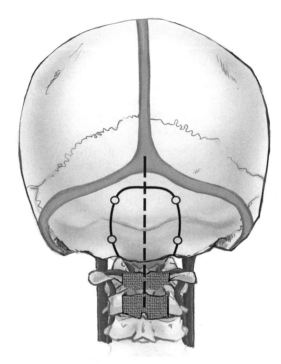

Fig. 14.24 Midline suboccipital craniotomy. C1 and C2 laminectomies can be performed as necessary.

Surgical Anatomy Pearl

Stay midline to minimize blood loss. If a more lateral exposure is required, an L or hockey-stick–shaped extension, or even an inverted U-shaped incision, is helpful in reflecting the large mass of occipital muscles and widening the surgical access.

◈ Mediolateral subperiosteal displacement of the muscles and their detachments from the spinous processes of C1 and C2, with skeletonization of the posterior arch and laminae.

◈ Make a suboccipital craniotomy/craniectomy and remove C1 posteriorly, getting a wide exposure on the foramen magnum. Careful subperiosteal dissection to avoid injury to the vertebral artery on the sulcus arteriosus of C1. The venous plexus around the vertebral artery (VA) is then apparent.

◈ Perform an occipital craniotomy or craniectomy. Bur holes in the midline and paramidline are connected with a craniotome or a rongeur. Once the craniotomy is fashioned, the atlanto-occipital membrane is carefully dissected and cleaned. The arch of C1 can be removed with a rongeur or high-speed drill, according to the surgeon's preference.

◈◈ Variation: For the infratentorial-supracerebellar approach, make a window-craniotomy centered over the external occipital protuberance, exposing on the superior one third the occipital lobes, with the torcular in the middle and the cerebellum hemispheres situated inferiorly.

◈ Open the dura below the lesion first to release the CSF, keeping in mind the possibility of finding venous lakes as well as a circular sinus at the foramen magnum. The dural incision is usually Y-shaped or L-shaped at the top and L- or I-shaped at the bottom. The dural margins are tacked up to the skin to avoid spillage of extradural blood into the CSF that may result in subsequent arachnoiditis.

Far Lateral Approach and Extreme Far Lateral Approaches

Position

The patient is placed in the lateral decubitus position with the head laterally flexed away from the lesion and with concomitant anterior flexion.

❖ Surgical Approach

◈ The skin incision varies between the possibility of a hockey stick or candy-cane inverted J-shaped incision starting either at the mastoid tip or just behind the external acoustic meatus. The long arm of the incision is usually carried over the spinous processes of the midcervical vertebrae.

◈ Proceed with the dissection of anatomic layers, with the muscles reflected to expose the lateral aspect of C1, C2, and the VA at the sulcus arteriosus. In particular, detach the sternocleidomastoid muscle and reflect it laterally. Detach and reflect medially the splenius capitis, longissimus capitis, semispinalis capitis, and splenius cervicis muscles. The rectus capitis major and the two oblique muscles are reflected medially as well. The VA is identified deep in the center of this muscle triangle.

◈ At this point, if mobilization of VA is necessary, open the transverse foramen of C1 and C2, to enable its reflection medially.

◈ Perform an occipital craniotomy as described above and take it as lateral as the occipital condyle. Depending on the lateral extent of the lesion, the procedure can also include a partial mastoidectomy and exposure of the sigmoid sinus.

◈◈ At the foramen magnum, several variants are possible, entailing dif-

> **Surgical Anatomy Pearl**
>
> The C2 nerve root is found just posterior to the VA and needs to be identified and spared if possible.

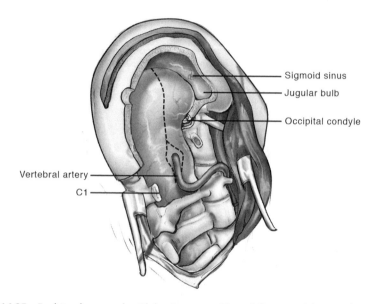

Sigmoid sinus

Jugular bulb

Occipital condyle

Vertebral artery

C1

Fig. 14.25 Far lateral approach with laminectomy C1, mobilization of the vertebral artery and drilling of the posteromedial part of the occipital condyle. (Adapted from George B. Clival Chordomas: Lateral Approaches. In: Nader R. et al. (Eds) Neurosurgery Tricks of the Trade. New York: Thieme; 2014:230.)

ferent extents of bony removal. All of these approaches (namely partial transcondylar, transcondylar, and transtubercular) have in common the drilling of the medial occipital condyle (one third in the partial transcondylar, half in the other two variants). Furthermore, the transcondylar approach enables opening the hypoglossal canal, and the transtubercular approach includes removal of the jugular tubercle to increase the intradural exposure (**Fig. 14.25** and **Fig. 22.18**, page 614).

■ References

Boldfaced references are of particular importance.

1. Raveh J, Laedrach K, Speiser M, et al. The subcranial approach for fronto-orbital and anteroposterior skull-base tumors. Arch Otolaryngol Head Neck Surg 1993;119:385–393

2. Raveh J, Turk JB, Lädrach K, et al. Extended anterior subcranial approach for skull base tumors: long-term results. J Neurosurg 1995;82:1002–1010

3. **Day JD, Koos WT, Matula C, Lang J. Color Atlas of Microneurosurgical Approaches. Stuttgart, New York: Thieme; 1997**

4. **Cusimano MD, Suhardja AS. Craniotomy revisited: techniques for improved access and reconstruction. Can J Neurol Sci 2000;27:44–48**

5. **Koos WT, Spetzler RF, Lang J. Color Atlas of Microneurosurgery. Microanatomy, Approaches, Techniques, 2nd ed. Stuttgart, New York: Georg Thieme Verlag; 1993**
6. **Day JD, Tschabitscher M. Microsurgical Dissection of the Cranial Base. New York: Churchill Livingstone; 1996**
7. Raveh J, Vuillemin T. The surgical one-stage management of combined cranio-maxillo-facial and frontobasal fractures. Advantages of the subcranial approach in 374 cases. J Craniomaxillofac Surg 1988;16:160–172
8. Mayfrank L, Gilsbach JM. Interhemispheric approach for microsurgical removal of olfactory groove meningiomas. Br J Neurosurg 1996;10:541–545
9. Mayfrank L, Reul J, Huffmann B, Bertalanffy H, Spetzger U, Gilsbach JM. Microsurgical interhemispheric approach to dural arteriovenous fistulas of the floor of the anterior cranial fossa. Minim Invasive Neurosurg 1996;39:74–77
10. Kadri PA, Al-Mefty O. The anatomical basis for surgical preservation of temporal muscle. J Neurosurg 2004;100:517–522
11. **Sekhar LN, Fessler RG. Atlas of Neurosurgical Techniques. New York: Thieme; 2006**
12. Gonzalez LF, Crawford NR, Horgan MA, Deshmukh P, Zabramski JM, Spetzler RF. Working area and angle of attack in three cranial base approaches: pterional, orbitozygomatic, and maxillary extension of the orbitozygomatic approach. Neurosurgery 2002;50:550–555, discussion 555–557
13. Alaywan M, Sindou M. Fronto-temporal approach with orbito-zygomatic removal. Surgical anatomy. Acta Neurochir (Wien) 1990;104:79–83
14. **van Furth WR, Agur AM, Woolridge N, Cusimano MD. The orbitozygomatic approach. Neurosurgery 2006;58(1, Suppl):ONS103–ONS107, discussion ONS103–ONS107**
15. Riina HA, Lemole GM Jr, Spetzler RF. Anterior communicating artery aneurysms. Neurosurgery 2002;51:993–996, discussion 996
16. Du R, Young WL, Lawton MT. "Tangential" resection of medial temporal lobe arteriovenous malformations with the orbitozygomatic approach. Neurosurgery 2004;54:645–651, discussion 651–652
17. Sindou M, Emery E, Acevedo G, Ben-David U. Respective indications for orbital rim, zygomatic arch and orbito-zygomatic osteotomies in the surgical approach to central skull base lesions. Critical, retrospective review in 146 cases. Acta Neurochir (Wien) 2001;143:967–975
18. Di Rienzo A, Ricci A, Scogna A, et al. The open-mouth fronto-orbitotemporozygomatic approach for extensive benign tumors with coexisting splanchnocranial and neurocranial involvement. Neurosurgery 2004;54:1170–1179, discussion 1179–1180
19. Youssef AS, Willard L, Downes A, et al. The frontotemporal-orbitozygomatic approach: reconstructive technique and outcome. Acta Neurochir (Wien) 2012;154:1275–1283
20. Campero A, Martins C, Socolovsky M, et al. Three-piece orbitozygomatic approach. Neurosurgery 2010;66(3, Suppl Operative):E119–E120, discussion E120
21. Conway JE, Raza SM, Li K, McDermott MW, Quiñones-Hinojosa A. A surgical modification for performing orbitozygomatic osteotomies: technical note. Neurosurg Rev 2010;33:491–500

22. Balasingam V, Noguchi A, McMenomey S, Delashaw JBJ. Frontotemporal-orbitozygomatic approach. Neurosurg Q 2005;15:113–121
23. Balasingam V, Noguchi A, McMenomey SO, Delashaw JB Jr. Modified osteoplastic orbitozygomatic craniotomy. Technical note. J Neurosurg 2005;102:940–944
24. Chang CW, Wang LC, Lee JS, Tai SH, Huang CY, Chen HH. Orbitozygomatic approach for excisions of orbital tumors with 1 piece of craniotomy bone flap: 2 case reports. Surg Neurol 2007;68(Suppl 1):S56–S59, discussion S59
25. **Aziz KM, Froelich SC, Cohen PL, Sanan A, Keller JT, van Loveren HR. The one-piece orbitozygomatic approach: the MacCarty burr hole and the inferior orbital fissure as keys to technique and application. Acta Neurochir (Wien) 2002;144:15–24**
26. MacCarty C. The Surgical Treatment of Intracranial Meningiomas. Springfield, IL: Charles C. Thomas; 1961
27. **Tubbs RS, Loukas M, Shoja MM, Cohen-Gadol AA. Refined and simplified surgical landmarks for the MacCarty keyhole and orbitozygomatic craniotomy. Neurosurgery 2010;66(6, Suppl Operative):230–233**
28. Al-Mefty O, Smith RR. Combined approaches in the management of brain lesions. In: Apuzzo M, ed. Brain Surgery: Complication Avoidance and Management. New York: Churchill Livingstone; 1993
29. **Tanriover N, Ulm AJ, Rhoton AL Jr, Kawashima M, Yoshioka N, Lewis SB. One-piece versus two-piece orbitozygomatic craniotomy: quantitative and qualitative considerations. Neurosurgery 2006;58(4, Suppl 2):ONS-229–ONS-237, discussion ONS-237**
30. Zabramski JM, Kiriş T, Sankhla SK, Cabiol J, Spetzler RF. Orbitozygomatic craniotomy. Technical note. J Neurosurg 1998;89:336–341
31. Zada G, Day JD, Giannotta SL. The extradural temporopolar approach: a review of indications and operative technique. Neurosurg Focus 2008;25:E3
32. Froelich S, Aziz KA, Levine NB, Tew JM Jr, Keller JT, Theodosopoulos PV. Extension of the one-piece orbitozygomatic frontotemporal approach to the glenoid fossa: cadaveric study. Neurosurgery 2008;62(5, Suppl 2):ONS312–ONS316, discussion ONS316–ONS317
33. Hayashi N, Hirashima Y, Kurimoto M, Asahi T, Tomita T, Endo S. One-piece pedunculated frontotemporal orbitozygomatic craniotomy by creation of a subperiosteal tunnel beneath the temporal muscle: technical note. Neurosurgery 2002;51:1520–1523, discussion 1523–1524
34. Bogaev CA. Osteotomy design and execution. Neurosurg Clin N Am 2002;13:443–474
35. Choudhry OJ, Christiano LD, Arnaout O, Adel JG, Liu JK. Reconstruction of pterional defects after frontotemporal and orbitozygomatic craniotomy using Medpor Titan implant: cosmetic results in 98 patients. Clin Neurol Neurosurg 2013;115:1716–1720
36. **Hernesniemi J, Ishii K, Niemelä M, et al. Lateral supraorbital approach as an alternative to the classical pterional approach. Acta Neurochir Suppl (Wien) 2005;94: 17–21**
37. Romani R, Elsharkawy A, Laakso A, Kangasniemi M, Hernesniemi J. Tailored anterior clinoidectomy through the lateral supraorbital approach: experience with 82 consecutive patients. World Neurosurg 2012;77:512–517

38. Romani R, Silvasti-Lundell M, Laakso A, Tuominen H, Hernesniemi J, Niemi T. Slack brain in meningioma surgery through lateral supraorbital approach. Surg Neurol Int 2011;2:167

39. **Reisch R, Perneczky A, Filippi R. Surgical technique of the supraorbital key-hole craniotomy. Surg Neurol 2003;59:223–227**

40. **Reisch R, Marcus HJ, Hugelshofer M, Koechlin NO, Stadie A, Kockro RA. Patients' cosmetic satisfaction, pain, and functional outcomes after supraorbital craniotomy through an eyebrow incision. J Neurosurg 2014;121:730–734**

41. Roche PH, Lubrano VF, Noudel R. How I do it: epidural anterior petrosectomy. Acta Neurochir (Wien) 2011;153:1161–1167

42. **Pieper DR, LaRouere M, Jackson IT. Operative management of skull base malignancies: choosing the appropriate approach. Neurosurg Focus 2002;12:e6**

43. Manolidis S, Jackson CG, Von Doersten PG, Pappas D, Glasscock ME. Lateral skull base surgery: the otology group experience. Skull Base Surg 1997;7:129–137

44. Fisch U, Mattox DE. Microsurgery of the Skull Base. Stuttgart, New York: Thieme Verlag; 1988

45. **Sanna M, Khrais T, Falcioni M, Russo A, Taibah A. The Temporal Bone: A Manual for Dissection and Surgical Approaches. New York: Thieme; 2005**

46. Day JD, Chen DA, Arriaga M. Translabyrinthine approach for acoustic neuroma. Neurosurgery 2004;54:391–395, discussion 395–396

47. **Chen JM, Fisch U. The transotic approach in acoustic neuroma surgery. J Otolaryngol 1993;22:331–336**

48. Fisch U, Chen JM. The transotic approach. In: Brackmann DE, Shelton C, Arriaga MA, eds. Otologic Surgery. Philadelphia: Saunders; 1994:Chapter 53

49. House WF, Hitselberger WE. The transcochlear approach to the skull base. Arch Otolaryngol 1976;102:334–342

50. **Sanna M, Saleh EA. Atlas of Microsurgery of the Lateral Skull Base. Stuttgart: Georg Thieme Verlag; 2007**

51. Samii M, Greganov V. Surgery of Cerebellopontine Lesions. Berlin, Heidelberg: Springer-Verlag; 2013

52. Russell SM, Roland JT Jr, Golfinos JG. Retrolabyrinthine craniectomy: the unsung hero of skull base surgery. Skull Base 2004;14:63–71, discussion 71

53. Wu CY, Lan Q. Quantification of the presigmoid transpetrosal keyhole approach to petroclival region. Chin Med J (Engl) 2008;121:740–744

54. Lustig LR, Jackler RK. The vulnerability of the vein of Labbé during combined craniotomies of the middle and posterior fossae. Skull Base Surg 1998;8:1–9

55. **Jackler RK. Atlas of Skull Base Surgery and Neurotology. Stuttgart, New York: Thieme Verlag; 2008**

56. Wang AC, Chinn SB, Than KD, et al. Durability of hearing preservation after microsurgical treatment of vestibular schwannoma using the middle cranial fossa approach. J Neurosurg 2013;119:131–138

57. Fisch U, Chen JM. Middle cranial fossa vestibular neurectomy. In: Brackmann DE, Shelton D, Arriaga MA, eds. Otologic Surgery. Philadelphia: Saunders; 1994:Chapter 39

58. House WF. Surgical exposure of the internal auditory canal and its contents through the middle, cranial fossa. Laryngoscope 1961;71:1363–1385

59. Garcia-Ibanez E, Garcia-Ibanez JL. Middle fossa vestibular neurectomy: a report of 373 cases. Otolaryngol Head Neck Surg 1980;88:486–490

60. Adunka OF, Buchman CA. Otology, Neurootology, and Lateral Skull Base Surgery. New York: Thieme; 2011

61. Matsushima K, Kohno M, Komune N, Miki K, Matsushima T, Rhoton AL Jr. Suprajugular extension of the retrosigmoid approach: microsurgical anatomy. J Neurosurg 2014;121:397–407

15 Transfacial/ Transmaxillary Approaches to the Skull Base

The paranasal sinuses and anterior skull base can be approached through external (transfacial/transmaxillary) or endonasal routes. Traditionally, external approaches were the only methods available, but in recent decades the expanded endoscopic approaches have been refined (see Chapter 16).

■ Main Indications

- External approaches generally afford excellent exposure of the nose, paranasal sinuses, and anterior skull base. However, despite the wide exposure, it is sometimes difficult to visualize further into the nose or the sinus cavities, which require additional illumination or magnification.
- The standard open transfacial and transmaxillary approaches provide access to the nose, sinuses, and anterior skull base.

■ Supraorbital Approaches (External Ethmoidectomy/Frontoethmoidectomy)[1,2]

Main Indications

- Chronic ethmoid or frontal sinusitis
- Persistent ethmoid/frontal sinusitis following endonasal sinus surgery
- Frontal sinus fractures
- Inflammatory complications of acute frontal sinusitis, including mucopyocele, or orbital or intracranial abscess
- Repair of anterior cranial cerebrospinal fluid (CSF) leaks
- Ligation of the anterior/posterior ethmoidal arteries (e.g., epistaxis)

❖ Incisions (Fig. 15.1; see also Chapter 20, Fig. 20.1, page 473)

◈ The incision is usually placed equidistant between the medial canthus and the midline of the nasal dorsum.

◈ For the ethmoid sinus, the incision is made between the medial canthus and nasal sidewall. It should be placed to preserve the medial palpebral ligament and the lacrimal sac.

◈ For frontal or frontoethmoidal work, the incision runs below the medial portion of the eyebrow and curves downward between the medial canthus and the nasal sidewall to approximately the level of the inferior orbital margin.

◈◈ Variation: The incision may be extended further laterally under the eyebrow or inferiorly along the nasofacial groove, depending on the need for exposure.

◈ Instead of a linear incision, a W-plasty type of incision along the nasal sidewall usually results in improved cosmesis postoperatively by reducing the risk of hypertrophic scarring.

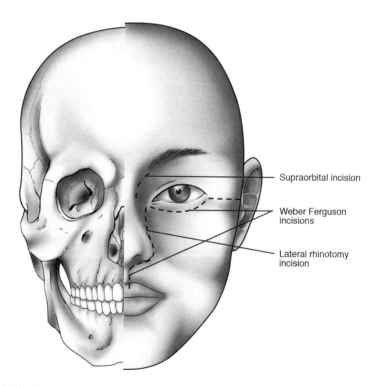

Supraorbital incision

Weber Ferguson incisions

Lateral rhinotomy incision

Fig. 15.1 The placement of various transfacial incisions: supraorbital, lateral rhinotomy, Weber-Ferguson.

◈ Bilateral supraorbital incisions connected by an incision across the nasal dorsum/glabella ("eyeglass" incision) provide further wide exposure of the undersurface and anterior wall of the frontal sinuses, but the incision across the nasal dorsum is not cosmetically optimal.

❖ Soft Tissue Dissection

◈ The skin, muscle layer, and periosteum are incised so the periosteum can be easily elevated from the bone.

◈ Bleeding from the angular arteries needs to be controlled by bipolar cautery or ligation.

◈ The soft tissues are elevated over the lacrimal bone.

◈ The lacrimal sac is preserved.

◈ If the ethmoid sinus is being accessed, the periorbita is elevated from the lamina papyracea, and the anterior ethmoid artery is identified and ligated as necessary.

❖ Bone Removal

◈ The ethmoid sinus can be entered through the lamina papyracea more inferiorly, staying inferior to the level of the previously identified anterior ethmoid artery.

◈ A complete ethmoidectomy can be performed along the skull base.

◈ The bony layer covering the anterior ethmoid cells is relatively thin and is easily removed with a punch or cutting bur.

◈ After the bone has been removed, the individual groups of ethmoid cells are removed piecemeal with standard sinus instruments under direct vision. Critical landmarks are the middle turbinate, the roof of the ethmoid, and laterally the orbital plate of the ethmoid bone.

◈ For the frontal sinus, the floor of the sinus and its junction with the anterior wall are removed, exposing the lumen of the frontal sinus. Further bone is removed depending on the exposure needed for the pathology. With the "eyeglass" incision, a small bone flap can be created and temporarily removed to provide wider exposure of the frontal sinus.

Complications

• Injury to the trochlea of the superior oblique (diplopia)
• Injury to the supraorbital nerve (temporary or permanent forehead numbness)
• Injury to the attachment of the medial palpebral ligament (telecanthus)
• Cerebrospinal fluid leak from injury to the roof of the ethmoid/cribriform plate (potential for intracranial infection)

- Orbital hematoma from bleeding from the anterior/posterior ethmoid artery being transected and retracting into the orbit (potential for permanent visual loss)
- Hypertrophic scarring (reduced with the W-plasty)

■ Osteoplastic Flap

The osteoplastic flap is used to approach the frontal sinus through down-fracturing or removal of the anterior frontal sinus wall. Down-fracturing and hinging the anterior frontal table forward is preferred with the periosteum still attached to the anterior table to maintain the blood supply.[3]

Main Indications[4]

- Large mucoceles eroding into the anterior fossa or orbit
- Benign or malignant neoplasms involving the frontal sinus
- Fractures of the frontal sinus/frontal bone
- Reconstruction of defects of the anterior or posterior frontal sinus walls
- Repair of frontobasal CSF leakage

❖ Incisions

There are three incisions for performing an osteoplastic flap. The bitemporal coronal incision is preferred.

- Bitemporal coronal incision
- ◈ Hair is removed for 1 to 2 cm along the line of incision.
- ◈ The incision starts anterior to the crus of the helix across the forehead to the contralateral side.
- ◈ The incision can be placed in front of the hair line (pre-trichal) or within the hair line.
- ◈ Bevel the direction of the scalpel in the direction of the hair follicles to avoid cutting across the hair follicles, which minimizes permanent alopecia postoperatively.
- ◈ Minimizing the use of electrocautery on the incision line helps to reduce the risk of alopecia. Bleeding is preferably controlled with bipolar cautery or hemostatic clamps (Raney clips).
- ◈ The lateral limbs of the incision should be placed sufficiently inferiorly to enable adequate mobilization and rotation of the soft tissue flap.
- ◈ Do not angle the incision anteriorly over the temple to avoid injury to the temporal branches of the facial nerve.

◈   The incision goes through the skin, subcutaneous tissue, and galea.
◈   The supraorbital and supratrochlear nerves are identified by a combination of blunt and sharp dissection near the supraorbital margins and protected.
◈   The outline of the bone cuts is marked on the anterior table (see below), and the periosteum is incised outside of the bone cut markings and elevated over the markings so that there is still periosteum intact on the anterior table. Some surgeons prefer to remove the anterior table, but this is not always necessary.
- Mid-forehead incision
◈   Ideally the mid-forehead incision is placed in a horizontal forehead rhytid.
◈   The remaining features are similar to those of the bitemporal coronal incision.
- Gull-wing incision
◈   The incision is placed superior to both eyebrows and joined across the glabella.
◈   The supratrochlear and supraorbital nerves are sacrificed.
◈   The remaining features are similar to those of the bitemporal coronal incision.

Advantages and Disadvantages of the Three Incisions

- The bitemporal coronal incision is preferred because of the wide exposure and the possibility of hiding the incision in the hair or hair line; however, it requires more dissection, and if there is preexisting alopecia (e.g., male pattern baldness), the incision may be noticeable postoperatively.
- Alopecia along the incision line postoperatively may occur if the incision is not beveled parallel to the hair follicles or excessive cauterization of the scalp edge is used.
- The mid-forehead incision is more direct to the anterior table and requires less dissection but has the potential to leave a visible scar and also has the disadvantage of leaving permanent numbness on the forehead superior to the incision.
- The gull-wing incision provides direct exposure to the anterior forehead, but permanently sacrifices the sensory nerve supply to the forehead, and the incision is very noticeable postoperatively. Patients would generally consider the gull-wing incision cosmetically unacceptable, particularly when the other two options are available.

❖ Bone Cuts: Surgical Approaches

There are several methods for outlining the limits of the anterior wall of the frontal sinus.[5]

◈ The traditional method is to use a nonmagnified anterior posterior (6-foot Caldwell) X-ray template; the X-ray is taken preoperatively, and the frontal sinus is cut out, oriented, sterilized, and placed on the anterior table during the operation. The outline of the template is marked on the anterior table (e.g., using methylene blue or a sterile marking pen).[6]

◈◈ An alternate method is to make a small frontal trephination and place an endoscope into the frontal sinus with the operating room lights dimmed. The resulting transillumination outlines the confines of the frontal sinus.

◈◈ A third method uses intraoperative image guidance to localize the frontal sinus walls.[7]

❖ Steps:

◈ The bone cuts are usually made with powered instruments such as an oscillating saw beveled in toward the frontal sinus to minimize the risk of inadvertent penetration of the posterior table and dura if the markings are slightly off.

◈ Osteotomes may help with the final elevation and down-fracturing of the anterior table of the frontal sinus.

◈ A horizontal osteotomy over the glabella helps to facilitate down-fracture of the anterior table and prevent inadvertent fracture of one or both orbital rims.

◈ Once the anterior table is down-fractured, the necessary surgery required is undertaken.

◈ The anterior table is secured back in position with miniplates.

◈ The pericranium is reapproximated followed by closure of the scalp.

◈ It is important to accurately reapproximate the galea, which is the strength layer in the closure.

◈ One or more drains may be placed as well as a compressive head dressing at the surgeon's discretion.

Complications

• Alopecia may occur along the bicoronal incision line, as discussed above.
• The supraorbital and supratrochlear nerves may be injured, resulting in transient or permanent numbness of one or both sides of the forehead.
• If the anterior table of the frontal sinus is significantly thinned or diseased preoperatively, the anterior table bone may necrose if removed completely. Ideally, the periosteum should be left on the anterior table to provide additional blood supply and minimize this complication. Postoperative infection may also result in bone loss and resultant cosmetic deformity.
• Infection of the soft tissue or bone may occur.
• Seroma may occur.

- Facial nerve paresis may occur (forehead/eye) if the temporal or zygomatic branches are injured.
- If dissection is taken over the supraorbital rim into the orbit, the trochlea may be injured, which could result in postoperative diplopia.
- Dural injury and resultant CSF leak may occur if the bone-cut outline is not exact or not beveled inward.

■ Sublabial Incision and Modifications

Main Indications[8]

- Operations in the maxillary sinus for inflammatory disease or neoplastic disease (Caldwell-Luc and Denker procedures)
- Approach to the pterygopalatine and infratemporal fossae
- Repair of orbital floor fractures
- Management of dental cysts affecting the maxillary sinus

❖ Placement of Incision

◈ The upper lip is retracted superiorly. The standard sublabial incision is placed in the oral vestibule just below the line of the gingivomucosal junction and it extends approximately from the canine tooth to the first molar but may be extended more laterally or medially as required for adequate exposure.

◈ The supramarginal incision along the gingival margin of teeth, similar to the above standard incision, is preferred by some surgeons in dentulous patients or if there is significant scarring from previous surgery in the area. It also creates a favorable scar for denture wearers.

❖ Soft Tissue Dissection

◈ The mucosa is incised to expose the periosteum on the anterior maxillary sinus wall.

◈ The periosteum is divided and elevated with the buccal soft tissues to expose the anterior maxillary wall up to the level of the infraorbital nerve, which is preserved.

◈ Care is taken not to put undue tension on the infraorbital nerve to prevent postoperative hypoesthesia or neuropathic pain. The location of the nerve can be approximated by drawing a vertical line through the level of the pupil and palpating the infraorbital rim and going 4 to 5 mm inferior to the rim.

❖ Bone Work

◈ Starting in the canine fossa, using osteotomes, bone punches, or powered instrumentation (e.g., oscillating saw, drill), an opening is made in the anterior maxillary wall and enlarged.

◈◈Alternatively, an anterior maxillary wall bone flap can be removed and reattached at the conclusion of the operation.

◈ The opening created has to be large enough to carry out the planned surgery.

◈ In dentulous patients, the inferior bone cuts need to stay above the dental roots so as to avoid devitalizing the teeth.

◈ The bony opening can extend superiorly up to the infraorbital nerve or around the nerve. The infraorbital rim is preserved, and in a Caldwell-Luc procedure, the medial buttress is preserved.

◈ The Denker's procedure extends the bone removal to include the medial anterior maxilla (medial buttress) for wider exposure.

Complications

- Hypoesthesia or neuropathic pain in the cheek from injury to the infraorbital nerve or associated branches of the second division of the trigeminal nerve may result in persistent pain/dysesthesia of the upper dentition/lower maxilla.
- Injury to the dental roots may occur.
- Loss of support/flattening of the nasal ala following Denker's procedure results in cosmetic deformity and possibly nasal obstruction.

■ Midfacial Degloving

Main Indications

- Procedures that require wide access to the midface, nasal pyramid, maxillary sinus, and orbit.
- Tumor resection involving the midface, nasal septum, paranasal sinuses, anterior skull base, or clivus.
- Most common use: management of large benign lesions of the sinonasal region and skull base (e.g., nasopharyngeal angiofibroma) or for selected malignancy in this area. For malignancy, the midfacial degloving approach has been used as the anterior transfacial exposure in anterior craniofacial resections when combined with an anterior craniotomy.
- Access to the nasopharynx and infratemporal fossa.
- Repair of extensive midfacial fractures.

❖ Placement of Incisions[9] (see Chapter 14, Fig. 14.4, page 347)

◈ Bilateral sublabial incision in the superior oral vestibule just below the gingivomucosal junction and centered on the frenulum extending from one maxillary tuberosity to the opposite maxillary tuberosity.
◈ Full nasal transfixion incision and continued laterally with bilateral intercartilaginous incisions continued along the floor of each nasal cavity and along the piriform apertures to produce circumferential incisions inside each nostril.
◈ The upper lateral cartilages are left in place connected over the anterior septal border.

❖ Soft Tissue Dissection

◈ Following completion of the sublabial incision, the soft tissues and periosteum are elevated over the anterior face of both maxillae up to the infraorbital margins and piriform aperture.
◈ The nasal soft tissues are sharply elevated over the upper and lower nasal cartilages, nasal bones, and frontal processes of the maxilla up to the glabella/nasal root.
◈ The infraorbital nerves are identified and preserved.

❖ Bone Removal

◈ Large bone openings are made in the anterior walls of the maxillary sinuses.
◈ The medial maxilla and piriform aperture on one or both sides can be removed; in many cases it may be possible to remove the anteromedial maxillary wall through osteotomies and replace these bone segments with miniplates at the conclusion of the operation to provide better nasal support and cosmesis.
◈ The extent of the bone and cartilage resection depends on the exact location, histopathology, and exposure required to remove the disease process.
◈ Removal of portions of the posterior nasal septum provides access to the nasopharynx, sphenoid, and clivus.
◈ The Le Fort I osteotomy is a variation of the sublabial incision with a horizontal osteotomy through the inferior maxilla and down-fracture of the maxilla for wide exposure to the central skull base.

Advantages and Disadvantages

• The main advantages are avoidance of external facial incisions and simultaneous exposure of the inferior and medial maxilla bilaterally (particularly helpful for tumors with bilateral involvement of the nasal cavity and maxillary sinus). In addition, if the exposure is found to be inadequate, a Weber-Ferguson or frontoethmoid incision can still be performed safely. The major disadvantages are limited exposure superiorly and posteriorly and the need for constant retraction of soft tissues for adequate exposure.

Complications

- Scar contracture (oral vestibule, nasal vestibules)
- Infraorbital nerve hypoesthesia
- Nasal deformity, especially around the nasal tip area, resulting from poor approximation of soft tissues or removal of cartilage/bone

■ Transoral Approach

Main Indications

- Removal of benign and malignant neoplasms of the nasopharynx
- External approach to the clivus/upper craniovertebral junction

Exposure

- For exposure of the clivus and sphenoid sinus, the soft palate is divided in the midline and the posterior hard palate and nasal septum usually require resection.
- For more inferior lesions (e.g., upper two cervical vertebrae or the anterior foramen magnum), division of the soft palate may be sufficient.

❖ Surgical Approach[10]

The patient is placed in the supine position with the head extended; as mentioned above, consider neck flexion/extension films in patients with possible neck instability.

- ◈ A suspension mouth gag, good illumination/magnification, or a microscope are used.
- ◈ A preformed dental palatal splint may aid in closure and protection of the palate postoperatively.
- ◈ Consider neck flexion/extension films in patients with possible neck instability.

◈ Divide the uvula and soft palate in the midline to the hard palate; the incision can continue over the hard palate, depending on the exposure required.

◈ The posterior pharyngeal wall mucosa and prevertebral fascia are incised from the superior nasopharynx inferiorly into the oropharynx as far as required for exposure of the pathology; lateral incisions from the midline superiorly and inferiorly may be required to elevate the soft tissues to expose the clivus and upper cervical spine.

◈ The soft tissues including the prevertebral musculature are reflected laterally to expose the ligaments and firm connective tissues around the dens of the axis and lower portion of the clivus.

◈ Portions of the posterior hard palate and posterior septum frequently require removal for adequate exposure.

◈ The anterior wall and rostrum of the sphenoid sinus are removed to provide adequate exposure if the pathology involves the sphenoid sinus or clivus.

◈ Kerrison rongeurs or other cutting instruments are useful for removal of the dense ligaments and connective tissue overlying the craniovertebral junction to provide adequate exposure.

◈ For lesions involving the sphenoid or clivus, great care and anatomic localization (e.g., image guidance or Doppler probe) are necessary to identify the carotid arteries and to avoid inadvertent injury.

Complications

• Infection (e.g., retropharyngeal abscess)
• Oronasal fistula if the soft tissues are not repaired well or dehisce secondary to wound infection postoperatively
• Velopharyngeal insufficiency from disturbance of soft palate closure against the posterior pharyngeal wall
• Atlantoaxial instability depending on the amount of bone removed and pathology in the region, which may require stabilization (see Chapter 24)
• Cerebrospinal fluid leak with the potential for intracranial infection
• Injury to the carotid arteries or basilar arteries

■ Lateral Rhinotomy and Extensions

Main Indications

• Resection of benign and some malignant tumors of the nose or paranasal sinuses

- As part of an anterior craniofacial resection combined with an anterior craniotomy

❖ Placement of Incisions

- Lateral rhinotomy (**Fig. 15.1**)
- ◈ The lateral rhinotomy incision runs along the nasofacial groove, usually starting superiorly below the medial end of the eyebrow.
- ◈ The incision is then placed approximately midway between the medial canthus and midline nasal bone, often with several W-plasties in the medial canthal region to prevent postoperative scar contracture.
- ◈ The incision runs inferiorly along the nasofacial groove around the alar base and then into the nasal cavity.
- ◈ It is important to stay several millimeters outside of the alar groove, as incisions placed directly in the groove are much more noticeable postoperatively.
- Weber-Ferguson (**Fig. 15.1**)
- ◈ The Weber-Ferguson incision extends under the eye, along the nasofacial groove, around the alar base to the upper lip philtrum, and then inferiorly through the philtrum.
- ◈ An upper gingivobuccal incision is made going posteriorly as far as is required (e.g., to the maxillary tuberosity) to develop a lip/cheek flap which usually includes sacrifice of the infraorbital nerve as it exits the maxilla, unless disease is clearly limited to the maxillary infrastructure. This incision affords exposure of the entire anterior maxilla and anterior zygoma.
- ◈ To gain greater exposure over the eye, the incision can be extended laterally from the lateral canthus but risks injury to the temporal ("frontal") branches of the facial nerve.
- ◈ The incision below the eye can be placed in a lower lid skin crease or along the infraorbital rim margin (infraorbital) or just below the inferior eyelashes (subciliary). The subciliary incision is generally more cosmetic but has a higher risk of postoperative ectropion.
- ◈ Similar to the lateral rhinotomy, the incision should stay just outside of the alar base groove, and the incision through the philtrum will heal more imperceptibly if one or more W-plasties are placed in this location.
- ◈ The Weber-Ferguson incision is the classic approach for radical maxillectomy, usually for malignancy of the maxillary sinus.
- Extended lateral rhinotomy
  - ○ The main advantage of the extended lateral rhinotomy over the Weber-Ferguson is that there is no infraorbital nerve sacrifice and no incision under the eye (which can lead to ectropion).
- ◈ There are several variations of the two main incisions (lateral rhinotomy and Weber-Ferguson).

◈◈ The most common variation is the extended lateral rhinotomy, which takes the lateral rhinotomy incision and combines it with the incision through the philtrum and upper gingivobuccal sulcus. The resulting exposure of the nasal cavity and anterior maxilla is good, but not as wide as with the incision under the eye.

◈◈ Another variation of the extended lateral rhinotomy carries the superior portion of the incision vertically on to the lower forehead to access the anterior cranial fossa from below.[11]

❖ Soft Tissue Dissection

◈ The incisions are made and deepened to the bone.

◈ The angular vessels near the medial canthus tend be problematic, so if they can be identified and ligated before injury/bleeding, it makes the procedure much smoother.

◈ The medial canthal tendon is sharply divided and tagged for reapproximation at the end of the procedure. Ideally, nonabsorbable suture is used to reapproximate the tendon to bone to minimize the risk of telecanthus postoperatively.

◈ The cheek flap is developed over the inferior orbicularis muscle.

◈ The periorbita is elevated from the lamina papyracea, the anterior ethmoid artery identified, and a decision is made about whether the artery requires ligation (which depends on the pathology, the exposure required, and the potential risk of inadvertent transection of the artery with resultant orbital hematoma).

◈ A cut is made below the frontoethmoidal suture line that marks the level of the cribriform plate.

◈ The lacrimal sac is typically preserved, but the nasolacrimal duct is transected. The duct may be left to drain into the nose; some authors recommend temporarily stenting the duct or marsupializing ("fish-mouthing") the duct open.[12]

❖ Bone Removal

The classic bone cuts for medial and total maxillectomy are described; however, there are many variations of subtotal maxillectomy possible, depending on the local extent of disease and pathology.

• Medial maxillectomy

◈ The lateral rhinotomy incision is usually combined with removal of the medial maxilla and ethmoid sinuses.

◈ The ipsilateral nasal bone is osteotomized (lateral osteotomy plus or minus lateral root osteotomy) and the nasal bone reflected medially.

◈ Bone removal or osteotomies are typically created in the anterior maxilla to remove the medial buttress with a vertical osteotomy from the medial orbital rim to the level of the nasal floor, and then a horizontal osteotomy at the level of the nasal floor.

◈ The posteromedial wall of the maxilla is osteotomized.

◈ An anterior buttress of frontal process of maxilla can remain to provide support postoperatively or it can be removed.

◈ Osteotomies are created along the frontoethmoid suture line and lamina papyracea.

• Total maxillectomy

◈ The nasal process of the maxilla is divided.

◈ The maxilla is separated from the zygomatic arch.

◈ Inferiorly the maxilla is divided through its alveolar process between the lateral incisor and canine tooth, through the midline palate to the posterior palate margin.

◈ Inferiorly and laterally, the maxilla is separated from the pterygoid plates.

◈ The method of reconstruction needs to be considered preoperatively. Classically, a split-thickness skin graft can be placed against the exposed cheek soft tissues and a prefabricated obturator placed. Where expertise exists, free tissue transfer and reconstruction of the defect with free vascularized bone and soft tissue provides superior function and cosmesis.[13]

Complications

• Telecanthus
• Ectropion
• Epiphora
• Enophthalmos (if a significant portion of the orbital floor is removed)
• Orbital hematoma
• Infraorbital nerve numbness
• Nasal deformity (if poor remaining bony support)

■ References

Boldfaced references are of particular importance.

1. Neal GD. External ethmoidectomy. Otolaryngol Clin North Am 1985;18:55–60
2. Dedo HH, Broberg TG, Murr AH. Frontoethmoidectomy with Sewall-Boyden reconstruction: alive and well, a 25-year experience. Am J Rhinol 1998;12:191–198
3. Maniglia AJ, Dodds BL. A safe technique for frontal sinus osteoplastic flap. Laryngoscope 1991;101:908–910
4. **Lee JM, Palmer JN. Indications for the osteoplastic flap in the endoscopic era. Curr Opin Otolaryngol Head Neck Surg 2011;19:11–15**

5. **Melroy CT, Dubin MG, Hardy SM, Senior BA. Analysis of methods to assess frontal sinus extent in osteoplastic flap surgery: transillumination versus 6-ft Caldwell versus image guidance. Am J Rhinol 2006;20:77–83**

6. Fung MK. Template for frontal osteoplastic flap. Laryngoscope 1986;96:578–579

7. **Volpi L, Pistochini A, Bignami M, Meloni F, Turri Zanoni M, Castelnuovo P. A novel technique for tailoring frontal osteoplastic flaps using the ENT magnetic navigation system. Acta Otolaryngol 2012;132:645–650**

8. **Barzilai G, Greenberg E, Uri N. Indications for the Caldwell-Luc approach in the endoscopic era. Otolaryngol Head Neck Surg 2005;132:219–220**

9. Traynelis VC, McCulloch TM, Hoffman HT. Craniofacial resection of the anterior skull base. In: Rengachary SS, Wilkins RH, eds. Neurosurgical Operative Atlas, 3rd ed. Baltimore: Williams & Wilkins; 1993:329–340

10. Maran AG. Surgical approaches to the nasopharynx. Clin Otolaryngol Allied Sci 1983; 8:417–429

11. Ketcham AS, Wilkins RH, Vanburen JM, Smith RR. A Combined intracranial facial approach to the paranasal sinuses. Am J Surg 1963;106:698–703

12. Smith O, Gullane PJ. Inverting papilloma of the nose: analysis of 48 patients. J Otolaryngol 1987;16:154–156

13. Shrime MG, Gilbert RW. Reconstruction of the midface and maxilla. Facial Plast Surg Clin North Am 2009;17:211–223

16 Endoscopic Transsphenoidal Approaches

■ Indications

1. Tumors and lesions involving the sella, parasellar regions, and suprasellar region
2. Lesions in the frontal fossa, clivus, petrous apex, and foramen magnum (extended approaches)
   - Considered the standard midline corridor for ventral endoscopic skull base approaches.
   - Combined with expanded approaches, the endoscopic transsphenoidal approaches provide access from the crista galli to the craniocervical junction[1-9] (**Fig. 16.1**).
   - The biportal four-handed technique, described by Cusimano and Fenton[1] in 1996, has become the standard approach and the basis for all the endonasal transsphenoidal and extended transsphenoidal approaches.

> **Surgical Anatomy Pearl**
>
> Sphenoid sinus: the gateway to the skull base.

■ Key Anatomical Considerations

- Anatomy of the nasal cavity including the presence of a deviated septum
- Pneumatization patterns of the sphenoid sinus (conchal, presellar, sellar, postsellar; see Chapter 2, **Fig. 2.14**, page 53)
- The relationship of the sphenoid intersinus septa and the internal carotid arteries (ICAs)
- The presence of a sphenoethmoidal cell (Onodi), which if unopened will limit access in the sphenoid and planum
- The lateral pneumatization of the sphenoid, which may provide further access in the coronal plane (including the cavernous ICA, middle cranial fossa)

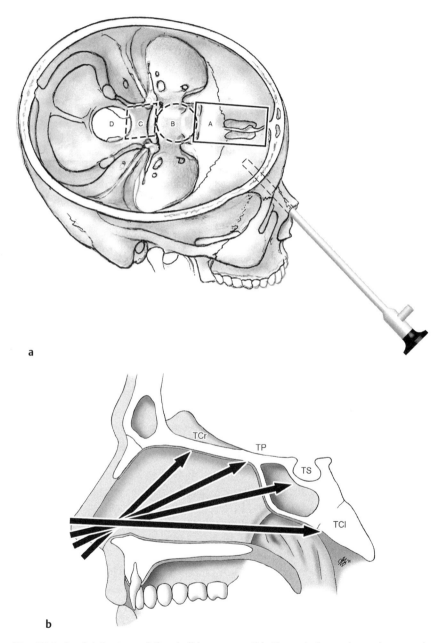

a

b

Fig. 16.1a,b **(a)** Regions of the skull base accessible through the endonasal approach: A, frontal fossa; B, sella; C, clivus; D, occipitocervical junction. **(b)** Endonasal approaches to the skull base. TCr, transcribriform; TP, transplanum; TS, transsphenoidal; TCl, transclival.

■ Patient Positioning

Typically the patient is placed in the supine position with the head neutral, the nose straight up, or with a slight amount of head extension. The bed should be in 10 to 15 degrees of reverse Trendelenburg to enable venous drainage.

- The head is typically fixed in a head frame (Sugita/Mayfield) to stabilize the head especially during bone removal near the critical structures (ICA, optic nerves).
- Stereotactic frameless navigation can be employed to help verify critical landmarks, but this must be regularly checked throughout the procedure on known visual landmarks (e.g., midline septum, nasal cavity floor, nasopharynx) to verify accurate registration.
- If a large cerebrospinal fluid (CSF) leak is expected as part of tumor removal (e.g., craniopharyngioma), a lumbar drain can be placed prior to surgery.
- Prepare and expose any areas of the body that may be required for skull base reconstruction (e.g., abdominal fat, tensor fascia lata).
- Adequately decongest the nasal cavity with ribbon gauze or pledgets soaked in topical 1:1,000 epinephrine at the beginning of the procedure.

■ Transnasal Approach

❖ Surgical Approaches

◈ All the of following steps are performed using a 0-degree endoscope. If a deviated septum is present, begin on the side opposite the deviation.

◈◈ Variation: Out-fracture the inferior turbinate to improve nasal access.

◈ Once the middle turbinate is visualized, there are two options to gain access to the posterior nasal space and the location of the superior turbinate:

◈◈ The middle turbinate can be lateralized with a freer elevator. Advantage: preservation of an anatomic structure, although it is distorted and crushed. Disadvantage: limited transnasal access for instrumentation and the potential for nasal synechiae.

◈◈ Amputate the inferior portion of the middle turbinate using endoscopic scissors. The base of the middle turbinate must be cauterized to minimize bleeding from branches of the sphenopalatine artery. Advantage: provides a greater freedom of movement of the instruments for tumor dissection and removal. Potential disadvantage: synechiae formation between remnant middle turbinate and the lateral nasal wall.

- The superior turbinate is the key anatomic structure that provides the location of the natural sphenoid ostium (**Fig. 16.2**).

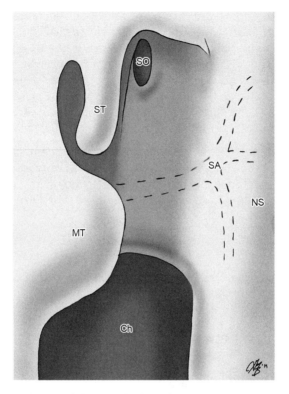

Fig. 16.2 Endoscopic view of the natural sphenoid ostium (SO), located just medial to the superior turbinate (ST) and above the nasal choana. MT, middle turbinate; SA, posterior septal artery; NS, nasal septum; Ch, choana.

- ○ The ostium is located just posteromedial to the superior turbinate and approximately 1.5 cm superior to the arch of the choana. *Tip*: Use a pledget soaked in topical 1:1,000 epinephrine to help vasoconstrict the mucosa in this area and visualize the natural ostium.
- ◈ Displace or resect the inferior half of the superior turbinate with straight-through cutting instruments.
- • A partial posterior ethmoidectomy can be completed to enhance visualization of the medial orbital wall.
- ◈◈ If a sphenoethmoidal (Onodi) cell is present, open the cell and expose the skull base, but recognize that the optic nerve can be dehiscent because of this pneumatization pattern.
- ◈◈ If the ostium cannot be easily visualized because of swollen mucosa, the blunt end of a Freer elevator can be used to probe the general location of

the natural sphenoid ostium (the tip of the Freer should easily fall into the sphenoid without any pressure); alternatively, an image guidance navigated pointer can be used to confirm the correct trajectory into the sphenoid sinus.

◈ Once the ostium is identified, open widely the sphenoid using forward- and backward-biting Kerrison punches. *Tip:* Open the sphenoid superiorly to the skull base and laterally to the medial orbital wall. This ensures that the surgeon will not have a restricted range of motion when working with longer curettes/suctions/dissecting instruments in the sella.

Be careful opening the sphenoid too inferiorly at this point in the operation, as the posterior septal branch of the sphenopalatine artery is located midway between the natural sphenoid ostium and the arch of the choana (this is the vascular pedicle to the nasoseptal flap).

- At this juncture of the endoscopic approach, there are three options for addressing the vascular pedicle:
  1. If no flap is anticipated to be required for the procedure, the artery and the surrounding mucosa may be cauterized with either monopolar or bipolar cautery.
  2. If a flap may not be required for the procedure but the surgeon wants to preserve the pedicle without having to harvest a flap, the mucosa may be reflected inferior to the sphenoid ostium (with the accompanying artery) with a Freer/Cottle elevator to expose the bony face of the sphenoid and sphenoid rostrum.
  3. If a flap is anticipated for part of the reconstruction at the end of the procedure, the surgeon may harvest the nasoseptal flap (see below). At this stage, the harvested nasoseptal flap can be placed in the nasopharynx for reconstruction at the end of the procedure.

◈ Posterior septostomy: perform the removal of mucosa and bone to enable using the bi-nostril, four-hand, two-surgeon technique; rather than drill and remove this portion of the bony septum, a large piece of the vomer can often be removed and saved for possible reconstruction of the sella/skull base.

◈ Resect the contralateral posterior septal mucosa using either a microdebrider or through-cutting forceps.

◈◈ Variation: An option at this stage is to use the contralateral posterior septal mucosa as a reverse flap and cover the exposed septal cartilage on the ipsilateral side if a nasoseptal flap was harvested (see below).

◈ Once this stage is completed, perform the same transnasal steps on the contralateral side.

- Any septal deviation can often be dealt with by bony or cartilaginous removal during the posterior septectomy.
  ○ The exception is if the septal deviation is significant and extends anteriorly to the nasal vestibule.

- ○ If this is the case, a traditional septoplasty with a hemi-transfixion incision may need to be performed at the beginning of the procedure to provide adequate transnasal access.
- Once both sphenoid sinuses are widely opened and the posterior septostomy is completed, the endoscopic view through one nostril should include both sphenoid sinuses and the remaining sphenoid rostrum **(Fig. 16.3)**.
- ◈ Remove most of the sphenoid rostrum with either backward-biting Kerrison punches or a high-speed cutting/diamond irrigating drill bit. Leave a small piece in the midline as a landmark.
  - ○ Depending on the shape, the bony sphenoid rostrum can occasionally be harvested as a piece of bone for sellar reconstruction.
  - ○ Do not twist and remove the sphenoid rostrum with grasping forceps, as it is often attached to the sphenoid intersinus septum (which, in turn, may be in close relationship with the ICA).

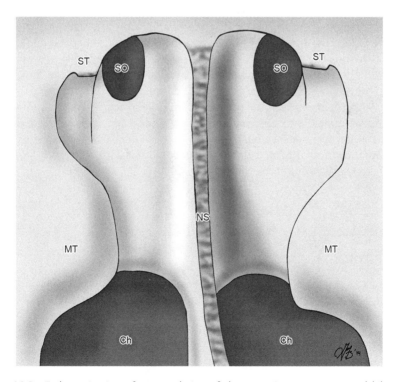

Fig. 16.3 Endoscopic view after completion of the posterior septectomy and bilateral sphenoidotomies. SO, sphenoid sinus/ostium; ST, cut edge of superior turbinate; NS, cut edge of posterior nasal septum; MT, middle turbinate; Ch, choana.

- The final transsphenoidal corridor often extends in a sagittal plane from the sphenoid floor to the planum sphenoidale and in a coronal plane from orbit to orbit.
  - This opening prevents any curved curettes/dissectors from being restricted at the sphenoid opening.
  - Furthermore, it provides sufficient room for instrument dissection within the sphenoid and sella.
- ◈ Once within the sphenoid, note all the relevant anatomy including the bulge of the sella, the carotid protuberances, the medial and lateral optico-carotid recesses, the clival recess, and the sphenoid bony septations (see Chapter 2, **Fig. 2.15**, page 54).
- For pathology confined to the sella, only the bony septations restricting access to the floor and the anterior face of the sella need to be removed (if these are thick, it is safest to use a high-speed diamond irrigating drill bit to remove the intersinus septa; otherwise, a large pituitary rongeur can be used).
  - If the intersinus septum is attaching to the midline sella, it must be removed until it is flush with the floor of the sella.
- ◈ Before performing the sellotomy/craniectomy, elevate the sphenoid mucosa overlying the sella with a Cottle elevator and displace it laterally.
- ◈◈ Variation: If a nasoseptal flap is anticipated to be used at the end of the procedure, the surgeon may remove the mucosa overlying the portions of the sphenoid sinus floor, which will be covered with the flap. This is done to prevent the possible future mucocele formation.
- ◈ At this stage, perform the sellotomy (resect the bone window en bloc by using chisels to save the small bone flap, which can be used for the reconstruction of the sellar floor).
- ◈◈ Variation: Drill the sellar floor away or remove it with curettes.
- ◈ Resect sellar/pituitary pathology (see Chapter 21.2, page 498).

■ Harvesting a Nasoseptal Flap

❖ Surgical Approaches[10,11]

- ◈ Inject the septum with 1% xylocaine with 1:100,000 epinephrine at multiple spots to help hydrodissect the mucosa from the underlying septal bone and cartilage.
- ◈◈ If a wider flap is required, the mucosa over the bony nasal cavity floor is also injected.
- Addressing the vascular pedicle:
  - The sphenoid ostium marks the superior margin of the horizontal incision line and can be extended medially over the bony sphenoid rostrum with either an insulated monopolar tip cautery or a sickle-shaped scalpel.

○ The inferior margin of the horizontal incision line is made at the arch of the choana. This incision is carried medially using either a cautery or a sickle-shaped scalpel to the posteroinferior aspect of the septum; the incision can be curved to follow the natural curvature of the posterior septum inferiorly.
○ With these two incisions, the vascular pedicle has been preserved (**Fig. 16.4**).

Tip: make the inferior incision of the nasoseptal flap first, leaving the superior attachment of the septal mucosa until the end to allow for easier elevation of the flap.

◈ Make the inferior incision line of the nasoseptal flap at the junction of the septum and the nasal cavity floor.
◈◈ If a wider flap is required, the incision line can be made to incorporate the mucosa of the nasal floor extending laterally to the inferior meatus.

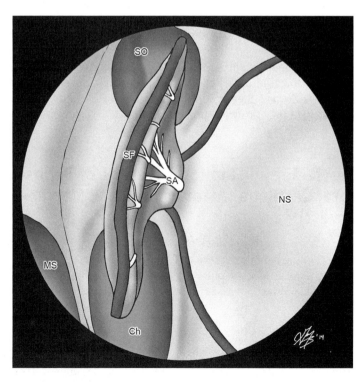

Fig. 16.4 Harvesting a right-sided nasoseptal flap. SO, sphenoid ostium, SF, nasoseptal flap; SA, posterior septal artery; NS, nasal septum; Ch, choana; MS, maxillary sinus.

- The incision line is brought anteriorly until the required length of the flap has been reached.
  - ○ The anterior limit of the flap can be extended as far as the mucocutaneous junction of the nasal vestibule.
  - ○ The length of the nasoseptal flap depends on two main factors:
    - ▪ The proposed area of reconstruction (e.g., sella, planum, cribriform plate, clivus, foramen magnum). Defects involving more anterior aspects of the skull base require the longest length of flap because of the distance from the sphenopalatine artery pedicle.
    - ▪ The pneumatization/depth of the sphenoid sinus as well as the bulge of the sella within the sphenoid.
      - □ A deeply pneumatized sphenoid may require a long length of the flap to lie properly within the sphenoid and cover the sellar defect.
      - □ A sella that bulges significantly into the sphenoid sinus may require a shorter flap because the distance from the pedicle to the sella is shortened.
- ◈ Make the superior horizontal incision with endoscopic scissors and connect it to the superior incision above the vascular pedicle. Preserve at least 1 cm of superior septal mucosa adjacent to the skull base, in order to preserve olfactory nerve fibers and minimize olfactory disturbance following surgery.
- ◈ Once the flap is harvested, place it into the nasopharynx for reconstruction at the end of the procedure. Be sure to inspect and achieve hemostasis from the cut edge of the superior septum as this can frequently bleed and obscure visualization during the procedure.

■ Reverse Septal Flap for Coverage of Exposed Septal Cartilage (After Nasoseptal Flap Harvest)[12]

- This flap is based on the anterior blood supply to the septal mucosa (branches of the descending palatine, anterior ethmoidal, facial artery).
- It is used to cover exposed septal cartilage after harvesting a nasoseptal flap, with the goal of reducing nasal crusting following surgery.

❖ Surgical Approaches

- ◈ After removing the posterior bony septum, make a vertical incision along the contralateral septal mucosa (usually at the level of the sphenoid rostrum).
- ◈ Make the superior and horizontal mucosal incisions parallel to the nasoseptal flap cuts on the contralateral side.

◈ Preserve the anterior pedicle to the flap and reverse the septal mucosa to cover the exposed septal cartilage on the contralateral side. This is held in place with 4-0 absorbable sutures to reapproximate the contralateral septal mucosa flap and the remaining free edge of the contralateral anterior septal mucosa.

■ Expanded Transplanum Approaches[5,13,14]

Indications

These approaches are indicated for lesions extending superiorly beyond the sella in the parasagittal plane (e.g., large macroadenomas, craniopharyngiomas, meningiomas, anterior circulation aneurysms) (**Fig 16.1**).

❖ Surgical Steps

◈ The same transnasal steps as described for a transsphenoidal approach are undertaken (including the harvest of a nasoseptal flap), with the following additional modifications:

- For adequate endoscopic exposure to the planum sphenoidale, a more complete anterior and posterior ethmoidectomy is usually required, as the anterior limit of bone removal often extends to the posterior ethmoidal arteries.
- If the skull base lesion extends far laterally to the plane of the medial orbital wall, bilateral maxillary antrostomies are first performed.
  - ○ The antrostomy facilitates identification of the orbital floor and the medial orbital wall (lateral boundaries of the ethmoid corridor).
  - ○ Additionally, it prevents iatrogenic maxillary sinus ostium obstruction if a more complete ethmoidectomy is performed.

◈◈ Variation: Using a 30-degree endoscope, skeletonize the skull base along the posterior ethmoid cavity by removing bony partitions with an up-biting, through-cutting instrument. This is an essential step.

- The posterior ethmoidal artery may be directly visualized if it is within a bony mesentery below the skull base.
- The anterior limit of bone removal during the transplanum approach is the posterior ethmoidal arteries, which may need to be cauterized with bipolar cautery.
- At this stage, there should be an unobstructed endoscopic view extending from the sella to the planum sphenoidale with a 30-degree endoscope.

◈ Use the image guidance pointer to confirm that there will be adequate endoscopic exposure to the anterior limit of the skull base tumor.

◈ Using a high-speed diamond irrigating drill bit, thin out a groove and then either use an osteotome to elevate and preserve the bone for reconstruction or just drill out the bone overlying the planum and then remove it with Kerrison rongeurs.
◈ Expose the dura overlying the planum. If the lesion is a meningioma, carefully cauterize the dura and then open it widely. Perform resection of the tuberculum/planum pathology using standard neurosurgical techniques.

■ Expanded Transcribriform Approaches[15–17]

Indications

These approaches are indicated for tumors involving the frontal lobe and the olfactory bulb (e.g., olfactory groove meningioma, esthesioneuroblastoma).

Surgical Steps

◈ Complete the transnasal portion of the transsphenoidal and transplanum steps.
  • For access to the cribriform plate and anterior cranial fossa, it is necessary to fully expose the floor of the skull base within the paranasal sinuses.
◈ Skeletonize the entire ethmoid skull base. Remove the anterior and posterior ethmoid partitions using up-biting, through-cutting instruments (a 30-degree endoscope may be required).
◈ Identify and expose the frontal sinus.
  • The frontal sinus outflow tract is usually identified posterior and medial to the agger nasi cell (the most anterior ethmoid air cell). Review the preoperative computed tomography (CT) imaging carefully to identify the frontal sinus outflow tract and the presence of additional frontal recess cells.
◈ With the frontal sinus identified, enlarge the opening widely so that the posterior table of the frontal sinus is adequately visualized.
  • An endoscopic modified Lothrop procedure (Draf III) is usually performed to remove the entire floor of the frontal sinus and create an interconnecting frontal sinus (which provides exposure to the anterior-most aspect of the anterior cranial fossa and the crista galli).
◈ Remove the superior portion of the nasal septum as well as the inferior portion of the frontal sinus intersinus septum. This may require a 70-degree endoscope and a curved irrigating drill bit.
  • With this step complete, the entire anterior skull base is exposed from the sella to the planum and cribriform plate (**Fig. 16.5**).

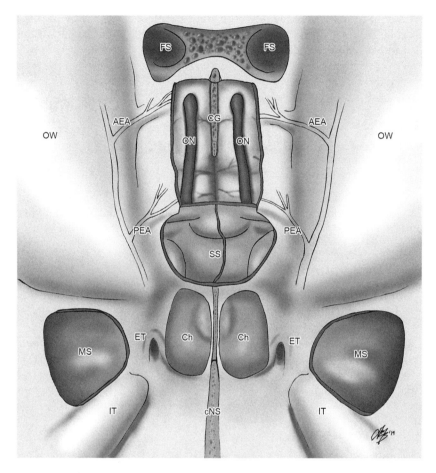

Fig. 16.5 Endoscopic view of the entire skull base from sella to the cribriform plate. FS, frontal sinus; OW, orbital wall; AEA, anterior ethmoidal artery; PEA, posterior ethmoidal artery; CG, crista galli; ON, olfactory nerve; SS, sphenoid sinus; Ch, choana; ET, eustachian tube; MS, maxillary sinus; IT, inferior turbinate; cNS, cut edge of nasal septum.

◈ Before performing a craniectomy around the tumor being resected, control and cauterize/ligate the anterior ethmoidal arteries.

◈◈ Variation: Cauterize these arteries with a bipolar cautery after the bone overlying the canal is skeletonized with a diamond drill bit.

◈◈ Variation: Remove the lamina papyracea and identify the anterior ethmoidal artery by retracting the periorbita laterally. The anterior ethmoidal artery can then be clipped under endoscopic visualization.

◈ Complete the craniectomy with either a high-speed drill or curved osteotome to expose the dura of the frontal lobe.

◈　Note that in the midline, the dura will be tented superiorly by the crista galli. This may need to be drilled away with an angled bur so that the dura can be accessible endonasally.

◈　Curved frontal sinus instruments are useful for the dissection of the lesion and its resection.

■ Endoscopic Transclival Approaches[18-22]

Indications

These approaches are indicated for lesions involving the clivus or posterior fossa (e.g., chordoma, chondrosarcoma, brainstem cavernoma, posterior circulation aneurysms).

Key Considerations

- The clivus is divided into a superior aspect that involves the posterior clinoid and dorsum sella and extends to the petrous apex; the inferior aspect extends to the level of the foramen magnum.
- Review the anatomy of the clivus and its close relationships to several neurovascular structures including the basilar artery (BA), superior cerebellar artery (SCA), anterior inferior cerebellar artery (AICA), posterior cerebral artery (PCA), and cranial nerves (CNs) III, IV, V, and VI (see Chapter 2).

❖ Surgical Steps

◈　Complete the transnasal portion of the transsphenoidal approach as previously described.
- The nasoseptal flap should be harvested because there is a high risk of CSF leak for tumors involving this region.

◈　Perform a wide maxillary antrostomy and total ethmoidectomy.

◈◈ For clival lesions that extend inferiorly and laterally, it may be necessary to complete an inferior turbinate resection, medial maxillectomy, and a possible transpterygoid approach for additional endoscopic access.

◈　Once a wide corridor has been obtained, it is at this stage that transsphenoidal access is extended inferiorly to expose the clivus.

◈　Reduce the floor of the sphenoid sinus and superior third of the clivus inferiorly with a high-speed cutting bur.

It is important to recognize the position of the internal carotid arteries in the lateral wall of the sphenoid sinus and maintain a midline corridor in the initial stages of the exposure (**Fig. 16.6**).

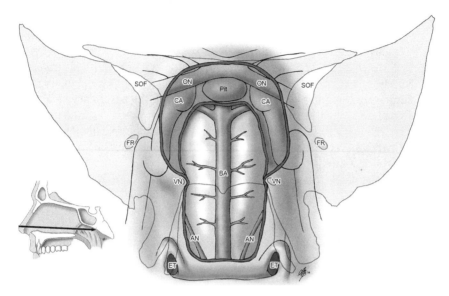

Fig. 16.6 The relevant critical anatomy during an extended endoscopic transclival approach. ON, optic nerve, CA, internal carotid artery; BA, basilar artery; VN, vidian canal/nerve; FR, foramen rotundum; SOF, superior orbital fissure; AN, abducens nerve; ET, eustachian tube.

The bone of the clivus can be quite vascular, which can be managed with either bone wax or a high-speed diamond drill bit.

- The vidian neurovascular bundle is an important landmark to identify the location of the petrous segment of the ICA.
    - It can be identified relatively easily in a well-pneumatized sphenoid sinus with a prominent vidian canal.
    - Alternatively, the vidian canal foramen can be identified in the pterygopalatine fossa.
        - The foramen sits in a coronal plane and is used to identify the vidian artery and nerve.
        - The vidian nerve is an important landmark as the anterior genu of the ICA is just posterior and lateral to the nerve.
        - Careful drilling of the bone of the vidian canal posteriorly and medially enables safe exposure of the anterior genu of the ICA.
- ◈ Identify the vertical component of the ICA by following its course from the posterior wall of the sphenoid sinus inferiorly.
    - In addition to image-guidance pointers, a microvascular Doppler probe is useful to follow and confirm the vertical course of the ICA.
    - The extent of skeletonization of the ICA depends on the extent of tumor extension laterally and posteriorly.

- However, exposure and identification of the ICA bony canal is an important step to enable safe drilling of the clivus posteriorly and avoid inadvertent vascular injury.

◈ Drill the clivus posteriorly until the clival pathology or dura is encountered.

◈◈ For clival lesions that extend inferiorly (including pathology involving the craniovertebral junction), it is necessary to open the nasopharyngeal mucosa and musculature. An extended tip monopolar cautery is used to incise the nasopharyngeal mucosa and an inferiorly based flap can be harvested for potential reconstruction at the end of the reconstruction.

◈◈ The mucosa can be incised and resected.

◈ Expose and split/resect the buccopharyngeal fascia and anterior muscles underneath the mucosa to expose the clivus. The paraclival soft tissue is incredibly fibrous and adherent. It can be slowly removed with persistence through various methods (cautery, microdebrider, coblation).

- The lateral boundaries of this tissue resection should not extend beyond the eustachian tubes, as the ICA is located posterolaterally in the nasopharynx **(Fig. 16.6)**.

◈ At this juncture, the bone of the clivus is encountered. It may be removed using high-speed irrigating drills until the pathology is encountered.

- Drilling away the clivus provides access to the brainstem and the posterior cranial fossa.
- If drilling proceeds inferiorly, the arch of C1 is encountered, providing an extended endoscopic approach to the craniovertebral junction.
- To reach even more inferiorly, the soft palate may need to be stitched and pulled down through the mouth to provide greater exposure.

■ Transpterygoid Approaches[8,23,24]

Indications

These approaches provide access to skull base lesions posterior to the maxillary sinus (e.g., middle cranial, pterygopalatine and infratemporal fossae, lateral sphenoid recess, petrous apex, cavernous sinus).

- Common pathologies include schwannomas, juvenile nasopharyngeal angiofibromas, sinonasal malignancy, and meningoencephaloceles.

Key Consideration

- If a pedicled nasoseptal flap is anticipated for skull base reconstruction, it will need to be harvested from the contralateral side, as this approach typically sacrifices the vascular pedicle on the ipsilateral side.

❖ Surgical Steps

◈ Complete the standard transsphenoidal approach as previously described.

◈◈ Variation: Depending on the location of the skull base lesion, a wide unilateral sphenoidotomy may be all that is required for access; however, the standard transsphenoidal corridor including posterior septectomy enables two-hand, four-instrument dissection.

◈ Perform a maxillary antrostomy and total ethmoidectomy on the ipsilateral side of the lesion in question. This provides access to the posterior wall of the maxillary sinus, which forms the anterior wall of the pterygopalatine fossa.

◈◈ If the lesion is large and involves a significant portion of the pterygopalatine fossa, perform also a medial maxillectomy with removal of the inferior turbinate to maximize exposure and access to this region.

◈◈ If the tumor extends into the intranasal space, debulk and remove this portion to expose the maxillary sinus and the lateral nasal wall.

◈ Elevate the mucoperiosteum from the lateral nasal wall immediately posterior to the surgically created maxillary antrostomy.

◈ Identify the bony spicule of the crista ethmoidalis, which marks the anterior wall of the sphenopalatine foramen.

◈ By gently elevating the mucosa from this region, identify the sphenopalatine and posterior nasal arteries. Ligate these vessels with bipolar cautery or surgical clips.

◈ To expose the anterior wall of the pterygopalatine fossa, remove the posterior wall of the maxillary sinus.

◈ Elevate the mucosa from the posterior maxillary sinus wall laterally. Resect the mucosa if it is involved with the tumor.

◈ Using the crista ethmoidalis as a guide, use the forward-biting Kerrison rongeurs to remove the anterior bony wall of the sphenopalatine foramen; this is then extended laterally to remove the ascending process of the palatine bone and the posterior wall of the maxillary sinus (**Fig. 16.7**).

◈◈ If the tumor involves the pterygopalatine fossa, the bone is removed laterally, superiorly, and inferiorly until the entire tumor is exposed.

• The limit is usually the floor of the maxillary sinus and the floor of the orbit where the infraorbital nerve is identified.

◈ Identify the periosteal fascia of the pterygopalatine fossa. The pulsations emanating from the maxillary artery should be visible.

◈ Carefully incise the fascia with a sickle-shaped scalpel. The fat of the pterygopalatine fossa will begin prolapsing into the surgical field.

◈ Use blunt instruments to tease out the maxillary artery. Once isolated, the artery is clipped at the midpoint of exposure; alternatively, the artery can be cauterized with bipolar cautery. Be careful not to clip the artery too far laterally, as it may tear and bleed. Proximal control of the maxillary artery can be difficult.

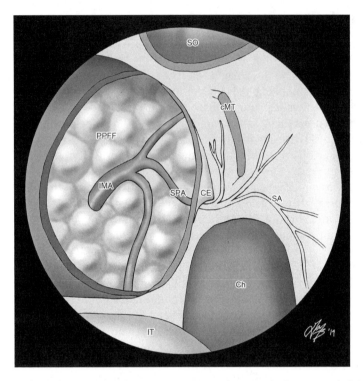

Fig. 16.7 The endoscopic view during a transpterygoid approach after removal of the posterior wall of the maxillary sinus. SO, sphenoid sinus/ostium; PPFF, pterygopalatine fossa fat; IMA, internal maxillary artery; SPA, sphenopalatine artery; CE, crista ethmoidalis; cMT, cut edge of middle turbinate; SA, sphenopalatine artery branches.

◈ Divide the artery to further expose the pterygopalatine fossa contents.
  • The vidian nerve can be identified more medially and followed to the vidian canal. This is an important landmark to identify the ICA (as previously described).
  • Superiorly, the pterygopalatine fossa (PPF) communicates with the foramen rotundum, where CN V$_2$ gives rise to branches of the sphenopalatine ganglion and the inferior orbital fissure (see page 39).
  • Laterally, the PPF communicates with the pterygomaxillary fissure, which leads into the infratemporal fossa (review the anatomy).
  • Depending on the location of the lesion in question, the tumor is now encountered and followed into the respective fossae.
◈ In a well-pneumatized sphenoid sinus that extends laterally and inferior to the middle cranial fossa, remove the posterior wall of the PPF. This is the anterior wall of the lateral sphenoid recess.

- This will provide an unobstructed view and access to the lateral sphenoid recess, middle cranial fossa, and lateral cavernous sinus.
- The skull base pathology can now be accessed by either removing the intrasinus component or carefully drilling the bone of the skull base.

■ Endoscopic Repair of Skull Base Defects

Key Considerations

- The risk of postoperative CSF leak from endonasal skull base surgery was considered a limiting factor during the growth and development of these approaches.
- The goal in reconstruction is to provide a durable separation between the intracranial and sinonasal cavity to minimize the chance of CSF leak and resultant meningitis.
- The best prevention of a postoperative CSF leak is to minimize the chance of an intraoperative CSF leak where possible.
- A multilayer closure is advisable, where possible, to reconstitute the different layers of the skull base and the sinonasal cavity **(Fig. 16.8)**.
  - Underlay graft to reconstitute the dural layer if absent
  - Rigid bone graft to reconstitute the bony skull base if possible
  - Only mucosal graft to reconstitute the sinonasal mucosa
- The repair should be durable to withstand the possibility of adjuvant treatment (e.g., external beam radiation) for skull base or sinonasal tumors.
- The reconstruction should minimize the risk of adverse sinonasal function and morbidity.
- Historically, defects < 1 cm in diameter have been successfully repaired (> 90% success rate) with multilayered free grafts of various materials (e.g., mucosa, fascia lata, synthetic derivatives[25]).
- Using free grafts alone, defects greater than 2 to 3 cm had been associated with an unacceptably high rate of CSF leak of greater than 20 to 30%.[26]
- With more experience and possibly the addition of local vascularized flaps harvested from the sinonasal cavity (especially the nasoseptal flap), the risks of CSF leak and associated intracranial complications are now reported to be less than 10% even for expanded endonasal approaches.[10,27–30]

❖ Surgical Steps

⊕ Whether free or vascularized pedicled grafts are being contemplated for the skull base repair, the sinonasal cavity should be inspected at the beginning of the procedure to ascertain whether local tissue is adequate or whether a remote donor site may be required.

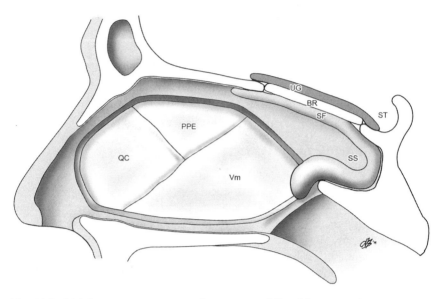

Fig. 16.8 Multilayer reconstruction with a nasoseptal flap following endoscopic cranial base approaches. QC, quadrangular cartilage; PPE, perpendicular plate of the ethmoid; Vm, Vomer; UG, underlay graft; BR, bone reconstruction; SF, nasoseptal flap; SS, sphenoid sinus; ST, sella turcica.

- Keep in mind the amount of sinonasal tissue that may need to be removed for both tumor extirpation and skull base access during the approach.
- Where possible, preserve the pedicle to the nasoseptal flap so that the option for a vascularized graft is preserved.
◈ Carefully inspect the skull base defect and ensure adequate hemostasis has been achieved both intracranially and also in the sinonasal cavity.

Small Bony Defect (< 1 cm) and CSF Leak Absent

◈ This is the most common scenario encountered in transsphenoidal pituitary surgery.
◈ The dura can be reconstructed with a bioabsorbable graft (e.g., Gelfoam) placed in an underlay fashion.
- For small bony defects (< 1 cm), formal bony reconstruction may not be necessary, and the sinonasal mucosal layer may be reconstructed with free mucosal graft harvested from the turbinate or the septum.

◈ Prior to placing the only mucosal graft, the mucosa around the edges of the bony defect are cauterized with bipolar cautery such that mucosa is not trapped (to prevent future mucocele formation).

◈ Mucosal grafts should always have the mucosal surface directed intranasally to prevent mucocele formation.

◈ Fibrin glue is then placed around the edges of the mucosal graft.

◈ Small pieces of Gelfoam can be placed into the sphenoid sinus to support the mucosal graft repair.

Small Defects (< 1 cm) and CSF Leak Present

◈ In the presence of a CSF leak, the multilayer closure has to be watertight.

◈ If there is a sizable dead space in the intracranial and extradural space, abdominal fat is useful to obliterate this potential reservoir of CSF.
  • Care has to be taken not to over-pack with fat, which may cause compression intracranially.

◈ A small amount of fibrin glue is used to secure the abdominal fat in place.

◈ The dural layer is reconstructed with either autologous fascia lata or a synthetic derivative—DuraGen® (Integra, Saint Priest, France), Durasis® (Cook Medical, Bloomington, IN), DuraMatrix® (Stryker, Kalamazoo, MI)—or other materials.
  • The key is to place the tissue in the subdural layer in an underlay fashion that extends beyond the border of the bony defect.

◈ It is an option for performing bony reconstruction for small defects.
  • If the bone cannot be placed with the possibility of its migration toward important intracranial structures (e.g., dehiscent carotid artery or optic nerve), no bony reconstruction is performed.
  • Bone can be harvested from the craniectomy or from the posterior septum.
  • The bone can be placed also in an underlay fashion to buttress the reconstructed dural layer ("bath-plug" technique).
  • Fibrin glue is then placed over the edges of the bony reconstruction.

◈ In small defects, the surgeon has the option of either placing a free mucosal graft to cover the defect or placing a nasoseptal flap.

◈ Fibrin glue is applied along the edges of the mucosal flap to secure it in place.

Large Skull Base Defects

◈ Larger skull base defects (> 1 cm) are encountered during extended endoscopic approaches (e.g., transclival, transtuberculum/planum, transcribriform) and are often associated with an intraoperative CSF leak, given the pathology of skull base lesions at these sites.

◈ Similar multilayer closure principles apply:
  • Abdominal fat to obliterate any significant dead space
    ○ Care must be taken if the defect communicates with the lateral ventricle, as the fat can migrate and cause obstructive hydrocephalus.
    ○ This is often not needed in transcribriform approaches where the frontal lobes will descend and obliterate the dead space after tumor removal.
◈ The dural layer is reconstructed preferably with an autologous fascia lata graft or a alternatively, a dural substitute (DuraGen, Durasis, DuraMatrix, or other materials) and placed in an underlay fashion (subdural plane).
◈ Where anatomically safe, the bone is reconstructed with either bone from the craniectomy or bone that is harvested from the posterior septum.
◈ A vascularized pedicled nasoseptal flap is routinely used for the mucosal layer of reconstruction.
  • See section on harvesting the nasoseptal flap (page 420).
  • If the nasoseptal flap is not available, alternative pedicled mucosal flaps from the sinonasal cavity have been described (e.g., inferior turbinate flap).
◈ Fibrin glue is placed over the edges of the nasoseptal flap.
◈ To support the nasoseptal flap in larger defects, a multilayered support buttress is recommended.
  • Gelfoam is first placed on the undersurface of the nasoseptal flap.
  • Finger cots composed of Merocel® sponges (Medtronic, Minneapolis, MN) wrapped in a latex free glove finger are then placed to support the flap, with the distal end of the Merocel sitting in the sphenoid sinus.
  • Bilateral nasal trumpets are then placed to support the finger cots.
    ○ In addition to providing an additional buttress, they enable patients to still breathe through the nose and enable the anesthesia team to potentially provide supplemental oxygen through the nasal cavity during extubation.
  • Alternatively, the use of an inflated Foley catheter has been described to support the nasoseptal flap.

■ Optional Pedicled Flap: Inferior Turbinate Flap[31,32]

❖ Surgical Steps

If a nasoseptal flap is not available, then an inferior turbinate flap is a reasonable alternative to repair a complex CSF leak.

◈ Inject the mucosa of the inferior turbinate in the submucoperiosteal plane.

◈ The superior incision of the flap is made with an insulated monopolar cautery or sickle-shaped scalpel and parallels the inferior turbinate at its attachment to the medial wall of the maxilla superiorly.

◈ The incision is carried to the head of the inferior turbinate.

◈ Using a Cottle or Freer elevator, the mucosa is carefully elevated away from the inferior turbinate bone.
   • This is followed inferiorly and then superiorly into the inferior meatus.

◈ Anteriorly, the superior incision must be connected to the elevated mucosa in the inferior meatus.
   • This frees the anterior edge of the flap.

◈ The inferior incision of the flap is then made at the apex of the inferior meatus and extended posteriorly.
   • Be careful not to cut across the pedicle of the inferior turbinate.

◈ The inferior turbinate flap can now be rotated for multilayer closure as previously described.

■ Postoperative Care

• To minimize sinonasal morbidity following endonasal skull base surgery, paying careful attention to postoperative care is paramount.

• For most endonasal bi-nostril approaches, bilateral Silastic sheets can be placed on each side of the septum and sutured at the end of the procedure to minimize synechiae formation in the nasal cavity.
   ○ They are removed 2 to 3 weeks following surgery.

• In the absence of any CSF leak, patients can leave the operating room with adrenaline-soaked gauze packing that is removed in the recovery room within 2 hours of the surgery.

• Alternatively, light nasal packing with Vaseline gauze in a well-lubricated latex-free finger glove can be placed in each nasal cavity to minimize nuisance bleeding from the nasal cavity overnight.
   ○ This packing is removed the morning following surgery, and antibiotics are maintained while the packs are in place.

• For patients who had an endoscopic repair requiring the use of Merocel sponges and the nasal trumpets to support the multilayer closure, the nasal trumpets are typically removed 48 hours after surgery.
   ○ The Merocel sponges are then removed 7 to 10 days following surgery.

• For the first 2 to 3 weeks postsurgery, all patients are instructed to use a saline spray for the nasal cavity; this is then followed by a high-volume saline squeeze bottle to optimize wound healing and help debride any residual crusting in the nasal cavity.

• Crusting that remains in the nasal cavity can be gently debrided in the clinic (usually beginning 2 to 3 weeks postsurgery).

■ References

Boldfaced references are of particular importance.

1. Cusimano MD, Fenton RS. The technique for endoscopic pituitary tumor removal. Neurosurg Focus 1996;1:e1, discussion 1p, e3
2. Jho HD, Carrau RL. Endoscopy assisted transsphenoidal surgery for pituitary adenoma. Technical note. Acta Neurochir (Wien) 1996;138:1416–1425
3. Carrau RL, Kassam AB, Snyderman CH. Pituitary surgery. Otolaryngol Clin North Am 2001;34:1143–1155, ix
4. Laws ER, Kanter AS, Jane JA Jr, Dumont AS. Extended transsphenoidal approach. J Neurosurg 2005;102:825–827, discussion 827–828
5. **Kassam A, Snyderman CH, Mintz A, Gardner P, Carrau RL. Expanded endonasal approach: the rostrocaudal axis. Part I. Crista galli to the sella turcica. Neurosurg Focus 2005;19:E3**
6. **Kassam A, Snyderman CH, Mintz A, Gardner P, Carrau RL. Expanded endonasal approach: the rostrocaudal axis. Part II. Posterior clinoids to the foramen magnum. Neurosurg Focus 2005;19:E4**
7. **Cavallo LM, Messina A, Cappabianca P, et al. Endoscopic endonasal surgery of the midline skull base: anatomical study and clinical considerations. Neurosurg Focus 2005;19:E2**
8. **Kassam AB, Gardner P, Snyderman C, Mintz A, Carrau R. Expanded endonasal approach: fully endoscopic, completely transnasal approach to the middle third of the clivus, petrous bone, middle cranial fossa, and infratemporal fossa. Neurosurg Focus 2005;19:E6**
9. Cappabianca P, Cavallo LM, Esposito F, De Divitiis O, Messina A, De Divitiis E. Extended endoscopic endonasal approach to the midline skull base: the evolving role of transsphenoidal surgery. Adv Tech Stand Neurosurg 2008;33:151–199
10. **Hadad G, Bassagasteguy L, Carrau RL, et al. A novel reconstructive technique after endoscopic expanded endonasal approaches: vascular pedicle nasoseptal flap. Laryngoscope 2006;116:1882–1886**
11. Pinheiro-Neto CD, Prevedello DM, Carrau RL, et al. Improving the design of the pedicled nasoseptal flap for skull base reconstruction: a radioanatomic study. Laryngoscope 2007;117:1560–1569
12. Caicedo-Granados E, Carrau R, Snyderman CH, et al. Reverse rotation flap for reconstruction of donor site after vascular pedicled nasoseptal flap in skull base surgery. Laryngoscope 2010;120:1550–1552
13. Cappabianca P, Cavallo LM, de Divitiis O, Solari D, Esposito F, Colao A. Endoscopic pituitary surgery. Pituitary 2008;11:385–390
14. **Barazi SA, Pasquini E, D'Urso PI, et al. Extended endoscopic transplanum-transtuberculum approach for pituitary adenomas. Br J Neurosurg 2013;27:374–382**
15. Greenfield JP, Anand VK, Kacker A, et al. Endoscopic endonasal transethmoidal transcribriform transfovea ethmoidalis approach to the anterior cranial fossa and skull base. Neurosurgery 2010;66:883–892, discussion 892
16. **Lee JM, Ransom E, Lee JY, Palmer JN, Chiu AG. Endoscopic anterior skull base surgery: intraoperative considerations of the crista galli. Skull Base 2011;21:83–86**

17. Liu JK, Christiano LD, Patel SK, Tubbs RS, Eloy JA. Surgical nuances for removal of olfactory groove meningiomas using the endoscopic endonasal transcribriform approach. Neurosurg Focus 2011;30:E3
18. Jho HD, Ha HG. Endoscopic endonasal skull base surgery: part 3—the clivus and posterior fossa. Minim Invasive Neurosurg 2004;47:16–23
19. Stamm AC, Pignatari SS, Vellutini E. Transnasal endoscopic surgical approaches to the clivus. Otolaryngol Clin North Am 2006;39:639–656, xi
20. Kassam AB, Vescan AD, Carrau RL, et al. Expanded endonasal approach: vidian canal as a landmark to the petrous internal carotid artery. J Neurosurg 2008;108:177–183
21. Stippler M, Gardner PA, Snyderman CH, Carrau RL, Prevedello DM, Kassam AB. Endoscopic endonasal approach for clival chordomas. Neurosurgery 2009;64:268–277, discussion 277–278
22. Fraser JF, Nyquist GG, Moore N, Anand VK, Schwartz TH. Endoscopic endonasal transclival resection of chordomas: operative technique, clinical outcome, and review of the literature. J Neurosurg 2010;112:1061–1069
23. Bolger WE. Endoscopic transpterygoid approach to the lateral sphenoid recess: surgical approach and clinical experience. Otolaryngol Head Neck Surg 2005;133:20–26
24. Kasemsiri P, Solares CA, Carrau RL, et al. Endoscopic endonasal transpterygoid approaches: anatomical landmarks for planning the surgical corridor. Laryngoscope 2013;123:811–815
25. Hegazy HM, Carrau RL, Snyderman CH, Kassam A, Zweig J. Transnasal endoscopic repair of cerebrospinal fluid rhinorrhea: a meta-analysis. Laryngoscope 2000;110:1166–1172
26. Kassam A, Carrau RL, Snyderman CH, Gardner P, Mintz A. Evolution of reconstructive techniques following endoscopic expanded endonasal approaches. Neurosurg Focus 2005;19:E8
27. Zanation AM, Carrau RL, Snyderman CH, et al. Nasoseptal flap reconstruction of high flow intraoperative cerebral spinal fluid leaks during endoscopic skull base surgery. Am J Rhinol Allergy 2009;23:518–521
28. Harvey RJ, Nogueira JF, Schlosser RJ, Patel SJ, Vellutini E, Stamm AC. Closure of large skull base defects after endoscopic transnasal craniotomy. Clinical article. J Neurosurg 2009;111:371–379
29. Cusimano MD, Kan P, Nassiri F, et al. Outcomes of surgically treated giant pituitary tumours. Can J Neurol Sci 2012;39:446–457
30. Juraschka K, Khan OH, Godoy BL, et al. Endoscopic endonasal transsphenoidal approach to large and giant pituitary adenomas: institutional experience and predictors of extent of resection. J Neurosurg 2014;121:75–83
31. Harvey RJ, Sheahan PO, Schlosser RJ. Inferior turbinate pedicle flap for endoscopic skull base defect repair. Am J Rhinol Allergy 2009;23:522–526
32. Yip J, Macdonald KI, Lee J, et al. The inferior turbinate flap in skull base reconstruction. J Otolaryngol Head Neck Surg 2013;42:6–0

17 Endoscopic Keyhole Approaches

Advances in anatomic knowledge, neuroradiological imaging, and endoscopic technology have evolved toward less invasive and less traumatizing surgical corridors to approach target lesions, as in the keyhole concept of *minimally invasive neurosurgery.*[1] Endoscopy plays an important role in the keyhole concept, thanks to its main advantages: (1) superb illumination; (2) high magnification; (3) panoramic view; and (4) the ability to "look around corners," even in deep surgical fields.

Endoscopic neurosurgery is when the endoscope is used solely as an optical device. All procedures are performed under endoscopic view. **Endoscope-assisted microneurosurgery** combines microscopic/endoscopic techniques.[2] The surgery is done with both techniques of visualization, with certain tasks assigned to certain stages of the procedure.

■ Keyhole Surgery

Advantages

Smaller incision, minimal brain exposure and retraction, and reduced blood loss with lower morbidity and mortality.

Disadvantages

Two-dimensional images (compensated by the advent of three-dimensional [3D] endoscopes); limitation of instrumentation; and learning curve for endoscopy.

Pearl

It is important to recognize that surgery involves more than just visualization. The principles of tumor access and resection as well as reconstruction remain the same as in more extensive openings.

Instruments

Because of the narrow corridor through the keyhole and coaxial manipulation under a straight or angled endoscope, intraoperative use of conventional micro-instruments becomes limited. Use of single-shaft instruments (e.g., scissors, grasping and coagulating forceps, and clip appliers) is mandatory.[1] Endoscopy may help make the approach *minimally invasive*, but the surgery itself should also be *minimally traumatizing*.[3]

◼ Supraorbital Keyhole Approach

The supraorbital keyhole approach is one of the most frequently used keyhole variants, and has been safely applied for accessing skull base neoplastic and/or vascular lesions **(Fig. 17.1)**. The supraorbital keyhole approach provides a less invasive alternative to more extensive skull base approaches such as coronal, pterional, and orbitozygomatic craniotomies.[1,4,5]

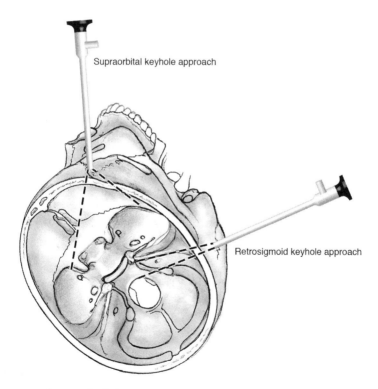

Supraorbital keyhole approach

Retrosigmoid keyhole approach

Fig. 17.1   Endoscopic keyhole approaches to the skull base with their potential angles of view.

Table 17.1   Indications for the Endoscopic Supraorbital Keyhole Approach

Meningioma (olfactory groove, tuberculum sellae, planum sphenoidale, anterior clinoid process)

Pituitary adenoma with suprasellar and lateral extension

Craniopharyngioma

Intra-axial tumor (glioma, metastatic brain tumor)

Anterior circulation aneurysms

Advanced indication:

Pathology at the medial temporal lobe in the middle skull base and around the upper brainstem in the posterior skull base

Indications

Indications for the supraorbital approach include most tumors of the anterior skull base and aneurysms of the anterior circulation[1,4-10] **(Table 17.1)**.

Supraorbital Keyhole Craniotomy

- The patient is placed in the supine position, and the head is rotated 0 to 60 degrees to the contralateral side. The degree of rotation is dictated by the location of the target area **(Fig. 17.2)**.
- ◈ Make the skin incision within the eyebrow, laterally to the supraorbital notch.
- ◈ Retract the skin flap and incise the pericranium superiorly to the orbicularis oculi muscle. Strip the temporalis muscle laterally from the superior temporal line.
- ◈ Make a bur hole laterally to the superior temporal line at the level of the anterior skull base.
- ◈ By means of the craniotome, make a straight-line cut from the bur hole parallel to the orbital rim, and then connect a C-shaped line from the bur hole to the medial edge of the previously made straight line.

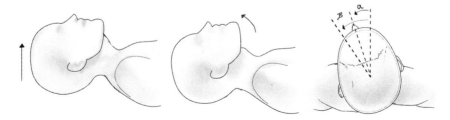

Fig. 17.2 Supraorbital keyhole craniotomy, and positioning of the head. Note the potentially different required angles, according to the surgical target.

- Use the intraoperative navigation system to localize and avoid the frontal sinus, whenever possible.
- The supraorbital craniotomy is performed with a width of approximately 2.5 cm and a height of 1.5 cm.
◈ Drill the inner bony edge of the craniotomy off in order to facilitate visualization, access, and free manipulation of the instruments.
◈ Incise the dura mater in a curved fashion and reflect it toward the skull base.[1,4,9]
◈ Introduce the endoscope into the surgical field.

Medial Variation of the Supraorbital Craniotomy

The paramedian supraorbital craniotomy is placed to obtain simultaneous exposure of the suprasellar and interhemispheric structures, although supraorbital neurovascular structures and opening of the frontal paranasal sinus are unavoidable in some cases.[1]

◈◈ Make an eyebrow incision with medial extension to the glabellar region.
◈◈ Retract the skin flap and incise the pericranium superiorly to the orbicularis oculi muscle, and then retract frontally to expose the frontal bone.
◈◈ Make a bur hole frontally in the paramedian plane.
◈◈ Using the craniotome, make a curved-line cut from the bur hole forming the medial and basal edges, and then connect another curved line defining the frontal and lateral edges from the bur hole to the lateral edge of the previously made basal line.
- Medial variation of the supraorbital craniotomy is performed with a width of approximately 2.5 cm and a height of 2.0 cm.
◈◈ Drill the inner bony edge of the craniotomy off to facilitate visualization, access, and free manipulation of the instruments.
◈◈ Incise the dura mater in a curved fashion and reflect it toward the skull base.
◈◈ Introduce the endoscope into the surgical field.

Application of the Endoscope

- Tumors and normal structures located around and behind the tuberculum sellae, sella turcica, optic apparatus, internal carotid artery, sphenoid ridge, and olfactory glove are well visualized by endoscopy.[4,5]
- In vascular neurosurgery, effective exclusion of the aneurysm and preservation of the parent artery and perforators, which cannot be visualized by microscope, are ensured by angled endoscopes in endoscope-assisted microscope surgery.[1,9]
- The endoscopic intracisternal navigation requires splitting of the arachnoid according to the same techniques and principles used in microneurosurgery.

■ Endoscopic Anterior Skull Base Reconstruction via a Supraorbital Keyhole

Dural defects resulting from surgical intervention must be reconstructed. A pedicled pericranial flap harvested endoscopically is an alternative option for reconstruction of the anterior skull base via a supraorbital keyhole.[11] The pedicled flap receives blood supply from the supraorbital artery.

◈ Make an eyebrow incision and dissect to the subperiosteal plane.
◈ Make two incisions around the coronal line and proceed with the endoscopic subgaleal dissection.
◈ Dissect down to the orbital rim. Connect this plane to the subperiosteal plane of the eyebrow incision. Identify vessels and protect a 3-cm pedicle.
◈ Incise the pericranial flap from the frontal bone and elevate in the subperiosteal plane.
◈ Rotate the pedicled pericranial flap and make a supraorbital keyhole.
◈ Overlay the pedicled pericranial flap over the skull base defect after management of the target regions.

Complications

- Skin incisions or retraction may damage the supraorbital branch (7.5%) and the frontal branch of cranial nerve (CN) VII (1–5.5%). Long-term sensory loss from neurapraxia of the supraorbital nerve is usually limited due to overlap of cutaneous innervation in that region of the scalp.[4,5]
- The frontal sinus may be opened by supraorbital keyhole craniotomy, and cerebrospinal fluid (CSF) leak may occur (4%). An opened frontal sinus needs to be packed with abdominal fat tissue or reconstructed using a pedicled galeal flap.[1,4,5,9]

■ Subtemporal Keyhole Approach

The subtemporal keyhole approach can be used as an alternative to the traditional subtemporal approach. This approach provides access to the posterolateral aspect of the suprasellar area, the upper half of the petroclival region, and the lateral aspect of the cavernous sinus with minimal invasiveness.[1,9,11]

Indications

The indications are listed in **Table 17.2**.[1,9,11]

Table 17.2   Indications for the Endoscopic Subtemporal Keyhole Approach

Intra-axial tumor (glioma, metastatic tumor, cavernoma, or hamartoma: located at
the medial temporal lobe, hypothalamus, midbrain, or pons)

Meningioma (petroclival, cavernous sinus, Meckel's cave)

Chordoma (upper or middle clivus, petroclival)

Posterior circulation aneurysms

Arachnoid cyst

Subtemporal Keyhole Craniotomy

The patient is placed in the supine position, and the ipsilateral shoulder is
raised with a cushion to facilitate head rotation. The head is rotated 60 to 100
degrees to the contralateral side, although a lateral position is preferable to
avoid excessive stretching of the neck muscles and blood vessels. The degree
of the rotation depends on the location of the lesion.

❖   Make a vertical linear skin incision with a length of 5 cm, from the inferior
    rim of the zygomatic arch anterior to the external auditory meatus.
❖   Incise the temporalis muscle fascia in a Y-shaped fashion with the basal
    leaflet reflected caudally over the zygomatic arch.
❖   Strip the inferior margin of the temporalis muscle and reflect it upward,
    exposing the squamous bone.
❖   Make a 2.5-cm craniotomy just above the zygomatic arch.
❖   Open the dura mater in an arched fashion and reflect it toward the skull
    base.[1,11]
❖   Introduce the endoscope into the surgical field.

Posterior Variation of Subtemporal Keyhole Craniotomy

A posterior subtemporal keyhole craniotomy facilitates visualization of the posterolateral prepontine, ambient, and quadrigeminal cisterns with less temporal
retraction, although the craniotomy needs to deal with the inferior anastomotic
vein of Labbé. Additional splitting of the tentorium provides access to the posterior skull base and exposure of the tentorial surface of the cerebellum and the
structures around the cerebellopontine angle (CPA).[1]

❖❖ Define the level of the subtemporal base according to the supramastoid
    crest and to the courses of the transverse and sigmoid sinuses.
❖❖ Make a straight incision with a length of about 5 cm, just behind the ear at
    the level of the mastoid process.
❖❖ Strip the inferior margin of the temporalis muscle and reflect it upward.

◈◈ Incise the subgaleal fascia and periosteum in the direction of the mastoid process with the basal leaflet of the fascia reflected caudally and the posterior flap of the fascia reflected posteriorly.

◈◈ Make a bur hole at the junction between the parietomastoidal and squamosal sutures, exposing the anterior border of the sigmoid sinus.

◈◈ Make a straight-line cut from the bur hole parallel to the temporal skull base, then connect a C-shaped line from the bur hole to the anterior edge of the previously made straight line.

◈◈ Drill the inner bony edge of the craniotomy off to facilitate visualization, access, and free manipulation of instruments.

◈ The posterior subtemporal craniotomy is performed with a width of approximately 2.5 cm and a height of 2.0 cm.

◈◈ Incise the dura mater in a curved fashion and reflect it toward the skull base.

◈◈ Introduce the endoscope into the surgical field.

Application of Endoscopy

The endoscope visualizes structures behind the trigeminal nerves in the cavernous sinus such as the internal carotid artery and abducens nerve. Anterior petrosectomy and incision of the tentorial edge and superior petrosal sinus provide access to the posterior skull base, and endoscopy demonstrates neurovascular structures around the parasellar area, petroclival region, and Meckel's cave with a panoramic view. An angled endoscope demonstrates structures at the level of jugular foramen inferiorly.[1,12,13]

Endoscopic Middle Skull Base Reconstruction via a Subtemporal Keyhole

Reconstruction of the middle skull base via a subtemporal keyhole is challenging. A pedicled deep temporal fascial flap harvested endoscopically is a potential alternative for reconstruction of the middle skull base via the subtemporal keyhole. The pedicled temporal fascial flap receives its blood supply from the middle temporal artery. The technique has been shown to be feasible in an anatomic study, but has not yet been applied clinically.[14]

◈ Make a subtemporal incision and dissect to the deep temporal fascia plane.

◈ Make two incisions in the superior temporal line and proceed with the endoscopic dissection between the superficial and deep temporal fascia.

◈ Dissect down to the zygomatic arch. Connect this plane to the deep temporal fascia plane of the subtemporal incision.

◈ Proceed with endoscopic dissection between the deep temporal fascia and temporal muscle to the zygomatic arch.

❖ Incise the deep temporal fascia with protection of a 1.5-cm pedicle, and reflect the pedicled deep temporal fascia caudally through the subtemporal incision.

❖ Incise the temporalis muscle and make a subtemporal keyhole.

❖ Overlay the pedicled deep temporal fascial flap over the skull base defect after managing target regions.

Complications

Approach-related complications include subdural hematoma, CSF leakage (4.6%), short-term memory disturbances (4.6%), and seizures.[1,9,11]

■ Retrosigmoid Keyhole Approach

The retrosigmoid keyhole approach is used to manage lesions in the posterior skull base. This approach provides access to the entire CPA and middle upper clivus, which do not extend beyond the tentorium superiorly and the foramen magnum inferiorly. The retrosigmoid keyhole approach offers an alternative option to more extensive approaches such as the traditional retrosigmoid, presigmoid transpetrosal, and translabyrinthine approaches.[1,15]

Indications

Indications for an endoscopic keyhole retrosigmoid approach are posterior skull base tumors including schwannomas, meningiomas (petroclival and tentorial), and dermoid/epidermoids of the CPA. Trigeminal neuralgia and hemifacial spasm can also be managed by this approach.[15-25]

Retrosigmoid Keyhole Craniotomy

The patient is placed in a lateral park-bench position with the head turned to the opposite side.

❖ Make a 3- to 5-cm straight skin incision within the retroauricular area.

❖ Incise the sternocleidomastoid muscle, and then separate the splenius capitis, longus capitis, and superior oblique muscles from their attachments to bone.

Emissary veins are usually exposed in the mastoid area, indicating a course close to the sigmoid sinus.

❖ Make a 2- to 3-cm keyhole craniotomy at the transverse-sigmoid sinus junction, in relation to the asterion.

◈ Open the dura mater in a curved fashion and reflect it toward the sigmoid sinus.[1,20,25]

Retrosigmoid Keyhole Craniotomy Caudal Variation

◈◈The skin incision and craniotomy should be placed caudally, with the anterior border close to the sigmoid sinus for the best visualization of the targeted neurovascular complex.[1]

Application of Endoscopy

A preliminary survey by endoscope is performed to visualize the neurovascular structures around the pathology; for example, identification of the facial nerve at the early stage of vestibular schwannoma is effective. The angled endoscope is available to inspect hidden structures such as tumors in the internal auditory meatus and ventral surface of the brainstem, and is thus useful to resect tumors located within corners.[15-20] For microvascular decompression of compression syndromes such as trigeminal neuralgia or hemifacial spasm, endoscopy secures views around the root entry zone of the trigeminal nerve or root exit zone of the facial nerve, contributing to inspection of the offending vessel and indentation. At the end of the procedure, the endoscope facilitates evaluation of the adequacy of the decompression.[21-25]

Complications

The mastoid air cell may be opened by retrosigmoid keyhole craniotomy, and CSF leakage may occur (3.2%). The opened air cell is packed with free muscle tissue or reconstructed using a pedicled galeal flap.[1,15,20] Dural sinuses injuries are also possible. Thermic injury of the cranial nerve have been reported; thus, the tip of the endoscope should also be held at a safe distance from the nerves and the illumination kept below the maximum level.

■ References

Boldfaced references are of particular importance.
1. **Perneczky RR, Kindel S, Kanno T, Tschabitscher M, Reisch R. Keyhole Approaches in Neurosurgery. Vol 1: Concept and Surgical Technique. Vienna, New York: Springer; 2009**
2. **Galzio RJ, Di Cola F, Raysi Dehcordi S, Ricci A, De Paulis D. Endoscope-assisted microneurosurgery for intracranial aneurysms. Front Neurol 2013;4:201**
3. **Tschabitscher M, Di Ieva A. Practical guidelines for setting up an endoscopic/skull base cadaver laboratory. World Neurosurg 2013;79(2, Suppl):16.e1–16.e7**

4. Zador Z, Gnanalingham K. Eyebrow craniotomy for anterior skull base lesions: how I do it. Acta Neurochir (Wien) 2013;155:99–106

5. **Wilson DA, Duong H, Teo C, Kelly DF. The supraorbital endoscopic approach for tumors. World Neurosurg 2014;82:e243–e256**

6. Fatemi N, Dusick JR, de Paiva Neto MA, Malkasian D, Kelly DF. Endonasal versus supraorbital keyhole removal of craniopharyngiomas and tuberculum sellae meningiomas. Neurosurgery 2009;64(5, Suppl 2):269–284, discussion 284–286

7. Reisch R, Stadie A, Kockro R, Gawish I, Schwandt E, Hopf N. The minimally invasive supraorbital subfrontal key-hole approach for surgical treatment of temporomesial lesions of the dominant hemisphere. Minim Invasive Neurosurg 2009;52:163–169

8. Berhouma M, Jacquesson T, Jouanneau E. The fully endoscopic supraorbital trans-eyebrow keyhole approach to the anterior and middle skull base. Acta Neurochir (Wien) 2011;153:1949–1954

9. Fischer G, Stadie A, Reisch R, et al. The keyhole concept in aneurysm surgery: results of the past 20 years. Neurosurgery 2011;68(1, Suppl Operative):45–51, discussion 51

10. Ditzel Filho LF, McLaughlin N, Bresson D, Solari D, Kassam AB, Kelly DF. Supraorbital eyebrow craniotomy for removal of intraaxial frontal brain tumors: a technical note. World Neurosurg 2014;81:348–356

11. Taniguchi M, Perneczky A. Subtemporal keyhole approach to the suprasellar and petroclival region: microanatomic considerations and clinical application. Neurosurgery 1997;41:592–601

12. **Komatsu F, Komatsu M, Di Ieva A, Tschabitscher M. Endoscopic approaches to the trigeminal nerve and clinical consideration for trigeminal schwannomas: a cadaveric study. J Neurosurg 2012;117:690–696**

13. **Komatsu F, Komatsu M, Di Ieva A, Tschabitscher M. Endoscopic extradural subtemporal approach to lateral and central skull base: a cadaveric study. World Neurosurg 2013;80:591–597**

14. **Komatsu M, Komatsu F, Di Ieva A, Inoue T, Tschabitscher M. Endoscopic reconstruction of the middle cranial fossa through a subtemporal keyhole using a pedicled deep temporal fascial flap: a cadaveric study. Neurosurgery 2012;70(1, Suppl Operative):157–161, discussion 162**

15. Li Z, Lan Q. Retrosigmoid keyhole approach to the posterior cranial fossa: an anatomical and clinical study. Eur Surg Res 2010;44:56–63

16. Magnan J, Barbieri M, Mora R, et al. Retrosigmoid approach for small and medium-sized acoustic neuromas. Otol Neurotol 2002;23:141–145

17. Shahinian HK, Eby JB, Ocon M. Fully endoscopic excision of vestibular schwannomas. Minim Invasive Neurosurg 2004;47:329–332

18. Kabil MS, Shahinian HK. A series of 112 fully endoscopic resections of vestibular schwannomas. Minim Invasive Neurosurg 2006;49:362–368

19. Mostafa BE, El Sharnoubi M, Youssef AM. The keyhole retrosigmoid approach to the cerebello-pontine angle: indications, technical modifications, and results. Skull Base 2008;18:371–376

20. Shahinian HK, Ra Y. 527 fully endoscopic resections of vestibular schwannomas. Minim Invasive Neurosurg 2011;54:61–67

21. Eby JB, Cha ST, Shahinian HK. Fully endoscopic vascular decompression of the facial nerve for hemifacial spasm. Skull Base 2001;11:189–197

22. El-Garem HF, Badr-El-Dine M, Talaat AM, Magnan J. Endoscopy as a tool in minimally invasive trigeminal neuralgia surgery. Otol Neurotol 2002;23:132–135
23. Jarrahy R, Eby JB, Cha ST, Shahinian HK. Fully endoscopic vascular decompression of the trigeminal nerve. Minim Invasive Neurosurg 2002;45:32–35
24. Cheng WY, Chao SC, Shen CC. Endoscopic microvascular decompression of the hemifacial spasm. Surg Neurol 2008;70(Suppl 1):S1, 40–46
25. Lang SS, Chen HI, Lee JY. Endoscopic microvascular decompression: a stepwise operative technique. ORL J Otorhinolaryngol Relat Spec 2012;74:293–298

18 Pearls of Skull Base Meningioma Surgery

Meningiomas are the among the most frequent skull base tumors, warranting some specific considerations, which are summarized here.

■ Epidemiological Pearls

- Thirty percent of meningiomas are skull base meningiomas (SBMs).[1] **Fig. 18.1** shows the localization of skull base meningiomas.
- The most frequent SBMs are at the medial sphenoid ridge (~ 30% of SBMs).[2]
- Eighty percent to 94% of SBMs are grade I, according to the World Health Organization (WHO) grading system.[2] WHO grade II and III SBMs are proportionately less common than those in the calvaria (~ 5–10% and 1.3%, respectively),[2] suggesting that SBMs may have important differences in tumor biology (e.g., mechanisms of tumorigenesis and progression).[3]
- Surgical mortality in all meningiomas in the United States is 1.8%.[4] Overall, SBMs have lower rates of complete resection than calvarial meningiomas and mortality of about 3 to 5%, with an overall morbidity of about 20 to 40%[2] **(Table 18.1)**.
- Mortality and morbidity are significantly related to the location and size. Risk groups can be stratified according to the CLASS acronym: comorbidities (C), tumor location (L), patient age (A), tumor size (S), and neurologic signs and symptoms (S)[5] **(Table 18.2)**. Risk assessment should take into consideration also the radioanatomic characteristics, such as attachment of the tumor, arterial and cranial nerve involvement, and brainstem relation.[6]
- Multiple meningiomas occur in fewer than 9% of meningiomas cases but in 50% of patients affected by neurofibromatosis type 2.
- Review pathology on page 138.

■ Clinical and Surgical Pearls

- Skull base meningiomas may grow less often and slower than meningiomas in other locations.[7]

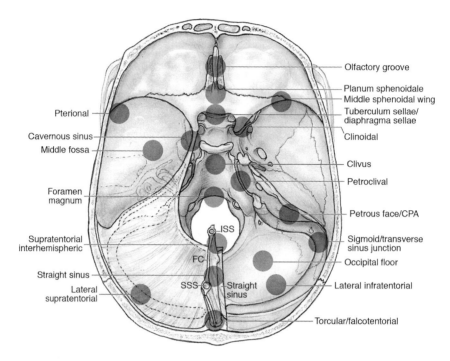

Fig. 18.1 Skull base meningioma localizations. CPA, cerebellopontine angle; FC, falx cerebri; ISS, inferior sagittal sinus; SSS, superior sagittal sinus.

Table 18.1 Surgical Morbidity in a Single Series of 226 Skull Base Meningiomas[2]

Intracranial hemorrhage	10.6%
Cerebrospinal fluid fistula	8.4%
Wound infection	6.6%
Pulmonary embolism	4.0%
Stroke	1.8%
Myocardial infarction	0.9%
New neurologic deficits	14.2% (permanent in 3.5%)

Table 18.2   CLASS Algorithm: Risk Groups Based on the Skull Base Location

Low risk	• Lateral and middle sphenoid wing
	• Posterior petrous bone
Moderate risk	• Olfactory groove/planum sphenoidale
	• Lateral/paramedian tentorium
	• Cerebellopontine angle
	• Posterior/lateral foramen magnum
High risk	• Clinoidal/medial sphenoid ridge
	• Cavernous sinus
	• Tuberculum sellae
	• Medial/incisural tentorium
	• Clivus

Source: Adapted from Joung H, Lee BS. The novel "class" algorithmic scale for patient selection in meningioma surgery. In: Lee JH, ed. Meningiomas: Diagnosis, Treatment, and Outcome. Berlin: Springer; 2008 Reprinted with permission.

- Meningiomas are surrounded by multiple arachnoidal layers, and their dissection should be intra-arachnoidal.[8] The fine dissection of the double arachnoid plane and "keeping the arachnoid with the patient" enables sparing neurovascular structures. This is my main rule of meningioma surgery.
- Arachnoidal planes are sometimes lost because the tumor origin is outside the arachnoid, and so the tumor growth is not invested with a layer of arachnoid. This enables the tumor to invade the adventitia of arteries or invade cranial nerves (e.g., types I and III clinoidal meningiomas, page 491).
- Attention to the presence or absence of the arachnoid plane and the presence or absence of brain edema on preoperative T2-weighted magnetic resonance imaging (MRI) is imperative in all meningioma surgeries.
- Surgical resectability of meningioma can also be related to their consistency. Hypointense tumors on T2-weighted MRI and fluid-attenuated inversion recovery (FLAIR) images are generally of harder consistency, whereas those showing hyperintense signals related to higher water content are of softer consistency.[9]
- Meningiomas calcifications are best diagnosed on computed tomography (CT) scan.
- Large tumors often require internal debulking, which enables decompression of the brain and facilitates identification of the arachnoid plane of dissection. The debulking can be performed with forceps or an ultrasonic aspirator.
- Meningiomas may cause hyperostosis by invasion in the haversian canals,[10] and the resection of the involved bone decreases the recurrence rate.[11] Skull base involvement is frequent (up to 70%), especially in the middle cranial fossa, and the bone drilling will decrease the risk of recurrence if it is feasible and safe to do so.

> **Surgical Pearl**
>
> The intraoperative use of 5-aminolevulinic acid (5-ALA) has been shown to be a somewhat useful technique (with a specificity of 100% and sensitivity of 89%) for identifying and then removing the bone infiltrated by the meningioma. Fluorescent bone is always infiltrated by the tumor, whereas nonfluorescent bone can contain meningiomatous components in 13% of cases.[12]

- The goal of meningioma surgery should be total resection in most cases; however, where it is judged to be of excess risk, a subtotal resection can be planned.
- Sixty percent of patients experience recurrence of these tumors after subtotal removal, so these patients must be watched with serial MRI or be offered adjuvant radiation in multiple or single fractions (radiosurgery)[13]; 28.5% of recurrent meningiomas may transform to a malignant variant.[14,15]
- The Simpson grading scale of resection, although described in 1957 (premicroscopic era), is still valuable in predicting recurrence of meningiomas[16] **(Table 18.3)**.
- A grade 0 has been added, for the resection of convexity meningiomas, meaning that a 2-cm margin of dura around the tumor is resected.[17–19] This is rarely attainable in SBM.

> **Surgical Pearl**
>
> Simpson grade I resection offers a definitive cure in more than 90% of cases.[16,20]

- The Kobayashi scale,[21] developed in the microscopic era, although probably more accurate, is rarely used and has not been validated in large studies.

Table 18.3   Simpson Grading Scale

Grade	Definition of Grade	1957	2014
I	Macroscopically complete tumor removal with excision of dural attachment and abnormal bone, including sinus resection whenever involved	9%	6.8%
II	Macroscopically complete tumor removal with coagulation of dural attachment	16–19%	9.6%
III	Macroscopically complete tumor removal without resection or coagulation of dural attachment or of its extradural extension (such as hyperostotic bone)	29%	19.2%
IV	Partial tumor removal	39–44%	28.8%
V	Simple decompression (biopsy)	100%	50%

Note: Definition of the grades takes into account the surgical removal of convexity and skull base meningiomas, and the overall risk of recurrence/progression in the original case series by Simpson[16] (1957) compared with a modern microsurgical series (2014).[2]

- A recent SBM series showed 5-year recurrence/progression-free survival of meningiomas undergoing Simpson grade I, II, III, and IV resection of 95%, 85%, 88%, and 81%, respectively.[22] The authors claimed no significant differences between the grades (no significant benefit performing more radical resection, also in skull base meningiomas, except for grade IV showing higher recurrence rates; however, the study has several limitations, such as short follow-up and limited sample size).[22] These findings, which involved several skull base meningiomas, have not been confirmed by other more recent studies, which involved more convexity meningiomas.[2,23,24]
- Some authors debate whether a Simpson grade I versus grade II resection is of relevance in recurrence and whether the added risk of a Simpson grade I resection in a SBM is worth the potential complications.[25] Nonetheless, most authors advocate performing gross-total resections whenever possible.[26]
- Complete resection of skull base meningioma (Simpson grade I–II) is feasible in almost 63% of all SBM cases.[2]
- The extent of SBM resection can be predicted according to the tumor attachment size, the arterial involvement, the brainstem contact, the "central cavity" location (skull base space delimited by the dural entry of cranial nerves [CNs] II to XII), and the cranial nerve group involvement.[6]
- The overall recurrence rate of SBMs is up to 16%.[2]
- A recent series (on convexity meningiomas) reported an overall recurrence rate of 4.3% for WHO grade I meningiomas (2.3% at 5 years and 4.3% at 10 years), 9.1% for grade II, and 50% for grade III, but other series report higher rates of recurrence for all WHO grades.[24,27]
- In petroclival and clivus meningiomas, brainstem compression/involvement is one of the most important factors related to outcome.
- The arachnoid plane between the meningioma and the brainstem (seen as a zone of low intensity on T1- and T2-weighted MRI) can be preserved (stage 1), lost but without edema (stage 2), or lost with associated brainstem edema on T2-weighted MRI (stage 3).[28] In stage 3 cases, branches from the basilar artery may supply the tumor, and if so, this may portend a higher risk of deficit, and a planned subtotal (rather than attempted gross total) resection of the tumor is recommended.[28]
- Devascularization of the tumor is one of the most critical steps in any meningioma surgery. Doing so will usually make for a bloodless surgical field and sometimes soften the tumor.[29] For this reason, knowing the main feeding arteries of meningiomas, as follows, is of value[30]:
  - Anterior and posterior ethmoidal arteries (and the variable middle ethmoidal arteries) together with the recurrent ophthalmic arteries and the lacrimal arteries and other smaller branches supply the dura of the anterior skull base, especially in the midline, and the one of the central skull base.
  - The middle meningeal artery (and all its branches) supplies the dura of the lateral portions of the three fossae.

- ○ Anterior and posterior meningeal arteries, occipital artery, ascending pharyngeal artery, subarcuate artery, coming from the vertebrobasilar system, vascularize the dura of the posterior fossa, above all in the midline zone (clivus, foramen magnum)[30] (see Chapter 22, **Fig. 22.8**, page 567).
- ○ The accessory meningeal artery supplies the middle fossa dura and the lateral wall of the cavernous sinus.
- ○ Tentorial arteries from the posterior cerebral artery and internal carotid artery (artery of Bernasconi-Cassinari) as well as some meningeal branches supply the tentorium.
- Preoperative embolization may be useful in some cases if the vessels supplying the tumor are easily accessible. A complete devascularization of the tumor may result in a lower blood transfusion requirement (reducing operative blood loss); however, the rate of major complications related to embolization is 0 to 5%, with a mortality of < 0.5%.[31-33]
- Because SBMs may involve the dural venous sinuses in up to 21% of cases,[2] it is important to assess this possibility preoperatively by means of angiogram, computed tomography venography (CTV) or magnetic resonance venography (MRV). In the event of sinus invasion, planned subtotal resection followed by radiosurgery on the tumoral components involving the sinuses is a valid option in selected case.[34] See also Chapter 26.

■ References

Boldfaced references are of particular importance.
1. Sutherland GR, Sima AAF. Incidence and classification of meningiomas. In: Schmidek HH, ed. Meningiomas and Their Surgical Management. Philadelphia: Saunders; 1991:10–21
2. **Scheitzach J, Schebesch KM, Brawanski A, Proescholdt MA. Skull base meningiomas: neurological outcome after microsurgical resection. J Neurooncol 2014;116: 381–386**
3. Sade B, Chahlavi A, Krishnaney A, Nagel S, Choi E, Lee JH. World Health Organization Grades II and III meningiomas are rare in the cranial base and spine. Neurosurgery 2007;61:1194–1198, discussion 1198
4. **Curry WT, McDermott MW, Carter BS, Barker FG II. Craniotomy for meningioma in the United States between 1988 and 2000: decreasing rate of mortality and the effect of provider caseload. J Neurosurg 2005;102:977–986**
5. Joung H, Lee BS. The novel "class" algorithmic scale for patient selection in meningioma surgery. In: Lee JH, ed. Meningiomas: Diagnosis, Treatment, and Outcome. Berlin: Springer; 2008
6. Adachi K, Kawase T, Yoshida K, Yazaki T, Onozuka S. ABC Surgical Risk Scale for skull base meningioma: a new scoring system for predicting the extent of tumor removal and neurological outcome. Clinical article. J Neurosurg 2009;111:1053–1061
7. Hashimoto N, Rabo CS, Okita Y, et al. Slower growth of skull base meningiomas compared with non-skull base meningiomas based on volumetric and biological studies. J Neurosurg 2012;116:574–580

8. Al-Mefty O, Al-Mefty R. Meningiomas: a personal perspective. In: De Monte F, Mc-Dermott MW, Al-Mefty O, eds. Al-Mefty's Meningiomas, 2nd ed. New York, Stuttgart: Thieme; 2011:3–12

9. Sitthinamsuwan B, Khampalikit I, Nunta-aree S, Srirabheebhat P, Witthiwej T, Nitising A. Predictors of meningioma consistency: a study in 243 consecutive cases. Acta Neurochir (Wien) 2012;154:1383–1389

10. Pieper DR, Al-Mefty O, Hanada Y, Buechner D. Hyperostosis associated with meningioma of the cranial base: secondary changes or tumor invasion. Neurosurgery 1999; 44:742–746, discussion 746–747

11. Bikmaz K, Mrak R, Al-Mefty O. Management of bone-invasive, hyperostotic sphenoid wing meningiomas. J Neurosurg 2007;107:905–912

12. Della Puppa A, Rustemi O, Gioffrè G, et al. Predictive value of intraoperative 5-aminolevulinic acid-induced fluorescence for detecting bone invasion in meningioma surgery. J Neurosurg 2014;120:840–845

13. Mathiesen T, Lindquist C, Kihlström L, Karlsson B. Recurrence of cranial base meningiomas. Neurosurgery 1996;39:2–7, discussion 8–9

14. Jääskeläinen J, Haltia M, Servo A. Atypical and anaplastic meningiomas: radiology, surgery, radiotherapy, and outcome. Surg Neurol 1986;25:233–242

15. Al-Mefty O, Kadri PA, Pravdenkova S, Sawyer JR, Stangeby C, Husain M. Malignant progression in meningioma: documentation of a series and analysis of cytogenetic findings. J Neurosurg 2004;101:210–218

16. Simpson D. The recurrence of intracranial meningiomas after surgical treatment. J Neurol Neurosurg Psychiatry 1957;20:22–39

17. Borovich B, Doron Y. Recurrence of intracranial meningiomas: the role played by regional multicentricity. J Neurosurg 1986;64:58–63

18. Borovich B, Doron Y, Braun J, et al. Recurrence of intracranial meningiomas: the role played by regional multicentricity. Part 2: clinical and radiological aspects. J Neurosurg 1986;65:168–171

19. Kinjo T, al-Mefty O, Kanaan I. Grade zero removal of supratentorial convexity meningiomas. Neurosurgery 1993;33:394–399, discussion 399

20. Mathiesen T, Kihlström L, Karlsson B, Lindquist C. Potential complications following radiotherapy for meningiomas. Surg Neurol 2003;60:193–198, discussion 199–200

21. DeMonte F, Smith HK, al-Mefty O. Outcome of aggressive removal of cavernous sinus meningiomas. J Neurosurg 1994;81:245–251

22. Sughrue ME, Kane AJ, Shangari G, et al. The relevance of Simpson grade I and II resection in modern neurosurgical treatment of World Health Organization grade I meningiomas. J Neurosurg 2010;113:1029–1035

23. Heald JB, Carroll TA, Mair RJ. Simpson grade: an opportunity to reassess the need for complete resection of meningiomas. Acta Neurochir (Wien) 2014;156:383–388

24. Hasseleid BF, Meling TR, Rønning P, Scheie D, Helseth E. Surgery for convexity meningioma: Simpson grade I resection as the goal: clinical article. J Neurosurg 2012;117:999–1006

25. Sekhar LN, Patel S, Cusimano M, Wright DC, Sen CN, Bank WO. Surgical treatment of meningiomas involving the cavernous sinus: evolving ideas based on a ten year experience. Acta Neurochir Suppl (Wien) 1996;65:58–62

26. Fukushima Y, Oya S, Nakatomi H, et al. **Effect of dural detachment on long-term tumor control for meningiomas treated using Simpson grade IV resection.** J Neurosurg 2013;119:1373–1379

27. Chen CM, Huang AP, Kuo LT, Tu YK. Contemporary surgical outcome for skull base meningiomas. Neurosurg Rev 2011;34:281–296, discussion 296

28. Sekhar LN, Swamy NK, Jaiswal V, Rubinstein E, Hirsch WE Jr, Wright DC. Surgical excision of meningiomas involving the clivus: preoperative and intraoperative features as predictors of postoperative functional deterioration. J Neurosurg 1994;81:860–868

29. Yasargil MG. Meningioma. In: Yasargil MG, ed. Microneurosurgery, vol 4B. Stuttgart, New York: Thieme; 1996:134–185

30. Martins C, Yasuda A, Campero A, Ulm AJ, Tanriover N, Rhoton A Jr. Microsurgical anatomy of the dural arteries. Neurosurgery 2005;56(2, Suppl):211–251, discussion 211–251

31. Borg A, Ekanayake J, Mair R, et al. Preoperative particle and glue embolization of meningiomas: indications, results, and lessons learned from 117 consecutive patients. Neurosurgery 2013;73(2, Suppl Operative):ons244–ons251, discussion ons252

32. Raper DM, Starke RM, Henderson F Jr, et al. Preoperative embolization of intracranial meningiomas: efficacy, technical considerations, and complications. AJNR Am J Neuroradiol 2014;35:1798–1804

33. Shah AH, Patel N, Raper DM, et al. The role of preoperative embolization for intracranial meningiomas. J Neurosurg 2013;119:364–372

34. Mathiesen T, Pettersson-Segerlind J, Kihlström L, Ulfarsson E. Meningiomas engaging major venous sinuses. World Neurosurg 2014;81:116–124

19 Anterior Skull Base Surgery

■ Tumors of the Anterior Skull Base

- The most common primary tumors in the anterior skull base (ASB) are meningiomas (~ 20% of intracranial tumors, ~ 40% when considered together with the sphenoid wing meningiomas).[1] Tuberculum sellae meningiomas are central skull base tumors, but they are discussed here in the differential diagnosis of olfactory groove and planum sphenoidale meningiomas.
- Among the malignant tumors of the sinonasal tract, esthesioneuroblastoma is the most common. In children, sarcoma is the most common malignant tumor of the ASB.
- Carcinoma of the ethmoid sinuses/nasal cavity with skull base involvement.
- Bony metastases (especially breast, lung, prostate, and myeloma).
- Very rare anterior cranial fossa schwannoma (most likely from the ethmoidal nerves or meningeal branches of the trigeminal nerve[2,3]).
- Other rarer conditions, such as sarcoidosis, tuberculosis, brown tumors, and mucoceles, can affect the region.

Malignant tumors have traditionally been treated with en-bloc resection of the ASB whenever possible. A malignant tumor that transgresses the dura and brain parenchyma has a poorer prognosis (see Chapter 23).

■ Olfactory Groove Meningiomas

- Olfactory groove meningiomas account for 9 to 18% of all meningiomas.[4,5]
- They originate in cribriform plate of the ethmoid bone and sphenoethmoidal suture.[6,7]
- They may involve any area from the crista galli to the planum sphenoidale, extending back into the pituitary fossa and laterally above the orbits.
- Because of frontal lobe compression, they often cause behavioral or mental status changes, which are subtle in the beginning and may go unrecognized

for years. Headache and anosmia are other common features. In posteriorly placed lesions such as those arising from or extending posterior to the planum or those extending posterior to the optic system, visual disturbances may be present. Historically, Foster Kennedy syndrome is considered a sign of a frontal fossa meningioma, but generally occurs only in the largest tumors (see page 183).

Olfactory groove meningiomas typically depress the optic chiasm as they extend backward, whereas tuberculum sellae meningiomas elevate it.[8] Olfactory groove meningiomas have the following attributes:

- Possible bone erosion, and ~ 20% of cases include ethmoid sinus invasion.[5,9,10]
- Possible displacement/involvement/encasement of the olfactory nerves. By definition, the olfactory groove meningioma starts at the level of the olfactory nerves.
- Blood to these tumors is supplied by the ethmoidal arteries and sphenoidal branches of the middle meningeal artery.

■ Tuberculum Sellae Meningiomas (Fig. 19.1)

- Tuberculum sellae meningiomas account for 5 to 10% of all intracranial meningiomas.
- They originate in the region of the chiasmatic sulcus and tuberculum sellae.
- In comparison with the other ASB meningiomas, lesions arising from the tuberculum give rise to visual disturbances earlier, typically causing bitemporal (or only superolateral) hemianopsia.[11]
- Tumors that start parasagittally or extend into one optic canal more than the other may present with asymmetric visual field loss, typically one-and-a-half syndrome, a relative afferent pupillary defect, and unilateral optic atrophy (see Chapter 10).
- The vascular supply comes from the posterior ethmoidal arteries and the meningeal vessels from the internal carotid artery (ICA). Preoperative embolization is often not feasible for these tumors.[12]
- Visual losses present sooner in patients with prefixed chiasms (i.e., shorter optic nerves) (see **Fig. 3.2b**, page 75).

■ Signs and Symptoms

Signs and symptoms include headache, olfactory disturbances/anosmia, visual field deficits (inferior or bitemporal visual field defects, depending on the size of the tumor and involvement of the optic chiasm, especially for tuberculum

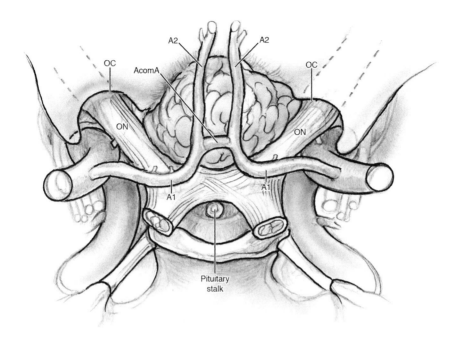

Fig. 19.1 Tuberculum sellae meningioma. AcomA, anterior communicating artery; OC, optic canal; ON, optic nerve.

sellae [TS] meningiomas), frontal lobe syndrome with mental deterioration, and short-term memory loss. Patients may also present with behavioral, personality, or psychiatric symptoms and may also appear depressed and apathetic. In older patients, these symptoms may be mistaken for dementia. Patients may also present with seizures, although this is rare.

- The more anteriorly placed the lesion, the more likely the patient will present with headache, anosmia, and behavioral change. The more posteriorly placed the lesion, the more likely the patient will present with visual complaints.
- Pain and nasal symptoms of obstruction and epistaxis are more common in lesions arising in the sinuses, which, as a group, are much more likely to be malignant.

■ Diagnostic Workup

Typical radiological work for meningiomas entails computed tomography (CT) and magnetic resonance imaging (MRI). CT is essential for defining hyperostosis and bone erosion. MRI is essential for defining localization and involvement of the optic chiasm and frontal lobe edema (T2 sequences). MRI with fat suppression is useful to identify tumor extension into the optic canal. Computed tomography angiography (CTA) or, rarely, angiogram may be required to define the relationships of the tumors with anterior cerebral arteries (see Chapter 5, page 114). The workup includes the following:

- Neuro-ophthalmologic testing (visual acuity, visual fields, color vision, optical coherence tomography [OCT]) (see Chapter 10)
- Endocrinologic testing for pituitary gland/hypothalamus hormonal functionality in tumors compressing the pituitary gland/stalk or hypothalamus (see Chapter 9)
- Neuropsychological testing (e.g., Montreal Cognitive Assessment, Folstein Mini–Mental State Examination, or other tests of cognitive abilities); particularly helpful as baselines for the long-term follow-up of patients

■ Treatment

Asymptomatic small meningiomas should be followed over time. Radiosurgery is an option for patients in whom surgery is contraindicated, although surgery remains the gold standard of treatment, especially for symptomatic patients who have signs of rapid visual deterioration.

■ Surgical Approaches

Surgical approaches are shown in **Fig. 19.2**. See also Chapter 14.

Bifrontal Craniotomy/Subfrontal Approaches

These approaches provide broad exposure of the anatomic region and tumor, with direct access to the anterior skull base if required.

- The pericranial flap can be easily used for reconstruction of the anterior fossa, if necessary (see **Fig. 14.3**, page 342).
- Depending on tumor size and extension, opening the frontal sinuses becomes inevitable in some cases.

Brain retraction should be avoided. Judicious use of lumbar drainage and performing the craniotomy as basal as possible are important caveats. Orbitozygomatic (OZ) osteotomy or simply an orbitocranial (OC) osteotomy in addition to the frontal craniotomy offers a more basal approach to the tumor, reduces the necessity to retract the frontal lobes, and particularly facilitates skull base reconstruction with pericranial flaps.

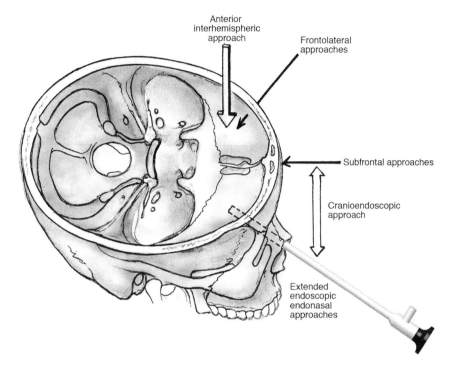

Fig. 19.2 Approaches to the anterior skull base.

- Extradural dissection with extensive devascularization of the tumor is particularly helpful. However, the anterior cerebral arteries should be left covered by arachnoid and not disturbed. The optic nerves and chiasm are usually visualized at later stages of dissection of the anteriorly placed tumors and should not be manipulated.
- Midline olfactory groove tumors, most of which are of considerable size, often require ligation and division of the superior sagittal sinus.
- For surgical approaches, see **Fig. 19.2**. For surgical steps, see Chapter 14, page 335.
- Orbital osteotomy may be used to enhance the exposure, reduce brain retraction, and facilitate repair.

Anterior Interhemispheric Approach

This approach has been described for resection of olfactory groove meningiomas[13,14] and TS meningiomas,[15,16] but it is limited by narrow corridors in reaching the tumor. The corridors can be enlarged only by the

Surgical Anatomy Pearl

Do not retract both frontal lobes.

mediolateral displacement/retraction of the frontal lobes, a process that entails the risk of injury to the bridging veins.

Frontolateral Approaches

Different frontolateral approaches can be used for asymmetric ASB tumors extending to one side. The side of the approach is generally the side of maximal extension of the tumor or of the visual field deficit. However, in TS meningiomas with visual impairment, a contralateral approach has been also suggested for providing potentially better visual outcomes.[17]

> **Surgical Anatomy Pearl**
>
> If the ICA is encased, perform the exposure on the side of the encased ICA itself.

Frontotemporal Craniotomy

In comparison with the bifrontal approach, the frontotemporal craniotomy spares the superior sagittal sinus and the cortical veins, and generally the frontal sinus does not have to be opened. This approach enables early dissection of the neurovascular complex.[18] The smaller unilateral pterional craniotomy can also be useful, but requires drilling of the anterior fossa floor and less flexibility to extend the exposure subfrontally for larger and contralateral tumors. However, it has been shown to be safe even when combined with a transsylvian exposure.[19,20]

One-and-a-Half-Fronto-Orbital Approach

This approach, with or without an orbital osteotomy, provides excellent basal exposure. See **Fig. 14.12**, page 362.

Lateral Supraorbital Approach

Olfactory groove meningiomas[21] and TS meningiomas[22] can be approached by means of this approach, with results comparable to those of the other more time-consuming approaches in terms of morbidity and mortality. However, the narrower approach may limit the ability to deal with the ICA.

■ Supraorbital Approach

This approach has been suggested for meningiomas of the anterior and central skull base,[23,24] although there is a limitation in the exposure of the tumor due to the restriction on available space intraoperatively. The visualization of the contralateral side of the tumor and anatomic structures is also more difficult.

Cerebrospinal fluid (CSF) drainage (by means of lumbar drainage or cisternal openings) is helpful in all approaches for minimizing brain retraction. However, in the event of a dissection of the subarachnoid space, the lumbar drain may make the arachnoid dissection more difficult because it may empty the cisterns of CSF.

- The risk of CSF leakage has to be evaluated with all approaches, and the surgeon must be prepared to repair any such leak.
- Frontal sinuses may often be avoided by means of these approaches. However, in cases where the frontal sinuses are transgressed, they should be repaired. If the opening is small (< 1 cm) and the mucosa intact, simple bone wax may suffice. For larger breaches of the sinus, the mucosa should be exenterated completely and the inner surface of the sinuses lightly drilled with a diamond bit. The frontal sinus ostium can be plugged with Gelfoam or fat, and then the sinus covered with a vascularized, pedicled pericranial flap harvested from the frontal scalp. Laying down the pedicled flap across the floor of an orbital cranial osteotomy avoids strangulating the flap that travels across a base of frontal bone left in place after a craniotomy. If orbital bony protuberances narrow the surgical corridor, drill them down.

Olfactory nerve preservation seems to be less successful in surgeries using a supraorbital approach than in more extended craniotomies.

■ Extended Endoscopic Transnasal Approach

Selected cases, such as olfactory groove or TS meningiomas (i.e., small midline lesions with no major vessel encasement, limited or no parasellar extension, or tumor extension into the sphenoid sinus) can be treated by means of an extended endoscopic transsphenoidal approach.[25–27] See also Chapter 16.

- The resection via a transsphenoidal route facilitates decompression of critical structures, such as the optic nerves and chiasm from below, rather than working on these structures from above and needing to work around them to get to the tumor. The approach also requires resection of involved bone and dura, but whether recurrences will be fewer as a result of using this approach has yet to be determined and requires an analysis of long-term follow-up data.
- It is a demanding technique, and surgeons should have considerable training and experience before attempting this approach. Close attention to whether the tumor extends or encases the optic nerve and major vessels requires high-resolution imaging.

■ Combined Approaches (Cranioendoscopic Approach)

The combination of the frontal craniotomy with a transnasal endoscopic approach can be used for large meningiomas or malignant tumors involving large areas of the brain cavity and the nasal cavity or paranasal sinuses, or for those where an en-bloc resection is considered essential.[28-30] The endoscopic endonasal approach enables the resection of the nasal/paranasal component of the tumors. On the other hand, the subfrontal approach enables the resection of the intracranial components, removal of the involved dura, and drilling of the cribriform plate. The technique is mostly used for the surgical resection of malignant sinonasal lesions.

- Some contraindications have been described for the use of this approach, such as lacrimal sac or orbital involvement, nasal pyramid or bony walls of the maxillary sinus involvement, and extension to the pterygopalatine or infratemporal fossa.[31]
- The endonasal endoscopic phase involves various combinations of the endoscopic approaches (e.g., transsphenoidal/transplanum/transcribriform approaches): lamina papyracea dissection, and further approaches such as medial maxillectomy, nasolacrimal duct exposure, removal below the lacrimal sac, and periorbital resection depending on tumor localization.[32]
- The transcranial phase involves a bifrontal craniotomy with a coronal incision for tailoring of a pedicled pericranial flap, which will be used in the reconstruction phase. The flap should be made as long as physically possible. Frontal lobe retraction can be avoided by using a low craniotomy with or without an orbital cranial osteotomy and with early CSF drainage. The anatomy of the lesion will determine the extent of bone resection. Reciprocating saws or fine drills can help facilitate en-bloc resection of bones.[32] Resection of dura and involved brain can be performed in subsequent steps based on preoperative imaging (look for enhancement and thickening of the meninges and edema or enhancement of the brain) and intraoperative "quick section" pathology.
- Working from different angles, head and neck surgeons and neurosurgeons can simultaneously visualize the margins of the resection.
- For cases with resection of dura, the dura can be reconstructed with a fascia lata free graft sutured in place. The pedicled pericranial flap is sutured down to the deepest aspects of the resection, just beyond the margins of the dural repair. Layered free fat grafts and fibrin glue may also be useful to support the repair. For defects adequately repaired by this technique via craniotomy, bone reconstruction is not necessary. The endonasal cavity can be reconstructed with a pedicled nasoseptal flap to aid in mucosal healing (see "Endoscopic Repair of Skull Base Defects," page 431).

- Synthetic cements such as methyl methacrylate should not be used with the opening of the sinuses because it will almost certainly become a site for infection.
- The overall complication rate depends on the patient population and the size of the lesions being treated. In one series, the overall complication rate was 16%,[30] and associated complications included CSF leakage (generally managed by lumbar drainage), frontal bone osteomyelitis, epistaxis, supraorbital anesthesia, and visual disorders.

■ Surgical Pearls

For any meningioma surgery, whether done from above or below the skull base, devascularization of the tumor should be performed prior to tumor resection. All hyperostotic bone should be removed.

- Imaging with CT or MRI should be carefully studied in every case to assess the transbasal extension. The goal of every surgical procedure should be gross total resection. Reconstruction should be an essential part of the planning phase in every case as well.
- Olfactory nerves should be anatomically preserved if possible. Dissect them from the tumor, open the olfactory cisterns, and avoid coagulation in this region. During resection of planum sphenoidale and olfactory groove meningiomas, both olfactory nerves are dissected and, if necessary, one is divided while leaving the other intact whenever possible.
- The anterior cerebral arteries should be left untouched behind the arachnoid membrane. If this is not possible, they must be dissected carefully from the posterior pole of the tumor from below in order to preserve all the perforating arteries and the recurrent arteries of Heubner.
- In tumors involving the optic nerves, extradural optic nerve decompression may be required. Optic canal involvement (above all in TS meningiomas) requires optic nerve decompression[33,34] by means of the unroofing of the optic canal, extradural anterior clinoidectomy with falciform ligament and optic nerve sheath opening, and endoscopic transnasal procedures.
- No coagulation is recommended in the vicinity of the optic nerves and chiasm. Preserve the perforators close to the chiasm; apply haemostatic material in case of bleeding rather than performing hemostasis with the bipolar forceps.
- Avoid frontal lobe retraction, considering that the frontal lobe may already be quite edematous, and retractors can make it worse.
- The tumor generally pushes the pituitary stalk backward, and it is usually possible to preserve the arachnoid membrane, the stalk, the basilar artery, and its branches.[1]

■ Outcome

The possibility of total resection depends on the patient and tumor characteristics such as tumor extension, invasiveness, and encasement of arteries of the anterior cerebral complex.[35] For confined meningiomas, gross total resection is often possible, whereas malignant tumors with brain invasion are rarely completed resected. Frontal basal syndromes can be prevented by avoiding brain retraction and preservation of all arteries and veins.

- In TS meningioma, when comparing different approaches, the frontolateral approaches have been shown to provide the best visual outcome in comparison with bifrontal approaches.[36]
- In olfactory groove meningiomas, olfaction may be preserved in the contralateral side of tumors less than 3 cm in diameter, whereas its preservation ipsilaterally to the tumor is extremely difficult.[37]
- **Table 19.1** summarizes outcome and complications of surgery for olfactory groove meningiomas[8,23,38,39] and **Table 19.2** for tuberculum sellae meningiomas.[26,40–42]

Table 19.1 Outcome and Complications of Transcranial Surgery for Olfactory Groove Meningiomas

Outcome		Complications	
Mortality	~ 0%	Visual loss	2%
		Visual disturbances	< 15%
Recurrence rate	< 10% (median of 8 years)	CSF leak	6%
Cognitive improvement	50–90%		
Improvement of visual acuity	26–83%	Infection	3%
Improvement of visual fields	29–100%	Seizure	5%
Olfaction	Lost ipsilaterally for tumor > 3 cm	Hematoma	3%
		Ischemia	1%
		Pit./Hypoth. injury	
		Tens. Pneumoc.	
		PE	

Abbreviations: CSF, cerebrospinal fluid; Hypoth., hypothalamus; PE, pulmonary embolism; Pit., pituitary gland; Tens. Pneumoc., tension pneumocephalus.

Table 19.2   Outcome and Complications of Transcranial and Endoscopic (*)
Surgery for Tuberculum Sellae Meningiomas

Outcome		Complications	
Mortality	~ 0%	Overall morbidity	11%
Gross total resection	88–92%	Visual worsening	12–17%
	~ 80%*		< 4%*
Improvement of visual acuity	57–63%	Infection	4%
	86–100%*		
		Pit./Hypoth. injury	
		Venous infarction/ischemia	
		Frontal sinus mucocele	
		Tens. Pneumoc.	

■ References

Boldfaced references are of particular importance.

1. **DeMonte F. Surgical treatment of anterior basal meningiomas. J Neurooncol 1996;29:239–248**

2. Figueiredo EG, Soga Y, Amorim RL, Oliveira AM, Teixeira MJ. The puzzling olfactory groove schwannoma: a systematic review. Skull Base 2011;21:31–36

3. Blake DM, Husain Q, Kanumuri VV, Svider PF, Eloy JA, Liu JK. Endoscopic endonasal resection of sinonasal and anterior skull base schwannomas. J Clin Neurosci 2014; 21:1419–1423

4. Chan RC, Thompson GB. Morbidity, mortality, and quality of life following surgery for intracranial meningiomas. A retrospective study in 257 cases. J Neurosurg 1984;60: 52–60

5. Solero CL, Giombini S, Morello G. Suprasellar and olfactory meningiomas. Report on a series of 153 personal cases. Acta Neurochir (Wien) 1983;67:181–194

6. Rubin G, Ben David U, Gornish M, Rappaport ZH. Meningiomas of the anterior cranial fossa floor. Review of 67 cases. Acta Neurochir (Wien) 1994;129:26–30

7. Spektor S, Valarezo J, Fliss DM, et al. Olfactory groove meningiomas from neurosurgical and ear, nose, and throat perspectives: approaches, techniques, and outcomes. Neurosurgery 2005;57(4, Suppl):268–280, discussion 268–280

8. **Hentschel SJ, DeMonte F. Olfactory groove meningiomas. In: De Monte F, McDermott MW, Al-Mefty O, eds. Al-Mefty's Meningiomas, 2nd ed. New York, Stuttgart: Thieme; 2011:196–205**

9. Bakay L, Cares HL. Olfactory meningiomas. Report on a series of twenty-five cases. Acta Neurochir (Wien) 1972;26:1–12

10. Maiuri F, Salzano FA, Motta S, Colella G, Sardo L. Olfactory groove meningioma with paranasal sinus and nasal cavity extension: removal by combined subfrontal and nasal approach. J Craniomaxillofac Surg 1998;26:314–317

11. Taylor SL, Barakos JA, Harsh GR IV, Wilson CB. Magnetic resonance imaging of tuberculum sellae meningiomas: preventing preoperative misdiagnosis as pituitary macroadenoma. Neurosurgery 1992;31:621–627, discussion 627

12. Chun JY, McDermott MW, Lamborn KR, Wilson CB, Higashida R, Berger MS. Delayed surgical resection reduces intraoperative blood loss for embolized meningiomas. Neurosurgery 2002;50:1231–1235, discussion 1235–1237

13. Mayfrank L, Gilsbach JM. Interhemispheric approach for microsurgical removal of olfactory groove meningiomas. Br J Neurosurg 1996;10:541–545

14. Mielke D, Mayfrank L, Psychogios MN, Rohde V. The anterior interhemispheric approach: a safe and effective approach to anterior skull base lesions. Acta Neurochir (Wien) 2014;156:689–696

15. **Curey S, Derrey S, Hannequin P, et al. Validation of the superior interhemispheric approach for tuberculum sellae meningioma: clinical article. J Neurosurg 2012; 117:1013–1021**

16. **Terasaka S, Asaoka K, Kobayashi H, Yamaguchi S. Anterior interhemispheric approach for tuberculum sellae meningioma. Neurosurgery 2011;68(1, Suppl Operative):84–88, discussion 88–89**

17. Jang WY, Jung S, Jung TY, Moon KS, Kim IY. The contralateral subfrontal approach can simplify surgery and provide favorable visual outcome in tuberculum sellae meningiomas. Neurosurg Rev 2012;35:601–607, discussion 607–608

18. **Bitter AD, Stavrinou LC, Ntoulias G, et al. The Role of the pterional approach in the surgical treatment of olfactory groove meningiomas: a 20-year experience. J Neurol Surg B Skull Base 2013;74:97–102**

19. **Fahlbusch R, Schott W. Pterional surgery of meningiomas of the tuberculum sellae and planum sphenoidale: surgical results with special consideration of ophthalmological and endocrinological outcomes. J Neurosurg 2002;96:235–243**

20. **Yasargil MG. Meningioma. In: Yasargil MG, ed. Microneurosurgery, vol 4B. Stuttgart, New York: Thieme; 1996:134–185**

21. **Romani R, Lehecka M, Gaal E, et al. Lateral supraorbital approach applied to olfactory groove meningiomas: experience with 66 consecutive patients. Neurosurgery 2009;65:39–52, discussion 52–53**

22. **Romani R, Laakso A, Kangasniemi M, Niemelä M, Hernesniemi J. Lateral supraorbital approach applied to tuberculum sellae meningiomas: experience with 52 consecutive patients. Neurosurgery 2012;70:1504–1518, discussion 1518–1519**

23. **Obeid F, Al-Mefty O. Recurrence of olfactory groove meningiomas. Neurosurgery 2003;53:534–542, discussion 542–543**

24. Telera S, Carapella CM, Caroli F, et al. Supraorbital keyhole approach for removal of midline anterior cranial fossa meningiomas: a series of 20 consecutive cases. Neurosurg Rev 2012;35:67–83, discussion 83

25. **de Divitiis E, Cavallo LM, Esposito F, Stella L, Messina A. Extended endoscopic transsphenoidal approach for tuberculum sellae meningiomas. Neurosurgery 2007;61(5, Suppl 2):229–237, discussion 237–238**

26. **de Divitiis E, Esposito F, Cappabianca P, Cavallo LM, de Divitiis O. Tuberculum sellae meningiomas: high route or low route? A series of 51 consecutive cases. Neurosurgery 2008;62:556–563, discussion 556–563**

27. **Bowers CA, Altay T, Couldwell WT. Surgical decision-making strategies in tuberculum sellae meningioma resection. Neurosurg Focus 2011;30:E1**

28. Yuen AP, Fung CF, Hung KN. Endoscopic cranionasal resection of anterior skull base tumor. Am J Otolaryngol 1997;18:431–433
29. **Castelnuovo PG, Belli E, Bignami M, Battaglia P, Sberze F, Tomei G. Endoscopic nasal and anterior craniotomy resection for malignant nasoethmoid tumors involving the anterior skull base. Skull Base 2006;16:15–18**
30. **Nicolai P, Battaglia P, Bignami M, et al. Endoscopic surgery for malignant tumors of the sinonasal tract and adjacent skull base: a 10-year experience. Am J Rhinol 2008;22:308–316**
31. **Batra PS, Citardi MJ, Worley S, Lee J, Lanza DC. Resection of anterior skull base tumors: comparison of combined traditional and endoscopic techniques. Am J Rhinol 2005;19:521–528**
32. Nicolai P, Yakirevitch A, Bolzoni Villaret A, Battaglia P, Locatelli D, Castelnuovo P. Combined cranioendoscopic approach. In: Stamm AC, ed. Transnasal Endoscopic Skull Base and Brain Surgery. Tips and Pearls. New York, Stuttgart: Thieme; 2011:350–354
33. **Mariniello G, de Divitiis O, Bonavolontà G, Maiuri F. Surgical unroofing of the optic canal and visual outcome in basal meningiomas. Acta Neurochir (Wien) 2013;155:77–84**
34. Sade B, Lee JH. High incidence of optic canal involvement in tuberculum sellae meningiomas: rationale for aggressive skull base approach. Surg Neurol 2009;72:118–123, discussion 123
35. **Goel A, Muzumdar D, Desai KI. Tuberculum sellae meningioma: a report on management on the basis of a surgical experience with 70 patients. Neurosurgery 2002;51:1358–1363, discussion 1363–1364**
36. Nakamura M, Roser F, Struck M, Vorkapic P, Samii M. Tuberculum sellae meningiomas: clinical outcome considering different surgical approaches. Neurosurgery 2006; 59:1019–1028, discussion 1028–1029
37. Welge-Luessen A, Temmel A, Quint C, Moll B, Wolf S, Hummel T. Olfactory function in patients with olfactory groove meningioma. J Neurol Neurosurg Psychiatry 2001;70: 218–221
38. Bakay L. Olfactory meningiomas. The missed diagnosis. JAMA 1984;251:53–55
39. **Bassiouni H, Asgari S, Stolke D. Olfactory groove meningiomas: functional outcome in a series treated microsurgically. Acta Neurochir (Wien) 2007;149:109–121, discussion 121**
40. **Sughrue ME, Sanai N, McDermott MW. Tuberculum sellae meningiomas. In: DeMonte F, McDermott MW, Al-Mefty O, eds. Al-Mefty's Meningiomas, 2nd ed. New York, Stuttgart: Thieme; 2011:206–213**
41. **Clark AJ, Jahangiri A, Garcia RM, et al. Endoscopic surgery for tuberculum sellae meningiomas: a systematic review and meta-analysis. Neurosurg Rev 2013;36: 349–359**
42. **Koutourousiou M, Fernandez-Miranda JC, Stefko ST, Wang EW, Snyderman CH, Gardner PA. Endoscopic endonasal surgery for suprasellar meningiomas: experience with 75 patients. J Neurosurg 2014;120:1326–1339**

20 Intraorbital Pathologies and Surgical Approaches

■ Intraorbital Diseases

- Intraorbital diseases have different age-related patterns of progress over different periods of time **(Table 20.1)**.
- Thyroid-associated orbitopathy is more frequent in Western countries and is the most common intraorbital disease in the Americas and Europe.
- In adults, the most frequently diagnosed malignant lesions involving the orbit are non-Hodgkin's lymphomas; extensions from basal cell carcinoma (BCC); and metastases, most commonly of BCC.[1,2] Choroidal melanoma is the most commonly diagnosed primary ocular malignant lesion, but it occurs less frequently than the other malignancies cited above. Cavernous hemangioma is the most common benign lesion involving the orbit.
  - The incidence and prevalence of various orbital pathologies vary geographically.
- Dermoid and epidermoid cysts are the most common benign lesions in children, whereas sarcomas (rhabdomyosarcomas) are the most common orbital malignant tumors (retinoblastoma is the most common intraocular malignancy in the pediatric population). Lymphoproliferative diseases are rare in children, accounting for less than 5 to 10% of orbital lesions.
- Orbital cellulitis: incidence: 1.6/100,000/year in children; 0.1/100,000/year in adults.[3] Orbital infections are more common in younger patients and more severe in older ones. Infectious orbital pathologies, although rare (about 2% of the pathologies affecting the orbit), are a serious condition with potentially life-threatening consequences.[4]
- Review anatomy in Chapter 2, page 43.

■ Orbital Approaches

- Basic principles of all surgery: bloodless field, adequate exposure and visualization, proper instrumentation, delicate manipulation. In benign expansive

Table 20.1 Orbital Pathologies Overview

Category			Description
Congenital and developmental			Dermoid cysts, fibrous dysplasia, hamartomas, meningoencephaloceles
Inflammatory and infective			Cellulitis/abscesses, parasitic (hydatid), granulomas (sarcoidosis, Wegener, fungal), amyloidosis, pseudotumor orbitae
Traumatic			Penetrating injuries, hematoma, foreign bodies
Neoplastic	Primary	Benign	Capillary hemangioma, hemangiopericytoma, neurinoma, neurofibroma, meningioma, lipoma, lacrimal gland pleomorphic adenoma
		Malignant	Lymphoma, leukemia, hemangiopericytoma, sarcomas (angio-, rhabdo-, lipo-, fibro-, etc.), neuroblastoma, Ewing's sarcoma, optic glioma, lacrimal gland adenoid-cystic carcinoma, melanoma
	Secondary		Extension from other sites (eyelid, paranasal sinuses, etc.)
	Metastatic		
Vascular	High-flow malformations		Aneurysm, arteriovenous malformations
	Low-flow malformations	Venous malformations	Distensible venous malformations, nondistensible venous malformations (cavernous hemangioma)
		Lymphatic malformations	Microcystic, macrocystic, or mixed (lymphangiomas)
		Combined venous-lymphatic malformations	Lymphatic dominant, venous dominant
Dysthyroid orbitopathy			
Miscellaneous			Osseous lesions (osteoma, etc.), mucoceles

Clinical Evaluation of Patients with Orbital Diseases: Practical Checklist

- *Vision acuity*: It is critical to measure visual acuity before any treatment is performed. Documentation for medicolegal issues is paramount. Reduced vision suggests involvement of the optic nerve or globe.
- *Pupils*: Evaluate the shape and symmetry of pupils. *Extraocular movements:* It is useful to note even minimal abnormal movements because a slight limitation in one eye may be the only evidence of orbital pathology.
- *Color vision*: Assessment of color vision is very important for evaluating optic nerve function. It can be done simply with Ishihara color plates; there is no need for more sophisticated tests.
- *Inspection:* Evaluate the entire face, focusing on proportion and symmetry.
- *Globe displacement*: Globe displacement does not always result in diplopia, but evaluating the position of the globe can be an important sign for many conditions (e.g., orbital trauma).
- *Palpation:* Palpate the upper and lower eyelid very carefully. Check the orbital rim for any step deformities or fractures.
- *Eyelid color*: Eyelid color can provide some information regarding orbital pathologies. In inflammatory disorders, eyelids are often erythematous. Spontaneous hemorrhage most frequently occurs with hemangioma and lymphangioma, which can also have bluish color.

Specialist Evaluation (see also Chapter 10)

- *Slit-lamp examination*: This exam is useful for evaluating the status of the cornea (and for evaluating exposure keratopathy). Several pathological conditions cause dilatation of conjunctival vessels and edema. In very severe cases the suspicion of a carotid-cavernous fistula should be raised.
- *Intraocular pressure*
- *Fundus examination*: This exam is necessary to assess the optic nerve. For example, tumors compressing the optic nerve produce disk edema or optic atrophy.
- *Pulsations*: Pulsations can be present in neurofibromatosis or in any other conditions in which brain pulsation can be transmitted to the orbital content. Extremely vascularized orbital tumors can also generate pulsations.
- *Exophthalmometry*: to evaluate proptosis.
- *Forced duction test*: to evaluate the movement of a given extraocular muscle.
- *Nasal endoscopy:* to evaluate the presence of sinonasal pathologies (inflammatory, neoplastic).

lesional surgery, keep the most intimate plane around the capsule of the lesion.
- The choice of the approach should be made based on the site, the anatomic relationships, and the suspected nature of the lesion; for example, a regional approach is appropriate for the orbit.[4] Each area can be reached by different approaches, with each providing a different angle of attack.

- Most orbital lesions, regardless of their origin within the orbit, extend freely through the intra- and extraconal spaces, especially in the apical region.
- The orbital skeleton and bony rim can limit surgical maneuvers in a narrow anatomic space. Sometimes bony work is necessary to increase operative space. Orbital or cranio-orbital bone segments may temporarily be removed and replaced in their original position without any morphological sequelae.
- Surgical access to orbital skeleton and periorbital structures through the eyelids and anterior orbit can be done using a wide range of skin and conjunctival incisions[5] (**Fig. 20.1**). The choice of the incision is greatly influenced by the surgeon's personal experience and the surgical target lesion.
- Orbital marginotomies available for surgical treatment of orbital diseases can be classified into four procedures based on the bony wall to be treated: inferior, lateral, superior, and medial.[6] Orbital bony disassembling can be performed as required (**Fig. 20.1**).
- Transcranial approaches can be used for orbital tumors located medially in the orbital apex, optic canal, and select orbital tumors with intracranial extension.

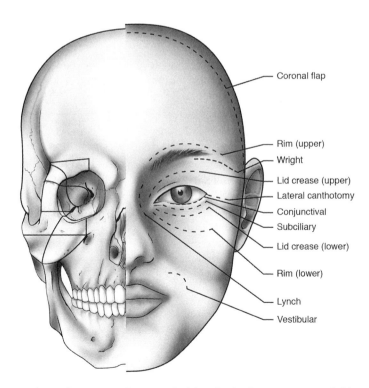

- Coronal flap
- Rim (upper)
- Wright
- Lid crease (upper)
- Lateral canthotomy
- Conjunctival
- Subciliary
- Lid crease (lower)
- Rim (lower)
- Lynch
- Vestibular

Fig. 20.1 Skin and conjunctival incision (*right*) and orbital marginotomies (*left*) to access orbital lesions.

Table 20.2   Surgical Approaches to the Orbit

Superior orbit	Coronal approach
	Superior eyelid approach
	Eyebrow approach
	Other neurosurgical approach (temporal, frontotemporal, etc.)
Lateral orbit	Lateral orbitotomy (Kronlein approach and variations)
	Superior eyelid approach
	Superior eyebrow approach
	Swinging eyelid approach
Inferior orbit	Swinging eyelid approach
	Transconjunctival approaches
	Inferior eyelid approach
	Transantral-transvestibular approach
Medial orbit	Trans-/precaruncular transconjunctival approach
	Transfacial approach (Lynch or paralateronasal incision)
	Transnasal approach

Among these approaches, the frontal, frontotemporal, and frontotemporal-orbitozygomatic (FTOZ) approaches, with or without preservation of the supraorbital rim, are very versatile **(Table 20.2)**.
- Endoscopic-assisted orbital approaches can offer improved visualization in select cases and minimize the amount of bone work required.

■ Coronal Approach

- Very versatile with multiple accessible areas: fronto-orbital region, upper and middle regions of the facial skeleton, anterior and middle cranial fossa
- Enables adequate management of the superolateral aspect of the whole orbit
- ◈ Dissect the lateral orbital rim in a subperiosteal fashion. Complete the exposure of lateral orbital rim and zygomatic regions.

> **Surgical Anatomy Pearl**
>
> In orbital dissection, be aware of the position of the medial canthal tendon.

■ Approaches to the Anterior Half of the Orbit (Fig. 20.2)

Medial Approaches

These approaches are used to access the roof and floor of the orbit, nasolacrimal region, ethmoidal complex, sphenoid sinus, and medial aspect of optic canal.

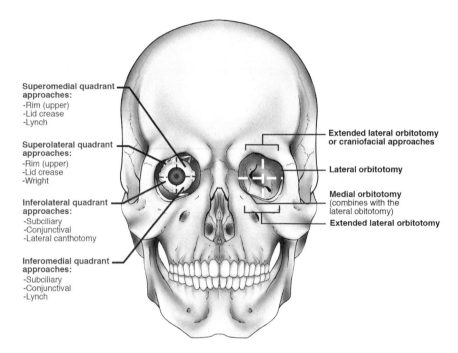

Superomedial quadrant approaches:
-Rim (upper)
-Lid crease
-Lynch

Superolateral quadrant approaches:
-Rim (upper)
-Lid crease
-Wright

Inferolateral quadrant approaches:
-Subciliary
-Conjunctival
-Lateral canthotomy

Inferomedial quadrant approaches:
-Subciliary
-Conjunctival
-Lynch

Extended lateral orbitotomy or craniofacial approaches

Lateral orbitotomy

Medial orbitotomy (combines with the lateral obitotomy)

Extended lateral orbitotomy

Fig. 20.2   Schematic representation of the approaches to the anterior *(left)* and posterior *(right)* compartments of the orbits.

◈   Transcutaneous approach—Lynch incision[7]: Make a slightly curved vertical incision down to the periosteum, beginning along the inferior aspect of the medial brow, midway between the medial canthus and the dorsum of the nose. Manage the local vessels (angular artery and vein). Once the periosteum is reached, dissect it in a subperiosteal plane. The medial canthal ligament may be elevated, but reapproximate it at the end of the procedure.

◈   Superior eyelid incision (medial half) and medial lid crease[4]: Used to access the medial wall and floor of the orbit as well as anterior orbital fat.

   •   Make the skin incision on a crease. Elevate the orbicularis muscle flap and identify the orbital rim. Laterally push the levator muscle. Expose the intraconal orbital fat. Trochlea and superior oblique muscle should be identified, and they can be temporarily detached (with limited functional impairment). Less scarring will occur postoperatively, but this approach provides a narrower window for deep work.[5] Incise and elevate the periorbita to gain access to the medial orbital wall.

   •   Potential risks: damage to lacrimal system and trochlea with subsequent diplopia.

   •   Limitations: limited access to orbital floor, and residual scarring (may be minimized with technical modifications).

◈ Paralateronasal incision: an inferior extension of the Lynch incision. It is performed when a wider window is needed and the lesion is not confined to orbital spaces.

◈ Transconjunctival approaches: include the "pericaruncular" approaches (precaruncular and transcaruncular), as well as the medial inferior fornix approach.

1. *Pericaruncular approaches (pre- and transcaruncular).* Induce vasoconstriction in the caruncle and semilunar fold region. Protect the cornea. Retract the upper and lower eyelid with sutures or retractors. Minimally retract the globe laterally with a malleable retractor and make a vertical incision. In the transcaruncular route, the incision is made in the region of the caruncle, whereas in precaruncular approaches, the incision is made just anterior to the caruncle.[8] Perform subconjunctival dissection. Identify the posterior limb of the medial canthal tendon and dissect it until the posterior lacrimal crest is reached (the posterior lacrimal crest can be identified with the surgical instruments). Identify the periorbita and incise it immediately posterior to the posterior lacrimal crest. Then, push the orbital content laterally in order to expose the medial wall of the orbit, from the floor to the roof, and from the posterior lacrimal crest to the optic canal/nerve. Identify and manage the anterior and posterior ethmoidal arteries. The following intraorbital dissection is based on the pathology to be treated. For example, orbital and optic nerve decompression can be performed by removing the lamina papyracea and medial aspect of the optic canal. If intraconal work is needed, the medial rectus muscle can be detached (it must be reattached at the end). If more space is needed, perform a lateral orbitotomy with lateral displacement of orbital content, in order to move the eyeball more laterally.[9] At the end of the procedure, closure of the conjunctiva is essential._

2. *Medial inferior fornix approach.* This approach provides access to the anterior intraconal space. Perform a medial 180-degree conjunctival incision close to the corneal limbus. Elevate the conjunctival flap and identify the anterior attachment of the medial rectus muscle. This approach eventually requires resection and medial retraction of the medial rectus muscle. Next, enter the tenon capsule. Intraconal fat is gently managed, and the anterior segment of the optic nerve can be exposed. Conjunctiva closure is essential following procedure completion.

   Potential risks: bleeding from vortex veins, and damage to the posterior ciliary vessels and central retinal artery.

   Complications: Disruption of the Horner muscle might allow the medial aspects of the eyelids to fall anteriorly away from the globe; lacrimal system damage.

Lateral Approaches

These approaches are used to access the lacrimal fossa region, lateral extra- and intraconal spaces, and anterior and middle cranial base.

◈ Superior eyelid incision (see Superior Approaches, below). This versatile route provides adequate exposure of the lateral wall of the orbit until the superior orbital fissure is reached. It is mostly utilized for extraconal work and cranial base approaches instead of for intraconal work. Endoscopic assistance is very helpful in deep work.

◈ Lateral rim approach/lateral canthal approach. Mostly dedicated to laterally placed, retrocanthal, anterior and mid-orbit lesions. Make a cutaneous incision from the lateral canthus toward the temporal fossa. Then perform a lateral canthotomy and superior and inferior lateral cantholysis. The superior and inferior palpebral limbs are tagged with stitches. Incise the periorbita and lift it from the lateral orbital wall to gain access to the superolateral extraconal space. At the end of the procedure, reapproximate the limbs of the lateral canthal tendons.[10,11] The lateral canthal tendon can sometimes be spared and not bisected by working just above and below it.[4]
  • Possible complications: eyelid retraction and lateral canthal tendon malfunction

◈ Lateral lid crease/lacrimal keyhole approach. Mostly dedicated to the lacrimal gland region. Make the incision as for the superior eyelid approach. Drill out the superolateral rim from a lateral direction and create a segmental superior rim opening. Spare the Whitnall tubercle region.

◈◈ Another option is drilling down the rim in order to visualize the lateral wall through the eyelid incision.[4]

◈ Transconjunctival approach/lateral inferior fornix approach. Mostly utilized for inferolateral orbital wall, anterior and mid-orbit inferolaterally located lesions.
  • Make an incision in the lateral inferior fornix and perform an inferior lateral cantholysis as well. Dissect the periorbita from the orbital wall. Skeletonize the orbital wall as needed and manage the intraorbital lesion. At the end, reattach the lateral portion of the inferior tarsal plate to the residual portion of the lateral canthal tendon (the suture should grasp the superior limb of the tendon in order to make the inferior eyelid adapt well to the globe).
  • Complications: pre-septal scarring with eyelid retraction, inferior eyelid malposition, bleeding.

Superior Approaches

These approaches are used to access the extra- and intraconal anterosuperior and superonasal spaces, lateral wall, anterior and middle cranial fossa. Various cutaneous incisions are possible: superior eyelid (which is more appealing cosmetically), brow, and sub-brow incisions.

◈ Brow and sub-brow approach. Make the incision to reach the periosteum of the orbital rim. Elevate the periorbit until the target area is reached, and open the periorbita for management of the intraorbital lesion. Drainage and closure in layers is essential following procedure completion.

◈ Superior eyelid approach. Make the skin incision on a lid crease. Identify the orbicularis muscle. Raise the suborbicularis flap and reach the superolateral orbital rim. The orbital septum can be spared or violated, depending on the target one wishes to reach. If it is violated, orbital fat invades the field and should be managed. If an intraconal target has to be reached, cut the levator aponeurosis and Müller's muscle. This maneuver can be done transversally or vertically. The latter option causes fewer postoperative problems. In the transverse maneuver, the superior aponeurotic system should be reapproximated at the end of the procedure.

Surgical Anatomy Pearl

Care should be taken to prevent damage to the superior oblique muscle tendon. The septum should not be closed, to avoid postoperative lagophthalmos.

In extra-periorbital approaches, dissect carefully the periorbita from the orbital bones, until reaching the superior and inferior orbital fissures. Resect bone (mainly on the greater wing of the sphenoid and orbital part of the frontal bone) as necessary. By means of a superior eyelid approach, you can reach the orbital roof (two thirds lateral), lateral orbital wall, and lateral aspect of the floor. Endoscopic assistance is advised for deep work.

Potential Risks

Risks include damage to the levator palpebrae muscle complex, and injury of the frontal, supraorbital, or supratrochlear nerves and vessels. In intraconal work, complications are related to the target areas. Keep in mind that the position of the central retinal artery is unpredictable.

The superior eyelid approach decreases many of the risks associated with more peripherally located incisions.[5] The incision heals well with minimal scarring.[12]

■ Inferior Approaches

These approaches are used to reach the inferior orbital rim, orbital floor, inferior intra- or extraconal space, lacrimal duct, and orbital apex.

◈   Transcutaneous approach/inferior eyelid approach. The lower eyelid route can be performed by means of subciliary or subtarsal incision. In subciliary incisions (2 mm below the free margin of the lower eyelid), dissection can be done either in the subcutaneous plane between the orbicularis and the skin, to the level of inferior orbital rim (the *skin technique),* or below the orbicularis (the *skin–muscle technique).*[11,13] In the typical skin–muscle technique, the flap is raised directly above the lower tarsus, detaching the orbicularis from the inferior tarsus. In the "step" technique,[14] the pretarsal orbicularis is preserved and the skin–muscle flap is raised below the pretarsal fibers. In the subtarsal incision (5 to 7 mm below the free margin of the lower eyelid), dissect below the orbicularis and raise a skin–muscle flap. Further dissection is advised in the preseptal plane. Regardless of the incision, the orbital rim is identified by palpation and, at this level, the periosteum is incised and a subperiosteal dissection is performed to increase working room. The anterior maxilla and orbital floor can be exposed as well. When intraorbital work is needed, the septum (or periorbita) is opened and the target area can be reached. At the end of the procedure, each layer should be reapproximated with sutures. Sometimes a lower eyelid suspensory suture (attached to the forehead) can be useful to avoid excessive shortening of the lower eyelid.
- Complications: ectropion, darkening of the skin, occasionally entropion (less likely with the "step" technique)

◈   Transconjunctival approach (inferior fornix approach). Indicated for extra- and intraconal inferior compartment work. Induce vasoconstriction under the conjunctiva and protect the eyeball using a corneal shield. Make an incision through the conjunctiva of the inferior fornix, midway between the lower border of the tarsus and the lowest point of the fornix.

◈   Make an incision along the capsulopalpebral fascia. Dissect in either a preseptal or a postseptal plane. A preseptal route is better in cases where the floor of the orbit must be accessed (this field is not invaded by fat). The postseptal (or retroseptal) route is easier and more direct. It is associated with fat invasion of the field, but this

Surgical Anatomy Pearl

Do not breach the inferior lacrimal punctum medially (as a general rule of thumb, do not disrupt the lacrimal system).

is generally a minor concern. In such a case, no eyelid dissection is required, as in the preseptal route. The floor is easily reached (easier in postseptal route). Make a periosteal incision and subperiosteal orbital dissection. Inferior fornix incisions can be associated with limited exposure. An associated lateral inferior cantholysis can also increase the working space.

◈◈ Variation: This incision can be combined with a lateral canthotomy incision—the so-called swinging eyelid approach. With this extended approach a wide exposure of the inferior orbit and zygoma is gained. When a lateral canthotomy is indicated, the whole procedure starts with this step. Closure (first inferior canthopexy suture and then conjunctival closure) follows procedure completion.

◈◈ Variation: An inferior marginotomy, with infraorbital nerve sparing, can be utilized alongside this technique, although it is rarely required.
  • Potential risks: damage to the inferior oblique muscle, lacrimal system, and infraorbital nerve
  • Possible complications: ectropion and increased scleral show with skin incisions,[15] although this is a controversial risk.[16] With swinging eyelid approach: ectropion, entropion, and tearing of the lid margin.[5]

◈ Transoral approach/transantral approach. Mostly indicated for inferomedial orbit and medial orbital apex. Make a mucosal incision in the vestibular area and perform a subperiosteal dissection. The infraorbital nerve has to be identified and spared. Expose the anterior maxillary wall and perform an anterior maxillotomy with a complete or partial ethmoidectomy. Remove the orbital floor (medial to the infraorbital nerve) and lamina papyracea. Expose the periorbita for management of the orbital pathology.
  • Possible complications: damage to infraorbital nerve, sensory disturbances

■ Approaches to Posterior Orbit and Orbital Apex (Fig. 20.2)

In these approaches, the removal of one or more orbital walls is usually required.

Lateral Orbitotomy

A lateral orbitotomy is indicated mainly for lateral and superior lesions, from anterior to the orbital apex. It is also known historically as the Kronlein technique, first reported in 1889.

• Skin incision options:
  1. An extended sub-brow incision, directed inferiorly toward the lateral canthus and posteriorly on the superior border of the zygomatic arch
  2. An elongated S-shaped incision starting from the superior eyelid and running inferolaterally toward the lateral canthal region and upper edge of the zygomatic arch
  3. An extended lateral canthotomy incision

4. Coronal approach, which is useful in cases when additional exposure or adjunctive procedures are required

◈ Expose the periosteum of the frontal and lateral orbital rim and zygomatic bones. Make an incision in the periosteum 2-mm posterior and parallel to the orbital margin. Inferior/posterior reflection of the temporalis muscle is also necessary. Dissect the periorbit from the inner surface of the lateral orbital wall. Use a malleable retractor and push the orbit contents medially. Osteotomies are performed as needed. Temporarily mobilize the lateral orbital rim and wall, and expose the periorbita for management of the orbital pathology. Perform replacement/reconstruction of bony structures, ensure proper drainage, and close in layers.

• Possible complications: related to different skin incisions (e.g., superior eyelid vs coronal) and orbital work done

Transnasal Endoscopic Approach

This approach is used in selected lesions of the medial orbital compartment, medial aspect of the superior orbital fissure, and optic canal. It is also very suitable for extraconal lesions. However, using it is more complex for intraconal lesions, for which it can be combined with a superior eyelid approach using a "pushing technique."

◈ Perform a complete spheno-ethmoidectomy and wide maxillary antrostomy. Drill the superior aspect of the palatine bone (orbital process) and manage the sphenopalatine vessels. Drill the lamina papyracea covering the Zinn's annulus, and expose the periorbita. Sometimes a septal window may be required to work contralaterally through the opposite nostril to gain a better angle to the target pathology.

• Possible complications: diplopia, nasal crusting, and sinusitis

Endoscope-Assisted Transorbital Approach

This approach can be done via the following approaches:

1. Superior eyelid approach (see Superior Approaches, above). With endoscopic assistance, the management of select lesions is possible without lateral orbitotomy. Even very select intraorbital lesions can be managed with this approach. The superior eyelid approach can also be combined with other approaches, typically the transnasal one, yielding a combined multiportal approach.

2. Inferior eyelid approach (see Inferior Approaches, above). The inferior eyelid approach can be used for posteriorly and inferolaterally located lesions. It can also be combined with other approaches, typically the transnasal one, yielding a combined multiportal approach.

Coronal Approach

See Chapter 14, on page 337.

Transfacial Approaches

These approaches include the facial disassembling and Le Fort approaches. They are very rarely performed for isolated orbital disease.

■ Selected Procedures

Optic Nerve Decompression

The endonasal approach is used for optic neuropathy. Perform a complete spheno-ethmoidectomy (a wide antrostomy is not necessary). After identification of the sphenoidal landmarks, partially remove the sphenoid mucosa. Drill the annulus of Zinn region and optic canal. The opening of the dura of the optic nerve can be performed but is not always considered necessary; it is best done along the superomedial aspect of the nerve.

Surgical Anatomy Pearl
The ophthalmic artery, in rare cases, can extend into the inferomedial quarter of the optic canal, and thus an incision in this area may damage the artery.

- Possible alternatives: transorbital or transcranial route

Orbital Decompression

A number of different procedures are included under this description. A surgical plan should be designed according to the patient's needs. Endoscopic visualization or visual magnification can be helpful.

- **The medial wall and medial aspect of the inferior wall** can be managed via the caruncular approach or transnasally.
- ◈ Perform a complete spheno-ethmoidectomy and a wide antrostomy. Identify and remove the lamina papyracea (leave it intact at the level of the frontal recess to decrease the risk of frontal sinus disease). Drill the infero-

Surgical Anatomy Pearl
One to four walls can be removed, but keep in mind that after one wall is removed, there is a tendency for the orbital structures to expand into that space, causing a degree of muscle disturbance.

medial angle posteriorly, around the palatine bone. Open the periorbita and gently exert pressure on the eyeball. **The inferior wall** can be managed via inferior eyelid or inferior transconjunctival approaches (see the inferior eyelid approach under Endoscope-Assisted Transorbital Approach, above). Once exposure is complete, remove the areas of the floor both medial and lateral to the infraorbital nerve. With a swinging eyelid approach, inferior and lateral walls can be managed. **The lateral wall and lateral aspect of the orbital roof** can be managed via the superior eyelid approach (or lateral canthal, coronal, and sub-brow; see superior eyelid approach under Superior Approaches, above). Once the superolateral orbit is identified, perform a careful subperiosteal dissection until the superior and inferior orbital fissures are reached. Retract the orbital content medially. A Silastic sheet can be useful to spare periorbital and orbital content.[17] Remove the lateral aspect of the frontal bone and the greater wing of the sphenoid until the anterior and middle cranial base dura are exposed. Open the periorbita and carefully disrupt the orbital septa. Partially remove the inferolateral fat (if necessary). At the end of the procedure, properly drain the area and close the opening in layers.

• Isolated fat removal, usually performed as part of a number of different expansion techniques, can also be done as an isolated procedure. The inferolateral and superomedial compartments are safe areas to decompress. Isolated fat removal can be performed by means of different transconjunctival approaches or even a superior eyelid approach (in this case, fat from the eyelid can also be removed).

Lateral Canthotomy and Inferior Cantholysis

Indicated for a rapid decompression of the orbital contents.

◈ Make a canthotomy incision (cut horizontally through the lateral palpebral fissure). The lower eyelid is still tethered to the lateral orbital rim by the inferior limb of the lateral canthal tendon. Cut the inferior limb, taking care to respect the palpebral skin. After inferior cantholysis, the lower eyelid is freed from the lateral rim. With inferior cantholysis, a partial incision in the inferior orbital septum is made. The orbital content is then free to expand.

Orbital Exenteration

Total Exentaration

◈ Total exenteration is indicated for lesions extending or close to the eyelids.
◈ Make an incision around the orbital rim; the medial part of the incision should be performed at the end. The incision includes skin and subcutaneous tissue. Identify the orbital rim and cut the periosteum.

◈ Elevate the periorbita up to the superior and inferior orbital fissures. Coagulate and cut their contents. Also coagulate and cut the ethmoidal arteries, followed by distraction and excision of the lacrimal sac. Coagulate/ligate and cut the optic nerve and ophthalmic artery at the orbital apex.

◈◈ In cases with very posteriorly located lesions, a lateral orbitotomy can also be performed to adequately control the orbital apex.[4] Endoscopic assistance eliminates the need for a lateral orbitotomy while still providing the surgeon with adequate visualization of the area surrounding the orbital apex. Reconstruction can also be performed, if necessary (temporalis muscle, fat-skin graft). See Chapter 27.

Lid Sparing Exenteration

Used for lesions not involving lid structures.

◈ Make the incision above the ciliary margin superiorly and below the ciliary margin inferiorly. Raise the skin–muscle (palpebral) flap (above orbital septum) until the orbital rim is reached. Make the incision along the periosteum in a circumlinear fashion. The remainder of the procedure is the same as for a total exenteration. A free fat graft or orbital implant is utilized to fill the cavity, and the lids are sutured.

Lid- and Conjunctiva-Sparing Exenteration[4]

◈ Make a lateral canthal incision that reaches to the lateral orbital rim. Dissect the periorbita from the lateral orbital rim. Perform a 360-degree peritomy; isolate and retract the rectus muscles anteriorly with sutures. Cut the levator aponeurosis and lower eyelid retractor from the tarsal plates. Extend the dissection peripherally, until reaching the orbital rim. Surgery proceeds as previously described. The temporalis muscle is transferred inside the orbit through a lateral orbitotomy. Insert a free fat graft to fill the remaining empty spaces.

Surgical Anatomy Pearl

Oversize the free fat graft. Conjunctiva is secured to the free edges of free graft.

• Reconstruction options for exenteration:[4]
  ○ Total exenteration: free grafts, primary healing, myocutaneous graft and flaps
  ○ Lid-sparing exenteration: primary healing, orbital implant, free fat graft, myocutaneous flap (temporalis muscle)
  ○ Lid and conjunctiva sparing exenteration: free fat grafts, dermis–fat graft with temporalis muscle flap
  ○ Extended exenteration: free flaps, myocutaneous flaps

Orbital Traumas

Orbital traumas in which the midface, skull base, and orbit are involved together should be managed by a multidisciplinary team that includes a maxillofacial surgeon, head and neck surgeon, neurosurgeon, and ophthalmoplastic surgeon, for optimal results. When dealing with these patients, first determine if they are conscious or not.

If the patient is unconscious: (1) inspect the face, orbital contours, and lids; (2) inspect the globe for position, integrity, hemorrhage, and lacerations; (3) inspect shape of pupils, pupil reaction, and the blink reflex; (4) if possible, inspect the fundus oculi.

If the patient is conscious, perform the same evaluation as above, but in addition evaluate visual acuity of both eyes, ocular movement, and supra- and infraorbital nerve sensation as well.

When examining the eyelids, be careful to never force the eyelid open if there is evidence of laceration. Two criteria are used for surgical intervention: ocular motility and orbital volume.

Other indications for surgery: wide orbital floor fracture with evident displacement and disruption of more than 40 to 50% of the floor; persistent diplopia with radiological evidence of muscle entrapment; enophthalmos > 2 mm at 2 weeks after trauma; early enophthalmos (in such cases surgery should be performed in 1 to 3 days).

Usually, combined fracture of the medial and inferior wall of the orbit requires surgery because of evident volume increase. Orbital rim fractures usually require surgical management, via osteosynthesis.

Contraindications to surgery include patients with eyeball damage (that should be treated first) or only one functional eye.

Goals of surgery: prevent visual impairment, minimize diplopia and eyeball displacement. Surgical approaches depend on the extension and type of the fractures and the involvement of several subunits (e.g., facial skeleton fractures). It is mandatory to evaluate and document visual function prior to surgical intervention. Take extra caution when operating on the only functional eye. Key surgical concept: the edge of the fracture site should be isolated from all margins and the prolapsed orbital content is gradually returned into the orbit.

Blowout fractures: One or more walls of the orbit are fractured, leaving the orbital rim intact. The following clinical features suggest the presence of a blowout fracture:

Diplopia
Enophthalmos
Orbital emphysema
Periorbital hematoma
Conjunctival hematoma or chemosis
Globe displacement
Abnormal motility
Anesthesia (V_1 and V_2 areas)

In the acute presentation, enophthalmos is frequently obscured by the presence of edema.

Orbital Floor Fracture

◈ Approaches: skin incision (skin crease/inferior eyelid, subtarsal, etc.), transconjunctival (inferior fornix), transnasal/transantral (endoscopically assisted).
 • The inferior eyelid approach is one of the most versatile.
◈ Regardless of the approach chosen, find the orbital rim and dissect it in a subperiosteal plane to gain adequate fracture exposure.
◈ Use implants if defects > 5 mm. Otherwise, replace fractured bones.
◈ The endoscopic transantral approach is another good option in the case of isolated orbital floor fractures (not well suitable for wide bony defects).

Medial Wall Fractures

◈ If isolated (rare), they usually do not require surgery unless diplopia is present.
◈ Most of the time this kind of fracture is associated with an orbital floor fracture.
◈ Check for cerebrospinal fluid (CSF) leak or lacrimal system damage.
◈ Approaches: skin incision (Lynch; see above), transconjunctival (pre- or transcaruncolar), transnasal (endoscopic assisted)

Orbitozygomatic Fractures

These fractures usually affect the facial contour as well. If so, also check for visual impairment, dystopia, and trismus. Inferior displacement of lateral canthal tendon and orbital rim step deformities are commonly seen. Surgical goals: regain adequate eyeball position and facial contour, and minimize diplopia and trismus. If there is no bone displacement, surgery is not indicated.

◈ These fractures are usually treated via the transoral approach through a *vestibular incision* (can be combined with superior eyelid approach to control the frontozygomatic area).
◈ Alternatively, an entry wound incision can be used to access the fracture.

Orbital Roof

The orbital roof is very rarely isolated. In most cases, it is associated with other craniofacial fractures and intracranial damage. In more than 90% of cases, frontal sinus wall fractures are present. Clinically, patients have orbital rim step deformities and focal tenderness, forehead depression, and vertical diplopia if the trochlea is damaged. A large blow-in fracture may cause pulsatile exophthalmos.

◈ Managed via entry wound, superior eyelid, or coronal approach.
◈ Rim fractures should be fixed.
◈ Neurosurgical injuries are usually more prominent and take priority in management.

Orbital Apex Fractures

These fractures are rarely isolated. They are usually managed via the craniotomic route, given the presence of intracranial damage. In selected cases without intracranial damage, the transnasal approach can be used. Optic nerve decompression can be attempted. Regardless of the approach, the goal of treatment is to remove compressive bone fragments and decompress the canal. Controversy still exists regarding the exact role of optic nerve decompression due to limited published data.

Nasoethmoidal Fractures

Management includes the attempt to restore the normal intercanthal distance and position of the posterior insertion of the medial canthal tendon to the posterior lacrimal crest.

◈ Managed via Lynch incision or coronal approach
◈ Fixation of any bony fragments

Craniofacial and Cranio-Orbital Approaches

See Chapter 14.

Frontal and Frontotemporal Craniotomy with or Without Supraorbital Rim Preservation

See Chapter 14, page 348.

Frontotemporal-Orbitozygomatic Approach

See Chapter 14, page 353.

■ References

Boldfaced references are of particular importance.

1. **Bonavolontà G, Strianese D, Grassi P, et al. An analysis of 2,480 space-occupying lesions of the orbit from 1976 to 2011. Ophthal Plast Reconstr Surg 2013;29:79–86**
2. Khandekar RB, Al-Towerki AA, Al-Katan H, et al. Ocular malignant tumors. Review of the Tumor Registry at a tertiary eye hospital in central Saudi Arabia. Saudi Med J 2014;35:377–384
3. Murphy C, Livingstone I, Foot B, Murgatroyd H, MacEwen CJ. Orbital cellulitis in Scotland: current incidence, aetiology, management and outcomes. Br J Ophthalmol 2014;98:1575–1578
4. Rootman J. Orbital Surgery. A Conceptual Approach, 2nd ed. Philadelphia: Lippincott & Williams; 2014
5. Sesenna E, Poli T, Magri AS. Orbital approaches. In: Cappabianca P, Iaconetta G, Califano L, eds. Cranial, Craniofacial and Skull Base Surgery. New York: Springer-Verlag; 2010:259–280
6. Sesenna E, Raffaini M, Tullio A, Moscato G. Orbital marginotomies for treatment of orbital and periorbital lesions. Int J Oral Maxillofac Surg 1994;23:76–84
7. Lynch RC. The technique of a radical frontal sinus operation which has given me the best results. Laryngoscope 1921;31:1–5
8. Moe KS. The precaruncular approach to the medial orbit. Arch Facial Plast Surg 2003;5:483–487
9. McCord CD Jr. A combined lateral and medial orbitotomy for exposure of the optic nerve and orbital apex. Ophthalmic Surg 1978;9:58–66
10. Wojno TH. Surgical approaches to orbital disease. Ophthalmol Clin North Am 1996;9:581–599
11. **Khan AM, Varvares MA. Traditional approaches to the orbit. Otolaryngol Clin North Am 2006;39:895–909, vi**
12. Eppley BL, Custer PL, Sadove AM. Cutaneous approaches to the orbital skeleton and periorbital structures. J Oral Maxillofac Surg 1990;48:842–854
13. Wilson S, Ellis E III. Surgical approaches to the infraorbital rim and orbital floor: the case for the subtarsal approach. J Oral Maxillofac Surg 2006;64:104–107
14. Ellis EI, Zide MF. Surgical Approaches to the Facial Skeleton, 2nd ed. Philadelphia: Lippincott Williams & Wilkins; 2005
15. Holtmann B, Wray RC, Little AG. A randomized comparison of four incisions for orbital fractures. Plast Reconstr Surg 1981;67:731–737
16. Manson PN, Ruas E, Iliff N, Yaremchuk M. Single eyelid incision for exposure of the zygomatic bone and orbital reconstruction. Plast Reconstr Surg 1987;79:120–126
17. Sellari-Franceschini S. Balanced orbital decompression in Grave's orbitopathy. Oper Tech Otolaryngol--Head Neck Surg 2012;23:219–226

21 Middle Skull Base Surgery

■ 21.1 Meningiomas Involving the Sphenoid Bone

■ General Information

Incidence

Meningiomas involving the sphenoid bone account for 11 to 18% of all intracranial meningiomas.[1–3]

Definitions and Classifications

The classification of the sphenoid meningiomas is based on their anatomic localization on the sphenoid wings (**Fig. 21.1**). The most common ones arise from the lesser wing; those on the greater wing are referred to as lateral sphenoid wing meningiomas and middle fossa meningiomas, although the size often blurs the distinction. Colloquially, the wings are incorrectly referred to as one wing, and the tumors are classified as those that occupy the medial, middle, or lateral component of the wing, or they may involve the orbit as spheno-orbital meningiomas. Other nomenclature:

- Outer third meningiomas, middle third sphenoidal wing meningiomas, clinoidal, and spheno-orbital meningiomas. **Outer third of the sphenoidal ridge meningiomas**: "pterional" meningiomas are essentially convexity meningiomas.
- **Middle sphenoidal wing meningiomas**: also called "alar" meningiomas.
- **Clinoidal meningiomas**: in the region of the anterior clinoid process (ACP) or the "medial" sphenoid wing. For the anatomic complexity of the ACP, clinoidal meningiomas have been classified separately[4] (see below).
- **Spheno-orbital meningiomas**: Prominent bone invasion and hyperostosis characterize these tumors that essentially involve the orbital walls, giving rise to neuro-ophthalmologic or cosmetic problems (e.g., exophthalmos,

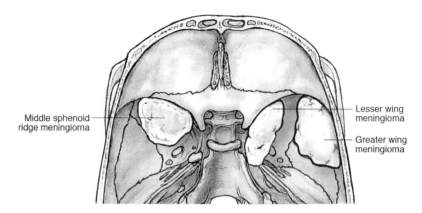

Fig. 21.1   Localizations of the sphenoid meningiomas.

proptosis). The subdural component of the tumor may be globular or may be quite thin and almost nonapparent in an "en-plaque" growth pattern. In any patient with exophthalmos and hyperostosis of the orbital walls, look for an en-plaque tumor; there will usually be one. The en-plaque growth pattern is defined as follows:

○ **En-plaque meningiomas**: The definition is related to the growth pattern of the meningioma, which enables differentiation from the most typical "globular mass" meningioma. En-plaque meningiomas infiltrate the dura mater in a diffuse, sheet-like appearance, giving rise to marked hyperostosis. Microscopically, they are identical to other meningiomas. This growth pattern is seen in 2 to 9% of all meningiomas.[5-7] The sphenoid wing is the typical localization of en-plaque meningiomas, although they have been described also in other skull regions. Their extensive origins can make them difficult to resect completely. The differential diagnosis includes other hyperostosis conditions: osteoma, Paget's disease, fibrous dysplasia.

Classification Systems of Sphenoidal Meningiomas (Fig. 21.1)

- Five categories[8,9]: A, clinoidal tumors; B, en plaque meningiomas with hyperostosis of the sphenoid bone; C, large invasive tumors of the sphenoid ridge; D, middle sphenoid ridge; E, lateral sphenoid ridge.
- According to the invasion of the surrounding structures [10]: A, lateral sphenoid wing, middle sphenoid wing, medial sphenoid wing with or without cavernous sinus (CS) infiltration; B, en-plaque meningiomas with or without CS infiltration; C, purely intraosseous tumors.

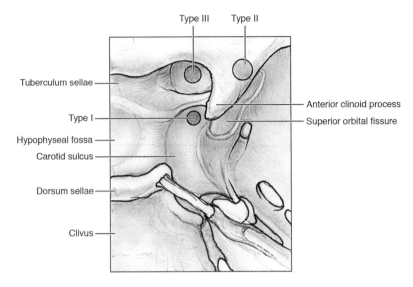

Fig. 21.2   Clinoidal meningioma types. (Adapted from Kristh AF. Clinoidal meningiomas. In: DeMonte F, McDermott MW, Al-Mefty O, eds. Al-Mefty's Meningiomas, 2nd ed. New York, Stuttgart: Thieme; 2011:228–236.)

Classification of the Clinoidal Meningiomas (Fig. 21.2)

Three types[4]:

- **Type I:** medial to the ACP, extra-arachnoidal, arising from the subclinoidal dura at the level where the internal carotid artery (ICA) from its subdural component enters into the arachnoidal cisternal space.
- **Type II:** arising superolaterally to the ACP; growing in the arachnoidal plane around the carotid cistern; separated then from the ICA and optic nerve by arachnoid membranes. This is the most common type.
- **Type III:** arising from the optic foramen region and extending into it (giving rise to early ophthalmologic disturbances because of invasion of the pial layer). Be aware of the risk of visual loss and ICA injury when complete resection is attempted.

Classification of the Spheno-Orbital Meningiomas[11]

Four types, based on the intraorbital tumor localization:

- I, superolateral; II, inferomedial; III, orbital apex; IV, diffuse[11]

Signs and Symptoms

The signs and symptoms are related to the size of the meningioma and the anatomic relationships.

- Exophthalmos: spheno-orbital tumors, hyperostosis of the orbital walls
- Often only headache or vertigo for asymptomatic tumors
- Blindness, optic nerve atrophy, visual field deficits (more typical for the clinoidal and spheno-orbital meningiomas)
- Diplopia, oculomotor or trigeminal deficits: in cases of involvement of the CS and/or orbital fissures or intraorbital invasion
- Cosmetic disturbances: pterional tumors invading the bone or temporal muscle
- Major and minor neurologic deficits (e.g., aphasia, hemiparesis, personality changes, memory loss, seizures) due to large tumors compressing the surrounding brain (especially in large pterional meningiomas)
- Seizures

Diagnostic Workup

Computed tomography (CT) is essential for defining hyperostosis. Magnetic resonance imaging (MRI) with fat suppression is necessary for detecting intraorbital extension of the tumor. Computed tomography angiography (CTA), or angiogram, may be required to define the relationships of the tumors with the ICA and the middle cerebral artery (MCA). Balloon test occlusion may be required when involvement of the ICA is observed and a more aggressive surgical treatment is planned.

Sphenoid meningiomas always require a strict pre- and postoperative neuro-ophthalmologic follow-up. The medial ones should have an endocrinologic assessment, especially in patients of childbearing age.

Treatment

Radiological follow-up ("scan and see") is appropriate in asymptomatic patients with small tumors. In symptomatic patients, surgery is recommended especially for healthy and younger patients. Early and aggressive surgical treatment has been advocated in medial sphenoid wing meningiomas for maximizing the outcome and for vision preservation.[12]

- Radiotherapy (RT) and/or radiosurgery (RS) are valid alternatives, as well as subtotal/partial resection followed by RT/RS. RS is only used in those cases with at least 2 to 3 mm between the lesion and the optic nerve and chiasm so as to keep doses below 8 Gy. See also Chapter 30.

Intraoperative Neuromonitoring

Intraoperative neuromonitoring is not always required or useful, but electro-myogram (EMG) of the oculomotor muscles may be of help for tumors with intraorbital or CS involvement (see page 90).

■ Surgical Approaches (Fig. 21.3)

1. Pterional/frontotemporal craniotomy is performed based on the size of the tumor, with an additional orbitocranial (OC) or orbitozygomatic (OZ) oste-otomy in order to further expose the anterior and middle cranial fossa, and to avoid brain retraction (see also **Fig. 14.8**, page 354).
2. Lateral supraorbital approach may be indicated.
3. Lateral transzygomatic approach may be indicated in some cases, such as for mobilization of the entire zygoma, leaving it pedicled on the masseter muscle.[13]

Lateral sphenoid bone and temporal bone can be hypertrophic and hypervas-cular. Performing a craniotomy on these bones is often dangerous and difficult. In such situation, drilling the bones is a valid alternative to the craniotomy.[14]

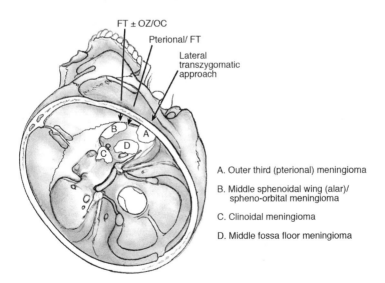

FT ± OZ/OC

Pterional/ FT

Lateral transzygomatic approach

A. Outer third (pterional) meningioma

B. Middle sphenoidal wing (alar)/ spheno-orbital meningioma

C. Clinoidal meningioma

D. Middle fossa floor meningioma

Fig. 21.3 Surgical approaches to the sphenoid tumors. FT, frontotemporal; OC, orbitocra-nial; OZ, orbitozygomatic.

❖ Surgical Step

◈ Perform an extradural dissection lateromedially to devascularize the tumor. Coagulation and division of the middle meningeal artery early are helpful in devascularizing the tumor.

Lateral and Middle Sphenoidal Ridge Meningiomas

◈◈ Drilling invaded/hyperostosis bone may be performed after dura dissection to further devascularize the meningioma.

◈ A curvilinear incision may be performed on the dura. Avoid early incision of the mediobasal dura in order to avoid epidural oozing in the subdural space.[15]

◈ An initial debulking of the tumor, also by means of the ultrasonic surgical aspirator, may be required for large tumors.

◈ Identify and preserve all the branches coming from the MCA, which may appear "engulfed" by the tumor; the arachnoid layer is often preserved.

Surgical Anatomy Pearl

Study meticulously the preoperative images for assessing the relationships. A true invasion of the MCA wall is very rare.[4] Because the arachnoid is usually preserved by the tumor, stay outside the arachnoid and do not disturb the MCA or its branches. If the subarachnoid space must be opened, follow the branches of the MCA from the lateral aspect to the medial aspect. Try to preserve each of the small lenticulostriate arteries, which are very fragile and can be encased and stretched by the tumor.

◈ After debulking, whenever required, perform a dissection of the tumor, keeping the arachnoid with the patient. This is mandatory in primary surgery, but it is more demanding (or not possible at all) in invasive meningiomas, recurrences, or after radiation therapy.

◈ Any dura involved with the tumor (showing nodules, thickening, or dura looking invaded) should be resected. If available, do intraoperative histological analysis of dural margins to identify invasion.

◈◈ For tumors involving the base of the middle cranial fossa, the dissection also has to be done around the foramina of the fossa. In cases of infratemporal invasion, the middle cranial fossa can be drilled as well.

◈◈ For the involvement of the CS, leave the tumor in situ and treat the residual with Gamma Knife or fractionated radiation if there is any concern about regrowth.

Pearl

Portions of the tumor involving the CS are better treated by RS/RT, which have better results for ophthalmoparesis and carotid artery preservation.[10,15–19]

◈◈ In cases of invasion of the orbit, dissect and strip the periorbita from the tumor. Generally, the opening of the periorbita is not necessary, except in cases where the tumor is infiltrated by tumor nodules.[15]

◈◈ In cases of involvement of the superior orbital fissure, avoid excessive resection of the bony structures around it or transgression of the annulus of Zinn.

Surgical Anatomy Pearl

In general, the tumors are extraconal and extra-periorbital.

Clinoidal Meningiomas

• Types I and III are the most difficult to remove due to their tight relationship with the internal carotid artery and the lack of a true arachnoidal plane.
• Type II has a higher chance to be totally removed with less risk of injuring the ICA and the optic nerve.
◈ In such tumors, extradural anterior clinoidectomy may be indicated.
◈ The optic canal can be decompressed at this stage or after intradural debulking/resection of the tumor. If needed, resect the optic strut and the optic roof with drill (under copious irrigation) or with ultrasonic bone aspirator (see page 321).

Surgical Anatomy Pearl

Do not coagulate around the optic nerve; every small oozing has to be controlled with Gelfoam or other hemostatic materials.

◈ Open the dural layer over the optic nerve (compulsory in type III clinoidal meningiomas).
◈ After the extradural part, open the dura in curvilinear fashion, and perform arachnoid dissection to expose the margins of the tumor.
• The goal of surgery in type II and III clinoidal meningiomas is total resection, but subtotal resection may be required in type I (and III, in some cases) clinoidal meningiomas, in order to avoid excessive risk of injury of the ICA.[20]

Spheno-Orbital Meningiomas

Complete resection of these tumors may not be feasible, if the optic nerve dura propria is breached. The goal of surgery is tissue diagnosis, decompression to relieve proptosis and visual deficits, and resection of as much of the tumor as is safe to perform.[21]

◈ These cases are ideal for the two-piece OZ approach after a frontotemporal craniotomy. Alternatively, one can simply drill through the hyperostotic superior and/or lateral wall(s) of the orbit after a frontotemporal craniotomy and access the orbital tumor from this approach.
◈ Resect the lateral and superolateral orbital walls invaded by the tumor.

◈   Resect all the intraorbital–extra-periorbital components of the tumor. Nodules invading the periorbita may require opening of the periorbita. Invasion of the annulus of Zinn should not be approached aggressively in order to avoid the risk of cranial nerves injury.

◈   Perform a wide opening of the optic canal for tumors extending medially and affecting the optic nerve.

◈◈ For the rare tumor invading the inferior part of the orbit and/or nasoethmoidal cells, an anterior approach (either in a second surgical step),[9] a combined infratemporal approach,[22] or a transmalar or transzygomatic subciliary approach may be performed.[23]

◈◈ Combined approaches requiring transcranial approach and endonasal endoscopic approach may be required for multicompartmental sphenoid meningiomas.[24]

◈◈ For the rare tumors invading the maxillary/malar bones, craniofacial approaches have to be performed, and bone reconstruction is performed for cosmetic reasons.

■ Reconstruction

Resected dura should be replaced by fascia lata, temporalis muscle fascia, or rarely pericranium. According to several neurosurgeons, these biological tissues remain the best material for duraplasty. Synthetic materials for duraplasty may be used as well.

• Reinforce the closure with fibrin glue if there is a risk of cerebrospinal fluid (CSF) leak.

• Periorbital defects should be repaired, with stitches or fascia lata/pericranium.

• Orbital reconstruction is required only for massive destruction of the orbital walls (by the tumor and/or after surgery), causing enophthalmos.

• Non-watertight duraplasty without orbital reconstruction is often satisfactory.[14]

■ Outcome

Alar and pterional sphenoid meningiomas have a higher rate of total resection and better outcome in comparison with clinoid meningiomas (which have a higher risk of new or worsened neurologic deficits, occurring in 19%).[25] Gross total resection is performed in 65 to 100% of alar sphenoid meningiomas[3,25] versus 43 to 65% of clinoidal meningiomas.[12,26]

Visual improvement occurs in up to 64 to 80% of clinoidal meningiomas.[12]

■ Complications

- Worsening cranial neuropathy, especially in tumors invading the optic canal or CS (20% of cases)[25]
- CSF leakage: consider also the extremely rare iatrogenic CSF orbitorrhea (CSF leakage into the orbit) or oculorrhea (CSF leakage through the orbit to the exterior side)[27]
- Neurologic deficits: aphasia, hemiparesis (< 9%)
- Seizures, especially with the alar meningiomas
- Hydrocephalus (< 7%), stroke, wound infection, pneumonia

■ Middle Fossa Floor Meningiomas

These meningiomas arise from the fossa of the middle skull base, with no connection (or less than 25% connection) to the surrounding more typical localizations (sphenoid wing, CS, tentorium, lateral convexity).[28–31]

Incidence

They account for 1.4% of all intracranial meningiomas.[28]

Classification

These meningiomas can be classified based on their connection/dural attachment.[28]

Signs and Symptoms

Signs and symptoms include headache, seizures, trigeminal deficits/neuralgia, cognitive decline, gait disturbances, hearing loss, and diplopia.

Surgical Approaches

The approaches include a frontotemporal craniotomy with or without OZ osteotomy, and a temporal craniotomy with or without a zygomatic osteotomy.

Outcome

Generally, these tumors are diagnosed when they become symptomatic due to their large size (> 3 cm), and the described overall surgical morbidity is 33%

(new neurologic deficit in 20% of patients, worse neurologic deficit in 20%).[28] Simpson grade 1 or 2 resection was achieved in 67% of patients in the only published series on purely middle fossa meningiomas.[29,30]

■ 21.2 Sellar/Parasellar Tumors

■ General Information

Review topographic anatomy, page 13.

Sellar/Parasellar Tumors

These tumors are listed in **Table 21.1.**

Signs and Symptoms

The signs and symptoms include headache (generally nonspecific, sometimes localized to the vertex or fronto-orbital region) and visual abnormalities (blurred vision, decreased visual acuity, decreased night vision, tunneling of vision, campimetric deficits, papilledema).[1]

In giant tumors, the following signs are seen: compression of the frontal lobe, frontal lobe syndrome with mental deterioration, short-term memory loss, anosmia, and generalized seizures. Hypothalamus involvement is indicated by thermoregulatory imbalances. Cavernous sinus involvement is indicated by facial pain, oculomotor deficits and diplopia, and ptosis. Sphenoidal sinus erosion

Table 21.1   Lesions of the Sellar/Parasellar Region

Benign tumors	Pituitary adenomas, meningiomas (tuberculum sellae, diaphragma sellae, from other surrounding anatomic structures), craniopharyngiomas, schwannomas, lipomas
Malignant tumors	Lymphomas, germ cell tumors, chordomas, chondrosarcomas, pituitary carcinomas, pituitary blastomas, metastases
Infiltrative processes	Lymphocytic hypophysitis, sarcoidosis, tuberculosis, histiocytosis X
Cysts	Rathke cleft cyst, arachnoid cyst, dermoid cyst
Other lesions	Abscesses, arteriovenous fistulas, germinomas, hemangiomas, granular cell tumors, gangliocytomas, astrocytomas, hamartomas, aneurysms

is indicated by CSF leak and epistaxis. Endocrinologic signs and symptoms are described in Chapter 9.

Diagnostic Workup

Computed tomography is essential for defining the sellar-parasellar and nasal anatomy, and above all for surgical planning. X-ray may show enlargement/erosion of the sellar region due to pituitary macroadenomas or meningiomas. MRI is essential for defining localization and involvement of the optic chiasm and frontal lobe edema (T2 sequences). MRI with fat suppression is useful for identifying tumor extension into the optic canal. CTA or, rarely, angiogram may be required to define the relationships of the tumors relative to anterior cerebral arteries, or to rule out the presence of aneurysms (see Chapter 5).

- Perform a neuro-ophthalmologic workup (see Chapter 10).
- Perform an endocrinologic workup for pituitary gland/hypothalamus functionality. Check for adiposity, subnormal temperature, slow pulse, and increased sugar tolerance, indicative of hypothalamic dysfunction.
- If an endoscopic transsphenoidal approach is planned, a full otolaryngological assessment with nasal endoscopy is needed to assess the sinonasal cavities for any concurrent pathologies (e.g., nasal polyps), anatomic variants from prior surgery (e.g., septal perforation), or any relative contraindications to endonasal surgery (e.g., narrow surgical corridor because of nasal vestibule stenosis or untreated sinusitis).
- Perform neuropsychological tests as well: Montreal Cognitive Assessment (MOCA), Mini–Mental State Examination (MMSE), or other tests for frontal lobe functionality and memory, which are useful above all for follow-up over time.

Treatment

Asymptomatic small tumors should be followed over time. Radiosurgery is an option for patients in whom surgery is not indicated or for tumor remnants/recurrences, especially in the case of pituitary adenomas that are clinically aggressive. Surgery remains the gold standard of treatment, particularly for symptomatic patients with signs of rapid visual deterioration.

■ Pituitary Tumors

Epidemiology and Pathology

For epidemiology and pathology, see page 143; for endocrinology, see page 222.

Classification

Endocrinologic Classification

Pituitary tumors are classified as functional (secreting) or nonfunctional (non-secreting).

Size-Related classification

Microadenomas are less than 10 mm in size, and macroadenomas are 10 mm or larger. Giant adenomas have a size > 40 mm or volume > 10 cm³.[2]

Histological and Immunohistochemistry Classification

See **Table 6.2**, page 133.

Anatomic Classification

Pituitary tumors can be sellar, suprasellar and/or parasellar. They can invade the surrounding spaces, such as the sphenoid sinus and/or the CS (as shown radiologically or histologically).

- The Hardy classification system[3,4] is described in **Fig. 21.4.**

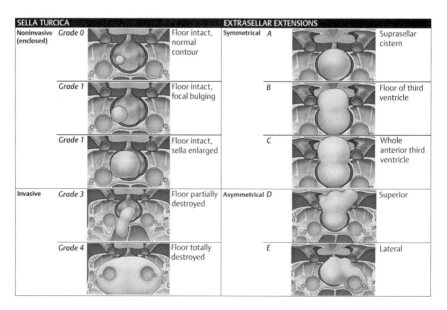

Fig. 21.4   The Hardy classification for evaluating pituitary tumor extension.

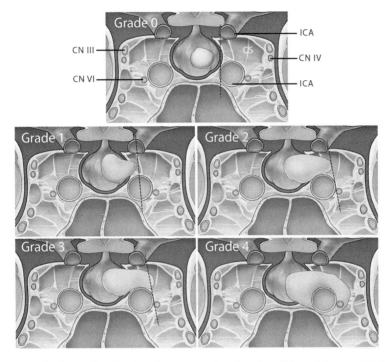

Fig. 21.5   The Knosp classification of cavernous sinus invasion. CN, cranial nerve; ICA, internal carotid artery. The dashed line shows the lateral extension of the pituitary adenoma in regard of the ICA.

The suprasellar extension of the tumor is not a criterion of invasiveness, because such extension may be related to the position of the adenoma within the normal pituitary gland, the size of the opening of the diaphragma sellae,[5] or the presence or size of the arachnoidal subdiaphragmatic cistern.[6]

- A grade five has been added for distant spread via CSF or blood (pituitary carcinoma).[7] The asymmetrical parasellar extension type E refers to the extracranial extradural invasion (into the lateral CS).[7]
- The Knosp classification system[8] **(Fig. 21.5)** is based on the invasion of the CS, with grades 3 and 4 considered to be true cavernous invasion.

Clinical Classification

Tumors are classified as typical adenomas and aggressive pituitary adenomas, the latter showing earlier and more frequent recurrences and possible resistance to conventional treatments, including radiotherapy.[9]

Surgical Indications for Pituitary Tumors

Indications include Cushing's disease, acromegaly, prolactinoma not responsive to medical therapy, nonfunctioning tumors with mass effect on the optic system or beyond, and pituitary apoplexy with optic nerve or chiasm functional impairment.

- Pituitary tumors may require a multimodal treatment, especially the aggressive ones.
- See indications and outcomes of radiotherapy on pituitary tumors on page 774.

Approaches to Pituitary Tumors

Transcranial Surgery

Pituitary tumors, particularly the giant ones with large suprasellar components/ invasion of the surrounding structures, may be treated by the standard transcranial approaches: pterional or subfrontal craniotomies (± OZ osteotomy), or rarely a subtemporal approach. Many of these patients can be treated by means of transsphenoidal approaches, particularly endoscopic ones.[2]

Transcranial surgery may be helpful if transsphenoidal surgery is considered difficult or contraindicated. For example, many surgeons in the past considered the conchal-type sphenoid sinus (see **Fig. 2.14**, page 53) as a relative indication for a craniotomy. However, with neuronavigation, this indication is becoming rare. Infections of the nose/paranasal sinuses, asymmetric extension of giant tumors around the parasellar compartments, some hourglass tumors (constrained into small openings of the diaphragm), and tumors with a very firm or fibrous consistency may still benefit from a craniotomy approach.

Endonasal Submucosal with Sublabial or Transseptal Approaches

See page 345.

Endoscopic Transsphenoidal Approach

In several centers, this approach is considered the gold standard, although not universally accepted as such.

Combined Approaches

Very stiff sellar tumors with large suprasellar components may require a combined approach, such as transsphenoidal approach for intrasellar component resection followed by the transcranial route. Also, giant multicompartmental tumors may require combined approaches (such as the pterional approach for lateral extension of the tumor, and the interhemispheric transventricular approach for resection of the intraventricular components).

❖ Endoscopic approach, technical nuances (see also Chapter 16):

◈ A nasoseptal vascularized mucosal pedicled flap can be used in patients at risk for postoperative CSF leakage. It can also be used for bone coverage and to avoid excessive postoperative crusting.

◈ The approach may be performed via a single nostril or by using the four-hand bi-portal technique,[10] although the biportal technique with a posterior septostomy and sphenoidotomy is used more commonly.

◈ The sphenoid sinus anatomic landmarks must be recognized (see **Fig. 2.15**, page 54). Removal of the sphenoidal septa enables wider surgical access. It is important to note the location of the septa on preoperative imaging and to connect these locations to intraoperative findings in order to clearly correlate and validate the intrasphenoidal surgical anatomy, including the position of the ICA. Stripping of the mucosa may also help in recognizing the landmarks.

◈ The bone of the sellar floor may be (1) thinned by using a diamond drill and then fractured; (2) removed with punches; or (3) removed en bloc by using chisels and a mallet if the sellar floor is thin in the periphery of the bony margins. Save the bony flap for reuse in the reconstruction of the sellar floor after the tumor resection. The margins of the sellar opening may be widened using punches, in order to identify the "four blues", that is, the two CSs bilaterally and the superior and inferior intercavernous sinuses (the latter, whenever present) on the superior and inferior margins. If available, use a micro-Doppler probe for detecting the ICA. Doppler may also identify the superior and inferior intercavernous sinuses.

◈◈ Whenever present and required, coagulate the inferior intercavernous sinus.

◈ Open the dura-periosteum of the sellar floor to expose the tumor. The dura can be opened by making a quadrangular incision, a T incision, or a stellate incision (star shaped), in order to have access to the tumor.

◈ Debulking of the tumor may be performed, especially in macroadenomas; otherwise an extracapsular dissection is suggested for an en-bloc resection, sparing the normal gland parenchyma. Start the dissection on the floor of the sella, proceeding laterally toward the CSs. The superior dissection has to reach the normal arachnoid of the diaphragma sellae. Use microcurettes of different sizes and angles to approach all the sides and components of the tumor (including the intracavernous components, whenever possible).

❖ Try to save a sufficient amount of tumor for pathology analysis (including electron microscopy). In cases of a very soft or very small tumor, which can be easily aspirated, a "suction trap" connected to the surgical suction tubing may be useful.

❖ Use angled optics (≥ 30 degrees) for suprasellar components of the tumor.

• Suprasellar components of the tumor might fall downward with the Valsalva maneuver.

• Control intratumoral bleeding with a hemostatic agent such as methylcellulose; local coagulation is generally not required. In large tumors, leaving a superior remnant may be risky because the remnant can hemorrhage postoperatively and cause hypothalamic compression. Usually, the bleeding from the tumor stops when the entire tumor has been removed. If it does not, look for more tumor or for injury to critical structures such as the venous sinus, the ICA, or a branch of the ICA, and consider packing it or ordering an angiogram when the bleeding is controlled.

> **Surgical Anatomy Pearl**
>
> The best way to avoid CSF leak is to keep the arachnoid intact. This can be achieved in over 95% of first-time surgeries.

Outcome

In microadenoma and non-giant macroadenoma, it is often possible to perform a total resection of the tumor. In giant pituitary adenoma, gross total resection has been achieved in 24% of patients, near-total resection in 17%, subtotal resection in 36%, and partial resection in 23%.[11] A case series has shown a higher reduction of the volume of giant pituitary adenoma treated by means of the endoscopic transsphenoidal surgery than by means of a microscopic transsphenoidal or transcranial approach[2] (**Table 21.2**).

• Visual deficit improvement in giant pituitary adenomas resection occurs at rates of 60 to 90%.[2,11]

• In pituitary adenomas with CS invasion, endoscopic endonasal resection is a feasible technique[12,13] that enables resection of 85% of tumors with Knosp grade 1 or 2 and 67% of tumors with Knosp grade 3 or 4.[14] The endonasal medial-to-lateral approach enables good resection of tumors in the medial aspect of the CS, but is not satisfactory in the lateral compartment. In fact, total/subtotal resection of the tumor in the most lateral part of the CS is generally not feasible by means of the endoscopic approach. In patients with acromegaly, CS invasion is the most significant predictor of unfavorable outcome, and aggressive removal of the invading tumor and of the medial wall of the CS, whenever feasible, is advocated by some authors to increase the remission rate.[15] Remnants/recurrences in the CS after debulking endoscopic

Table 21.2   Outcomes of Surgical Resection of Giant Pituitary Adenomas (Volume > 10 cm³) in a Series of 72 Patients[2]

Outcome	BETS	MTS	Craniotomy
Gross total removal	20.7% Y	14.3% Y	
	79.3% N	85.7% N	100% N
Visual improvement	96.2% Y	85.7% Y	72.4% Y
	3.8% N	14.3% N	27.6% N
Headache improvement	100% Y	100%	81.8% Y
			18.2% N
General complications*	7.0 %Y	7.1% Y	31.0% Y
	93.0% N	92.8% N	69.0% N
Days of hospitalization	6.58	5.57	16.57
(mean, range)	(2–52)	(0–13)	(2–184)

Abbreviations: BETS, binasal endoscopic transsphenoidal approach; DI, diabetes insipidus; MTS, microscopic transsphenoidal approach; Y, yes; N, no.
*Pulmonary embolism, deep vein thrombosis, hydrocephalus, subdural hygroma, vasospasm, postoperative hematoma, bacteremia, death. Of such complications: death in 0% of the BETS and MTS group vs 3.4% in the craniotomy group.
Note: Only some of the significant results are reported.

surgery should be evaluated for their hormonal production, growth, or potential for neurologic deficit. Despite the presence of remnants, many patients can still show endocrine remission.[16] For those without a medical or surgical option, radiosurgery remains an effective alternative for tumor control and is also reasonable for endocrinologic control.

- The outcomes of transsphenoidal and microsurgical approaches for pituitary tumors are likely equivalent for experienced surgeons,[17] although in some studies the endoscopic approach seems to provide an improved likelihood of tumor removal, and it is safer,[18] especially for tumors within the CS.[2,19,20] Some authors believe that vascular complications may be more prevalent in the endoscopic transsphenoidal technique,[21] whereas others find no difference.[5] The microscopic and endoscopic techniques provide similar outcomes in the treatment of nonfunctioning pituitary adenomas (at least in Knosp grade 0 to 2 tumor types).[22]

Complications of Pituitary Tumor Surgery

- The overall complication rate is 9%[23]; the surgical mortality is < 1%.
- CSF leakage occurs in 5% or less.[23] A series has shown a higher intraoperative rate with the endoscopic technique than with the microscopic technique, with no difference in the incidence of postoperative CSF rhinorrhea.[22] The risk of meningitis is < 2%.

- Visual deterioration occurs in 2%.
- Hypothalamic injury, hypopituitarism, diabetes insipidus (transient in < 5%, permanent in < 1%),[24] CS nerves injury, brain/brainstem injury.
- Pneumocephalus (especially in the endoscopic approaches).
- Vascular complication (< 2% ICA injury; it is possible to lower it to 0% by using the intraoperative Doppler probe and micro-hook blade[25]). Rare cases of postoperative ICA vasospasm have been described in the event that subarachnoid bleeding is encountered.[26]

Surgical Pearl

Rescue in case of ICA injury: pack the defect with hemostatic material (Gelfoam, Surgicel), and transfer the patient to the endovascular suite for cerebral angiogram and endovascular repair. Proximal control of the cervical ICA in the neck is rarely required but can be lifesaving in the even that it becomes necessary to control bleeding.

- The endonasal approaches are related also to rhinological complications (epistaxis, hyposmia/anosmia, nasal crusting/synechiae, mucocele/pyocele, septal deviation).

■ Craniopharyngioma

This is a benign epithelial tumor, World Health Organization (WHO) grade I, that is often totally or partially cystic, and typically is located in the sellar-suprasellar region. It arises along the vestiges of the stomodeal diverticulum, mostly at the level of the infundibulum, where squamous epithelial rests occur,[27-29] or along the remnants of the primitive craniopharyngeal duct (nasopharynx, sphenoid bone, or predominantly intraventricular).[27,30-33]

Epidemiology and Pathology

Craniopharyngioma accounts for 1.2 to 5% of all intracranial tumors. The incidence is 0.5 to 2.5 cases per one million people per year.[34] Craniopharyngioma is the most common tumor in children (5–10%).[35] The incidence peaks between the ages of 5 and 15 years and between the ages of 45 and 60 years.[36] The papillary subtype is more common in adults than in children. (See also Chapter 6, page 148).

Pearl

Malignant transformation is very rare and has a poor prognosis.[37]

Vascularization

Craniopharyngioma is vascularized by perforators from the ICA, posterior cerebral artery (PCA), anterior cerebral artery (ACA), and anterior communicating artery (AComA).

Clinical Presentation

- Endocrinologic dysfunction:
  - Children: delay in puberty onset, short stature
  - Children/adults: diabetes insipidus, hypothyroidism
  - In cases of intrasellar invasion with pituitary involvement: hypopituitarism, amenorrhea, galactorrhea, infertility
- Neurologic deficits:
  - Visual deficits: decreased vision, bitemporal hemianopia, optic nerve atrophy, papilledema (especially in hydrocephalus)
  - Signs and symptoms related to obstructive hydrocephalus/raised intracranial pressure: headache, nausea, vomiting
    - Hydrocephalus is present in up to 48% of children[38] and 13% of adults,[39] and is generally caused by tumors with retrochiasmatic localization.
  - Craniopharyngioma is often diagnosed based on the related obstructive hydrocephalus, which is a surgical priority, above all in children. Behavioral disturbances: frontal lobe syndrome, memory loss, apathy, incontinence, hypersomnia, and Korsakoff syndrome (involvement of mammillary body and limbic system; rare)
- Seizures are rare, but have been described after surgery.

Preoperative Assessment

Magnetic resonance imaging with and without gadolinium is essential to see the nature of the tumor, its cystic components, and the relations with the diencephalic structures. Magnetic resonance angiography (MRA) or CTA and rarely digital subtraction angiography (DSA) are used for demonstrating displacement/encasement of arteries. See also **Table 5.4** on page 119.

- CT scan is performed to identify intralesional calcifications (present in 50% of adults and 100% of children)[40,41] as well as the bony anatomy of the skull base in preoperative planning.
- Preoperative endocrinologic evaluation and postoperative follow-up assess pituitary gland and hypothalamus function/dysfunction and determine the need for replacement therapy. Diabetes insipidus is a presenting symptom in up to 38% of patients, rising to 70% after surgery. It has to be corrected in either case with vasopressin (see Chapter 9).

- Neuro-ophthalmological evaluation and postoperative follow-up are indicated.
- Neurobehavioral assessment and neuropsychological testing are indicated, particularly in children.

Differential Diagnosis

The differential includes sellar and suprasellar tumors, such as pituitary adenomas, Rathke cleft cysts, meningiomas, dermoids/epidermoids, arachnoid cysts, more rarely germinoma, hamartoma, abscess, inflammatory diseases, suprasellar aneurysms, and optic nerve or hypothalamic gliomas.

Anatomy-Based Classifications

- Based on the relationship with the diaphragma sellae, craniopharyngioma can be sellar (infradiaphragmatic), suprasellar (supradiaphragmatic), or both.
- Relative to the optic chiasm, craniopharyngioma can be prechiasmatic, subchiasmatic, or retrochiasmatic.
- Relative to the third ventricle, craniopharyngioma can be intra- or extraventricular, or below the ventricle.[42]
- There are six types[43]: (1) purely intrasellar-infradiaphragmatic; (2) intra- and suprasellar, infra- and supradiaphragmatic; (3) supradiaphragmatic, parachiasmatic, extraventricular; (4) intra- and extraventricular; (5) paraventricular in relation to the third ventricle; and (6) purely intraventricular.
- Craniopharyngioma can be classified based on the suprasellar extension and infundibulum as follows[44] **(Fig. 21.6)**:
  - Type I: preinfundibular
  - Type II: transinfundibular (with extension into the stalk)
  - Type III: retroinfundibular (extending behind the pituitary gland and stalk)
    - IIIa: extending into the third ventricle
    - IIIb: extending into the interpeduncular cistern
  - Type IV: isolated to the third ventricle and/or optic recess

Surgical Approaches

Surgery is the primary treatment for the management of craniopharyngiomas. Debates exist regarding the advantages and disadvantages of minimal or maximal surgery. Proponents of the minimalist approach argue that total resection is associated with too high a risk, and it is best to treat only the symptomatic component as many times as is necessary to deal with the patient's symptoms. Maximalists argue that the best approach in the long term is the safe removal of as much of the tumor as possible during the first operation, to decompress and to minimize recurrences. The maximalists also argue that this is safer than

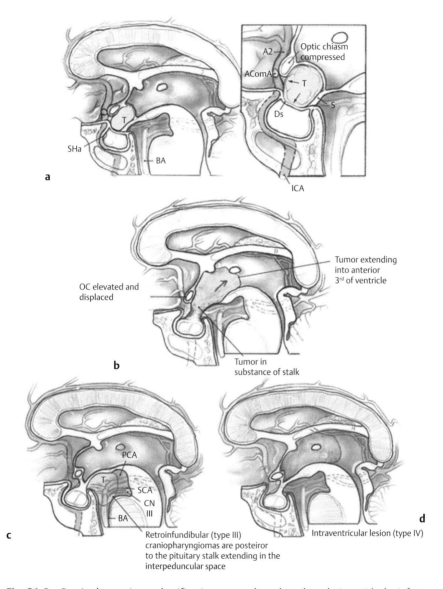

Fig. 21.6 Craniopharyngioma classification system based on the relation with the infundibulum. A, preinfundibular; B, transinfundibular; C, retroinfundubilar; D, purely intraventricular. AComA, anterior communicating artery; BA, basilar artery; CN, cranial nerve; Ds, diaphragma sellae; ICA, internal carotid artery; OC, optic chiasm; PCA, posterior cerebral artery; Pg, pituitary gland; S, stalk; SCA, superior cerebellar artery; SHa, superior hypophyseal artery; T, tumor. (From McLaughlin N, et al. Endoscopic Approach to Craniopharyngioma. In: Nader R. et al. Neurosurgery Tricks of the Trade. New York: Thieme; 2014:277.)

many repeated surgeries. Gross total, near total, or subtotal resection may be complicated by recurrences, particularly the development of cysts, which may be minimized with fractionated radiotherapy.[45] Radiotherapy after resection is advocated because, after gross total resection, a mean of 21% recurrence has been described (65% in subtotal resection, 42% after partial resection[46]), which is decreased to 17% after gross total resection followed by radiotherapy (see also Chapter 30, page 791).[45,47]

Subfrontal Approach

This approach is indicated especially for suprasellar tumors in the presence of a postfixed chiasm. A translamina terminalis extension of the approach may be required to deal with the retrochiasmatic or intraventricular components[48,49] and to facilitate access to the vertical components of the tumors. An OZ osteotomy may also be very helpful in reaching superiorly placed components of the tumor.

Frontolateral Approaches

The pterional or frontotemporal approach is one of the most used, often with its lateral supraorbital or supraorbital variants, giving access to the triangles of the sellar-parasellar region for removal of tumors between the optic nerves and the opticocarotid triangle or between the ICA and cranial nerve (CN) III. Although these triangles may be quite narrow, the tumor may widen the space between the ICA and optic nerve, thus providing access in certain cases. The frontolateral approaches enable doing a clinoidectomy and optic nerve unroofing, but if the tumor extends widely in a contralateral direction, the visualization of the optic nerve can be difficult. For small asymmetric tumors, the supraorbital keyhole approach has been suggested as well, but the approach is limited by the size of the frontal sinus, and there is limited vertical exposure.

Anterior Interhemispheric Approach

This approach is indicated for prechiasmatic tumors or those with large extensions into the third ventricle but that are primarily midline in nature.

Surgical Pearl

The frontolateral approaches may be extended with an OZ osteotomy, in order to give more basal access and less frontal lobe retraction to reach the superior aspects of the tumor. Some surgeons advocate the eyebrow approach using a mini-craniotomy and endoscope assistance for resection of the tumor.[50–53]

Subtemporal Approach

This approach is indicated for retrochiasmatic tumors with inferior or lateral extension to the middle fossa.[54]

Transpetrosal Approach

This approach is suggested for retrochiasmatic craniopharyngiomas, because it provides an upward projection to dissect the upper pole of the tumor and it facilitates visualization of the hypothalamus and pituitary stalk.[55–57] Prolonged temporal lobe retraction is one of its limitations.

Extended Endoscopic Endonasal Approach

This approach is indicated for sellar/suprasellar tumors, with a larger component in the sella.[58–61] It has the advantage of approaching the chiasm and AComA complex from below rather than from above. It requires meticulous dissection and patience but can be very effective.

Transcallosal and Transcortical Approaches

These approaches are used for pure intraventricular craniopharyngiomas or extraventricular tumors with large intraventricular components.

Intracavitary Therapy, Cyst Drainage

Purely cystic craniopharyngiomas may undergo sole intracystic aspiration via a catheter connected to an Ommaya reservoir, which is used for aspiration of the cystic liquid over time. A single aspiration is not suggested, considering the high likelihood of the cyst refilling. Moreover, the intracystic catheter can be used for the instillation of radioisotopes (32 phosphorus, 90 yttrium, 123 iodine, 198 aurum, 186 rhenium) to deliver a high local dose (~ 150 Gy) of radiation to the epithelial layer of the cyst, for sclerosing drugs (bleomycin),[62] or for interferon-α.[63] The catheter may be positioned by means of stereotactic- or endoscope-assisted guidance.

Surgical Pearls of the Transcranial Approaches

- Cerebrospinal fluid drainage may be required at the beginning of the operation, via ventricular or lumbar drain, above all in subfrontal approaches.
- An early debulking of the tumor and/or puncture of the cystic component may help in the dissection of the arachnoidal plane around the capsule of the tumor, especially at the level of the optic nerves, taking care to preserve the suprasellar vascularization (perforators to the optic chiasm and hypothalamus).

- The tumor can be resected by accessing the space between the optic nerves, the opticocarotid triangle, the caroticosylvian space, or through the lamina terminalis (retrochiasmatic/intraventricular components).

Surgical Pearl

Avoid bipolar coagulation in the suprasellar cistern, whenever possible, in order to preclude vascular damage to the hypothalamus or the optic apparatus.

- In cases of anatomic variants of pre- or postfixed optic chiasm, or for displacement of the chiasm by the tumor, the planum sphenoidale can be drilled to create a larger space. In cases of violation into the sphenoid sinus from the planum, the skull base defect is sealed by suturing the pericranial flap (prepare it beforehand in the frontobasal approach) and by using fibrin glue and fascia lata.
- Every attempt to preserve the pituitary stalk should be made. The stalk can be difficult to visualize because of stretch/compression by the tumor, but the characteristic longitudinal striae of purplish portal blood vessels and the brownish tinge of the stalk are characteristic. In some cases the stalk has to be sacrificed for complete removal of the tumor. In such a case, transect the stalk as distally as possible in order to reestablish antidiuretic hormone (ADH) production.

Other Surgical Approaches

Transbasal Subfrontal Translamina Terminalis Approach

This approach provides midline visualization of the optic chiasm and third ventricle, avoiding the blind spots of the supra- and retrosellar regions, as can occur in the frontolateral approaches.

- The subfrontal approach can be extended to transbasal or transglabellar via an orbitocranial osteotomy, with resection of the anterior wall of the frontal sinus, in order to provide more basal exposure with less retraction of the frontal lobes.[48]
- ◈ The tumor component in the third ventricle can be identified by opening the lamina terminalis. After opening, debulk the central part of the tumor (also by means of ultrasonic aspirator or by aspiration of the cystic components) and gently dissect the capsule from the ventricular walls, removing it through the lamina terminalis. Next, dissect and remove the components of the tumor in the infrachiasmatic and interpeduncular cisterns.

Extended Endoscopic Approaches

The endonasal route can be used for intrasellar subdiaphragmatic tumors[64,65] as well as with supradiaphragmatic components (by means of extended approaches), for the management of remnants or recurrences.[47] The extended endoscopic technique can be used also for intraventricular components, providing more direct access to subchiasmatic, retrosellar, and intraventricular components than with the transcranial approaches.[47,66]

- The transsphenoidal endoscopic approach is especially suggested for tumors with prechiasmatic or preinfundibular growth.[44,67]
- The position of the tumor in relation to the infundibulum may suggest extension of the approach.[44] Type I lesions require a transplanum/transtubercular approach. Type II lesions require the superior intercavernous sinus split[68] for an improved angle of attack. In type III tumors the infundibulum limits direct approach, which is why the pituitary gland and the stalk, according to some authors, have to be mobilized (pituitary transposition), in order to avoid neurovascular manipulation.[44] Posterior clinoidectomy/superior clivectomy may be performed as well.
- A wide exposure in the extended approach is required for preserving the superior hypophyseal artery complex, which can be displaced from the tumor.
- Reconstruction techniques are mandatory for reducing the risk of postoperative CSF leak (see Chapter 16).

Disadvantages

Tumors isolated to the third ventricle or optic recess (type IV)[44] may not be amenable to endoscopic resection. Moreover, recurrences/remnants of tumor previously treated by endonasal route may be more difficult to manage due to the presence of scars (i.e., vessels adherent to fascia lata, if previously used for the repair). As in all the transsphenoidal techniques, a relative contraindication is the presence of acute/subacute sinusitis.

Nuances of the Endoscopic Technique

- Lumbar drainage and the pedicled nasoseptal flap are highly recommended to reduce the risk of CSF leakage, above all the potential high-flow CSF leakages (i.e., opening of the ventricles).
- The superior intercavernous sinus is coagulated and divided to open the dura and access the suprasellar space.

Outcome

In a retrospective series of 100 craniopharyngiomas (79% purely infradiaphragmatic and 66% involving the supradiaphragmatic space), the endoscopic endonasal approach provided an overall gross-total removal of the craniopharyngioma in 70% of cases.[69] Improvement to visual disturbances was observed in 75% of cases.

Surgical Complications

- Injury to the pituitary stalk
- Diabetes insipidus, which may occur in 47 to 93%[39,70–72]
- Panhypopituitarism: generally present before surgery; occurs in 50 to 100%, depending on tumor localization (there is a higher risk of panhypopituitarism in sellar tumors) and the preoperative pituitary function.[72–74] In the case of normal preoperative pituitary function, new pituitary deficits occur in 58% of cases.[72]
- Hypothalamic injury: 40%[75]
- Vascular injury, blindness (which can be caused by optic nerve/chiasm direct injury or occlusion of the chiasmatic perforators): < 2%
- New cranial nerve palsy
- Pneumocephalus (especially in the endoscopic approaches)
- Infective or aseptic meningitis, the latter due to leakage of cystic material in the cisterns

Surgical Pearl

Leakage of cystic material in the cisterns may be avoided by aspiration of the intracystic fluid and continuous irrigation of the surgical cavity, for dilution of the tumor fluid.

- The endoscopic technique is related to CSF leakage rate in the range of 15%[47,69] (up to 28% in cases of tumors involving the third ventricle),[69] although improvement in reconstruction techniques can decrease the rate to 4%.[69]
- Mortality rate: < 4%[69]

Surgical Pearl

All the endoscopic endonasal techniques have a steep learning curve. Extensive experience is required in order to reduce the risk of complications.

Prognosis

At 10-year follow-up, 70 to 90% of patients are recurrence-free. The overall 10-year survival ranges from 30 to 70%, depending on the treatment modality used.[28,43,76] Predictors of recurrences are a large postsurgical remnant, and, according to some authors, the histological subtype, as follows: adamantinomatous tumors have higher rates of recurrence (due to the higher invasiveness of the pia),[77-80] although this is debatable. In endoscopic case series, 22 to 34% of recurrences require further surgery.[69,72] In these second operations, the endoscopic endonasal approach can also be used, although in some cases a transcranial route may be chosen.

Visual outcomes have been reported to improve in 70 to 100%[81] and to worsen in 2.5 to 10% of patients.[69,82]

■ Rathke Cleft Cysts

These are cystic remnants of the embryological Rathke pouch, mostly located in the sellar and suprasellar regions.[83,84]

Incidence

They are found in 22% of the general population's autopsy specimens, and are often incidentally found. Rathke cleft cysts account for less than 9% of all resected sellar tumors.[84-86] The incidence peaks between 40 and 50 years of age.[85-87]

- These cysts are generally asymptomatic; when symptomatic, they can cause headaches in up to 80% of patients; endocrine dysfunction; visual loss (11–67%); intracystic bleeding; and chemical meningitis due to spilling of cystic fluid, although this is rare.[86]
- The differential diagnosis includes other sellar/parasellar cystic lesions, such as craniopharyngiomas, dermoid/epidermoid cysts, xanthogranulomas, and sellar arachnoid cysts.[84]

Treatment

When symptomatic, the cysts should be surgically drained via a transsphenoidal approach. Generally, a partial resection of the cyst is considered to be sufficient, and the total removal of the cyst wall is not required. Aggressive and complete resection of the cyst wall yields a lower recurrence rate but a higher rate of CSF leakage and endocrinological dysfunction.

◈ Failure to reconstruct the sellar floor may result in the cyst draining into the sphenoid sinus, which entails a minimal risk of meningitis.

Outcome

Postoperatively, 70% of patients demonstrate neurologic or endocrinologic improvement. Headache can resolve in 80 to 90% of patients. There is a 20% recurrence rate after cyst drainage.

■ Diaphragma Sellae Meningiomas

Incidence

These are rare meningiomas, originating from the leaves of the diaphragma sellae. They are often considered similar to tuberculum sellae meningiomas, and are generically defined as suprasellar meningiomas.[88]

Classification

- These meningiomas are classified based on the site of origin[88]:
  - Type A, from the upper leaf of the diaphragm sellae, anteriorly to the pituitary stalk
  - Type B, from the upper leaf of the diaphragm sellae, posteriorly to the pituitary stalk
  - Type C, from the inferior leaf of the diaphragm sellae, with subdiaphragmatic/intrasellar expansion
- It is possible to speculate that subdiaphragmatic meningiomas originate from the arachnoid of the so-called subdiaphragmatic cistern.[6]
- The pattern of growth and the site of origin are related to the specific clinical findings, with more neurohypophysis/hypothalamus deficits in type B, and hypopituitarism and eventually visual deficits in type C, as in nonfunctioning pituitary adenomas.
- Type C diaphragma sellae meningiomas and tuberculum sellae meningiomas should be differentiated from pituitary adenomas; look for a tapered dural base, a tumor epicenter, and bright homogeneous enhancement after gadolinium (brighter than in pituitary adenomas). Generally, in pituitary adenomas, the pituitary gland and the diaphragma sellae are not highly detectable on MRI, whereas the pituitary stalk can be undetected in diaphragma sellae meningiomas.[89] Thus, the differential diagnosis can be difficult.
- Headache is more present in the types A and C.[88]

Surgical Approaches Based on Type

Extended transsphenoidal approaches are possible for all three types. Transcranial approaches (pterional, frontotemporal-orbitozygomatic [FTOZ], subfrontal) are preferred for types A and B, but type C may be better accessed by the transsphenoidal route given their downward growth pattern. Visual function preservation and improvement are a main goal of surgery, and both transcranial approaches and transsphenoidal approaches can achieve optic nerve decompression.[89]

■ 21.3 Cavernous Sinus Surgery

■ Pathology of the Cavernous Sinus

Cavernous sinus tumors account for 1% of intracranial tumors, with meningiomas as the most frequent one (40%).[1]

- The pathologies involving the CS include meningiomas, pituitary adenomas with parasellar extension, schwannomas of the parasellar nerves (primarily, trigeminal schwannoma), dermoids/epidermoids, CS hemangiomas, chordomas and chondrosarcomas, chondroblastomas and osteoblastomas, craniopharyngiomas, hemangiopericytomas, neurofibromas, angiofibromas, adenoid cystic carcinomas and adenocarcinomas, metastases, squamous cell carcinomas, intracavernous aneurysms, cavernous-carotid fistulas, dural arteriovenous fistulas, and infections such as mucormycosis or aspergillosis.
- Tumors originating from surrounding structures may invade the CS as well, such as middle cranial fossa/sphenoid meningiomas, petroclival tumors, and others.

■ Diagnoses

Meningioma of the Cavernous Sinus

- Incidence: 0.5 per 100,000[2]
- 60% of patients may have quiescent tumors, whereas neurologic worsening, growth rates, and radiographic progression have been variably reported in the literature (27% worsening neurologically over time, average of 8 years of time for radiographic doubling of the size)[2-4]

Trigeminal Schwannoma

See page 525.

Cavernous Sinus Hemangioma

This is a rare extra-axial vascular neoplasm accounting for less than 3% of CS tumors.[5] Typically hypervascular and presenting with CN VI palsy. These lesions enhance brightly with nuclear red blood cell labeling.

■ Signs and Symptoms of the Cavernous Sinus Tumors

Signs and symptoms include numbness, neuralgia, anesthesia/hypoesthesia in the involved trigeminal branch (predominantly in V_1 and V_2), numb cheek syndrome (in differential diagnosis with infraorbital neuropathy), headache, and chewing deficits. Compression of the intracavernous nerves may cause diplopia. Tumors with posterior extension can give rise to brainstem compression, with related neurologic signs and symptoms. See also Chapter 7.

■ Preoperative Assessment

Assessment includes a detailed history and physical examination, including vision (to distinguish these tumors from an orbital apex lesion), as well as standard neuroradiological assessment by CT and MRI. CT is important also to define the bone erosion/hyperostosis, the pneumatization of the sphenoid sinus as well as of the ACP, intratumoral calcifications, and the presence of a middle clinoid process and a bony bridge between it and the ACP (forming a bony canal around the ICA).

• MRI assesses the nature of the lesion. MRI/MRA and DSA are essential to define the caliber of the ICA. A balloon test occlusion with single photon emission computed tomography (SPECT) and acetazolamide test is used for assessing the collateral circulation, which may help to determine the cerebrovascular reserve in the event of ICA occlusion/sacrifice (see balloon test on page 301).

■ Classification of Cavernous Sinus Tumors

Based on the degree of CS invasion and the involvement of the intracavernous ICA, tumors can be classified as follows[6]:

• Grade 1: one area involved, with no ICA encasement
• Grade 2: two or more areas involved, with partial ICA encasement
• Grade 3: all the areas involved, with ICA totally encased but with no ICA stenosis
• Grade 4: same as grade 3, but the ICA is narrowed or occluded
• Grade 5: bilateral CS involvement, ± ICA encasement/stenosis/occlusion

---

A Note About Cavernous Sinus Meningiomas

Meningiomas that start in an area where no arachnoid plane exists (e.g., within the CS proper) will grow into the adventitia of the ICA and narrow it once it is circumferentially involved. Meningiomas that arise from the lateral wall of the CS will not infiltrate or narrow the ICA but rather displace it medially. This will occur in medial sphenoid wing tumors that arise from the lateral wall. In most cases, the lateral wall remains intact. Thus, the appearance of the ICA on preoperative imaging (not involved, displaced, partially or totally encased, or occluded) is very useful in determining resectability of the lesion.[6]

Identify the involvement of the ICA and the other intracavernous sinus structures.

- Based on the size and extension of the tumor[7]:
  - < 2.5 cm, confined to the CS and areas around it
  - ≥ 2.5 cm, extending into multiple regions
- CS tumors can be purely intracavernous, intra- and extracavernous, or extracavernous with secondary involvement of the CS.

■ Treatment

Treatment is based on the natural history of the disease.

■ Surgical Approaches

The approach should be defined by whether the CS lesion displaces the ICA (e.g., schwannoma) or is infiltrative (e.g., meningioma). Because the lesions that displace structures maintain a good plane with the CS nerves and ICA, they are amenable to resection. The infiltrative ones grow into structures that lack an arachnoid plane, such as the cavernous segment of the ICA, and do infiltrate them. Thus, these lesions demonstrate a narrow ICA on MRI and cause a progressive permanent cranial neuropathy. Resection of these lesions is difficult and requires excision of the ICA and cranial nerves. In cases of infiltrative pathologies and patterns on MRI, Gamma Knife radiosurgery or fractionated radiation may better preserve function than surgery (see page 772).

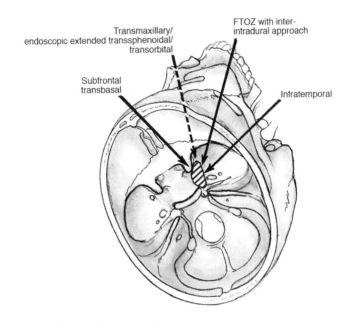

Fig. 21.7 Surgical approaches to the CS.

The CS can be approached as follows (**Fig. 21.7**):

1. Medially/anteromedially: via an endoscopic extended transmaxillary approach or transcranial transbasal approach. Combined transfacial/transsphenoidal approaches as well as transorbital approaches are valid alternatives in selected cases.
2. Anterolateral transcranial approaches:
    *   Infratemporal approach
    *   OZ approach with an interdural or intradural approach if subdural tumor exists

In transcranial surgery for CS lesions, the interdural approach via a FTOZ or extended pterional approach can be considered as the gold-standard technique.[8,9] Several modifications of the OZ approach have been described (see Chapter 14). The zygomatic approach is more restricted than the OZ approach and it gives access only to the posterior part of the CS and the petrous apex[10] and is best for patients with very small temporalis muscle (otherwise, access is much improved with the full OZ approach).

*   Tumors with components in Meckel's cave, parasellar space, and petroclival region may require more posterior approaches, such as the transpetrous approach or the supratentorial-infratentorial combined approaches.

■ Surgical Positions

- Transcranial approaches: patient supine, minimal anti-Trendelenburg position of the body, head rotated in the head-holder 30 degrees to the contralateral side.
- Endoscopic approaches: patient supine, head in neutral position

■ Surgical Pearls

- In transcranial approaches, place a lumbar drain preoperatively, and drain at least 100 cc of CSF for brain relaxation.
- Place the patient in the anti-Trendelenburg position to enable blood outflow from the CS to the jugular veins.
- Drape the neck to gain proximal ICA control.
- Drape the abdomen or the thigh for fat graft harvest.

> **Pearl**
>
> Check the turgor of the veins in the neck to adjust the position.

■ Steps of the Anterolateral Approach to the Cavernous Sinus

FTOZ Approach

See page 353.

❖ Interdural approach:

Originally indicated for intracavernous aneurysms, it may be indicated for any CS surgery for access to all the intracavernous compartments.

- ◈ An osteoplastic or free flap is possible. Preserve a pedicled pericranial flap.
- ◈ Extradural osteotomy: by use of an irrigated drill, flatten the sphenoid wing and the protuberances of the orbital roof, skeletonize the superior orbital fissure, or perform an OZ osteotomy.
- ◈ Coagulate the meningo-orbital artery.
- ◈ Open the falciform ligament and the dura overlying the anterior clinoid process.
- ◈ Drill the ACP. Make it thinner, and drill its medial component (optic strut) if the lesion is anteriorly placed.

Surgical Anatomy Pearls

- Be cognizant of the position of the optic nerve and preserve it. Check the preoperative CT scan for the presence of a middle clinoid process.
- Avoid opening the sphenoid/ethmoid sinuses, unless it is a planned component of the operation. If it is, pack the opening with fat or muscle, and cover it with a fascial graft and fibrin glue to avoid CSF leakage.
- Perform a careful extradural approach for mobilization of the optic nerve and ICA, if the lesion is anterior.

◈ After the extradural steps, if the lesion is extending into the subdural space, open the dura, and, if necessary, the sylvian fissure can be split and the cisterns accessed.

❖ Surgical steps for reaching the superior part of the CS:

◈ Drill the lesser wing, unroof the optic nerve, and perform anterior clinoidectomy (see page 366).

◈ Open the dura and reflect it over the orbit. For maximal exposure, depress the orbital contents, especially any infraorbital fat breached out of the periorbita.

◈ Elevate the dura of the middle fossa in the posterior-to-anterior direction.

◈ Identify the foramen spinosum, coagulate the middle meningeal artery, and plug the foramen to avoid bleeding.

◈ Identify and carefully dissect CN V_2 and V_3.

Surgical Anatomy Pearl

If it is necessary to expose the petrous portion of the ICA (which is not always required), it should be done prudently, to prevent ICA bleeding. Proximal control of the ICA at the neck is much easier and faster.

◈ Identify and dissect the greater superficial petrosal nerve (GSPN) from the dura at its emergence at the facial hiatus.

◈ Identify the Glasscock triangle, which overlies the carotid artery (see **Table 2.4**, page 20).

◈ Drill the space, noting the landmarks of the Glasscock triangle, and expose the petrous ICA. The tensor tympani muscle is the posterior limit of the exposure.

Surgical Anatomy Pearl

Avoid traction on the GSPN, because it can lead to facial palsy via traction on the geniculate ganglion.

Surgical Anatomy Pearl

Make enough space for potential clipping of the ICA, if required, or for inflating a catheter balloon in the carotid canal, in order to temporarily occlude it.[11]

◈ Open the dural rings for access at the superoanterior portion of the CS.

◈ Open the dura of the superior CS, from the anterior to the posterior clinoid process.

◈ The intracavernous ICA should be carefully mobilized, and the tumor debulked or resected. CN VI and the intracavernous arteries should be respected.

Surgical Anatomy Pearl

The opening of the dura requires careful visualization of the CN III and the ICA, in order to avoid lesioning these structures.

◈ Further subperiosteal dissection and drilling of the bone (ACP or posterior clinoid process [PCP], dorsum sellae, clivus, planum sphenoidale) may be required, based on the extent of the pathology.

Surgical Anatomy Pearl

Anterior clinoidectomy and medial extension of the drilling may put the CS and the middle cranial fossa in communication with the sphenoid sinus. Obliterate carefully the communication (with Gelfoam, muscle, and/or glue).

❖ Surgical steps for lateral exposure of the entire CS:

◈ Use the OZ approach ± subtemporal/infratemporal approach.

❖ Surgical steps for extradural or intradural exposure:

◈ The intradural approach gives access to the CS via its dural roof, whereas the extradural is based on the dissection of the two layers of the lateral wall of the CS.[12]

◈ Peel the lateral wall of the CS, starting in the area of the sphenoparietal sinus[12] and proceeding lateromedially in the regions of V_2 and V_3 and from anterior to posterior, toward the tentorial edge and Meckel's cave, as required by the location of the pathology.

◈ Identify the CS triangles and nerves, such as CNs IV and V_1, delimitating Parkinson's triangle (see Chapter 2, **Fig. 2.6**, page 22). However, pathology may change the shape of the anatomical triangles.

Surgical Anatomy Pearl

Bleeding from the CS can be managed by using hemostatic material, such as Gelfoam or Surgicel. The windows between V_1 and V_2 and posterior to the clinoidal ICA can be injected with fibrin glue (0.5–1 mL using a blunt needle), so that the CS compartments are filled with glue and the bleeding controlled.[13]

◈ In the extradural dissection, more bone can be drilled (e.g., around the foramina of the trigeminal nerve), in order to gain access to the infratemporal fossa, whenever required.

◈◈ Variation: The opening of the foramina rotundum and ovale enables the mobilization of the trigeminal nerve. The drilling of the petrous apex provides access into the posterior fossa.

❖ CS as a surgical corridor to reach the posterior fossa:

◈ The CS can be accessed to reach the posterior fossa, e.g., for basilar aneurysms (above all for low-lying located aneurysms).

◈ After the FTOZ/extradural frontotemporal approach: (1) remove the ACP, (2) section the distal and proximal dural rings for CS opening, and (3) drill the dorsum sellae and clivus for access into the interpeduncular and prepontine cisterns.

❖ Surgical modifications:

◈ Pretemporal transcavernous approach,[14] pretemporal transzygomatic transcavernous approach[15]: after OZ craniotomy, (1) dissect the dura of the middle and anterior fossa to expose the superior orbital fissure (SOF); (2) dissect the sylvian fissure and basal cisterns; and (3) perform interdural dissection by proceeding medially to reach the ACP.

• All the described variants have common points: exposure of the middle cranial fossa and drilling of the sphenoid wing and lateral and superior orbital walls to achieve a wide pre- and subtemporal corridor.

• The meningo-orbital artery is the landmark where the dura propria of the temporal lobe can be dissected from the lateral wall of the CS. The dissection along the intradural space enables anatomic preservation of the intracavernous nerves.

• The opening of the CS, primarily its roof, involves manipulation of the CN III, causing temporary palsy (in general, subsiding after 2 to 12 weeks).[16]

◈◈ When it is required and when it can be done, as in presence of anatomic variants (e.g., hypoplastic posterior communicating artery, PcomA), the PComA can be cut to provide more access to the posterior fossa cisterns.[15]

❖ **Endoscopic extended endonasal approach to the CS**

◈ See surgical steps on page 428.

■ Surgical Outcomes

Gross total resection of meningiomas has been described in 12 to 92% of cases,[2] with a recurrence rate of 12% in patients who underwent gross total resection versus 26% in patients undergoing subtotal resection.[17]

■ Surgical Complications

- Ischemic complications: occurring in 5% of patients[6,17,18]
- Intraoperative injury of the ICA:
  - Options of treatment: temporary clipping and direct repair with 6-0 or 8-0 sutures; vein graft repair; occlusion of the ICA, in the presence of collateral circulation; endovascular treatment.[19,20]

■ 21.4 Trigeminal Schwannoma
■ Anatomy

Review the topographic anatomy of the trigeminal nerve on page 80.

The trigeminal nerve begins intradurally, and is quickly surrounded by the pre-pontine and then the trigeminal cistern in the posterior fossa. In Meckel's cave, the trigeminal ganglion remains in the subarachnoid space, and then the three branches V_1, V_2, and V_3 become interdural. This is the anatomic basis of the interdural surgical approaches.

Trigeminal schwannomas are also known as trigeminal neurinomas, neurilemomas, or neuromas. They are benign tumors arising from the Schwann cells of the trigeminal nerve.

■ Incidence

- Trigeminal schwannomas account for less than 0.4% of intracranial tumors, and 0.8 to 8% of intracranial schwannomas.[1–3]
- Although rare, it is the second most common intracranial schwannoma, after the vestibular schwannoma.

Surgical Pathology

Generally, trigeminal schwannomas are soft, yellowish, and may have several small or large cysts lined by tumor cells. The vascularity can vary from avascular to highly vascular, but most tumors are relatively avascular. Trigeminal schwannomas typically displace structures such as other cranial nerves and the carotid artery, but can occasionally be adherent, or fibrous, and engulf nerves and vessels, particularly if they have been exposed to prior irradiation such as that delivered by Gamma Knife.

Surgical Anatomy Pearls

- In the CS/Meckel's cave, trigeminal schwannomas tend to push medially rather than engulfing the ICA and intracavernous nerves.
- Structures at major risk during surgery: PCA and SCA in posterior fossa approaches, ICA and intracavernous nerves in middle fossa approaches.

- Trigeminal schwannomas can be solid, cystic, or mixed.
  - The cystic component of the tumors is more difficult to resect because the tumors engulf the neurovascular peritumoral structures more often and are more adherent to vessels and nerves. Cystic tumors have been described as occurring in 6.5% of cases.[4]
  - As in vestibular schwannoma, the cystic component of trigeminal schwannoma can be more difficult to remove because it is closely adhered to surrounding neurovascular structures.
- Trigeminal schwannomas may arise from each segment of the trigeminal nerve, in its ganglionic or postganglionic segments; they can be confined in a single compartment or can be multicompartmental, and have a typical "dumbbell" or "hour-glass" shape, with one component in the posterior fossa and one in the middle fossa. The tumor may extend to the infratemporal fossa, but if it does, a plexiform neurofibroma should be suspected.
- These tumors can arise from the following[4]: (1) the cisternal portion of CN V (21%) (in the intradural/subarachnoid space); (2) around the ganglion in Meckel's cave (36%); (3) the peripheral divisions (13%). Types 2 and 3 are in the interdural compartment. In addition to these three types, these tumors can also be multisegmental/multicompartmental (30%).
  - In the middle cranial fossa, trigeminal schwannomas lie in the interdural space, between the apparent inner and the true outer layer of the lateral walls of the CS. For this reason, the ideal surgical technique for their resection is the middle fossa interdural approach.[5–7]
  - Posterior fossa trigeminal schwannomas rarely arise from the motor root.
- Giant trigeminal schwannomas may extend to all the compartments.

- Dumbbell-shaped tumors may develop from the cisternal portion into the CS segment, or from the CS/Meckel's cave into the peripheral divisions, reaching the infratemporal fossa.

Signs and Symptoms

- The duration of the symptoms before surgery ranges from 2 months to 17 years (average 3 years).[4] Commonly, the signs and symptoms include headache, facial hypoesthesia, facial pain (tingling sensation, trigeminal neuralgia-like pain, trigeminal neuropathic pain, dysesthesia), facial weakness and numbness, neuralgia, anesthesia/hypoesthesia in the involved trigeminal branch, numb cheek syndrome (in differential diagnosis with infraorbital neuropathy), and chewing deficits.
- Meckel's cave/intracavernous schwannomas can compress the other cranial nerves, causing diplopia; this is a rare and later finding in larger tumors.
- Cisternal trigeminal schwannomas can give rise to brainstem compression, with related neurologic signs and symptoms.

Preoperative Assessment

Assessment includes a detailed history and physical exam, including the corneal reflex, and standard neuroradiological assessment by CT and MRI. CT is also important in defining the bone erosion, whereas magnetic resonance venography (MRV) is essential for monitoring venous drainage and patency of the dural sinuses. MRA, CTA, or angiogram may be useful for delineating the tumor's relationships with the arteries.

Differential Diagnosis

The differential includes meningiomas, neurofibromas, metastases, schwannomas of the other intracavernous nerves, facial or petrosal nerve schwannomas, epidermoids, hemangiopericytomas, and dermoids.

Anatomy-Based Classifications

Several classification systems are anatomically based; they are listed in **Table 21.3**.

Treatment

Surgery is the first step in the majority of cases for tissue diagnosis, decompression, and complete oncological surgical resection.[5,12,13]

Table 21.3   Anatomically Based Classification Systems for Trigeminal Schwannomas

Classification and References

Type[8]	Location
1	Mainly middle fossa
2	Mainly posterior fossa
3	Both middle and posterior fossae

Type[9]	Location
M	Middle cranial fossa, in the interdural space
P	Posterior cranial fossa, intradural or interdural space
E	Extracranial, further subdivided[10]: E1: in the orbit E2: in the pterygopalatine fossa E3: in the infratemporal fossa
MP	Multicompartmental, dumbbell-shaped tumor that follows the trigeminal nerve between the middle and posterior cranial fossae
ME	Between the middle cranial fossa and the extracranial space
MPE	Middle and posterior fossae and extracranial space

Type[4]	Location
1	Peripheral
2	Ganglion cavernous (Meckel's cave), originating from the gasserian ganglion and abutting the inferior lateral wall of the cavernous sinus
3	Posterior fossa root
4	Dumbbell shaped, which can be either: Subtype 1: cavernous root extending along the trigeminal root proximal to the porus trigeminus Subtype 2: from the gasserian ganglion to the extracranial portion of the nerve

Group[2, 11]	Location	Subgroups
A	Predominantly middle cranial fossa	A1: Anterior paracavernous ± extension into the superior orbital fissure or orbit A2: Posterior paracavernous and Meckel's cave A3: Both anterior and posterior paracavernous
B	Predominantly posterior cranial fossa	–

Table 21.3 (*continued*)

Group[2, 11]	Location	Subgroups
C	Major components in both middle and posterior cranial fossa	C1: Middle fossa component in posterior paracavernous and Meckel's cave C2: Middle fossa extension beyond posterior paracavernous region
D	Major extracranial component	D1: Major extracranial component without remarkable intracranial extension D2: Major extracranial component with remarkable intracranial extension

- Complete resection is the goal whenever possible. It is associated with increased long-term, recurrence-free survival, whereas subtotal excision may result in recurrence.[14]
- Total resection has been described as feasible in almost 75% of cases.[4]
- Preservation of the neurovascular structures around the tumor is a crucial point for the outcome, and often a subtotal resection is the compromise to avoid new neurologic deficits.

As is typical in schwannomas, the tumor arises from one of the fascicles of the nerve, expanding and compressing the surrounding fascicles. The goal of surgery is to remove the tumor and preserve the anatomic integrity and function of the other fascicles.[5,11]

■ Surgical Approaches (Fig. 21.8)

Except for the cisternal tumor, which may require a transpetrosal or a retrosigmoid lateral suboccipital approach, tumor resection may require a frontotemporal craniotomy with or without an OZ osteotomy (complete or partial), based on its specific extension. Posterior fossa components can also be approached using middle fossa or infratemporal approaches, although they can be more challenging.[15–17]

- Based on the segment of the trigeminal nerve involved in the tumor, the following surgical approaches are feasible:
  1. Posterior fossa/cisternal segment: retrosigmoid lateral suboccipital approach and/or translabyrinthine presigmoid approach.[2]
  2. Meckel's cave/CS location: interdural middle fossa approach, extradural fronto-temporopolar approach[2,18] or basal lateral subtemporal via peri-

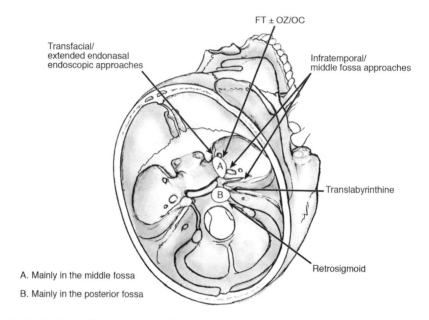

FT ± OZ/OC

Transfacial/
extended endonasal
endoscopic approaches

Infratemporal/
middle fossa approaches

Translabyrinthine

Retrosigmoid

A. Mainly in the middle fossa

B. Mainly in the posterior fossa

Fig. 21.8 Surgical approaches to the trigeminal schwannomas, based on their main localization. FT, frontotemporal; OC, orbitocranial; OZ, orbitozygomatic.

cavernous lateral loop approach.[4] The lateral loop refers to the lateral triangle, that is, the space formed between the lateral border of V_2 and the medial border of V_3 (see **Table 2.4**, page 20).[19,20] The approach provides the shortest and shallowest corridor to Meckel's cave, elevating the outer layer of dura mater and keeping the inner layer intact to expose the tumor, without peeling the two layers of dura at the level of CNs III and IV. There is a low risk of injury to the abducens nerve and accompanying ophthalmoparesis.[4,8,15] The infratemporal fossa approach has been described for such tumors as well.[3]

3. Peripheral V_1: temporopolar transorbital approach.
4. Peripheral V_2 and/or V_3: anterior infratemporal fossa approach, transfacial approach, or extended lateral transmaxillary endoscopic approach.
5. Posterior and middle cranial fossa dumbbell-type tumors: extended middle fossa approach or combined petrosal approach. The middle fossa and/or infratemporal fossa exposures also facilitate accessing the posterior fossa component.[15]

In posterior fossa tumors with a component within Meckel's cave, the cave itself often becomes expanded. Sometimes it is possible to perform a single approach, such as a posterior fossa approach, without doing a combined approach, and removing the component in Meckel's cave:

◈   Introduce an angled curette into Meckel's cave and gently remove any soft ganglionic components under endoscopic visualization. The assisted-retrosigmoid intradural suprameatal approach has been shown to be feasible and safe for radical resection of dumbbell-shaped trigeminal schwannoma.[11]

   Middle cranial fossa approaches are essentially based on the interdural dissection of the CS, which is an anatomic-based technique for approaching parasellar tumors, such as trigeminal schwannomas and cavernous hemangiomas.[6] Tumors with large middle and posterior fossa components can be resected fully via the middle fossa approach by following the tumor through Meckel's cave into the posterior fossa.[16]

◈   Consider lumbar drainage in those cases with minimal risk of herniation. After a frontotemporal craniotomy, with drilling of the sphenoid ridge or an OZ osteotomy, perform an extradural dissection of the floor of the middle cranial fossa, from lateral to medial and from posterior to anterior, identifying the foramina and arcuate eminence.

◈   Coagulate and divide the middle meningeal artery and vein, and then plug the foramen spinosum with hemostatic material and/or bone wax.

◈◈ Variation: Drain the CSF to facilitate temporal lobe relaxation, in order to avoid its excessive retraction during the extra- and interdural approaches.

◈   Expose the tumor by means of the interdural approach, incising the CS wall at the level of the superior orbital fissure, or in the lateral loop, and peeling away the dura from CNs III, IV, V_2, and V_3. Perform the interdural dissection with a subperiosteal elevator or a Penfield dissector.

◈   Preserve the adjacent nerves and then internally debulk the tumor. Once the bulk is diminished, dissect the walls free from the surrounding structures.

◈   Control bleeding from the CS with Gelfoam, methylcellulose, Surgifoam® (Ethicon, Bridgewater, NJ) or drops of fibrin glue, while also trying to avoid packing it too densely.

Surgical Anatomy Pearls

• Excessive packing in the CS may cause ICA stenosis or intracavernous nerves compression.
• The ICA can always be checked by means of an intraoperative Doppler probe.
• Depending on the localization of the tumor, the most sensitive structures that may be inadvertently injured during the resection of a trigeminal schwannoma are CNs IV and VI, as well as the PCA and SCA (these injuries are more common than injuries to the ICA).

❖ **Transfacial approach:** see Chapter 15.

❖ **Extended endoscopic approach:** In selected cases, the extended endonasal endoscopic approach is a feasible technique to remove trigeminal and other nonvestibular skull base tumors.[6] For such purpose, the transposition of the vidian nerve has been suggested as well.[21]

❖ **Combined approach:** Multicompartmental trigeminal schwannomas may require combined approaches, such as the middle cranial fossa approach with petrosectomy, the retrosigmoid approach for tumors involving the posterior and middle cranial fossae, or the transcranial and transfacial/endonasal approaches for tumors involving the middle cranial fossa and pterygopalatine/subtemporal fossae.

■ Surgical Outcome

- A mortality rate close to 0% is reported in the most recent literature.
- Facial pain resolved in > 90% of patients.[4]
- Total resection was performed in 75% of patients, near-total removal in 7%, and subtotal removal in 17%.[4]

■ Complications

Complications include infections, ischemic complications, CSF leakage, temporary temporal lobe swelling, trismus, diplopia (generally transitory), intracavernous cranial nerves deficits, exophthalmos, ICA injury or stenosis (excessive packing of hemostatic material into the CS), facial pain, problems in jaw opening, and atrophy of the temporal muscle. Corneal anesthesia can occur, so special care of the eyes is required preoperatively and postoperatively. An ophthalmology consultation is recommended in cases of corneal anesthesia.

Hypoesthesia with or without dysesthesia is very common in trigeminal schwannomas (65% of patients), and it can also worsen after surgery in 12% of cases. Anesthesia dolorosa is very rare.

■ Radiation Therapy

Gamma Knife radiosurgery can be used for the primary treatment of the lesion or for treatment of any residual tumor mass left behind following subtotal resection (useful for a tumor residual up to 3 cm in diameter as long as the distance from the optic pathways is greater than 2 to 3 mm) (see Chapter 30).

- After Gamma Knife radiosurgery, 85 to 100% of patients have their tumor growth under control, but the control rates depend on duration of follow-up.[14,23–25]
- Facial pain may improve in two thirds of patients.[24]
- Up to 27% of patients may have worsening of the cranial neuropathies following radiosurgery, so fractionated radiation therapy is also an option, particularly for large tumors without brainstem compression, or for those unable to undergo surgery.[24]

■ 21.5 Osseous Lesions of the Skull Base

- Systemic skeleton disorders or localized lesions can give rise to a variety of presentations ranging from cranial nerve compression with focal neurologic deficit (e.g., visual loss), to pain, raised intracranial pressure, seizures, systemic features, or deformity. The lesions can involve any of the bones of the skull base, and may be primary or secondary and focal or diffuse in nature.
- More typical lesions are fibrous dysplasia, ossifying fibroma, osteopetrosis, and osteoma.[1] Other lesions described as involving the skull base are osteoblastoma, osteosarcoma, Ewing's sarcoma, giant cell tumor, Paget's disease, and hyperostosis frontalis interna.[2] Rare lesions in the skull base include intraosseous hemangioma, osteoid osteoma, brown tumor associated with hyperparathyroidism, and eosinophilic granuloma **(Table 21.4)**.

> **Pearl**
>
> Every bone tumor in the skull base should be assumed to represent a metastasis until proven otherwise.

■ Fibrous Dysplasia

Fibrous dysplasia is a rare disease (2.5% of all bone tumors) characterized by fibrous tissue replacing the normal bone (arrest of new bone formation at the woven bone stage). Vascularized fibrous stroma surrounds the disorganized osteoid trabeculae.

- Osteocalcin is a typical marker of fibrous dysplasia (deficient/absent in ossifying fibromas).
- It can be part of the McCune-Albright syndrome (fibrous dysplasia, café-au-lait spots, and hyperfunctioning endocrinopathies) or it can be associated with neurofibromatosis type 2.

Table 21.4 Epidemiology and Outcomes of Osseous Lesions of the Skull Base

Disease, Reference	Epidemiology		Outcomes	
Fibrous dysplasia[3–8]	Male/female ratio	1:1	Recurrence rate	18–50%
	Proportion of all bone tumors	2.5–7%	Loss of vision	5%
	Craniofacial localization:		Malignant transformation:	
	Monostotic	10–25%	Monostotic	0.5%
	Polyostotic	50–90%	McCune-Albright syndrome	4%
	Polyostotic fibrous dysplasia in McCune-Albright syndrome	3%	Mortality rate	53.6%
Ossifying fibroma	Case reports in the sphenoid bones, paranasal sinuses, and orbits			
Osteopetrosis[9,10] (Albers-Schönberg disease)	Autosomal recessive	1/250,000		
	Autosomal dominant	1/20,000		
Osteomas[11]	Peripheral	48%	Recurrence rate	9%
	Central	29%		
	Paranasal sinuses	21%		
Osteoblastoma[12–15]	Male/female ratio	3:1	Recurrence rate	16–21%
	Proportion of primary bone tumors	5%		
	Craniofacial localization	1–4%		

Osteosarcoma[16,17]	Proportion of osteosarcomas that affect head and neck	< 10%
	Localization:	
	Maxilla	24%
	Overall survival:	
	5 years	63–74%
	10 years	55%
	Disease-specific survival:	
	5 years	67%
	10 years	61%
	Recurrence rate:	
	Local recurrence	37%
	Distant metastases	21%
	Rate of complications at 5 years:	
	Surgical	28%
	Radiotherapy	40%
Ewing's sarcoma[18]	Prevalence that affects cranium	1–6%
	Recurrence rate	7%
	Overall survival at 5 years	57.1%
Giant cell tumor[19–23]	Proportion of all bone tumors	< 5%
	Proportion affecting craniofacial region	1%
	Malignant transformation	7%
	Recurrence rate	14.3–25%
Paget's disease[24]	Polyostotic involvement	63.9%
	Complication rate	63%
	Malignant transformation into osteosarcoma	50%
Hyperostosis frontalis interna[25,26]	Prevalence:	
	General population	5–12%
	Women < 40	< 10%
	Postmenopausal women	40–65%
Intraosseous hemangioma[27,28]	Male/female ratio	1:3
	Proportion of all bone tumors	< 1%
	Recurrence rate:	
	Partial resection	40%
	Complete resection	< 1%

- 90% of craniofacial lesions present by 3.4 years of age.[5]
- 70 to 85% of patients with fibrous dysplasia have a monostotic form of the disease (involvement of a single bone, such as the jaw), whereas others have multiple localizations.[6,29,30] The monostotic form typically affects the fronto-orbital region, with the polyostotic form affecting multiple bones, mostly the splanchnocranium and orbital areas.[29]
- On a CT scan fibrous dysplasia has a typical ground-glass density. The lesions can be associated with mucoceles, which are identifiable on MRI.
- There is a 0.5% incidence of malignant transformation.[31]
- The differential diagnosis includes hyperostosis related to meningioma (look for the en-plaque meningioma on contrast-enhanced MRI, especially in patients presenting with exophthalmos) in younger patients and in older adults; other expansile bony lesions such as prostate carcinoma may mimic fibrous dysplasia.
- The lesions may be enormous and involve multiple bones, but are typically asymptomatic or minimally symptomatic as opposed to lesions such as a hyperostosing meningioma.
- Lesions can present with deformity in childhood and occasionally optic nerve compression if involving the optic canal. The deformity rarely progresses after adolescence, but the patient may require optic nerve decompression.
- Indications for surgery:
  - Tissue diagnosis (though the ground-glass appearance and minimal symptomatology is typical). Rapid change and new onset of pain in previously quiescent lesion may signify malignant degeneration.
  - Decompression of cranial nerves (e.g., optic compressive neuropathy).
  - Cosmetic deformity (e.g., exophthalmos).

■ Ossifying Fibroma

Ossifying fibroma with osteoblasts and lamellar bone occasionally occurs in the sphenoid bones, paranasal sinuses, and orbits. It usually presents as a focal mass. It is rarely as extensive as, but is often more calcified than fibrous dysplasia. It may cause symptoms by local mass effect or by obstruction of a paranasal sinus with secondary mucocele formation. Treatment requires resection of the lesion to reestablish sinus drainage.

Surgical Indications

These diseases are rare and can be incidentally found on radiological imaging, not based on indications. Patients require a radiological and clinical follow-up over time, particularly a neuro-ophthalmology follow-up in cases of orbit/sphenoid wing/optic canal involvement.

- Pain related to fibrous dysplasia and other bone lesions can be successfully managed with bisphosphonates.
- Surgical decompression is the treatment of choice for acute/progressive cranial neuropathy, particularly in cases of optic nerve compression with visual deficits/blindness.

> **Pearl**
>
> Visual evoked potentials (VEPs) are indicated postoperatively and for follow-up, especially in infants.

- The indications vary based on the craniofacial zone that is involved by the lesions. A total excision of the dysplastic bone with bony reconstruction is suggested for zone 1 (fronto-orbital, zygomatic, upper maxillary regions) if there is progression, deformity, or concern about malignant change, whereas a more conservative approach is advocated in the other three zones: zone 2, hair-bearing skull; zone 3, central skull base; zone 4, tooth-bearing maxilla and mandible.[32] If there is progression, a possible malignant change, or a progressive cranial nerve deficit, surgery is indicated regardless of location.

❖ Surgical Approaches

◈ The approach selected depends entirely on the bone and location affected along with the surgical goal. For example, if the goal is optic nerve decompression, then an extradural frontotemporal approach (or also supraorbital approach) to the optic canal will suffice. Rarely is the whole lesion removed. Some cases (e.g., bilateral optic nerve compression) may require a bifrontal approach via a coronal incision.
  - Localization of the disease in the sinuses, clivus, tuberculum sellae, or other midline structures can be treated by means of endoscopic transsphenoidal approaches. Endoscopy can also be used for biopsy, when indicated for diagnosis.

◈ Perform extradural drilling of the orbital roof and sphenoid bone.

◈ Remove the lateral and superior orbital rims for complete decompression of the optic canal and orbital fissures.

◈ Perform optic nerve decompression, 180 degrees circumferentially around the optic nerve.

> **Pearl**
>
> The primary goal of surgery is nerve decompression, not complete resection of the lesion itself.

> **Surgical Anatomy Pearl**
>
> To reach the optic canal via a supraorbital or frontolateral approach, it is often necessary to drill the highly irregular and thick orbital roof, in order to smooth it down and minimize the frontal lobe retraction and risk of iatrogenic injury.[33]

◈ Orbital decompression requires orbital osteotomies.
◈ Extensive bone resections may require custom implants for the orbital reconstruction.
◈ Exenterate sinus mucosa and pack the sinus in cases entailing entry into a nasal sinus.

Complications

CSF leakage, cranial nerve injury, blindness.

■ Osteopetrosis

Osteopetrosis is also known as marble bone disease or Albers-Schönberg disease.

- Osteoclast dysfunction gives rise to a defective balance of bone turnover and thickening of bone.
- Typical involved are CNs II, VII, and VIII.[34]
- Radiologically it is possible to see thickening and sclerosis of the calvaria, with other specific findings: ventriculomegaly, tonsillar herniation, proptosis, dural venous sinus stenosis, and optic nerve sheath dilatation.[35]
- Mild forms can be asymptomatic; otherwise, skull base involvement can give rise to blindness, facial paralysis, and deafness.[35]
- The autosomal recessive form is defined as malignant osteopetrosis.
- Infantile osteopetrosis (malignant osteopetrosis) can cause occlusion/narrowing of all the skull base foramina, giving rise to compression of blood vessels. Venous drainage occlusion may give rise to secondary hydrocephalus. Carotid canal stenosis may give rise to brain infarction.

■ Osteomas

Osteomas are slow-growing osteoblastic tumors that are the commonest bone tumors of the craniofacial skeleton. Because they arise in bones formed by intramembranous ossification, they are commonly seen in the parietal and frontal bones. They may present uncommonly by obstruction of the frontal sinus and the ensuing development of a mucocele.

- Treatment requires resection of the lesion and reestablishment of sinus function.

■ References

Boldfaced references are of particular importance.

21.1 Meningiomas Involving the Sphenoid Bone

1. Jääskeläinen J. Seemingly complete removal of histologically benign intracranial meningioma: late recurrence rate and factors predicting recurrence in 657 patients. A multivariate analysis. Surg Neurol 1986;26:461–469
2. Rohringer M, Sutherland GR, Louw DF, Sima AA. Incidence and clinicopathological features of meningioma. J Neurosurg 1989;71(5 Pt 1):665–672
3. Stafford SL, Perry A, Suman VJ, et al. Primarily resected meningiomas: outcome and prognostic factors in 581 Mayo Clinic patients, 1978 through 1988. Mayo Clin Proc 1998;73:936–942
4. **Al-Mefty O. Clinoidal meningiomas. J Neurosurg 1990;73:840–849**
5. De Jesús O, Toledo MM. Surgical management of meningioma en plaque of the sphenoid ridge. Surg Neurol 2001;55:265–269
6. **Mirone G, Chibbaro S, Schiabello L, Tola S, George B. En plaque sphenoid wing meningiomas: recurrence factors and surgical strategy in a series of 71 patients. Neurosurgery 2009;65(6, Suppl):100–108, discussion 108–109**
7. **Shrivastava RK, Sen C, Costantino PD, Della Rocca R. Sphenoorbital meningiomas: surgical limitations and lessons learned in their long-term management. J Neurosurg 2005;103:491–497**
8. Bonnal J, Thibaut A, Brotchi J, Born J. Invading meningiomas of the sphenoid ridge. J Neurosurg 1980;53:587–599
9. Brotchi J, Pirotte B. Sphenoid wing meningiomas. In: Sekhar L, Fessler R, eds. Atlas of Neurosurgical Techniques: Brain. New York: Thieme; 2006:623–632
10. Roser F, Nakamura M, Jacobs C, Vorkapic P, Samii M. Sphenoid wing meningiomas with osseous involvement. Surg Neurol 2005;64:37–43, discussion 43
11. **Mariniello G, Bonavolontà G, Tranfa F, Maiuri F. Management of the optic canal invasion and visual outcome in spheno-orbital meningiomas. Clin Neurol Neurosurg 2013;115:1615–1620**
12. **Chaichana KL, Jackson C, Patel A, et al. Predictors of visual outcome following surgical resection of medial sphenoid wing meningiomas. J Neurol Surg B Skull Base 2012;73:321–326**
13. Langevin CJ, Hanasono MM, Riina HA, Stieg PE, Spinelli HM. Lateral transzygomatic approach to sphenoid wing meningiomas. Neurosurgery 2010;67(2, Suppl Operative):377–384
14. **Oya S, Sade B, Lee JH. Sphenoorbital meningioma: surgical technique and outcome. J Neurosurg 2011;114:1241–1249**
15. **Simon M, Schramm J. Lateral and middle sphenoid wing meningiomas. In: De Monte F, McDermott MW, Al-Mefty O, eds. Al-Mefty's Meningiomas, 2nd ed. New York, Stuttgart: Thieme; 2011:214–227**
16. **Cusimano MD, Sekhar LN, Sen CN, et al. The results of surgery for benign tumors of the cavernous sinus. Neurosurgery 1995;37:1–9, discussion 9–10**

17. Sekhar LN, Patel S, Cusimano M, Wright DC, Sen CN, Bank WO. Surgical treatment of meningiomas involving the cavernous sinus: evolving ideas based on a ten year experience. Acta Neurochir Suppl (Wien) 1996;65:58–62

18. Russell SM, Benjamin V. Medial sphenoid ridge meningiomas: classification, microsurgical anatomy, operative nuances, and long-term surgical outcome in 35 consecutive patients. Neurosurgery 2008;62(3, Suppl 1):38–50, discussion 50

19. Bassiouni H, Asgari S. Tentorial meningiomas. In: DeMonte F, McDermott MW, Al-Mefty O, eds. Al-Mefty's Meningiomas, 2nd ed. New York, Stuttgart: Thieme; 2011: 168–176

20. **Krisht AF. Clinoidal meningiomas. In: DeMonte F, McDermott MW, Al-Mefty O, eds. Al-Mefty's Meningiomas, 2nd ed. New York, Stuttgart: Thieme; 2011:228–236**

21. Ringel F, Cedzich C, Schramm J. Microsurgical technique and results of a series of 63 spheno-orbital meningiomas. Neurosurgery 2007;60(4, Suppl 2):214–221, discussion 221–222

22. Mickey B, Close L, Schaefer S, Samson D. A combined frontotemporal and lateral infratemporal fossa approach to the skull base. J Neurosurg 1988;68:678–683

23. Basso AJ, Carrizo A. Sphenoid ridge meningiomas. In: Schmiedek HH, ed. Meningiomas and Their Surgical Management. Philadelphia: WB Saunders; 1991:233–241

24. Attia M, Patel KS, Kandasamy J, et al. Combined cranionasal surgery for spheno-orbital meningiomas invading the paranasal sinuses, pterygopalatine, and infratemporal fossa. World Neurosurg 2013;80:e367–e373

25. **Sughrue ME, Rutkowski MJ, Chen CJ, et al. Modern surgical outcomes following surgery for sphenoid wing meningiomas. J Neurosurg 2013;119:86–93**

26. Nakamura M, Roser F, Jacobs C, Vorkapic P, Samii M. Medial sphenoid wing meningiomas: clinical outcome and recurrence rate. Neurosurgery 2006;58:626–639, discussion 626–639

27. Chi M, Kim HJ, Koktekir BE, Vagefi R, Kersten RC. Iatrogenic cerebrospinal fluid oculorrhea. J Craniofac Surg 2014;25:469–470

28. Sughrue ME, McDermott MW. Meningiomas of the middle fossa floor. In: De Monte F, McDermott MW, Al-Mefty O, eds. Al-Mefty's Meningiomas, 2nd ed. New York, Stuttgart: Thieme; 2011:331–335

29. Graziani N, Bouillot P, Dufour H, et al. [Meningioma of the floor of the temporal fossa. Anatomo-clinical study of 11 cases]. Neurochirurgie 1994;40:109–115

30. **Sughrue ME, Cage T, Shangari G, Parsa AT, McDermott MW. Clinical characteristics and surgical outcomes of patients presenting with meningiomas arising predominantly from the floor of the middle fossa. Neurosurgery 2010;67:80–86, discussion 86**

31. Vaghi MA, Bruzzone MG, Visciani A, Passerini A. Intracranial tumors arising from the floor of the middle fossa. Ital J Neurol Sci 1985;6:469–475

21.2 Sellar/Parasellar Tumors

1. Krisht AF, Tindall GT. Pituitary Disorders. Comprehensive Management. Baltimore: Lippincott Williams & Wilkins; 1999

2. **Cusimano MD, Kan P, Nassiri F, et al. Outcomes of surgically treated giant pituitary tumours. Can J Neurol Sci 2012;39:446–457**

3. Hardy J. Transsphenoidal surgery of hypersecreting pituitary tumors. In: Kohler P, Ross G, eds. Diagnosis and Treatment of Pituitary Tumors. Amsterdam: Excerpta Medica; 1973:179–194

4. Hardy J. The transsphenoidal surgical approach to the pituitary. Hosp Pract 1979;14: 81–89

5. **Campero A, Martins C, Yasuda A, Rhoton AL Jr. Microsurgical anatomy of the diaphragma sellae and its role in directing the pattern of growth of pituitary adenomas. Neurosurgery 2008;62:717–723, discussion 717–723**

6. **Di Ieva A, Tschabitscher M, Matula C, et al. The subdiaphragmatic cistern: historic and radioanatomic findings. Acta Neurochir (Wien) 2012;154:667–674, discussion 674**

7. Wilson CB. Neurosurgical management of large and invasive pituitary tumors. In: Tindall G, Collins W, eds. Clinical Management of Pituitary Disorders. New York: Raven Press; 1979:335–342

8. **Knosp E, Steiner E, Kitz K, Matula C. Pituitary adenomas with invasion of the cavernous sinus space: a magnetic resonance imaging classification compared with surgical findings. Neurosurgery 1993;33:610–617, discussion 617–618**

9. **Di Ieva A, Rotondo F, Syro LV, Cusimano MD, Kovacs K. Aggressive pituitary adenomas—diagnosis and emerging treatments. Nat Rev Endocrinol 2014;10:423–435**

10. **Cusimano MD, Fenton RS. The technique for endoscopic pituitary tumor removal. Neurosurg Focus 1996;1:e1, discussion 1p, e3**

11. **Juraschka K, Khan OH, Godoy BL, et al. Endoscopic endonasal transsphenoidal approach to large and giant pituitary adenomas: institutional experience and predictors of extent of resection. J Neurosurg 2014;121:75–83**

12. Frank G, Pasquini E. Endoscopic endonasal cavernous sinus surgery, with special reference to pituitary adenomas. Front Horm Res 2006;34:64–82

13. **Ceylan S, Koc K, Anik I. Endoscopic endonasal transsphenoidal approach for pituitary adenomas invading the cavernous sinus. J Neurosurg 2010;112:99–107**

14. **Woodworth GF, Patel KS, Shin B, et al. Surgical outcomes using a medial-to-lateral endonasal endoscopic approach to pituitary adenomas invading the cavernous sinus. J Neurosurg 2014;120:1086–1094**

15. Nishioka H, Fukuhara N, Horiguchi K, Yamada S. Aggressive transsphenoidal resection of tumors invading the cavernous sinus in patients with acromegaly: predictive factors, strategies, and outcomes. J Neurosurg 2014;121:505–510

16. Oldfield EH. Editorial: management of invasion by pituitary adenomas. J Neurosurg 2014;121:501–503

17. **Starke RM, Raper DM, Payne SC, Vance ML, Oldfield EH, Jane JA Jr. Endoscopic vs microsurgical transsphenoidal surgery for acromegaly: outcomes in a concurrent series of patients using modern criteria for remission. J Clin Endocrinol Metab 2013;98:3190–3198**

18. Gao Y, Zhong C, Wang Y, et al. Endoscopic versus microscopic transsphenoidal pituitary adenoma surgery: a meta-analysis. World J Surg Oncol 2014;12:94–97

19. Wagenmakers MA, Boogaarts HD, Roerink SH, et al. Endoscopic transsphenoidal pituitary surgery: a good and safe primary treatment option for Cushing's disease, even in case of macroadenomas or invasive adenomas. Eur J Endocrinol 2013;169: 329–337

20. Fathalla H, Cusimano MD, Di Ieva A, et al. **Endoscopic versus microscopic approach for surgical treatment of acromegaly. Neurosurg Rev 2015;38:541-549**

21. Ammirati M, Wei L, Ciric I. **Short-term outcome of endoscopic versus microscopic pituitary adenoma surgery: a systematic review and meta-analysis. J Neurol Neurosurg Psychiatry 2013;84:843-849**

22. Dallapiazza R, Bond AE, Grober Y, et al. **Retrospective analysis of a concurrent series of microscopic versus endoscopic transsphenoidal surgeries for Knosp Grades 0-2 nonfunctioning pituitary macroadenomas at a single institution. J Neurosurg 2014;121:511-517**

23. Halvorsen H, Ramm-Pettersen J, Josefsen R, et al. **Surgical complications after transsphenoidal microscopic and endoscopic surgery for pituitary adenoma: a consecutive series of 506 procedures. Acta Neurochir (Wien) 2014;156:441-449**

24. Paluzzi A, Fernandez-Miranda JC, Tonya Stefko S, Challinor S, Snyderman CH, Gardner PA. Endoscopic endonasal approach for pituitary adenomas: a series of 555 patients. Pituitary 2014;17:307-319

25. Dusick JR, Esposito F, Malkasian D, Kelly DF. **Avoidance of carotid artery injuries in transsphenoidal surgery with the Doppler probe and micro-hook blades. Neurosurgery 2007;60(4, Suppl 2):322-328, discussion 328-329**

26. Mansouri A, Fallah A, Cusimano MD, Das S. **Vasospasm post pituitary surgery: systematic review and 3 case presentations. Can J Neurol Sci 2012;39:767-773**

27. Jane JA Jr, Laws ER. Craniopharyngioma. Pituitary 2006;9:323-326

28. Karavitaki N, Cudlip S, Adams CB, Wass JA. Craniopharyngiomas. Endocr Rev 2006; 27:371-397

29. Prabhu VC, Brown HG. The pathogenesis of craniopharyngiomas. Childs Nerv Syst 2005;21:622-627

30. Brunel H, Raybaud C, Peretti-Viton P, et al. [Craniopharyngioma in children: MRI study of 43 cases]. Neurochirurgie 2002;48:309-318

31. Crotty TB, Scheithauer BW, Young WF Jr, et al. Papillary craniopharyngioma: a clinico-pathological study of 48 cases. J Neurosurg 1995;83:206-214

32. Pan J, Qi S, Lu Y, et al. Intraventricular craniopharyngioma: morphological analysis and outcome evaluation of 17 cases. Acta Neurochir (Wien) 2011;153:773-784

33. Pascual JM, González-Llanos F, Barrios L, Roda JM. Intraventricular craniopharyngiomas: topographical classification and surgical approach selection based on an extensive overview. Acta Neurochir (Wien) 2004;146:785-802

34. Haupt R, Magnani C, Pavanello M, Caruso S, Dama E, Garrè ML. Epidemiological aspects of craniopharyngioma. J Pediatr Endocrinol Metab 2006;19(Suppl 1):289-293

35. Adamson TE, Wiestler OD, Kleihues P, Yaşargil MG. Correlation of clinical and pathological features in surgically treated craniopharyngiomas. J Neurosurg 1990;73: 12-17

36. Bunin GR, Surawicz TS, Witman PA, Preston-Martin S, Davis F, Bruner JM. The descriptive epidemiology of craniopharyngioma. J Neurosurg 1998;89:547-551

37. Sofela AA, Hettige S, Curran O, Bassi S. Malignant transformation in craniopharyngiomas. Neurosurgery 2014;75:306-314, discussion 314

38. Hoffman HJ, De Silva M, Humphreys RP, Drake JM, Smith ML, Blaser SI. Aggressive surgical management of craniopharyngiomas in children. J Neurosurg 1992;76: 47–52

39. **Fahlbusch R, Honegger J, Paulus W, Huk W, Buchfelder M. Surgical treatment of craniopharyngiomas: experience with 168 patients. J Neurosurg 1999;90:237–250**

40. Hald JK, Eldevik OP, Brunberg JA, Chandler WF. Craniopharyngiomas—the utility of contrast medium enhancement for MR imaging at 1.5 T. Acta Radiol 1994;35:520–525

41. Harwood-Nash DC. Neuroimaging of childhood craniopharyngioma. Pediatr Neurosurg 1994;21(Suppl 1):2–10

42. Steno J, Malácek M, Bízik I. Tumor-third ventricular relationships in supradiaphragmatic craniopharyngiomas: correlation of morphological, magnetic resonance imaging, and operative findings. Neurosurgery 2004;54:1051–1058, discussion 1058–1060

43. **Yaşargil MG, Curcic M, Kis M, Siegenthaler G, Teddy PJ, Roth P. Total removal of craniopharyngiomas. Approaches and long-term results in 144 patients. J Neurosurg 1990;73:3–11**

44. **Kassam AB, Gardner PA, Snyderman CH, Carrau RL, Mintz AH, Prevedello DM. Expanded endonasal approach, a fully endoscopic transnasal approach for the resection of midline suprasellar craniopharyngiomas: a new classification based on the infundibulum. J Neurosurg 2008;108:715–728**

45. Masson-Cote L, Masucci GL, Atenafu EG, et al. Long-term outcomes for adult craniopharyngioma following radiation therapy. Acta Oncol 2013;52:153–158

46. Karavitaki N, Brufani C, Warner JT, et al. Craniopharyngiomas in children and adults: systematic analysis of 121 cases with long-term follow-up. Clin Endocrinol (Oxf) 2005;62:397–409

47. **Cavallo LM, Prevedello DM, Solari D, et al. Extended endoscopic endonasal transsphenoidal approach for residual or recurrent craniopharyngiomas. J Neurosurg 2009;111:578–589**

48. Liu JK, Christiano LD, Gupta G, Carmel PW. Surgical nuances for removal of retrochiasmatic craniopharyngiomas via the transbasal subfrontal translamina terminalis approach. Neurosurg Focus 2010;28:E6

49. **Liu JK. Modified one-piece extended transbasal approach for translamina terminalis resection of retrochiasmatic third ventricular craniopharyngioma. Neurosurg Focus 2013;34(1, Suppl):Video 1**

50. Wiedemayer H, Sandalcioglu IE, Wiedemayer H, Stolke D. The supraorbital keyhole approach via an eyebrow incision for resection of tumors around the sella and the anterior skull base. Minim Invasive Neurosurg 2004;47:221–225

51. **Reisch R, Perneczky A. Ten-year experience with the supraorbital subfrontal approach through an eyebrow skin incision. Neurosurgery 2005;57(4, Suppl):242–255, discussion 242–255**

52. McLaughlin N, Ditzel Filho LF, Shahlaie K, Solari D, Kassam AB, Kelly DF. The supraorbital approach for recurrent or residual suprasellar tumors. Minim Invasive Neurosurg 2011;54:155–161

53. Wilson DA, Duong H, Teo C, Kelly DF. The supraorbital endoscopic approach for tumors. World Neurosurg 2014;82:e243–e256

54. Symon L, Pell MF, Habib AH. Radical excision of craniopharyngioma by the temporal route: a review of 50 patients. Br J Neurosurg 1991;5:539–549

55. **Al-Mefty O, Ayoubi S, Kadri PA. The petrosal approach for the total removal of giant retrochiasmatic craniopharyngiomas in children. J Neurosurg 2007;106(2, Suppl):87–92**

56. **Al-Mefty O, Ayoubi S, Kadri PA. The petrosal approach for the resection of retro-chiasmatic craniopharyngiomas. Neurosurgery 2008;62(5, Suppl 2):ONS331–ONS335, discussion ONS335–ONS336**

57. Hakuba A, Nishimura S, Inoue Y. Transpetrosal-transtentorial approach and its application in the therapy of retrochiasmatic craniopharyngiomas. Surg Neurol 1985;24: 405–415

58. Jagannathan J, Dumont AS, Jane JA Jr. Diagnosis and management of pediatric sellar lesions. Front Horm Res 2006;34:83–104

59. Norris JS, Pavaresh M, Afshar F. Primary transsphenoidal microsurgery in the treatment of craniopharyngiomas. Br J Neurosurg 1998;12:305–312

60. de Divitiis E, Cappabianca P, Gangemi M, Cavallo LM. The role of the endoscopic transsphenoidal approach in pediatric neurosurgery. Childs Nerv Syst 2000;16:692–696

61. **Teo C. Application of endoscopy to the surgical management of craniopharyngiomas. Childs Nerv Syst 2005;21:696–700**

62. Steinbok P, Hukin J. Intracystic treatments for craniopharyngioma. Neurosurg Focus 2010;28:E13

63. Cavalheiro S, Di Rocco C, Valenzuela S, et al. Craniopharyngiomas: intratumoral chemotherapy with interferon-alpha: a multicenter preliminary study with 60 cases. Neurosurg Focus 2010;28:E12

64. Honegger J, Buchfelder M, Fahlbusch R, Däubler B, Dörr HG. Transsphenoidal microsurgery for craniopharyngioma. Surg Neurol 1992;37:189–196

65. Laws ER Jr. Transsphenoidal microsurgery in the management of craniopharyngioma. J Neurosurg 1980;52:661–666

66. **Cavallo LM, de Divitiis O, Aydin S, et al. Extended endoscopic endonasal transsphenoidal approach to the suprasellar area: anatomic considerations—part 1. Neurosurgery 2007;61(3, Suppl):24–33, discussion 33–34**

67. Wang KC, Kim SK, Choe G, Chi JG, Cho BK. Growth patterns of craniopharyngioma in children: role of the diaphragm sellae and its surgical implication. Surg Neurol 2002; 57:25–33

68. Kaptain GJ, Vincent DA, Sheehan JP, Laws ER Jr. Transsphenoidal approaches for the extracapsular resection of midline suprasellar and anterior cranial base lesions. Neurosurgery 2001;49:94–100, discussion 100–101

69. **Cavallo LM, Frank G, Cappabianca P, et al. The endoscopic endonasal approach for the management of craniopharyngiomas: a series of 103 patients. J Neurosurg 2014;121:100–113**

70. Tomita T, McLone DG. Radical resections of childhood craniopharyngiomas. Pediatr Neurosurg 1993;19:6–14

71. Sanford RA. Craniopharyngioma: results of survey of the American Society of Pediatric Neurosurgery. Pediatr Neurosurg 1994;21(Suppl 1):39–43

72. Koutourousiou M, Gardner PA, Fernandez-Miranda JC, Tyler-Kabara EC, Wang EW, Snyderman CH. Endoscopic endonasal surgery for craniopharyngiomas: surgical outcome in 64 patients. J Neurosurg 2013;119:1194–1207

73. De Vile CJ, Grant DB, Kendall BE, et al. Management of childhood craniopharyngioma: can the morbidity of radical surgery be predicted? J Neurosurg 1996;85:73–81

74. Kalapurakal JA, Goldman S, Hsieh YC, Tomita T, Marymont MH. Clinical outcome in children with recurrent craniopharyngioma after primary surgery. Cancer J 2000;6: 388–393

75. Yang I, Sughrue ME, Rutkowski MJ, et al. Craniopharyngioma: a comparison of tumor control with various treatment strategies. Neurosurg Focus 2010;28:E5

76. Rajan B, Ashley S, Gorman C, et al. Craniopharyngioma—a long-term results following limited surgery and radiotherapy. Radiother Oncol 1993;26:1–10

77. Weiner HL, Wisoff JH, Rosenberg ME, et al. Craniopharyngiomas: a clinicopathological analysis of factors predictive of recurrence and functional outcome. Neurosurgery 1994;35:1001–1010, discussion 1010–1011

78. Tavangar SM, Larijani B, Mahta A, Hosseini SM, Mehrazine M, Bandarian F. Craniopharyngioma: a clinicopathological study of 141 cases. Endocr Pathol 2004;15:339–344

79. Pierre-Kahn A, Recassens C, Pinto G, et al. Social and psycho-intellectual outcome following radical removal of craniopharyngiomas in childhood. A prospective series. Childs Nerv Syst 2005;21:817–824

80. **Frank G, Pasquini E, Doglietto F, et al. The endoscopic extended transsphenoidal approach for craniopharyngiomas. Neurosurgery 2006;59(1, Suppl 1):ONS75–ONS83, discussion ONS75–ONS83**

81. **de Divitiis E, Cappabianca P, Cavallo LM, Esposito F, de Divitiis O, Messina A. Extended endoscopic transsphenoidal approach for extrasellar craniopharyngiomas. Neurosurgery 2007;61(5, Suppl 2):219–227, discussion 228**

82. Kanter AS, Sansur CA, Jane JA Jr, Laws ER Jr. Rathke's cleft cysts. Front Horm Res 2006;34:127–157

83. **Zada G, Lin N, Ojerholm E, Ramkissoon S, Laws ER. Craniopharyngioma and other cystic epithelial lesions of the sellar region: a review of clinical, imaging, and histopathological relationships. Neurosurg Focus 2010;28:E4**

84. **Aho CJ, Liu C, Zelman V, Couldwell WT, Weiss MH. Surgical outcomes in 118 patients with Rathke cleft cysts. J Neurosurg 2005;102:189–193**

85. Kim JE, Kim JH, Kim OL, et al. Surgical treatment of symptomatic Rathke cleft cysts: clinical features and results with special attention to recurrence. J Neurosurg 2004; 100:33–40

86. Benveniste RJ, King WA, Walsh J, Lee JS, Naidich TP, Post KD. Surgery for Rathke cleft cysts: technical considerations and outcomes. J Neurosurg 2004;101:577–584

87. **Kinjo T, al-Mefty O, Ciric I. Diaphragma sellae meningiomas. Neurosurgery 1995; 36:1082–1092**

88. Cappabianca P, Cirillo S, Alfieri A, et al. Pituitary macroadenoma and diaphragma sellae meningioma: differential diagnosis on MRI. Neuroradiology 1999;41:22–26

89. **Mortini P, Barzaghi LR, Serra C, Orlandi V, Bianchi S, Losa M. Visual outcome after fronto-temporo-orbito-zygomatic approach combined with early extradural and**

intradural optic nerve decompression in tuberculum and diaphragma sellae meningiomas. Clin Neurol Neurosurg 2012;114:597–606

21.3. Cavernous Sinus Surgery

1. Radhakrishnan K, Mokri B, Parisi JE, O'Fallon WM, Sunku J, Kurland LT. The trends in incidence of primary brain tumors in the population of Rochester, Minnesota. Ann Neurol 1995;37:67–73
2. **Dunn IF, Al-Mefty O. Cavernous sinus meningiomas. In: De Monte F, McDermott MW, Al-Mefty O, eds. Al-Mefty's Meningiomas, 2nd ed. New York, Stuttgart: Thieme; 237–247**
3. Bindal R, Goodman JM, Kawasaki A, Purvin V, Kuzma B. The natural history of untreated skull base meningiomas. Surg Neurol 2003;59:87–92, discussion 92
4. **Nakamura M, Roser F, Michel J, Jacobs C, Samii M. The natural history of incidental meningiomas. Neurosurgery 2003;53:62–70, discussion 70–71**
5. Bansal S, Suri A, Singh M, et al. Cavernous sinus hemangioma: a fourteen year single institution experience. J Clin Neurosci 2014;21:968–974
6. **Cusimano MD, Sekhar LN, Sen CN, et al. The results of surgery for benign tumors of the cavernous sinus. Neurosurgery 1995;37:1–9, discussion 9–10**
7. **Raso J, Sekhar LN, Tzortzidis F. Anatomy of the cavernous sinus. In: Sekhar LN, Oliveira ED, eds. Cranial Microsurgery: Approaches and Techniques. New York: Thieme; 1999:176–181**
8. **Dolenc VV. Anatomy and Surgery of the Cavernous Sinus. Vienna, New York: Springer-Verlag; 1989**
9. **Dolenc VV. Microsurgical Anatomy and Surgery of the Central Skull Base. New York: Springer-Verlag; 2003**
10. al-Mefty O, Anand VK. Zygomatic approach to skull-base lesions. J Neurosurg 1990; 73:668–673
11. Wascher TM, Spetzler RF, Zabramski JM. Improved transdural exposure and temporary occlusion of the petrous internal carotid artery for cavernous sinus surgery. Technical note. J Neurosurg 1993;78:834–837
12. **Yasuda A, Campero A, Martins C, Rhoton AL Jr, de Oliveira E, Ribas GC. Microsurgical anatomy and approaches to the cavernous sinus. Neurosurgery 2005;56(1, Suppl):4–27, discussion 4–27**
13. Krayenbühl N, Hafez A, Hernesniemi JA, Krisht AF. Taming the cavernous sinus: technique of hemostasis using fibrin glue. Neurosurgery 2007;61(3, Suppl):E52, discussion E52
14. Day JD, Giannotta SL, Fukushima T. Extradural temporopolar approach to lesions of the upper basilar artery and infrachiasmatic region. J Neurosurg 1994;81:230–235
15. **Krisht AF, Kadri PA. Surgical clipping of complex basilar apex aneurysms: a strategy for successful outcome using the pretemporal transzygomatic transcavernous approach. Neurosurgery 2005;56(2, Suppl):261–273, discussion 261–273**
16. Samson DS, Hodosh RM, Clark WK. Microsurgical evaluation of the pterional approach to aneurysms of the distal basilar circulation. Neurosurgery 1978;3:135–141

17. Sindou M, Wydh E, Jouanneau E, Nebbal M, Lieutaud T. Long-term follow-up of meningiomas of the cavernous sinus after surgical treatment alone. J Neurosurg 2007;107:937–944
18. Pichierri A, Santoro A, Raco A, Paolini S, Cantore G, Delfini R. Cavernous sinus meningiomas: retrospective analysis and proposal of a treatment algorithm. Neurosurgery 2009;64:1090–1099, discussion 1099–1101
19. O'Sullivan MG, van Loveren HR, Tew JM Jr. The surgical resectability of meningiomas of the cavernous sinus. Neurosurgery 1997;40:238–244, discussion 245–247
20. Sekhar LN, Patel S, Cusimano M, Wright DC, Sen CN, Bank WO. Surgical treatment of meningiomas involving the cavernous sinus: evolving ideas based on a ten year experience. Acta Neurochir Suppl (Wien) 1996;65:58–62

21.4. Trigeminal Schwannoma

1. Konovalov AN, Spallone A, Mukhamedjanov DJ, Tcherekajev VA, Makhmudov UB. Trigeminal neurinomas. A series of 111 surgical cases from a single institution. Acta Neurochir (Wien) 1996;138:1027–1035
2. Samii M, Migliori MM, Tatagiba M, Babu R. Surgical treatment of trigeminal schwannomas. J Neurosurg 1995;82:711–718
3. Goel A, Shah A, Muzumdar D, Nadkarni T, Chagla A. Trigeminal neurinomas with extracranial extension: analysis of 28 surgically treated cases. J Neurosurg 2010;113:1079–1084
4. Wanibuchi M, Fukushima T, Zomordi AR, Nonaka Y, Friedman AH. Trigeminal schwannomas: skull base approaches and operative results in 105 patients. Neurosurgery 2012;70(1, Suppl Operative):132–143, discussion 143–144
5. Dolenc VV. Frontotemporal epidural approach to trigeminal neurinomas. Acta Neurochir (Wien) 1994;130:55–65
6. Kobayashi M, Yoshida K, Kawase T. Inter-dural approach to parasellar tumors. Acta Neurochir (Wien) 2010;152:279–284, discussion 284–285
7. Muto J, Kawase T, Yoshida K. Meckel's cave tumors: relation to the meninges and minimally invasive approaches for surgery: anatomic and clinical studies. Neurosurgery 2010;67(3, Suppl Operative):ons291–ons298, discussion ons298–ons299
8. Jefferson G. The trigeminal neurinomas with some remarks on malignant invasion of the gasserian ganglion. Clin Neurosurg 1953;1:11–54
9. Yoshida K, Kawase T. Trigeminal neurinomas extending into multiple fossae: surgical methods and review of the literature. J Neurosurg 1999;91:202–211
10. Komatsu F, Komatsu M, Di Ieva A, Tschabitscher M. Endoscopic approaches to the trigeminal nerve and clinical consideration for trigeminal schwannomas: a cadaveric study. J Neurosurg 2012;117:690–696
11. Samii M, Alimohamadi M, Gerganov V. Endoscope-assisted retrosigmoid intradural suprameatal approach for surgical treatment of trigeminal schwannomas. Neurosurgery 2014;10(Suppl 4):565–575, discussion 575
12. Goel A, Muzumdar D, Raman C. Trigeminal neuroma: analysis of surgical experience with 73 cases. Neurosurgery 2003;52:783–790, discussion 790

13. Liu XD, Xu QW, Che XM, Yang DL. Trigeminal neurinomas: clinical features and surgical experience in 84 patients. Neurosurg Rev 2009;32:435–444

14. Huang CF, Kondziolka D, Flickinger JC, Lunsford LD. Stereotactic radiosurgery for trigeminal schwannomas. Neurosurgery 1999;45:11–16, discussion 16

15. Goel A. Infratemporal fossa interdural approach for trigeminal neurinomas. Acta Neurochir (Wien) 1995;136:99–102

16. Goel A, Nadkarni T. Basal lateral subtemporal approach for trigeminal neurinomas: report of an experience with 18 cases. Acta Neurochir (Wien) 1999;141:711–719

17. King J, Cusimano M, Hawkins C, Dirks P. Extradural middle fossa approach to a clear cell meningioma in a child. Can J Neurol Sci 2009;36:257–261

18. Day JD, Giannotta SL, Fukushima T. Extradural temporopolar approach to lesions of the upper basilar artery and infrachiasmatic region. J Neurosurg 1994;81:230–235

19. Fukushima T. Manual of Skull Base Dissection. Pittsburgh, PA: AF-Neurovideo Inc.; 2004

20. Wanibuchi M, Friedman HA, Fukushima T. Photo-Atlas of Skull Base Dissection: Technique and Operative Approaches. New York: Thieme; 2009

21. Shin SS, Gardner PA, Stefko ST, Madhok R, Fernandez-Miranda JC, Snyderman CH. Endoscopic endonasal approach for nonvestibular schwannomas. Neurosurgery 2011;69:1046–1057, discussion 1057

22. Prevedello DM, Pinheiro-Neto CD, Fernandez-Miranda JC, et al. Vidian nerve transposition for endoscopic endonasal middle fossa approaches. Neurosurgery 2010;67(2, Suppl Operative):478–484

23. Pan L, Wang EM, Zhang N, et al. Long-term results of Leksell gamma knife surgery for trigeminal schwannomas. J Neurosurg 2005;102(Suppl):220–224

24. Phi JH, Paek SH, Chung HT, et al. Gamma knife surgery and trigeminal schwannoma: is it possible to preserve cranial nerve function? J Neurosurg 2007;107:727–732

25. Sheehan J, Yen CP, Arkha Y, Schlesinger D, Steiner L. Gamma knife surgery for trigeminal schwannoma. J Neurosurg 2007;106:839–845

21.5. Osseous Lesions of the Skull Base

1. Patel SJ. Fibrous dysplasias, osteopetrosis, and ossifying fibromas. In: Sekhar LN, Fessler RG, eds. Atlas of Neurosurgical Techniques. New York, Stuttgart: Thieme; 2006:618–622

2. Tucker WS, Nasser-Sharif FJ. Benign skull lesions. Can J Surg 1997;40:449–455

3. Chapurlat RD, Meunier PJ. Fibrous dysplasia of bone. Best Pract Res Clin Rheumatol 2000;14:385–398

4. Lee JS, FitzGibbon E, Butman JA, et al. Normal vision despite narrowing of the optic canal in fibrous dysplasia. N Engl J Med 2002;347:1670–1676

5. Hart ES, Kelly MH, Brillante B, et al. Onset, progression, and plateau of skeletal lesions in fibrous dysplasia and the relationship to functional outcome. J Bone Miner Res 2007;22:1468–1474

6. MacDonald-Jankowski D. Fibrous dysplasia: a systematic review. Dentomaxillofac Radiol 2009;38:196–215

7. **Rahman AM, Madge SN, Billing K, et al. Craniofacial fibrous dysplasia: clinical characteristics and long-term outcomes. Eye (Lond) 2009;23:2175–2181**

8. Ricalde P, Magliocca KR, Lee JS. Craniofacial fibrous dysplasia. Oral Maxillofac Surg Clin North Am 2012;24:427–441

9. Loría-Cortés R, Quesada-Calvo E, Cordero-Chaverri C. Osteopetrosis in children: a report of 26 cases. J Pediatr 1977;91:43–47

10. Bollerslev J, Andersen PE Jr. Radiological, biochemical and hereditary evidence of two types of autosomal dominant osteopetrosis. Bone 1988;9:7–13

11. Larrea-Oyarbide N, Valmaseda-Castellón E, Berini-Aytés L, Gay-Escoda C. Osteomas of the craniofacial region. Review of 106 cases. J Oral Pathol Med 2008;37:38–42

12. Adler M, Hnatuk L, Mock D, Freeman JL. Aggressive osteoblastoma of the temporal bone: a case report. J Otolaryngol 1990;19:307–310

13. Bilkay U, Erdem O, Ozek C, et al. Benign osteoma with Gardner syndrome: review of the literature and report of a case. J Craniofac Surg 2004;15:506–509

14. Lucas DR, Unni KK, McLeod RA, O'Connor MI, Sim FH. Osteoblastoma: clinicopathologic study of 306 cases. Hum Pathol 1994;25:117–134

15. Lucas DR. Osteoblastoma. Arch Pathol Lab Med 2010;134:1460–1466

16. Jasnau S, Meyer U, Potratz J, et al; Cooperative Osteosarcoma Study Group COSS. Craniofacial osteosarcoma Experience of the cooperative German-Austrian-Swiss osteosarcoma study group. Oral Oncol 2008;44:286–294

17. Guadagnolo BA, Zagars GK, Raymond AK, Benjamin RS, Sturgis EM. Osteosarcoma of the jaw/craniofacial region: outcomes after multimodality treatment. Cancer 2009; 115:3262–3270

18. **Desai KI, Nadkarni TD, Goel A, Muzumdar DP, Naresh KN, Nair CN. Primary Ewing's sarcoma of the cranium. Neurosurgery 2000;46:62–68, discussion 68–69**

19. Dahlin DC. Caldwell Lecture. Giant cell tumor of bone: highlights of 407 cases. AJR Am J Roentgenol 1985;144:955–960

20. Feigenberg SJ, Marcus RB Jr, Zlotecki RA, Scarborough MT, Berrey BH, Enneking WF. Radiation therapy for giant cell tumors of bone. Clin Orthop Relat Res 2003;411:207–216

21. Borges BB, Fornazieri MA, Bezerra AP, Martins LA, Pinna FdeR, Voegels RL. Giant cell bone lesions in the craniofacial region: a diagnostic and therapeutic challenge. Int Forum Allergy Rhinol 2012;2:501–506

22. **Zhang Z, Xu J, Yao Y, et al. Giant cell tumors of the skull: a series of 18 cases and review of the literature. J Neurooncol 2013;115:437–444**

23. **Prasad SC, Piccirillo E, Nuseir A, et al. Giant cell tumors of the skull base: case series and current concepts. Audiol Neurootol 2014;19:12–21**

24. Gumà M, Rotés D, Holgado S, et al. [Paget's disease of bone: study of 314 patients]. Med Clin (Barc) 2002;119:537–540

25. Hershkovitz I, Greenwald C, Rothschild BM, et al. Hyperostosis frontalis interna: an anthropological perspective. Am J Phys Anthropol 1999;109:303–325

26. May H, Peled N, Dar G, Abbas J, Hershkovitz I. Hyperostosis frontalis interna: what does it tell us about our health? Am J Hum Biol 2011;23:392–397

27. **Heckl S, Aschoff A, Kunze S. Cavernomas of the skull: review of the literature 1975–2000. Neurosurg Rev 2002;25:56–62, discussion 66–67**

28. Park BH, Hwang E, Kim CH. Primary intraosseous hemangioma in the frontal bone. Arch Plast Surg 2013;40:283–285

29. Nager GT, Kennedy DW, Kopstein E. Fibrous dysplasia: a review of the disease and its manifestations in the temporal bone. Ann Otol Rhinol Laryngol Suppl 1982;92:1–52

30. Beuerlein ME, Schuller DE, DeYoung BR. Maxillary malignant mesenchymoma and massive fibrous dysplasia. Arch Otolaryngol Head Neck Surg 1997;123:106–109

31. Chen YR, Noordhoff MS. Treatment of craniomaxillofacial fibrous dysplasia: how early and how extensive? Plast Reconstr Surg 1990;86:835–842, discussion 843–844

32. Al-Mefty O, Fox JL, Al-Rodhan N, Dew JH. Optic nerve decompression in osteopetrosis. J Neurosurg 1988;68:80–84

33. Johnston CC Jr, Lavy N, Lord T, Vellios F, Merritt AD, Deiss WP Jr. Osteopetrosis. A clinical, genetic, metabolic, and morphologic study of the dominantly inherited, benign form. Medicine (Baltimore) 1968;47:149–167

34. Curé JK, Key LL, Goltra DD, VanTassel P. Cranial MR imaging of osteopetrosis. AJNR Am J Neuroradiol 2000;21:1110–1115

35. Tolar J, Teitelbaum SL, Orchard PJ. Osteopetrosis. N Engl J Med 2004;351:2839–2849

22 Posterior Skull Base Surgery

■ Posterior Skull Base

Review the anatomy of the posterior fossa and cerebellopontine angle (CPA) in Chapter 2 and see **Fig. 2.9**, page 30.

Surgical conditions of the posterior fossa include the following:

- Vestibular schwannomas (the most common CPA tumor)
- Clival, petroclival, and CPA meningiomas (2% of intracranial meningiomas), foramen magnum meningiomas (3% of meningiomas)[1,2]
- Dermoids/epidermoids of the CPA (7% of CPA tumors)
- Chordoma and chondrosarcoma of the clivus
- Tentorial meningiomas
- Jugular foramen paraganglioma, schwannomas, meningiomas
- Schwannomas of the facial, trigeminal, and lower cranial nerves
- Microvascular decompression of cranial nerves (CNs) V, VII, VIII, IX, and X (see Subchapter 22.8, below)
- Other CPA and posterior fossa lesions: arachnoid cysts, lipomas, neurenteric cysts
- Vertebrobasilar system and dural sinuses vascular neurosurgery

Preoperative Assessment

The anatomic complexity of the posterior fossa and CPA tumors gives rises to a wide range of signs and symptoms. A detailed neurologic exam, with particular attention to the cranial nerves and to cerebellar and brainstem function is essential before surgery.

- It is recommended to refer the patient for dedicated audiogram tests to assess the patient's hearing function.

Symptoms

Symptoms include headaches, gait disturbances, cranial nerve palsies, cerebellar and brainstem compression signs, and possible hydrocephalus.

The majority of studies report tumor sizes ranging from 2 to 4 cm at the time of first diagnosis of CPA meningiomas.[3-5]

Radiology

- Computed tomography (CT) for bone anatomy and degree of bone pneumatization, presence of tumor calcification, neuronavigation.
- Magnetic resonance imaging (MRI) for tumor characterization, presence of edema, integrity of the arachnoid plane (in T2, regarding meningiomas), consistency of the tumor (hyperintensity in T2 indicates a softer tumor); magnetic resonance angiography (MRA)/magnetic resonance venography (MRV) recommended for peritumoral vascularization and sinus patency.
- Angiography: venous and arterial anatomy, for eventual embolization. Check preoperatively, in MRI/MRV or angiogram, the size and shape of the transverse and sigmoid sinuses, the position of the jugular bulb, the position of the vein of Labbé, anastomotic circles, and the size and pattern of the dural sinuses.

Intraoperative Monitoring

Monitoring should include somatosensory evoked potentials, motor evoked potentials (including lower cranial nerves), facial nerve monitoring, brainstem auditory evoked response, and electroencephalogram (EEG). CN VI monitoring is not usually done.

■ 22.1 Vestibular Schwannoma

- Benign, slowly growing tumor (also called acoustic neurinoma, neurilemoma, or neuroma, but these terms should no longer be used)
- Very rarely may undergo malignant change[6]

Epidemiology

- Vestibular schwannomas (VSs) account for 8 to 10% of intracranial tumors and 85% of CPA tumors.

- The annual incidence is 0.78 to 1.15 cases per 100,000 population.
- Vestibular schwannomas are generally symptomatic after age 30.
- 90 to 95% are unilateral; 4% are bilateral in neurofibromatosis type 2 (NF2).

Risk Factors

There have been no definite risk factors identified. An increased risk of VS has been shown to positively correlate with mobile phone use of at least 5 years' duration,[7] but this finding is still controversial.[8]

Pathology

See Chapter 6, page 135.

- In 70 to 90% of the cases, VSs arise from the inferior vestibular branch at the Obersteiner-Redlich junction,[9,10] which is between the peripheral and central myelin and is 8 to 12 mm distal from the brainstem.
- Approximately 6 to 30% of VSs originate from the superior vestibular nerve.[9,10]
- Rarely, cases have been reported in which the origin of the VS is the cochlear or facial nerve (1% each), whereas some cases have reported the origin arising from the nervus intermedius.
- Growth rate: average 1 mm/year (range 0 to more than 10 mm/year). Three patterns: no or very slow growth; slow growth (1–2 mm/year); and fast growth (> 8 mm/year, often in cystic VSs). The volume doubles in 1.6 to 4.4 years.[11]
  - In a study of 197 patients, 66.3% had no growth, 23.9% had slow growth, 4.1% had fast growth, and 3% had smaller tumors. Follow-up ranged from 12 to 180 months.[12] These data should be considered in deciding on conservative versus surgical/radiosurgical treatment.

Clinical Signs and Symptoms

Clinical signs and symptoms most often occur as an insidious and progressive triad of hearing loss, tinnitus, and disequilibrium **(Table 22.1)**. Hearing loss occurs at a rate of 7% at higher frequencies, and sudden hearing loss may occur in 10% of cases. Depending on the size of the tumor and the extent of brainstem compression, more symptoms may arise, such as numbness, limb weakness, facial twitching, and brainstem symptoms. Obstructive hydrocephalus is rarely the presentation of the tumor. Hydrocephalus may be also caused by elevated

Table 22.1   Signs and Symptoms of Vestibular Schwannomas[14]

Sign or Symptom	%
Hearing loss	98
Tinnitus	70
Dysequilibrium/vertigo	67
Headache	32
Facial numbness	29
Facial weakness	10
Diplopia	10
Nausea and vomiting	9
Change of taste	6

cerebrospinal fluid (CSF) protein secondary to tumor presence. Tumor resection also may be the treatment of the hydrocephalus itself, avoiding the use of a ventricular shunt.[13]

Diagnostic Tools: Investigations and Imaging

- Audiogram, check auditory function: new Hannover classification:[15]
  - H1, normal hearing, 0–20 dB and 95–100% speech discrimination score (SDS)
  - H2, useful hearing, 21–40 dB and 70–94% SDS
  - H3, moderate hearing, 41–60 dB and 40–69% SDS
  - H4 poor hearing, 61–80 dB and 10–39% SDS
  - H5 nonfunctional hearing > 80 dB and 0–9% SDS
- Brainstem auditory evoked potentials (BAEPs): See pages 92 and 191. Intraoperative BAEPs are very helpful, giving feedback every 30 to 90 seconds.[15,16] A wave V loss is generally associated with deafness, but changes in waves I and III may predict it before the injury occurs via manipulation/traction of the nerve.
- CT, MRI, and, for giant tumors (> 4 cm), computed tomography angiography (CTA) or, rarely, a digital substraction angiogram are used when a transpetrosal approach is planned (vascular and sinuses anatomy).
- MRI with three-dimensional (3D) spin echo sequences provides detail on the cranial nerves (see also **Table 5.4**, page 117).

Grading

Grading is demonstrated in **Table 22.2** and **Fig. 22.1**.

Table 22.2   Grading of Vestibular Schwannomas

Tumor extension classification system[15-17]

    T1 Purely intrameatal

    T2 Intra- and extrameatal

    T3 a Filling the cerebellopontine cistern

        b Reaching the brainstem

    T4 a Compressing the brainstem

        b Severely dislocating the brainstem and compressing the fourth ventricle

Size- and anatomy-related classification system[9,18]

    Grade 1 Diameter 1–10 mm, intracanalicular

    Grade 2 < 20 mm, intracanalicular and intracisternal

        2a Tumor does not extend more than 10 mm into the CPA*

        2b Tumor extends 11–18 mm into the CPA from the porus acusticus**

    Grade 3 < 30 mm, reaching the brainstem

    Grade 4 ≥ 30 mm, indenting and displacing the brainstem

Abbreviation: CPA, cerebellopontine angle.

*Measured from the lip of the porus acusticus.

**Leaving 5 to 8 mm between the tumor and the brainstem.

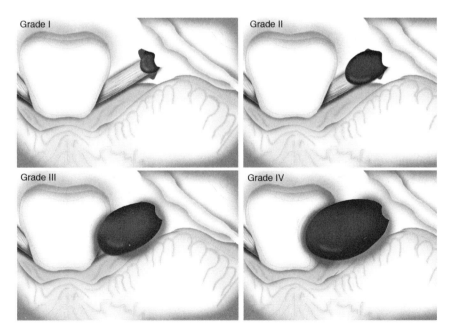

Fig. 22.1   Vestibular schwannomas grading based on the Koos et al classification system. (Adapted from Koos WT, Matula C, Lang J. Color Atlas of Microneurosurgery of Acoustic Neurinomas. New York, Stuttgart: Georg Thieme Verlag; 2002.)

Surgical Anatomy Pearls

- Grade 4 tumors are associated with a higher incidence of hydrocephalus.
- In fewer than 10% of cases and especially in patients with NF2, the tumor can be purely extracanalicular, growing in the CPA. The rare entity of an extrameatal vestibular schwannoma has been defined as "medial acoustic neuroma," in which the clinical characteristics are quite different from the other vestibular schwannomas. Medial acoustic neuromas result in preserved hearing and more severe cerebellum, brainstem, and trigeminal impairment.[19] Medial acoustic neuromas are often cystic, hypervascular, large, and highly adherent to the brainstem for focal lack of the typically-found duplicated arachnoidal layer.[20]

Surgical Pathology

It is important to recognize the patterns of displacement of the CPA cranial nerves when approaching the tumor. Review CN VII and VIII anatomy in Chapter 3, see also **Fig. 3.3** on page 86.

Facial Nerve

See **Table 22.3**.

- The nerve can be recognizable in the form of a thin bundle, but in one third of cases it may be splayed out into multiple projections adherent to the capsule (this occurs in two thirds of cases of VS in patients affected by von Recklinghausen's disease).

Vestibulocochlear Nerve

See **Table 22.4**.

- In tumors grade 3 and 4, the hearing is lost in 90% of cases. In the few cases when the hearing is functional, such as in cases with a displaced normal nerve, every attempt should be made to preserve it.

Table 22.3   Pattern of Displacement of Cranial Nerve VII[9]

Pattern	Percent of Cases
Anterior displacement	70
Superior displacement	10
Posterior course around the tumor	7
Inferior course	13

Table 22.4   Pattern of Displacement of Cranial Nerve VIII[9]

Type	Pattern	Percent of Cases
I	The nerve is involved in the tumor, making the separation virtually impossible	50
II	The nerve begins as a bundle from the brainstem, but it splays out in the tumor	40
III	The nerve is spared in its anatomic integrity	10*

*It runs medially (18%), laterally (2%), or inferiorly (80%) to the tumor.

- **Arterial supply to the tumor**: branches from the anterior inferior cerebellar artery (AICA), meningeal branches from internal carotid artery (ICA) and external carotid artery (ECA). In contrast, the rarer variant of hypervascular VSs is supplied by the vertebrobasilar system, presenting several intratumoral arteriovenous shunts.[21]

Treatment

- The type of treatment depends on the size of the tumor, its growth pattern, the neurologic symptoms (cranial nerves or brainstem compression), and patient age and comorbidities **(Fig. 22.2)**.
- Small tumors or those found at follow-up that have not shown any growth might be managed conservatively[22] **(Fig. 22.3)**, but treatment is suggested when the tumor shows growth over time, there is a worsening of the neurologic symptoms, or new neurologic deficits arise.
- Gamma Knife radiosurgery is suggested for controlling the growth (with hearing preservation ranging from 64 to 85% and facial nerve preservation in > 95%

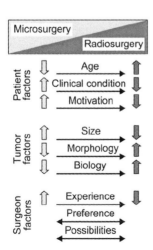

Fig. 22.2 Factors to evaluate in determining the treatment for vestibular schwannomas. (From Koos WT, Matula C, Lang J. Color Atlas of Microneurosurgery of Acoustic Neurinomas. New York, Stuttgart: Georg Thieme Verlag; 2002.)

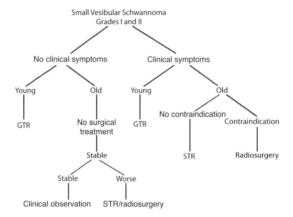

Fig. 22.3 Small vestibular schwannomas: algorithm of treatment. GTR, gross total resection; STR, subtotal resection. (Adapted from Koos WT, Matula C, Lang J. Color Atlas of Microneurosurgery of Acoustic Neurinomas. New York, Stuttgart: Georg Thieme Verlag; 2002.)

of cases)[11] of tumors smaller than 3 cm or for the treatment of recurrences/residuals of tumors after surgery (see also Chapter 30, page 782). The possible radiosurgical complications, such as hearing loss, facial and trigeminal deficits, hydrocephalus, and potential malignant transformation, must be considered. Other possible complications, such as delayed severe headache, severe facial pain, new motor deficits, or hydrocephalus requiring ventriculoperitoneal shunt, should be considered as well.[23] As with surgery, patients with a tumor volume > 5 cm³ have increased rates of complications.[24] Regardless of size, Gamma Knife yields better facial nerve results than does open surgery. Surgical resection is still the best treatment modality[25] for those healthy patients who are younger than 60 years and have mass effect causing ataxia, severe vertigo or dizziness, brainstem compression, or tumors that are mostly cystic (**Figs. 22.3** and **22.4**).

Surgical Approaches (Fig. 22.5)

• Approaches are tailored to the patient, the tumor, and the surgeon's preferences and experience.
• Surgery is indicated for tumor grades 1 and 2a[9] or smaller than 2.5 cm,[26] with no functional hearing; a petrosal translabyrinthine approach or retrosigmoid paracerebellar (RSPC) approach may be appropriate.
• For small tumors (grades 1 and 2a) with good hearing, a middle fossa approach (extradural subtemporal approach) or suboccipital transmeatal approach may be appropriate.
• For grade 2, 3, and 4, an RSPC approach may be appropriate.

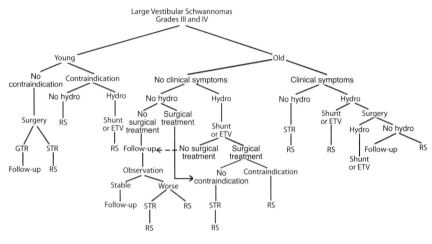

Fig. 22.4 Large vestibular schwannoma, algorithm of treatment. ETV, endoscopic third ventriculocisternostomy; GTR, gross total resection; Hydro, hydrocephalus; RS, radiosurgery; STR, subtotal resection. (Adapted from Koos WT, Matula C, Lang J. Color Atlas of Microneurosurgery of Acoustic Neurinomas. New York, Stuttgart: Georg Thieme Verlag; 2002.)

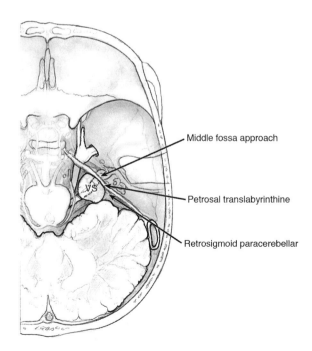

Fig. 22.5 Surgical approaches to a vestibular schwannoma (VS).

- Retrosigmoid and translabyrinthine (TL) approaches can be used virtually for all sizes of tumors, with the important difference being that hearing preservation is possible in the retrosigmoid approach and not possible in the translabyrinthine approach, but the latter has potentially a lower risk of brain retraction, and according to some authors, a lower risk of facial palsy. A high-riding jugular bulb can limit TL approaches, whereas this is not a limitation with the RSPC approach. Any but the smallest tumors still require the removal of bone posterior to the sigmoid sinus either via drilling or a craniotomy/craniectomy. This enables retraction of the sigmoid to gain access to the periphery of the tumor. The transcochlear approach is used for extensive prepontine tumors, but it is technically demanding and has a high risk of facial palsy.
- A complementary view from an otoneurological surgeon perspective suggests the following algorithm for the selection of the surgical approach[22,27]: the translabyrinthine approach for tumors > 1.5 cm or for tumors smaller than this size in patients with nonserviceable hearing. Tumors ≤ 1.5 cm in patients with serviceable hearing and tumors < 0.5 cm in patients younger than 65 might be approached via a middle cranial fossa approach; otherwise via a retrosigmoid approach.

> **Surgical Pearl**
>
> Avoid use of a muscle relaxant for the facial muscles monitoring. Electric stimulation of the facial nerve and evoked muscular responses may be used for prognostication.

- Intraoperative monitoring may be helpful.
- Some surgeons perform a temporary tarsorrhaphy prior to surgery (after anesthesia), and remove it after surgery if there is no facial nerve palsy.

> **Pearl**
>
> Transthoracic echocardiography is recommended with the patient in the sitting/semi-sitting position for monitoring air embolism, particularly in patients with a known patent foramen ovale.

- Combined approaches, such as a combined retro- and presigmoid approach or retrosigmoid and middle fossa approaches, may be required for management of giant multicompartmental tumors.

❖ Surgical Approaches

- Surgical steps of the translabyrinthine approach: see Chapter 14, page 371
- Surgical steps of the retrosigmoid paracerebellar approach: See also Chapter 14, page 385

Surgical Anatomy Pearls

- All RSPC approaches should expose the sigmoid and transverse sinuses sufficiently so that the view of the surgeon is flush parallel with the petrous face. By drilling the posterior margin of the mastoid (in the so-called extended retrosigmoid approach), the complete exposure of the sigmoid sinus and removal of the mastoid process provides an increase in the angle of work by almost 25 degrees. The mastoid cortex flap can be resected by using chisels instead of being drilled, so that it can be used for reconstruction.[28]
- Always wax the holes of the mastoid, or pack it by using small pieces of muscle/fat, in order to avoid a CSF leak.

◈◈ A cruciate dural opening is also possible but it tends to dry out more than a C-shaped opening (see dural opening options in Chapter 14, **Fig. 14.23**, page 389).

◈ Dissect and explore the CPA, and check and coagulate the bridging veins between the cerebellar cortex and the tentorium.

◈ Preserve the petrosal veins whenever possible.

◈ Make an interlayer dissection between the two layers of arachnoid: the peripheral layer of the posterior fossa and the layer enveloping the tumor.

Surgical Anatomy Pearl

Check for anatomic variants during dissection **(Tables 22.3** and **22.4)**.

- Check the lateral position of the facial or vestibulocochlear nerves. Perform a stimulation of the posterior and lateral capsule of the tumor to check the position of CN VII, particularly in cases of NF2.
- Check the position of the AICA and its branches, especially the subarcuate artery (going into the subarcuate fossa superiorly to the porus acusticus). Rare variant of AICA: the subarcuate type loops into and out of the dura mater posterior to the internal auditory canal (IAC). In such a case, the dura must be incised around the artery and reflected medially along with the vessel.

◈ Protect the other cranial nerves by using a gelatin sponge.

◈ Debulk the tumor's posterior and central portions (by ultrasonic aspirator, pituitary forceps, and/or a curved cutting instrument).

◈ Separate the capsule of the tumor from the brainstem, and elevate the inferior pole to find the arachnoid plane separating the tumor from the lower cranial nerves.

◈ Drill the IAC 180 degrees around. Open the dural envelope in the IAC.

◈ Dissect the tumor from AICA and CN VIII. Dissect the tumor from the brainstem and cerebellum, starting from the origin of the trigeminal root. Try to remain between the two arachnoid layers, whenever possible. Dissect the lateral pole **(Fig. 22.6)**.

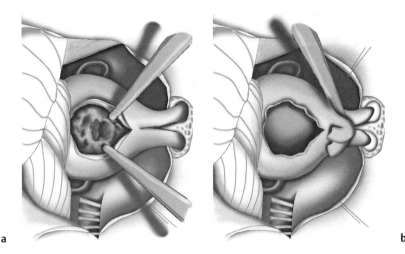

a   b

Fig. 22.6a,b   Resection of right-sided vestibular schwannoma. **(a)** Tumor debulking. **(b)** Section of the vestibular nerves for the total removal of the tumor.

Surgical Anatomy Pearls

- Always check for the anatomic position of the facial nerve. You may use stimulation with low-intensity current (0.1–0.2 mA) to distinguish the facial nerve fascicle from arachnoid bundles and other nerves.
- Facial nerve stimulation at the end of the operation at the brainstem: 0.2 mA, normal function; if no stimulation, with up to a stimulus of 2 mA, the nerve must be inspected. If anatomically interrupted, repair it with microsutures, graft, or hypoglossal-facial anastomosis if the brainstem stump cannot be found (see Chapter 28).[29]
- Use angled-endoscopes for exploring the CPA and searching for potential remnants, especially in the IAC and around the nerves.

Closure

Closure includes dura mater closure, graft of pericranium, and/or fibrin glue. If craniotomy has been performed, reimplant the bone flap with titanium microplates. Use cement or titanium mesh for gaps or in cases of a craniectomy.

❖ Surgical steps of the middle approach:

◈ Make the craniotomy as low as possible to reach the middle cranial fossa, otherwise, extend it by drilling the inferior bone margin.

◈ Elevate the dura over the petrosal surface from posterior to anterior, preserving the greater superficial petrosal nerve.

◈ Identify the edge of the petrous ridge, and drill Kawase's area to the superior semicircular canal and to the IAC.

◈◈ Variation: The drilling can be performed according to the Garcia-Ibanez technique by identifying the arcuate eminence and the greater superficial petrosal nerve, and then by drilling between the lines created by these structures for access to the IAC. It is like the Fish technique, and avoids resecting the greater superficial petrosal nerve (GSPN).[30] A complete unroofing exposing the geniculate ganglion and the origin of the GSPN may be performed according to the House technique,[31] which requires much more time.

◈ Continue the drilling medial to the cochlea, by using a 2-mm diamond drill, exposing the facial nerve. Open the dura of the IAC, divide the vestibular nerve, and dissect the tumor from its superior aspect. At the end of the resection, fill the space with fat graft.

Vestibular Schwannomas in Neurofibromatosis Type 2

- These tumors can be more challenging because of the multiple surgeries these patients may require and the potential for cumulative neurologic morbidity.[32,33] In 40% of cases, these tumors are multilobular, with neurovascular structures passing between the lobules. The tumors can even infiltrate the nerve fibers. Total resection with function preservation is much more demanding, and the morbidity is greater.
- Small tumors should be surgically removed, whereas remnants or recurrences may also be managed by radiotherapy. Surgical removal gives the best outcome, especially in terms of hearing preservation.[15] Loss or alteration of waves I and III may be an indication for performing a partial or subtotal resection of the tumor with IAC opening for cochlear nerve decompression.[34] Hearing restoration in patients who are already deaf may be attempted with auditory brainstem (midbrain) implants.[35–37]
- Consider cochlear implants in specific cases (see Chapter 14 on page 383).
- Radiosurgery or fractionated radiotherapy may control the tumor in 81% of patients at 10 years' follow-up,[38,39] with a hearing preservation rate of 33 to 43% (with some deterioration possible also in a delayed fashion over several years).[40] Patients with just one side affected could benefit more from surgery, with radiotherapy reserved for older patients or for patients with medical contraindications to major surgery.[32,34,41]

Outcome

- The overall total removal rate is 70 to 90%.
- The recurrence rate of the tumor (recurring between 1 and 13 years after the first surgery) has been shown to be 0.05% with the enlarged translabyrinthine approach, 0.7% with the retrosigmoid approach, and 1.8% with the middle cranial fossa approach.[42]

- The retrosigmoid approach is very versatile, most general neurosurgeons are familiar with it.[43]

Facial Nerve Preservation

Facial nerve preservation depends on the size of the tumor and the preoperative dysfunction, but overall preservation occurs in 82% of cases 1 week after surgery, and 91% of cases 12 to 18 months after surgery.[9] The mean preservation is 92 to 96%.[21,44] Facial nerve preservation is nearly always possible for tumors smaller than 1 cm.[45]

- Severe facial nerve palsy (House-Brackmann grade III–VI) may occur in up to 10% of cases for each centimeter in diameter of the tumor.[46] It can be temporary (up to 60% of these patients improve over the follow-up). In such cases, tarsorrhaphy is required as soon as possible after surgery. Otherwise, taping the eye for several days and moistening it every 2 hours should be sufficient.

Hearing Preservation

Hearing preservation depends on the size of the tumor as well on the anatomic variant of CN VIII, with an overall rate of 87% in grade 2 tumors[18] and 10% in large tumors.

Complications[46–48]

On a analysis of more than 6,500 patients, the overall complication rate was 28% (26.2% nervous system complications versus 5.1% non–nervous system complications, such as pneumonia, venous thrombosis, acute myocardial infarction, and pulmonary embolism).[48]

- Overall mortality: < 0.5%
- Facial nerve palsy (see above in the "Facial Nerve Preservation" paragraph)
- Cerebellar contusion/infarction with ataxia: < 1%
- Hematoma: 1%
- Brain infarction/edema (e.g., following occlusion of the vein of Labbé): < 1%
- Brainstem injury: < 1%
- Hydrocephalus: < 4%
- Venous sinus injury/transverse/sigmoid sinus thrombosis: up to 4.5%. It may be related to retraction/manipulation of the sinus during surgery, direct trauma during craniotomy/craniectomy, desiccation of the sinus in long operations, or migration of bone wax.[49–51]
- CSF leakage: < 7%, pseudomeningocele

- ○ Management options:
  1. Reinforcing the wound (more stitches, compressive dressing)
  2. Lumbar drainage for 3 to 5 days, draining 5 to 15 cc/h
  3. Surgical repair (also waxing the air cells of the mastoid bone)
- Wound infections: 2%
- Meningitis: 1%
- Trigeminal deficit: 2%
- CN IV or VI palsy (diplopia): < 1%
- Lower cranial nerve paralysis (dysphagia, aspiration pneumonia): 0.5%. Arytenoid adduction and thyroplasty for unilateral vocal cord paralysis, nasogastric (NG) tube, and feeding jejunostomy may be required in such cases. See Chapter 8.
- Seizures: up to 7%[49]
- In cases entailing the harvesting of abdominal fat, a complication rate of 3% for abdominal subcutaneous hematoma has been reported.[47]
- The postoperative quality of life of patients can be reduced by headache, wound problems, dural irritation, and spasms of the neck muscles related to the surgical position.

> **Pearl**
>
> Patient surveys suggest that the complications with open surgery are worse than those reported by surgeons.

■ 22.2 Clival, Petroclival, and Petrous Meningiomas

- Posterior fossa meningiomas account for 10% of intracranial meningiomas. Clival and petroclival meningiomas account for 3 to 10% of posterior fossa meningiomas and less than 2% of intracranial meningiomas.[1] Meningioma is the second most frequent tumor of the CPA, after vestibular schwannoma (up to 15% of CPA tumors).[2,3]
- It is rare to see tumors confined to solely one area. Most tumors extend from the clivus to the petrous bone and so are most accurately termed "petroclival." However, those that take their origin more medially present a greater challenge to the surgeon.
- The petrous face can be divided into three areas: an area medial to Meckel's cave, a middle area between Meckel's cave and the IAC, and an area lateral or posterior to the IAC. Tumor localizations are shown in **Fig. 22.7**. Tumors originating in each of these areas displace cranial nerves and vessels in different ways, and so understanding the origin helps the surgeon to plan the approach and to minimize complications.

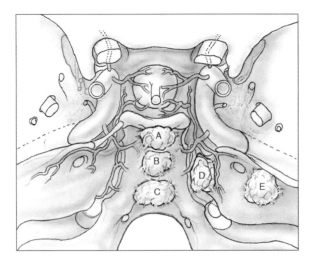

Fig. 22.7   Localizaiton of clival (A, upper clivus; B, mid-clivus; C, lower clivus), petroclival (D), and cerebellopontine angle (E) meningiomas.

- Some of these tumors also extend upward into Meckel's cave and into the cavernous sinus or the middle fossa. The surgeon must decide which components of the tumor are most responsible for the patient's symptoms and most amenable to safe surgical extirpation.
- *Clival meningiomas* have a dural attachment in the midline along of the clivus. Their origin arises medial to the entrance to Meckel's cave. They displace the brainstem posteriorly.[4]
- *Petroclival meningiomas,* or, as they are more appropriately described, medial petrous meningiomas, have a dural attachment at the petroclival junction, medial to the IAC, and lateral to the entrance to Meckel's cave, posterior to the gasserian ganglion. They displace the brainstem posteriorly and contralaterally.[4]
- *Petrous face meningiomas* or *CPA meningiomas* arise from the dura of the posterior surface of the petrous bone, lateral to the entrance of the trigeminal nerve into Meckel's cave.[5]

■ Blood Supply of the Tumor

The blood supply is from the clival branches of the meningohypophyseal trunk, branches of the external carotid artery (e.g., ascending pharyngeal), the meningeal artery of the vertebral arteries, or arteries of the vertebral and basilar arteries in the case of pial invasion[6] **(Fig. 22.8)**.

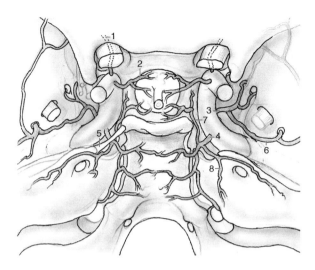

Fig. 22.8   Meningeal arteries involved in the vascularization of the clival, petroclival, and CPA meningiomas. 1, ophthalmic artery; 2, superior hypophyseal artery; 3, lateral carotido-cavernous artery; 4, meningohypophyseal trunk; 5, Gruber's ligament; 6, anterior petrosal branch of the middle meningeal artery; 7, inferior hypophyseal artery; 8, tentorial artery.

■ Signs and Symptoms

The signs and symptoms vary based on the position and size of the tumor, with headache and cranial nerve palsies (especially hearing loss, facial numbness/pain, followed by double vision, dysarthria, and dysphagia) occurring most commonly. Tinnitus, ataxia, motor/sensory signs and symptoms, and hydrocephalus are also common.

■ Classifications

Clival Meningiomas

Anatomic classification of clivus tumors[6] (**Fig. 22.7**):

- Upper clivus: above the trigeminal nerve root
- Mid-clivus: between the trigeminal root and CN IX
- Lower clivus: from CN IX to the foramen magnum

Petroclival Meningiomas

Petroclival meningiomas are often diagnosed when they have a large or giant size (≥ 4–5 cm in diameter), involving more anatomic compartments.

Surgical Anatomy Pearl

Petroclival meningiomas are limited to the petroclival region in only 10% of cases. More frequently they involve the Meckel's cave, and/or the CPA, middle fossa, and foramen magnum.[7]

Cerebellopontine Angle Meningiomas[5,8]

Based on the relation of the tumor to the internal acoustic meatus, CPA meningiomas can be:

- postmeatal (± extension into the meatus);
- premeatal (medial and superior extension ± extension into Meckel's cave, or into the meatus, or medial and inferior extension ± extension into the jugular foramen/meatus, or a combination of these patterns); or
- with a pre- and postmeatal extension.

Petrous face meningiomas can also be classified based on their location relative to the meatus.

■ Treatment

Surgery should be the first-line treatment in young patients and for tumors larger than 3 cm, particularly in patients with significant local mass effect or increased intracranial pressure. Otherwise, careful monitoring, radiosurgery, and fractionated radiation therapy are also options to consider. **Fig. 22.9** provides an algorithm of treatment for petroclival meningiomas.[9] Surgery is also a very good option for younger patients with smaller tumors and impending neurologic compromise or neurologic symptoms. A total removal in conjunction with excellent long-term control maintains the possibility of preserved function in these patients.[10]

- Some surgeons have moved to combined-treatment paradigms with more conservative local resections followed by radiosurgery of the remnant. As a result, the total excision rate in some series have dropped recently (from 78–91% in the 1990s to 32–43% in 2007[1,11–13]). Whether this paradigm will achieve better long-lasting control, improved survival, and less overall morbidity remains to be seen.

Pearl

For very small or asymptomatic tumors, observation or radiosurgery alone is also an acceptable option.

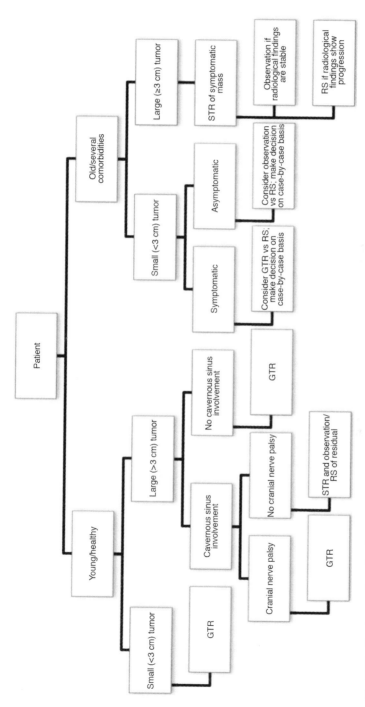

Fig. 22.9 Treatment algorithm for petroclival meningiomas. GTR, gross total resection; RS, radiosurgery; STR, subtotal resection. (Adapted from Coopens JR, Couldwell WT. Clival and petroclival meningiomas. In: DeMonte F, McDermott MW, Al-Mefty O, eds. Al-Mefty's Meningiomas, 2nd ed. New York, Stuttgart: Thieme; 2011:270–282.)

■ Surgical Approaches

The main goals of surgery are tissue diagnosis; decompression of the brainstem, cerebellum, and cranial nerves; and oncological maximal safe resection. Simpson grade I resection is not always feasible due to the desire to minimize potential neurologic morbidity. Subtotal/partial resection followed by imaging follow-up and/or radiotherapy often can be considered adequate for a prolonged good clinical outcome.

- A number of surgical approaches are possible for these tumors (**Table 22.5** and **Fig. 22.10**). The approach should be tailored to the patient and the actual extent of the tumor. For those tumors that extend through the tentorial incisura into the middle fossa, a combined transtentorial infra-supratentorial approach with or without a posterior or anterior petrosectomy is helpful. For those lesions that are confined within the posterior fossa, a laterally placed posterior fossa craniotomy flush with the face of the petrous bone with or without a retrolabyrinthine posterior petrosectomy often provides a wide and efficacious corridor. The extended transtemporal exposures (extended

Table 22.5   Approaches Used for Clival, Petroclival, and Cerebellopontine Angle (CPA) Meningiomas

Approach	Variant/Extension
Retrosigmoid paracerebellar	• Presigmoid exposure* • ±Partial/total labyrinthectomy • ±Transcochlear/total petrosectomy
Frontotemporal-orbitozygomatic	• Alone or in combination with other approaches • Transcavernous approach
Posterior petrosal	• Partial/total labyrinthectomy • Transcochlear/total petrosectomy
Subtemporal transtentorial	• Extended middle fossa (anterior petrosectomy) • ± Retrosigmoid paracerebellar • ± Transtentorial
Far lateral/extreme lateral	• Transcondylar • Retrocondylar
Extended transsphenoidal	• Transclival • Posterior clinoidectomy, pituitary transposition
Transbasal	
Transoral	
Suboccipital	

*For all but the smallest tumors, all the approaches with presigmoid exposures are combined with exposure of the dura posterior to the sigmoid via a posterior fossa craniotomy or craniectomy.
Note: See text for indications. Several combinations of these approaches can be performed.

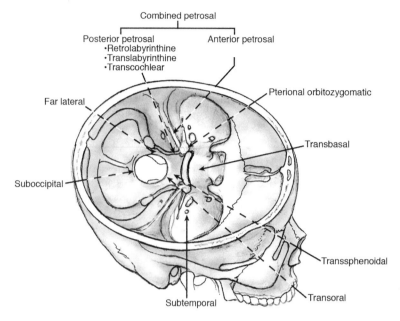

Fig. 22.10 Petrosal approach for resection of petroclival meningiomas. In: Badie B, ed. Neurosurgical Operative Atlas 2E: Neuro-oncology. New York: Thieme, 2006:170–179.

retrolabyrinthine, transcochlear) approaches are also excellent ways to access these lesions. Occasionally, an isolated lesion presents purely anteriorly along the clivus and an extended transsphenoidal approach may be appropriate. For **posterolateral approaches,** see Chapter 14, page 384.

■ Surgical Positions

The patient is placed in the supine position with a large roll used to elevate the ipsilateral shoulder. The head is fixed in pins and turned 70 degrees to the contralateral side. A lateral position or park-bench position can also be used. Some surgeons prefer placing the patient in the sitting position. The extended transtemporal procedures are done with the patient in the supine position with the head turned, with or without a shoulder roll. All pressure points should be carefully padded.

The space between the shoulder and the ear should be maximized by a number of maneuvers: tilting the ipsilateral shoulder inferiorly and anteriorly away from the ear, padding it, and taping it there; and tilting the vertex of the head down toward the floor. This can be facilitated by allowing the dependent arm, in the lateral or park-bench position, to hang below the level of the bed on a well-padded arm board. Once the patient is positioned and carefully secured in place, the operating table should be tilted laterally and in the Trendelenburg/ anti-Trendelenburg position before starting the operation to ensure that the patient is stable and will not move during bed repositioning intraoperatively and that any lines or the endotracheal tube will not be at risk of disruption during movements of the bed. Prepare and drape the patient's abdomen or the lateral thigh for fascia lata and fat graft, which are later required for closure.

- Intraoperative monitoring is useful for the dissection of cranial nerves.
- Note that all retrosigmoid paracerebellar approaches should carry the craniotomy far lateral enough so as to clearly expose the transverse and sigmoid sinuses. The CSF should also be drained from the cisterna magna routinely in all cases for posterior fossa meningioma prior to the main opening of the dura. This usually requires drilling away some of the mastoid. This technique brings the surgeon parallel with the petrous face and avoids the need to retract the cerebellum.
- With appropriate brain relaxation, an approach flush parallel with the petrous face, and extensive initial internal debulking of the mass, the RSPC posterior fossa craniotomy approach can access most of the lesions without brain retraction.
- The RSPC approach can be combined with a variety of extensions medial to the sigmoid sinus—the so-called **presigmoid exposure**. The smallest of these involves removing the bone in Trautmann's triangle medial and anterior to the sigmoid sinus by a simple mastoidectomy that preserves the labyrinth and otic capsule. More extensive bone removal can include removal of a part of the labyrinth (partial labyrinthectomy) or all of it (total labyrinthectomy, or doing a total labyrinthectomy with removal of the cochlea and anterior medial petrous apex (transcochlear and total petrosectomy).
- For small or medium-size, laterally located tumors of the petrous face or mid-clivus or larger tumors of the lateral petrous face or CPA: retrosigmoid paracerebellar approach or a presigmoid petrosal approach without labyrinthectomy (retrolabyrinthine petrosal approach).
- For small or medium-size, centrally located tumors of the upper or mid-clivus (when hearing is unaffected): retrosigmoid paracerebellar approach, posterior petrosal presigmoid approach, or posterior petrosal partial labyrinthectomy approach.
- For small or medium-size, centrally placed tumors of the upper or mid-clivus (when hearing is not preserved): retrosigmoid paracerebellar approach or translabyrinthine petrosal approach, providing additional exposure to the IAC.
- For retro-meatal petrous face tumors: retrosigmoid paracerebellar approach.

- For giant-size, purely midline clival tumors, when the brainstem is tilted away from the side with no hearing: total petrosectomy or combined approaches (retrosigmoid paracerebellar approach with presigmoid extension ± partial or complete labyrinthectomy and subtemporal transtentorial approach if there is supratentorial tumor).
- For tumors located at the lower clivus: retrosigmoid paracerebellar approach or extreme lateral transcondylar approach if the surgical corridor is small.[14]
- For lateral tumors of the petrous ridge or tumors in the CPA: retrosigmoid paracerebellar approach[15] or retrosigmoid suprameatal approach. Rarely, a retrosigmoid craniotomy and intradural resection of the petrous apex with drilling and removal of the suprameatal tubercle can be used to manage CPA meningiomas when there is difficulty reaching the suprameatal components.
- Combined approaches may be required for tumors with extension above and below the dorsum sellae.
- The frontotemporal-orbitozygomatic (FTOZ) approach may be performed for tumors extending superiorly to the dorsum sellae, alone or alongside other approaches, as indicated by the size and localization of the tumor.
- Clival/petroclival meningiomas can also be approached by means of the endoscopic extended endonasal transclival approach.[16] An endoscopic endonasal transcavernous posterior clinoidectomy with interdural pituitary transposition has been suggested as well.[17]
- Further approaches to the clival and petroclival tumors: transbasal, transoral, subtemporal, suboccipital, and far lateral.
- Retrosigmoid intradural suprameatal and retrosigmoid transtentorial approaches provide adequate exposure to the petroclival regions.
- The anterior upper third of the posterior fossa can also be reached by a transcavernous approach for the treatment of selected petroclival meningiomas, trigeminal schwannomas, and clival chordomas, but it is rarely used.[18]

❖ Posterior Petrosal Approach Technique

◈ **Incision.** A number of incisions are acceptable. The most common is likely a C-shaped incision along or below the superior temporal line to reach the retroauricular region. For orbitozygomatic (OZ) combined approaches, the incision should come down anterior to the tragus and an extension to the frontal region is added to provide access to the orbital margin (see Chapter 14, **Fig. 14.22**, page 388).

◈ Elevate the pericranium and the temporal muscle, and reflect the muscle anteriorly.

◈ The sternocleidomastoid muscle can be reflected anteriorly with the trapezius, semispinalis capitis, and splenius capitis muscles inferiorly and posteriorly, for optimal exposure and reconstruction at the end of the operation.

Surgical Anatomy Pearls

- For all but the smallest tumors, all the approaches with presigmoid exposures are combined with exposure of the dura posterior to the sigmoid sinus via a posterior fossa craniotomy or craniectomy.
- Many authors call the posterior petrosal approaches simply the "petrosal approaches." Here the term *posterior petrosal* is used to distinguish these approaches from the anterior petrosal approach popularized by Kawase et al,[19] which are performed from a middle fossa exposure. These petrosal approaches include exposure of the dura anterior and medial to the sigmoid sinus, and then varying amounts of removal of the otic capsule (labyrinth, cochlea) and ultimately the petrous apex in a total petrosectomy.[20]

◈ Expose the temporal, retrosigmoid, and mastoid areas, as well as the root of the zygoma.

◈ Identify the position of the venous sinuses.

◈ Craniectomy and craniotomy (using one or more bur holes) are two viable alternatives. Bur holes can be placed on the transverse sinus, taking care not to injure the mastoid emissary vein.

Surgical Anatomy Pearl

Extension of the craniotomy: it should be larger (at least ~ 1 cm) anteriorly and posteriorly to the extent of the tumor (as seen in preoperative neuronavigation).

◈◈ Variation: Perform retrosigmoid craniotomy, mastoidectomy, and/or further exposures according to the planned approach.

❖ Retrolabyrinthine presigmoid approach:

◈ Perform mastoidectomy and partially unroof the sigmoid sinus, semicircular canals, vestibular aqueduct, jugular bulb, and mastoid segment of the facial nerve in order to leave these structures in a partial bone "shell" for protection. The sinodural angle must be exposed.

◈◈ **Variation:** Partial labyrinthectomy/petrous apicectomy:

- Perform a complete cortical mastoidectomy; see the position of the semicircular canals (blue line).
- Prior to opening the canals, wax them to avoid loss of endolymphatic fluid and hearing loss. Despite taking this step, however, the majority of patients will still lose hearing.
- Perform a partial labyrinthectomy for the petrous apicectomy, between the ampulla of the superior semicircular canal and the entrance of the vestibular aqueduct into the petrous dura.[21]
- Skeletonize the superior wall of the IAC.

◈◈ Variation with **translabyrinthine approach:** faster than the partial labyrinthectomy/petrous apicectomy approach, it also provides more exposure of the IAC.

Surgical Anatomy Pearl

Exposure of the presigmoid dura should be maximized while also removing as few temporal bone structures as possible.

◈ After the mastoidectomy, resect the semicircular canals and open the vestibule.
◈ Skeletonize the facial nerve from its genu to the stylomastoid foramen.
◈ Resect the bone of the IAC.
  • At the end of these surgical steps, the visible walls in the surgical corridors are the sigmoid sinus posteriorly, the tegmen dura superiorly, the facial nerve anteriorly, and the jugular bulb inferiorly (see Chapter 14, **Fig. 14.20**, page 374).
◈◈ Variation with **total petrosectomy:** reserved for giant midline tumors. It can be useful in those cases with prior surgery or radiation, bilateral extension of the tumor, or extensive vascularization. Often the procedure can be multistaged.
◈ The exposure is similar to that of the other petrosal approaches, but transecting and over-sewing the external auditory canal is required.[22]
◈◈ Variation: Dissect the temporomandibular joint capsule from the glenoid fossa.
◈ Perform a labyrinthectomy with exposure of the facial nerve.
◈ For lesions with significant supratentorial extension, a temporal craniotomy with or without a zygomatic osteotomy including the condylar fossa, with further resection of the condyle and neck of the mandible, may be required if access to the horizontal petrous segment of the ICA is needed.[22]
◈ Identify and resect the greater superficial petrosal nerve and the middle meningeal artery.
◈ Expose, pack with autologous fat, and suture the cartilaginous eustachian tube.[22]
◈◈ Variation: Unroof the petrous ICA. Divide the fibrocartilaginous ring around the cervical carotid at its entrance into the skull base for anterior mobilization of the ICA.
◈◈ Variation: Remove the cochlea and bone medial to the mastoid segment and posteriorly mobilize the facial nerve.
◈ Perform a medial petrous apex and lateral clivus resection.
◈◈ In multistaged operations, at this point, the first step could be stopped, and the facial nerve should be covered with Gelfoam before closure and reopening for tumor resection in the second stage of the operation.

❖ Dural opening

Begin with the cisterna magna or in the presigmoid region, from the inferior part of the sigmoid sinus, parallel to the jugular bulb.

◈ The presigmoid incision should come up to the superior petrosal sinus. The temporal dura should be opened parallel to the floor of the middle fossa.

> **Surgical Anatomy Pearl**
>
> Open the basal cisterns for CSF drainage.

◈ When the incisions join the superior petrosal sinus, the latter should be suture ligated and divided **(Fig. 22.11a)**.

◈ Next, divide the tentorium.

◈ Put sutures on the dural edges for the augmentation of the space.

> **Surgical Anatomy Pearl**
>
> Be mindful of the vein of Labbé and ensure that it sustains no damage.

◈ Cauterize the superior petrosal veins, whenever required.

◈ Open Meckel's cave to mobilize and visualize the trigeminal root. Open the arachnoid between the nerves.

◈ Start tumor debulking between CNs IV and V and CNs V and VII to VIII, to minimize the manipulation of the nerve complexes.[6]

◈ Proceed toward the base and inferior pole of the tumor and identify CN VI, disconnecting and coagulating the petroclival dura.

◈ Dissect the other nerves and the basilar artery and its branches.

◈ Resect any potential intracavernous extension of the tumor (although for intracavernous tumor components it

> **Surgical Anatomy Pearl**
>
> Preserve the arachnoid plane for the brainstem decompression.

> **Surgical Anatomy Pearls**
>
> • Be mindful of the superior cerebellar artery (SCA) and CN IV and ensure that they sustain no damage **(Fig. 22.11b)**.
>
> • Tentorial detachment is an important requirement in combined petrosal approaches in order to provide access to medium-to-large petroclival tumors and to facilitate their resection. The preoperative understanding of the anatomic relationships between the tentorium and the temporal bridging veins as well as with CNs IV to VI is of paramount importance.[23]
>
> • A petrosal approach with tentorial resection generally requires sectioning of the superior petrosal sinus, although the dura may be opened more anteriorly to it, in order to preserve it, by means of further drilling of the medial wall of the petrous bone, to reach anteriorly up to the suprameatal area. The separation of the tentorium from Meckel's cave in fact enables a connection between the middle and posterior cranial fossa with a partial opening of the tentorium and preservation of the superior petrosal sinus.[24]

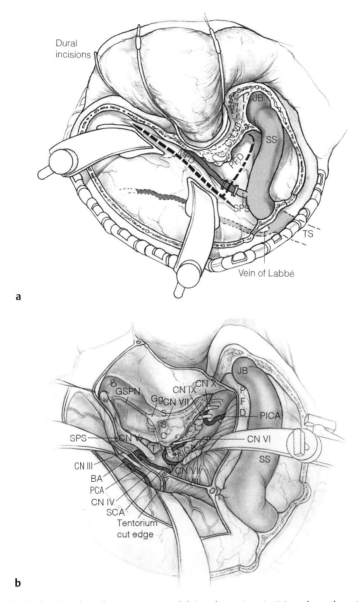

Fig. 22.11a,b Combined petrosectomy. **(a)** Dural opening: incision along the middle fossa dura (MFD) and posterior fossa dura (PFD). **(b)** Intradural exposure. BA, basilar artery; CN, cranial nerve; Gg, geniculate ganglion; GSPN, greater superficial petrosal nerve; JB, jugular bulb; PCA, posterior cerebral artery; PICA, posterior inferior cerebellar artery; SCA, superior cerebellar artery; SPS, superior petrosal sinus; SS, sigmoid sinus; SSC, semicircular canal; TS, transverse sinus. (From Baaj AA, Agazzi S, van Loveren H. Combined Anterior and Posterior Petrosectomy. In: Nader R. et al. (Eds). Neurosurgery Tricks of the Trade. New York: Thieme; 2014:34–35.)

is better to combine this approach with a subtemporal approach and OZ osteotomy).

❖ Closure

Wherever possible, perform primary dural closure. Pack the eustachian tube well. However, the presigmoid exposure often requires duraplasty with autologous tissue such as fascia lata and fat graft.

◈ Fill the presigmoid space or the space of the total petrosectomy with autologous fat.

◈ Reinforce it with fibrin sealants.

◈◈ Some surgeons add a titanium mesh cranioplasty, miniplates, or hydroxyapatite cement to improve cosmesis.

◈◈ Some surgeons use the "split technique" to cover the mastoid defect **(Fig. 22.12)**.

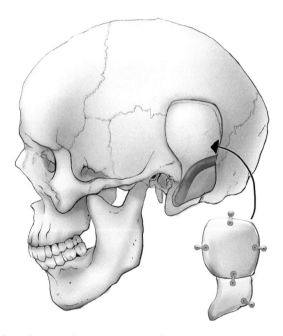

Fig. 22.12 Split technique. The temporal bone flap can be split with a reciprocating saw, providing a split calvarial bone to cover the mastoidectomy defect. (Adapted from Bogaev C, Sekhar LN. Petroclival meningiomas. In: Sekhar LN, Fessler RG, eds. Atlas of Neurosurgical Techniques. New York: Thieme; 2006:695–710.)

◈   Suture the temporal and retroauricular muscles.

◈◈ Variation: Microplate-Bridge technique: a fascial graft fixed with a long micro-titanium plate over the presigmoid-subtemporal defect may help prevent CSF leak.[25]

■ Outcome

Surgical radicality and morbidity are related to the different tumor types (**Table 22.6**).

Clival and Petroclival Meningioma

Gross total resection: 20 to 85% survival,[7,26–29] dependent on tumor size, consistency, invasion of the cavernous sinus, and cranial nerve involvement.[30] Skull base approaches enable a Simpson grade I or II resection (total removal) with good outcome and functional status in 76% of patients.[31] The recurrence rate is dependent on the degree of resection, as well as on later radiotherapy. Recurrence-free survival has been reported up to 96% at 3 years and 79.5% at 12 years.[1] As a result, the recurrence rate ranges from 0 to 42%.[32] Recurrence at 8 years after surgery followed by radiosurgery has been reported as less than 22%.[1,7,26,32]

Cerebellopontine Angle Meningioma

Overall gross total removal (Simpson grade I and II) is possible in up to 86% of patients,[33] although the degree of resection correlates with the tumor topographic location. The degree of resection is highest in the suprameatal and retromeatal subtypes, and lowest in the premeatal and inframeatal types.[8]

Mortality

The mortality rate in clival-petroclival meningioma is 0 to 9%, largely caused by brainstem stroke,[7,29,30,32] and below 5% in CPA meningiomas.[33]

Morbidity

Morbidity entails cranial nerve palsies (new or worsening of preexisting conditions), which can be transitory or permanent, especially of CNs II, IV, and VI in clival and petroclival meningiomas.[29,30] Cranial nerve deficits occur at a rate of 30 to 76%[29] in petroclival meningioma surgery, according to the different published series. A preoperative low Karnofsky performance score, age ≥ 60,

Table 22.6 Summary of the Epidemiological and Outcome Data of Clival, Petroclival, and CPA Meningiomas

Type	Occurrence	Resection Rate	Survival	Recurrence	Morbidity	Mortality
Clival	Overall incidence: < 2% of intracranial tumors collectively	GTR with good outcome and functional status reportedly possible in 76% of patients	20–85% survival with GTR	0–42%; dependent on degree of tumor resection and later radiotherapy; recurrence-free survival reported to be 96% at 3 years and 79.5% at 12 years postop; recurrence 8 years postop followed by radiosurgery reportedly <22%	Cranial nerve palsies, transitory or permanent (especially of CNs II, IV, VI)	Lower cranial nerve injuries (namely CN X deficits; reported in 12% of cases) in cases of large meningiomas; stroke; temporal lobe infarction; brainstem injury; CSF leak (occurs in 15% of cases); hematoma, wound infection, tongue swelling	0–9%; typically related to the occurrence of brainstem stroke
Petroclival					Cranial nerve palsies, transitory or permanent (especially of CNs II, IV, VI) occurring at rates of 30–76%		

| CPA | Overall GTR possible in up to 86% of patients but largely varies by tumor location | | Up to 9.5% | | Cranial nerve palsies, transitory or permanent (overall rate of 35%, permanent damage in 23.5% of cases); very good facial nerve function in almost 90% of cases postop; hearing is preserved in 90% of cases | | < 5% |

Abbreviations: CN, cranial nerve; GTR, gross total resection.

brainstem edema, absence of the arachnoidal plane, vessel/CNs encasement, and hard consistency of the tumor are among the factors contributing to a worse outcome.[7,28]

- CPA meningiomas: The overall CN deficit rate is approximately 35% (permanent in 23.5% of cases).[34] Some series report very good facial nerve function (House-Brackmann grades 1 to 2) in almost 90% of cases of CPA meningiomas after resection, especially in the retromeatal types,[33] with a preservation of hearing in 90% of cases.[8]

> **Pearl**
>
> CPA meningiomas have a recurrence rate up to 9.5%,[3,35,36] thereby providing impetus for regular radiological follow-up.[33]

- Lower cranial nerve injuries can occur in large meningiomas.[37–39] CN X deficit has been reported in up to 12% of cases.[34]
- Stroke, temporal lobe infarction, brainstem injury, and CSF leak (occurrence rate up to 15%) are also possible, especially in combined approaches. Other reported complications include hematoma, wound infection, and tongue swelling.

> **Pearl**
>
> Petroclival meningioma surgery significantly affects patients' health and quality of life for several years, suggesting that patients' psychosocial support and rehabilitative measures should also be improved.[1,39]

■ 22.3 Epidermoid and Dermoid Tumors

- These tumors account for 1% of intracranial tumors, with an epidermoid/dermoid ratio of 4:1, and account for 7% of CPA tumors (they can also arise in the parasellar region or other locations). In the posterior fossa, another typical localization is the fourth ventricle (more common for dermoids).

- Epidermoid tumors at the CPA are also called cholesteatomas, although this definition is used more for middle ear lesions, with chronic middle ear infections giving rise to entrapped epithelium, forming a kind of pocket that may or may not extend into the posterior fossa.

> **Surgical Anatomy Pearl**
>
> Typically, epidermoids occupy the lateral position (CPA) and the dermoids the midline **(Table 22.7)**. Other skull base locations include the petrous apex.

Table 22.7   Comparison of Epidermoids and Dermoids

Feature	Epidermoid	Dermoid
Frequency	0.5–1.5% of brain tumors	0.3% of brain tumors
Lining	Stratified squamous epithelium	Also include dermal appendage organs (hair follicles and sebaceous glands)
Contents	Keratin, cellular debris, and cholesterol; occasional hair	Same as epidermoids + hair and sebum
Location	More common laterally (e.g., CPA)	More commonly near midline
Radiology	High signal on DW-MRI, for differentiation from CSF	Variable intensities and calcium from dental elements
Associated anomalies	Tend to be isolated lesions	Associated with other congenital anomalies in up to 50% cases
Meningitis	May have recurrent aseptic meningitis (including Mollaret's meningitis)	May have repeated bouts of bacterial meningitis

Abbreviations: CPA, cerebellopontine angle; CSF, cerebrospinal fluid; DW-MRI, diffusion-weighted magnetic resonance imaging.
Source: Adapted from Greenberg MS. Handbook of Neurosurgery, 7th ed. New York: Thieme; 2010.

- Very few cases of malignant transformation of an epidermoid cyst into carcinomas have been reported.[1]

■ Pathology

Epidermoids or so-called pearly tumors (because of their shiny white pearl–like appearance) grow due to the accumulation of keratin and cholesterol, expanding and filling the subarachnoid spaces. Dermoids are made up of stratified squamous epithelium, containing dermal elements, including hair, sebaceous glands, or even teeth. See also Chapter 6, page 153.

■ Radiology

Epidermoids show high signal on diffusion-weighted (DW) MRI, for differentiation from CSF; dermoids may show variable intensities and calcium from dental elements. See also Chapter 5, page 126.

■ Signs and Symptoms

The signs and symptoms depend on the location of the lesion. In the CPA, cranial neuropathies are noted: CN V, isolated trigeminal neuralgia; CN VII, hemifacial spasm; CN VIII, sudden hearing loss. Cranial nerve palsies are related to the tumor size and position, with possible involvement of the lower cranial nerves as well, and hydrocephalus/intracranial hypertension. A rare cause of aseptic meningitis (Mollaret's meningitis) is related to spilling of intracystic components within the CSF.[2,3] These patients present with a sudden severe headache reminiscent of a subarachnoid hemorrhage, but MRI shows fat density globules in the subarachnoid space. Patients usually recover over days to weeks.

■ Treatment

Conservative treatment with clinical and radiological follow-up is an option in asymptomatic/debilitated patients, but surgery remains the gold standard of treatment, with no role for radiotherapy. Tumors are very soft and avascular, and can be debulked piecemeal.

■ Surgical Approaches for CPA Epidermoids

The retrosigmoid approach is most commonly used for the resection of CPA epidermoids. Transpetrous approaches are generally reserved for specific cases of petrous apex epidermoids, or large cholesteatomas involving the middle ear and temporal bone.

Surgical Anatomy Pearls

- The capsule of the tumor should be carefully dissected and removed, except in cases when it is too tightly adhered to cranial nerves, blood vessels, and/or the brainstem. Blood vessels and cranial nerves are generally engulfed, and therefore the resection has to be done carefully, in piecemeal, and often incompletely to avoid vascular damage and/or neurological dysfunction. An ultrasonic aspirator is rarely needed but may also speed up tumor debulking.
- Try to avoid spilling of intracystic contents within the CSF, so as to preclude chemical meningitis or hydrocephalus. To contain any spillage of contents, protect the surrounding structures with cottonoids. Use copious saline irrigation of the surgical field. Some authors advise utilizing hydrocortisone or perioperative steroids but without evidence.[4]

- Intraoperative cranial nerves monitoring is helpful.
- Angled endoscopes can help in the microsurgical approach (or in pure endo-scopic approaches) to ensure a greater degree of tumor resection by looking around the vessels and cranial nerves in areas that cannot be otherwise observed.[5-7]

■ Outcome

Resection can be total or subtotal and in cases in which the cyst or some com-ponent of the tumor is stuck to the brainstem/nerves/vessels, these adherent sections are left in order to avoid/decrease the risk of morbidity.[8] Symptoms such as trigeminal neuralgia and headache are often relieved for years due to the effective debulking. MRI every year or every other year with diffusion se-quences is used to monitor possible regrowth of the lesion, which may occur even beyond a decade.[9] Symptomatic recurrences, occurring after subtotal re-moval, may require further surgery after an extended period of time because of their slow growth rate. Mortality is rare and recurrences are related to the amount of tumor remnant from the initial surgery.

■ 22.4 Chordoma and Chondrosarcoma

■ Epidemiology

Chordoma and chondrosarcoma each account for 0.15% of intracranial tumors. Chordomas occur at an incidence rate of 0.5 to 8 cases per million persons per year,[1-4] 32% of which have cranial localization.[3] In general, chordomas are lo-cated at the midline of the skull base (i.e., clival chordoma), whereas chondro-sarcoma are paramedian (at the petrosphenoclival synchondrosis) **(Table 22.8)**.

■ Signs and Symptoms

These tumors can give rise to diplopia, proptosis, facial pain, headache, retro-orbital pain/pressure, cranial nerve palsy (above all in CN VI), visual loss, otal-gia, nasal obstruction, epistaxis, dysphonia, and dysphagia, depending on the tumor location and invasion of other anatomic structures.

- Occipitocervical pain may occur in cases of instability due to invasion of the occipitocervical joint.
- In cases of brainstem compression, long tract signs may be present.
- Signs of increased intracranial pressure are possible.

Table 22.8   Characteristics of Chordomas and Chondrosarcoma

Characteristic	Chordoma	Chondrosarcoma
Percent of brain tumors	0.15%	0.15%
Origin	Notochordal remnants	Embryonal mesenchymal remnants
Skull base location	Midline paramedian	Paramedian
Age range (years)	6–78	25–57
Median age	45	40
Male/female ratio	1.5:1	3.7:1
Pathological types	Chondroid Nonchondroid Dedifferentiated	Classical (grade I, II, III) Mesenchymal Dedifferentiated
Histopathological markers	EMA, cytokeratin, and brachyury +	EMA, cytokeratin, and brachyury –
MRI marker	Increase in ADC values	Decrease in ADC values

Abbreviations: ADC, apparent diffusion coefficient; EMA, epithelial membrane antigen.
Source: Adapted from Rostomily RC, Sekhar LN, Elahi F. Chordomas and chondrosarcomas. In: Atlas of Neurosurgical Techniques. Brain. Sekhar, L.N.; Fessler, R.G. ed. New York, Stuttgart: Thieme; 2006:778–810.

■ Gross Pathology

See Pathology, pages 164–165.

Chordoma and chondrosarcoma are lytic, expansile, and locally invasive into surrounding structures (clivus, cavernous sinuses, petrous bone, craniocervical junction). The extent of their invasion influences the surgical approach. The tumors are generally extradural and are also not very vascularized and generally quite soft (cartilaginous, similar to vertebral disks) or gelatinous. Calcifications make the resection more difficult.[5,6]

- Chordomas have a slow and progressive growth and tend to be very invasive locally. Some patients die due to local tumor effects, and not as a result of metastases.
- Chordomas are much more aggressive than chondrosarcomas of the skull base.[7–10]
- Chordomas and chondrosarcomas require a multidisciplinary team approach for increasing the survival time, improving the quality of life, and lowering the morbidity.[11]

■ Radiology

For lytic lesions, a CT scan is performed to demonstrate skull base erosions and tumoral calcifications.

On MRI, both tumors are iso-hypointense on T1- and hyperintense on T2-weighted images. Diffusion-weighted MRI may be useful in differentiating chordoma from chondrosarcoma, with chondrosarcoma having higher apparent diffusion coefficient (ADC) values.[12] See also Chapter 5.

- Chordomas may develop anteriorly, toward the sphenoid sinus; laterally, into the CPA; inferiorly toward the foramen magnum and spinal canal, with invasion of the retropharyngeal space also possible.
- Differential diagnosis with ecchordosis physaliphora (benign notochordal remnant at the dorsum sellae, generally asymptomatic, but can still cause headache, diplopia, pain). In ecchordosis, there is no gadolinium enhancement.[13]

■ Other Lesions Found in the Clivus Area

Other lesions include meningioma, metastasis, plasmacytoma, lymphoma, neuroenteric cyst, retroclival components of craniopharyngiomas and pituitary adenomas, mucocele of the sphenoid sinus, nasopharyngeal carcinoma and rhabdomyosarcoma, and chondromyxoid fibroma.

- The preoperative radiological workup includes CTA/MRA for assessment of the tumoral and peritumoral vascularization.

■ Treatment

Surgery is the main treatment for these lesions and is performed for tissue diagnosis, tumor debulking, and maximal safe oncological resection. Almost all cases of chordoma are followed by high-dose radiotherapy because of the radioresistance of the lesion. Despite aggressive surgical resection and radiation, 20% of chordoma cases recur within 1 year.[14] Debate exists over whether low-grade chondrosarcoma that is fully resected requires radiation, as the behavior of chondrosarcoma can be quite variable.

- Survival is related to the degree of resection: 5-year survival rate: 90% for chondrosarcoma and 65% for chordoma after gross total resection, with percentages decreasing in cases of partial resection.

■ Radiotherapy

See Chapter 30, pages 777 and 779 .

■ Surgical Approaches (Table 22.9)

Given the size of the tumor, patient signs and symptoms, and general condition of the patient, the surgical options are biopsy followed by observation or radiation, or surgical resection with or without radiation. In symptomatic patients, the best treatment is surgery (as extensive as possible) followed by radiation. Radical resection of chordomas and chondrosarcoma improves the long-term prognosis.[15-17]

- Eroded/infiltrated bones as well as infiltrated dura should be resected as well. Intratumoral calcifications may occur, especially in chondrosarcoma, and should be drilled and removed.
- Intraoperative monitoring of lower cranial nerves can be useful in surgery. Preoperative balloon test occlusion of the carotid or vertebral artery may be useful if surgical sacrifice might be needed, but the rate of false negatives is high and the test itself entails a risk of stroke.
- The approach depends on the exact location and extent of the tumor. The approaches can be anterior (e.g., transfacial, subfrontal, endoscopic transnasal/transoral, extended transsphenoidal or combined), anterolateral (e.g., FTOZ), lateral (e.g., subtemporal with anterior petrosectomy), posterolateral (e.g., retrosigmoid, translabyrinthine), or inferolateral (e.g., far-lateral approaches).
    1. **Transfacial approaches**: include facial translocation (and all its variants), Le Fort I transmaxillary transpterygoid approach,[18] transoral or extended transsphenoidal, and high anterior cervical retropharyngeal

Table 22.9 Approaches Used for Chordoma and Chondrosarcoma

Approach	Variant/Extension
Transfacial	• Facial translocation • Le Fort I transmaxillary transpterygoid approach • Transoral ± extended transsphenoidal • Cervical retropharyngeal
Extended subfrontal	
Frontotemporal-orbitozygomatic	• Transcavernous • ± Subtemporal
Subtemporal	• Extended middle fossa (anterior petrosectomy) • ± Retrosigmoid paracerebellar • ± Transtentorial
Far lateral/extreme lateral	• Transcondylar • Retrocondylar
Extended transsphenoidal	• Transclival • Posterior clinoidectomy, pituitary transposition

Note: See text for indications. Several combinations of these approaches can be performed.

approaches for midline-paramedial lesions (see Chapter 15). The use of retractors in natural cavities (nasal, paranasal, and mouth) widens the surgical corridors and provides direct ventral access to the target, without any brain manipulation. Postoperative facial swelling is generally tolerated by the patient, but there are risks of speech, swallowing, or airway dysfunction, cosmetic problems (with accompanying psychological problems and worse quality of life), and infections.

2. **Extended subfrontal approaches**: provide access to the midline clivus, medial cavernous sinus, petrous apex, occipital condyles, and foramen magnum.[19] Tumoral components too lateral or at the level of the dorsum sellae cannot be reached. For the technical steps, see page 343.

3. **FTOZ approach with transcavernous route**: used for management of intracavernous tumor components. Combined with a subtemporal approach, the upper clivus and petrous apex are accessible.

4. **Subtemporal transpetrous approach**: provides access to tumor components in the middle cranial fossa, upper clivus, and cavernous sinus.

5. **Subtemporal-infratemporal approach**: extends more inferiorly than the OZ approach in order to reach the horizontal segment of the petrous ICA,[20] the parapharyngeal space, orbit, and paranasal sinuses in the event of their involvement. The OZ approach would include the glenoid fossa. This approach also may be used in cases where ICA bypass is deemed necessary.

6. **Transpetrosal approach**: Determining the tumor extension (upper, middle, or lower clivus, and lateral extension) enables the surgeon to choose the type of petrosectomy (such as Kawase's approach in the subtemporal craniotomy, posterior petrosectomy, translabyrinthine, or transcochlear approach). For the technical steps, see Chapter 14 and page 573.

7. **Lateral transcondylar approach**: used for managing tumors in the upper ventral cervical spine, lower clivus, foramen magnum, and occipital condyles.[21] This approach requires extraperiosteal management of the vertebral artery, especially for tumors extending laterally to it.[15] In some cases, its transposition is necessary, providing wider exposure of the C0-C1 and C1-C2 joints. This approach and any posterior fossa approach can be complicated by cerebellar damage, vertebral artery injury, lower cranial nerve injury, or occipitocervical instability (occurring when > 50% of the condyle is resected).

◈◈The far lateral approach (dorsal transcranial transcondylar) may be associated with the ventral endoscopic endonasal transcondylar (far medial approach) for resection of extensive lesions involving both ventromedial and dorsolateral compartments.[22]

Surgical Anatomy Pearl

If more than 50% of the condyle is resected, occipital cervical fusion is usually advised.

8. **Endoscopic extended transclival approach**: the gold standard of treatment in several institutes, but its limitations have to be carefully considered (e.g., the large laterally extending tumor volume).[23] The endonasal approach can be used with the transoral approach for lower extensions of the tumor below the tip of the odontoid, if necessary. A more lateral extension of the tumor, toward the petrous apex or within the cavernous sinus, can be managed by the transpterygoid extension of the endoscopic approach (see page 428).[24]

❖❖ Variation: An endoscopic endonasal transcavernous posterior clinoidectomy with interdural pituitary transposition has also been reported,[24] but there are insufficient data regarding its use for the resection of chordomas and other tumors.

9. **Combined approaches**: As mentioned above, multicompartmental large tumors may be reached by combined approaches, such as transoral and transnasal. For tumors extending from the clivus downward toward the foramen magnum, extended transsphenoidal and transcranial approaches (retrosigmoid, subtemporal, or transcondylar) may be utilized depending on the location of the tumor components.

• Surgery for chordoma/chondrosarcomas is often necessary to alleviate symptoms that arise due to recurrences, after surgery and radiotherapy (RT). After RT, more adhesion and fibrosis make tumor resection more difficult and it entails greater morbidity, especially in terms of cranial neuropathy. This possibility must be discussed with patients and family before surgery.

• Chordoma/chondrosarcoma may be associated with a high potential for CSF leakage, so attention must be paid to reconstruction when a surgical resection is planned. The history must include information regarding prior surgical procedures, especially the prior use of radiation and the presence of pericranial flaps. Autologous fat can be used to fill dead spaces. Fascia lata or other dural substitute can be used for dural reconstruction, and vascularized pericranial or mucosal nasal-septal flap(s) can be used to cover and seal skull base defects.

■ Prognosis

Local control and overall survival is related to the degree of gross total resection. Initial attempts to safely resect as much tumor as possible are important. In chondrosarcoma, prognosis is related to tumor grading. The 5-year survival rates are as follows: grade I, 90%; grade II, 81%; grade III, 43%.[25] The presence of metastasis (occurring in 7–18% of cases) is associated with a poorer prognosis.

• The average overall survival of patients with chordoma is 7 to 9 years. In the different published series, the 5-year survival has been reported 68 to

72%, the 10-year survival rate 40 to 80%, and the 20-year survival rate 13 to 31%.[3-5,26-31] Older patients have a worse prognosis.

- Chordoma metastases occur in 4 to 43% of patients,[2] lowering the median survival to 12 months.
- Chordoma is notorious for spreading along the line of surgical access, so the surgeon should try to avoid tumor spillage, especially transsphenoidally if possible.

Prognosis in the Extended Endonasal Endoscopic Approach

A total resection in 71 to 95% of patients at first surgery has been reported,[32-34] with a global total resection rate (including the second surgery on recurrence) of 65%.[32] A review reported that patients treated by means of the endoscopic ventral approach have a higher percentage of gross total resection, fewer cranial nerve deficits, a lower incidence of meningitis, a lower mortality rate, and fewer local recurrences compared with patients treated with an open microscope-assisted surgical approach.[35]

Complications

The overall surgical morbidity rate is 23 to 69%, and the overall surgical mortality rate is 2 to 14%.[11,14,23,31,33,36-40]

- In endoscopic approaches, cerebrospinal fluid leakage occurred in 5 to 21% of patients.[31-33] This rate can decrease toward 0% with careful multilayered closures and the use of a nasoseptal flap; meningitis 3 to 14% of patients.[31,32] Other reported complications include new cranial nerve palsy and ICA injury with accompanying pseudoaneurysms (which can also be fatal if left untreated[32]).
- Trouble swallowing may require tracheostomy and percutaneous endoscopic gastrostomy.
- Patients with skull base chordomas have been shown to have a poorer quality of life and higher levels of depression than the general population, generally related to neurologic deficits (such as bowel/bladder dysfunction and sensory deficits) and pain medication or corticosteroid use.[40]

■ 22.5 Tentorial Meningiomas
■ Anatomy

Review the topographic anatomy of the tentorium on page 31.

- Meningiomas are the most common tumors involving the tentorium. Sporadic cases of tentorial schwannomas (most likely of the trochlear nerve), solitary fibrous tumors/hemangiopericytomas, dermoids and epidermoids, plasmacytomas, sarcomas, and metastases have been reported. Dural arteriovenous fistulas are discussed in Chapters 12 and 25.
- Thirty percent of posterior fossa meningiomas and about 6% of intracranial meningiomas originate from the tentorium.[1-4]
- Meningiomas of the falcotentorial angle are regarded as a specific subgroup, accounting for less than 1% of intracranial meningiomas, often extending into the pineal region, and they may attain a large size before their discovery.[5-9]
- Depending on the site of origin, the lesions can grow inferiorly, superiorly, across the tentorium, anteriorly, or posteriorly.

> Transtentorial approaches are also used for reaching the mediobasal temporal lobe, occipital lobes, cerebellum, pineal region, petroclival region, and posterior circulation.

■ Symptoms

The symptoms on presentation depend on the primary site of the lesion. Lesions in the incisura tend to present with cranial neuropathy and brainstem compression, whereas those in the broad leaves of the tentorium or falcotentorial region tend to present with mass effect. The most frequent symptoms of tentorial meningiomas, in order of frequency, are headache, dizziness, gait disturbance, mental changes, visual disturbances, and seizures. In less than 10% of patients, trigeminal neuralgia, hemihypesthesia, tinnitus, and dysphagia have been reported.[10] Occlusion of the transverse and/or sigmoid sinuses may lead to raised intracranial pressure and papilledema similar to a pseudotumor cerebri syndrome.

■ Signs

Signs include gait ataxia; deficits of CNs II, III, V, VIII, and IX; papilledema; mental deficits; hemiparesis; homonymous hemianopsia; hemihypesthesia; aphasia; and arterial hypertension.

- Tentorial meningiomas are incidentally discovered in about 4% of patients.[10]

■ Classification

Yasargil's classification system has eight types, based on the origin of the meningioma in relation to the tentorium,[6] later merged into five groups,[5] due to the lack of differentiation between T1 and T2, as well as T6 and T7 in neuroimaging (**Table 22.10** and **Fig. 22.13**).

- Specific classification systems have been proposed for the falcotentorial meningioma based on the origin of the tumor (**Table 22.11**).

■ Radiology

Besides the standard neuroimaging, computed tomography venography (CTV) or MRV is recommended for visualizing the drainage patterns and the patency of venous sinuses. A cerebral angiogram may be particularly helpful for incisural tumors with involvement of the galenic venous systems and arteries of the posterior circulation.

Table 22.10   Tentorial Meningioma Classifications Based on the Origin of the Tumor

Tentorium-Related Classifications		
Findings from Yasargil[6]		**Findings from Bassiouni et al[5]**
T1	Free tentorial notch (anterior)	Medial incisural
T2	Middle part	
T3	Posterior part	Falcotentorial
T4	Intermediate tentorial surface	Paramedian
T5	Torcular herophili	Peritorcular
T6	Lateral outer tentorial ring (posterior)	Lateral tentorial
T7	Anterior part	
T8	Falcotentorial	Falcotentorial
Tentorial Fold-Related Classification[11]		
Type 1	Origin in the dorsal portion of the tentorial fold	
Type 2	With extension into the anterior portion of the middle fossa	
Type 3	Combination of type 1 and 2	
Tentorial incisura-related classification[12]		
Lateral		Posteromedial

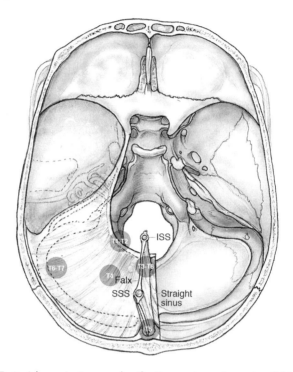

Fig. 22.13 Tentorial meningiomas: classification systems (see also **Tables 22.10** and **22.11**). ISS, inferior sagittal sinus; SSS, superior sagittal sinus.

■ Treatment

Treatment is tailored to the patient (physiological age, comorbidities, and neurologic status), the lesion (size, position, effect on surrounding brain, and prior treatment), and the experience and preferences of the surgical team. Options include (1) conservative monitoring with repeat scans and neurologic examinations, (2) radiotherapy, (3) radiosurgery, (4) surgery, and (5) surgery for biopsy/partial resection followed by radiotherapy (RT)/radiosurgery (RS).

■ Surgical Approaches

The surgical approach and patient positioning are determined based on the location and extent of the tumor.

Table 22.11   Falcotentorial Meningioma Classifications Systems

Source	Classification	Description
Asari et al[13]	Anterior	Between the inferior sagittal sinus and the great vein of Galen
	Inferior	Between the great vein of Galen and the straight sinus
	Posterior	Along the straight sinus
	Superior	Above the tentorium
Bassiouni et al[14]	Type I	Between the falx leaflets, above the junction of the great vein of Galen and the straight sinus; its growth displaces the vein of Galen and the internal cerebral veins inferiorly
	Type II	Below the tentorium, near the junction of the veins of Galen and the straight sinus, pushing the Galenic venous system superiorly
	Type III	From the paramedian tentorial incisura, with the vein of Galen medial to the tumor
	Type IV	From the falcotentorial junction along the straight sinus (as with T8 in Yasargil's classification); its growth displaces the Galenic venous system contralaterally

- Zygomatic extended middle fossa approach, transzygomatic or subtemporal approach, or frontotemporal craniotomy ± OZ osteotomy is used for the treatment of incisural or lateral supratentorial tumors.
- Supracerebellar infratentorial approach is used for infratentorial tumors.
- Petrosal approach is used for middle or posterior incisural tumors with extension in the petroclival area.
- Retrosigmoid approach is used for infratentorial tumors.
- (Bi)Occipital (and later transtentorial) approach is used for falcotentorial meningiomas.
- Combinations of all these approaches are used for complex multicompartmental tumors.
- In patients with obstructive hydrocephalus, consider pre- or intraoperative ventricular CSF drain or endoscopic third ventriculocisternostomy in cases where incomplete resection is anticipated.
- In torcular/peritorcular meningiomas, the craniotomy should be extended to encompass all the posterior sinuses[15] (**Fig. 22.14**).
- For large falcotentorial meningiomas, a bilateral occipital transtentorial/transfalcine approach is used, with large exposure of the supra- and infratentorial compartments.[16]

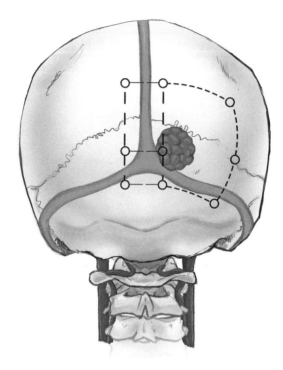

Fig. 22.14 Craniotomy for resection of peritorcular/falcotentorial meningiomas. (Adapted from Harsh GR. Peritorcular meningiomas. In: DeMonte F, McDermott MW, Al-Mefty O, eds. Al-Mefty's Meningiomas, 2nd ed. New York, Stuttgart: Thieme; 2011:177–186.)

- In cases involving the (lateral and sagittal) sinuses, the options are as follows (see also Chapter 26):
  - ○ Division/resection of the sinus, in cases of complete occlusion by the tumor, as shown in preoperative venogram.
  - ○ In cases of inadequate visualization of the occlusion in preoperative studies, trial occlusion of the sinus may be performed.
  - ○ In cases of partial involvement of the sinus, the tumor can be peeled away, with repair of the sinus wall, whenever possible. Alternately, the tumor remnant can be left and followed over time, or the patient can undergo radiosurgery. Preservation of the infiltrated sinus has lower morbidity, but it entails a recurrence rate of up to 26%,[2,5] although more aggressive surgical resection of the involved sinus has been associated with a recurrence rate of 16 to 21%.[4,17,18] Radiosurgery may help in managing residuals remaining in the sinus.
  - ○ Shunting of the sinuses using blood-diverting shunts has been reported.[19,20]

- The drainage of the galenic venous system and the straight sinus should be preserved.
- Before the closure, the Valsalva maneuver is recommended to confirm that there is no bleeding from the involved sinuses.
- Surgical approaches suggested for the resection of the falcotentorial meningioma: occipital transfalcine/transtentorial for type I, infratentorial supracerebellar for type II, occipital transtentorial for type III, and occipital approach for type IV.[14]

■ Results and Outcome

Overall, total resection has been reported in up to 91% of patients.[21] Outcome depends on the factors related to the tumor, the patient, and the surgical team. The reported rates of surgical mortality are 0 to 3.7%, and the rates of surgical morbidity are 10 to 55%, with complications often resolving on follow-up.[2,12,17,21,22] Among the reported complications are hemiparesis, hemianopia, CN III to VII deficits, gait ataxia, hematomas, CSF leak, meningitis, and cortical blindness.

- Tumors located lateral to the tentorium have a better prognosis in comparison with the medially located ones, but the involvement of the sinuses carries further intra- (bleeding) or post- (bleeding or thrombosis) operative risks.
- Postoperative cranial nerve deficits may occur in incisural tumors, in about 10% of cases.[22]
- Careful closure is necessary in order to avoid the often reported postoperative complications of CSF leakage and pseudomeningocele.[23]
- Subtotal removal of tentorial tumors has been associated with a longer progression-free period and higher quality-of-life scores in comparison with more radical resections.[24]

■ Postoperative Follow-Up

The extent of resection and the meningioma World Health Organization (WHO) grade direct the postoperative follow-up. Remnants of WHO grade I tumors may be followed over time, based on the symptoms and the age of the patient. Grade II meningiomas may be observed in the case of gross total resection, and patients should undergo radiation on any evidence of recurrence. Patients with grade III meningiomas should undergo radiation with fractionated doses or, in selected cases, radiosurgery.

■ 22.6 Jugular Foramen Tumors

■ Anatomy

Review topographic anatomy of the jugular foramen on page 31.

■ Incidence

The most common type of tumor within the jugular foramen is the paraganglioma, which affects 1 in 1.3 million people annually, with women more commonly affected than men. It occurs predominantly in patients between 40 and 70 years of age.[1,2]

■ Glomus Jugulare Tumors (Paragangliomas)

Pathology

See page 151.

Gross Pathology

- These are highly vascularized, nonencapsulated tumors.
- They are histologically benign and rarely malignant, but problematic due to mass effect and invasion of surrounding vasculature, dura, and cranial nerves in addition to bone erosion.
- The annual growth rate of glomus jugulare tumors is 0.79 mm/year.[3]
- Extensive vascularization can be attributed to angiogenesis driven by vascular endothelial growth factor and platelet-derived endothelial cell growth factor. Key vasculature associated with these tumors includes the external carotid artery from the inferior tympanic branch of the ascending pharyngeal artery and in some cases the occipital artery's and posterior auricular artery's meningeal branches.[4,5]
- These tumors are differentiated from other tumors by their tendency to follow the path of least resistance, such as vascular channels, the neural foramina, the eustachian tube, and mastoid air cell tracts.[6]
- They typically can be differentiated from smaller glomus tympanicum tumors that originate in the cochlear promontory by their propensity to extensively erode bone and severely damage the ossicular chain.[7] Nevertheless,

Table 22.12   Glomus Tumor Classification Systems

Grade	Tumor Location
Fisch classification[8,9]	
A	Glomus tympanicum, cleft of middle ear
B	Tympanomastoid area, no extension into infralabyrinthine compartment
C	Temporal bone infralabyrinthine compartment, petrous apex extension
C1	Begins to extend toward vertical part of carotid canal
C2	Vertical part of carotid canal invaded
C3	Horizontal part of carotid canal invaded
D1	Diameter less than 2 cm with intracranial extension
D2	Diameter more than 2 cm with intracranial extension
Glasscock-Jackson classification[10]	
I	Small size, jugular bulb, middle ear, mastoid affected
II	Potential intracranial involvement, extension under internal auditory canal
III	Potential intracranial involvement, extension into petrous apex
IV	Potential intracranial involvement, extension past petrous apex into intratemporal fossa/clivus

tumors may also be classified as glomus jugulotympanicum tumors under instances when the tumor involves both compartments, and the differentiating characteristics of glomus tympanicum and glomus jugulare tumors are not clearly distinguishable.

Classification

Glomus tumor classification systems are listed in **Table 22.12,** and examples are shown in **Figs. 22.15** and **22.16.**

■ Schwannomas

Incidence

Schwannomas are the second most common type of tumor within the jugular foramen, with 90% of jugular foramen schwannomas arising from the glossopharyngeal or vagus nerve.[11,12]

Pathology

See page 135.

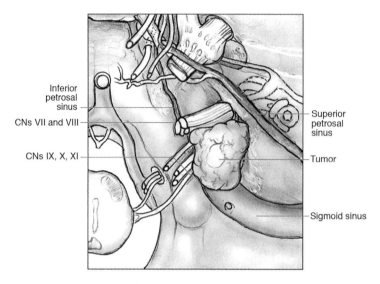

Fig. 22.15 Example of a tumor of the jugular foramen, extending under the internal auditory canal.

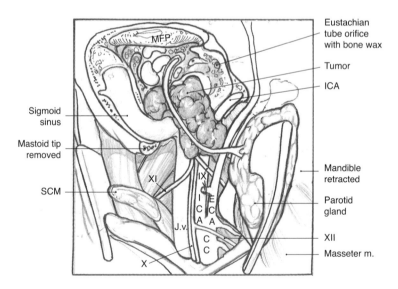

Fig. 22.16 Approach to a jugular foramen tumor paraganglioma with exocranial component, via the far lateral approach combined with transmastoid exposure and facial nerve skeletonization. CC, common carotid artery; ECA, external carotid artery; ICA, internal carotid artery; JV, jugular vein; MFP, Middle Fossa; SCM, sternocleidomastoid muscle. (From Sanna M, et al. Middle Ear and Skull Base Glomus Tumors: Tympanic and Tympanojugular Paragangliomas. In. Wiet MD. Ear and Temporal Bone Surgery. New York: Thieme; 2006:230.)

Table 22.13   Samii Classification System of the Schwannomas of the Jugular Foramen[14]

Subtype	Tumor Location
A	Cerebellopontine angle, minimal intracranial extension and jugular foramen involvement
B	Intracranial extension and significant jugular foramen involvement
C	Extracranial with jugular foramen extensions
D	Intra- and extracranial extensions, dumbbell-shaped

Gross Pathology

Schwannomas are well-defined, rubbery, off-white tumors characterized by smooth and well-corticated remodeling of the jugular foramen.

- Commonly undergo retrogressive alterations: hyalinization, necrosis, hemorrhage, calcification, and cystic degeneration[13]

Classification

A classification of the schwannomas of the jugular foramen is listed in **Table 22.13**.

■ Meningiomas

Incidence

Meningiomas are rare. Primary jugular foramen meningiomas have been reported in fewer than 100 cases; they are more frequent in women (2:1).[15,16] Only 4% of posterior fossa meningiomas are jugular foramen meningiomas.[17]

Pathology

See page 138.

Gross Pathology

Meningiomas are well-defined, solid, sessile, extra-axial tumors with a wide dural base.

- They originate near the jugular bulb, specifically from the arachnoid cap surrounding the bulb.

- They are highly invasive, have a centrifugal manner of growth, and entail significant skull base penetration, especially into the temporal bone and surrounding neurovascular entities.
- Jugular foramen remodeling results in a permeative-sclerotic look in the surrounding bone.
- Flow voids are not present, but dural tails are noted, enabling differentiation from jugular foramen tumors.

Imaging

See page also Chapter 5.

Imaging with a CT bone window is indicated. The CT findings include the following:

- Glomus jugulare tumor: "moth-eaten" form of temporal bone, jugular spine, and carotid crest erosion.
- Jugular foramen schwannoma: no bony invasion; scalloped, smooth, and sclerotic edges seen within the widened jugular foramen.
- Jugular foramen meningiomas: significant bone invasion and hyperostosis around jugular tubercle and jugular spine.

The MRI findings include the following:

- T1-weighted MRI of paragangliomas typically shows "salt and pepper" feature formed by the flow voids present in the well-vascularized glomus jugulare tumor, which are heterogeneously enhanced following gadolinium injection.[18]
- Indium octreotide (analogue of radiologic somatostatin) can be utilized to differentially diagnose paragangliomas.[19]
- T1-weighted imaging of schwannomas yields low-intensity signals, whereas T2-weighted imaging yields high-intensity signals. Enhancement with gadolinium injection is typically very bright, but heterogeneous if cystic degeneration or necrosis is present.[18]
- T1-weighted imaging of meningiomas: low to intermediate signal intensity, with significant enhancement following gadolinium injection.[18]

Cerebral angiography findings include the following:

- Characteristic hypervascularity seen around glomus jugulare tumors.
- Changes in ICA morphology (narrowing or other irregularities) are signs of invasion of the carotid wall by the tumor.
- Schwannomas and meningiomas do not show such extreme vascularity as glomus jugulare tumors.

Cerebral angiography is helpful when considering tumor venous outflow for preoperative planning (dominance of venous sinus, obstruction or occlusion of sinus).

> **Pearl**
>
> Dopamine-, norepinephrine-, and epinephrine-containing secretory granules may also be noted in the paraganglioma's ultrastructure. The effects of such catecholamine release should be assessed through preoperative studies.

Clinical Presentation

Glomus tumors are the most common tumor type to occur in the jugular foramen. As a result of this tumor's significant vascular involvement, patients often present with pulsatile tinnitus, swallowing difficulty, and conductive hearing loss along with pain around the ear and temporal bone.

- Systemic manifestations: if the tumor is catecholamine- or serotonin-secreting, other clinical symptoms such as intraoperative blood pressure and pulse fluctuations, bronchoconstriction, pulmonary stenosis, abdominal pain, among other endocrinopathies, may be present.
- In more severe cases of jugular foramen tumors, tumor growth may result in substantial damage to the ossicles, carotid crest, and compression of the brainstem, cerebellum, and cranial nerves, resulting in palsies and other neuropathies. Common symptoms accompanying such damage include dysphagia, hoarseness, vertigo, tongue weakness, paresis of the trapezius and sternocleidomastoid muscles, ataxia, nystagmus, hemiparesis, and obstructive hydrocephalus.[20]

Surgical Treatment

Gross total surgical resection is currently the gold standard for treating jugular foramen tumors. The goal of achieving complete resection, however, should be balanced by the need to preserve neurologic function; thus, several factors and appropriate surgical approaches must be considered. The choice of approach is dependent on the size, location, and extent of vascular involvement.

> **Pearl**
>
> Jugular foramen tumors are surgically challenging, but the recent advances in microsurgery, neuroimaging, and adjuvant treatments, such as radiotherapy, have greatly improved treatment success rates.[21,22]

Extended Far Lateral Transjugular Posterior Infratemporal Fossa Approach (Mastoid-Neck Approach)

Indications and Advantages

- Highly versatile (multidirectional), utilized for resection of most jugular foramen tumors.
- Combination of transmastoid, suprajugular, transjugular, extreme lateral infrajugular transcondylar transtubercular, and high cervical approaches.
- Intra- and extracranial portions of the tumor can be resected through one-stage total exposure of jugular foramen.
- No rerouting of facial nerve is needed to expose infratemporal internal carotid artery and lower clivus.

❖ Surgical Positioning

- Patient is placed in the supine position, with the head turned laterally away from the side with the lesion after placing the patient in a three-point Mayfield pin fixation system. Intraoperative monitoring of CNs VII to XII, auditory brainstem response (ABR), somatosensory evoked potentials (SSEPs), and motor evoked potentials (MEP) should be set up.[20,23]

❖ Surgical Steps

1. **Postauricular infratemporal incision:**
◈ At a 2- to 3-cm posterior to superior margin of the ear, make a C-shaped combined retroauricular–high cervical skin incision and continue the incision inferiorly to the neck, following the anterior border of the sternocleidomastoid muscle.
◈ Reflect the skin flap anteriorly to expose the posterior auricular muscle located behind the external ear canal, and locate and preserve (or harvest, if needed) the greater auricular nerve.
◈ Progressively dissect the muscular attachments of the mastoid tip to gain exposure.

2. **High cervical exposure:**
- Used to locate extracranial regions of ICA, internal jugular vein, and lower cranial nerves
- Posterior margin of angle of mandible is the anterior limit; mastoid tip posterior margin is the posterior limit (approach limits: crucial to preserve postoperative neck movement/mastication)
◈ Divide the subcutaneous tissue and platysma and retract the anterior margin of the sternocleidomastoid muscle posteriorly to gain visualization

of the posterior belly of the digastric muscle, which should be reflected superoanteriorly to protect the facial nerve.

◈ If required, open carotid sheath, and identify key structures: hypoglossal nerve, ansa cervicalis, vagus nerve, spinal accessory nerve, glossopharyngeal nerve, stylohyoid muscle, internal and external carotid arteries, and internal jugular vein.

3. Retrolabyrinthine mastoidectomy:

◈ To complete mastoidectomy, the body and tip of the mastoid, the spine of Henle, the posterior of the zygoma root, the supramastoid crest, and the asterion should be fully exposed.

◈ A retrolabyrinthine mastoidectomy is performed to expose the sigmoid sinus, jugular bulb, posterior fossa dura, and mastoid segment of the facial nerve (fallopian canal), with preservation of the semicircular canals.

◈◈ Variation: Transection of the ear canal with blind sac closure can be performed in cases where the tumor invades the middle ear and further exposure of the vertical segment of the petrous internal carotid artery is needed.

4. Anterior translocation of the facial nerve:

◈ Following skeletonization of the facial nerve in the fallopian canal, remove the mastoid tip to facilitate exposure of the jugular bulb at the site of the jugular foramen and where it encounters the superior portion of the internal jugular vein.

◈ Keep cartilage and soft tissue around the facial nerve to preserve blood supply to the facial nerve.

◈ Detach the styloid process and reflect the stylopharyngeus muscle anteriorly to see the upper cervical ICA.

◈◈ Variation: The mastoid segment of the facial nerve can be displaced anteriorly to further expose the vertical segment of the petrous ICA.

5. Far lateral transcondylar-transtubercular exposure:

◈ Perform a retrosigmoid craniectomy that includes the lip of the foramen magnum.

◈ After taking care to protect the vertebral artery, use a high-speed drill to remove the posteromedial portion (about one third) of the occipital condyle, with preservation of the occipital condyle–C1 joint articulation.

◈ Skeletonize the extradural hypoglossal canal and reduce the posteromedial jugular tubercle and open the posterior rim of the jugular foramen.

6. Removal of internal jugular vein, jugular bulb, and sigmoid sinus:

◈ Coagulate all arterial vasculature leading to the tumor, which can be felt underneath the venous systems. These structures need to be ligated and occluded to access the underlying tumor within the jugular bulb.

◈ Tie off the internal jugular vein with a suture ligature, and then tie off or occlude the sigmoid sinus (distal to the vein of Labbé).

◈ Open the lateral wall of the internal jugular vein to resect the tumor inside.

◈ Control back-bleeding from inferior petrosal sinus with gentle packing with Surgicel or Gelfoam.

◈ The tumor is resected with care to preserve the medial wall of the jugular bulb (intrabulbar dissection) to prevent damage to the lower cranial nerves.

7. Retrosigmoid intradural exposure:
• This exposure is necessary for a tumor that extends intradurally.

◈ Make a curvilinear dural incision behind the sigmoid sinus and jugular bulb toward the site at which the vertebral artery enters the dura.

◈ Remove intradural tumor and decompress brainstem and preserve cranial nerves and critical vasculature.

8. Reconstruction of skull base:
◈ Perform a thorough multilayer reconstruction of the cranial base, with watertight dural closure using a previously harvested autologous fascia lata or pericranial flap with fibrin glue.

◈ The mastoid defect and anatomic dead space are plugged with autologous fat.

◈ Cranial bony defects can be repaired with titanium mesh or Medpor® Titan (Stryker, Kalamazoo, MI), which consists of titanium sheets embedded within polyethylene.[24]

Outcomes

Glomus Jugulare Tumors

• Gross total resection: 73.3%; near-total resection: 20%; subtotal resection: 6.7%[23]
• Recurrence in 3.3%; mean time to recurrence: 82.8 months[25]

Schwannomas

• Recurrence in 8.9% of cases in a series of 81 patients[26]

Meningiomas

• Rarity of cases, thus limited data available regarding treatment, long-term follow-up, and recurrence.[15]
• Radical resection in all patients, 25% recurrence rate within a mean of 45 months of follow-up.[27]

- 75% recurrence rate within a mean of 8 years of follow-up[28]; clearly, a longer follow-up period postsurgery is associated with an increased recurrence of tumor.

Complications

Cranial Nerve Damage

- Most significant factor leading to postoperative morbidity (cranial nerve palsies)[29]
- Lower cranial nerves palsies following surgery in 9.8% of patients (permanent in more than half)[30]

Surgical Anatomy Pearls

- Intraoperative cranial nerve monitoring should be utilized to minimize additional damage.
- Avoid surgical resection of the medial wall of the jugular bulb to minimize or prevent damage to lower cranial nerves (intrabulbar dissection).

Vascular Injury

The ICA and other vessels may be damaged intraoperatively. All attempts to repair such damage should be made, but in extreme cases some vasculature may be sacrificed with or without a bypass (this consideration is dependent on the findings from the patient's preoperative balloon test occlusion study).[20]

Cerebrospinal Fluid Leakage and Other Complications

- A CSF leak occurs in 3.9% of patients.[30]
- Meningitis, aspiration pneumonia, and septicemia may occur as a result of CSF leakage or due to poor wound healing and ineffective wound closure.[30]
- Pneumonia, pulmonary embolism, wound infection, aspiration, and meningitis occur in 2 to 6% of patients.[31]

Surgical Pearl

A CSF leak can be avoided with meticulous multilayer cranial base reconstruction with watertight dural closure, fat grafting, vascularized flaps, dural sealants, and postoperative lumbar drainage. In some cases, it can be treated with postoperative CSF diversion (lumbar drainage, shunting).

■ 22.7 Foramen Magnum Tumors

■ Anatomy

Review topographic anatomy of the foramen magnum (FM) (page 30) and vertebral artery segments (page 65, **Fig. 2.21B**, page 67). The suboccipital triangle is a key anatomic structure for the surgical approaches to the region (see **Fig. 2.16**, page 58).

Surgical Anatomy Pearl

The third segment, V3 is the most important part of the vertebral artery (VA) in relation to the FM. V3 is the most mobile segment of the VA and can change position according to head movement. Therefore, this needs to be accounted for intraoperatively. The vertical and horizontal portions of V3 are positioned 90 degrees to each other in a patient lying in the supine position, but after head rotation, such as in a posterolateral approach, the vertical and horizontal parts of the vessel become almost aligned in the same direction, with the posterior arch of C1 in between. Branches of VA that arise in the V3 segment are often involved in the vascular supply of tumors in this region.[1]

■ Lesions of the Foramen Magnum

- Surgery of the FM encompasses the treatment of any lesion in the region between the lower aspect of the jugular foramen and the upper part of the C2 vertebra.
- Extra-axial tumors, congenital lesions, bony anomalies, or vertebral artery aneurysms are the most common lesions of the FM (**Table 22.14**).
- Masses in the FM can be classified as neoplastic or nonneoplastic. Tumors can be thought of anatomically as being either craniospinal (located above and extending caudally into the FM) or spinocranial (located below and growing rostrally toward the FM), or purely in the foramen magnum proper. Dural-based extramedullary tumors are usually slowly progressing, low-grade lesions such as meningiomas or schwannomas. When they are intramedullary, they tend to be astrocytomas or ependymomas. Tumors outside the dura are more likely to be chordomas and metastases.
- Other lesions of the foramen magnum region include aneurysms, glomus jugulare tumors, arteriovenous malformations (AVMs), craniovertebral junction anomalies, osseous tumors, hemangioblastomas, melanomas, angiolipomas, epidermoid cysts, and metastases.
- Intra-axial lesions at the level of the brainstem (e.g., gliomas, cavernous malformations) can also be treated via skull base approaches to the FM.

Table 22.14   Foramen Magnum Lesions

Extra-Axial Tumors	Nonneoplastic Lesions
• Meningioma • Neurofibroma • Chordoma • Chondrosarcoma • Epidermoid • Metastasis • Bone tumor	• Aneurysms or ectasia of the vertebral artery • Odontoid process in case of basilar invagination • Pannus from involvement of odontoid with rheumatoid arthritis or old nonunion fracture

■ Foramen Magnum Meningiomas

- Ten percent of meningiomas are located in the posterior fossa, and the FM is the second most common posterior fossa location for these tumors.[2,3]
- FM meningiomas are rare and account for only 1.8 to 3.2% of brain and spinal cord meningiomas.[4,5] Schwannomas are the second most common neoplastic lesion in this region.

■ Epidemiology

Like all meningiomas, FM-based meningiomas occur most commonly in women between 40 and 60 years of age.[4,5] In the pediatric population, FM meningiomas are associated with neurofibromatosis and can be more aggressive in terms of growth rate, size, malignant features, and recurrence compared with those in adults. Multiple meningiomas should trigger investigations for NF1 or NF2. Other risk factors include previous radiation exposure or genetic loss from chromosome 22.

■ Pathology

Review meningiomas pathology on page 138.

- FM meningiomas arise from the arachnoid at the craniovertebral junction (CVJ).
- In the FM, the meningothelial histological subtype is the most common occurring in 22 to 72% of patients, followed by the psammomatous (17–28%) and fibrous types.[2,3] The distinction between encapsulated or en-plaque tumors can be made intraoperatively. En-plaque meningiomas typically penetrate the dura, cross tissue planes, and have no arachnoid "capsule." Al-

though histological subtype does not correlate with the extent of resection for FM meningiomas, the presence of brain or transdural invasion, as well as higher proliferation indices and/or higher WHO grades may predict prognosis and risk of recurrence.

■ Clinical Presentation

- An analysis of more than 1,000 patients found an average of 26.5 months duration of symptoms; 54.5% of the patients presented with cervical and suboccipital pain/stiffness as the earliest and most common symptom.[6]
- Morning headaches are made worse by movement of the neck as well as stimuli that increase intracranial pressure, such as coughing or the Valsalva maneuver.
- Motor weakness is the second most common symptom, occurring in almost half of patients. The classic picture is that of wasting of the intrinsic muscles of the hand, accompanied by upper motor neuron deficit of the leg; however, any pattern of motor weakness can occur. The usual findings are (1) atrophy of small muscles of the hand; (2) spastic lower limbs; and (3) foramen magnum syndrome (also called rotating paralysis), in which symptoms start in the ipsilateral arm and then in the ipsilateral leg, followed by the contralateral leg and finally the contralateral arm) (see also Chapter 7).
- Sensory disturbances, such as numbness/paresthesia and tingling in the hands, and classically dissociated sensory loss (although any pattern may occur) are experienced by 30% of patients. Impingement of lower cranial nerves can occur, causing dysphagia in 10.3%.[6] Test the C2 dermatome.
- Gait disturbances are found in 18% of cases.

Examination Pearl

Look for lower cranial nerve palsies (inspect the tongue for atrophy or fasciculations; look for atrophy of the sternocleidomastoid and trapezius muscles), neurogenic bladder, and, less commonly, ataxia or cerebellar signs, downbeat nystagmus (usually indicating compression at the FM). Hoarseness, and ipsilateral Horner's syndrome as well as respiratory difficulties are usually a late finding and they may require a speech, language, and swallowing review to assess the perioperative risk of aspiration and need for percutaneous gastrostomy or tracheostomy.

■ Investigations and Imaging

- Computed tomography is the preferred imaging modality to distinguish bony structures as well as for the measurement of landmarks such as the occipital condyle and lateral mass of C1, which can help in planning the extent of bony resection required to access the tumor or enlarge the surgical access. CTA or conventional angiography is useful in defining vascular anatomy, vascular relationships, and tumor blood supply, but MRI and MRA are most useful in defining the relationships of the lesion to the neural and vascular anatomy.

■ Classification

Foramen magnum meningiomas are classified according to the dural infiltration, location, and involvement with the VA. Most lesions arise within the dural sheath (craniospinal, spinocranial) but they can spread across the dura (transdural) or be outside the dural sheath. The dentate ligaments (DLs) are the landmarks between the anterior and posterior compartments. Based on their dural insertion and position with respect to the DLs, the FM meningiomas will be anterior, lateral, or posterior.[7]

- In order of frequency, FM meningiomas are most commonly anterolateral (anterior to DL) (68–98%), then posterolateral (dorsal to DL), strictly posterior (on both sides of posterior midline), and rarely anterior (dural attachment on both sides of anterior midline).[5] The surgical approaches of the posterior and posterolateral cases are the same, and these are sometimes grouped into one category.[8]
- Foramen magnum meningiomas can also be classified according to their effect on neurovascular and surrounding structures such as the VA, cervicomedullary parenchyma, and cranial nerves. FM lesions found anterior to the neuraxis are technically challenging, as surgeons will encounter the brainstem, cranial nerves, and VA and have very narrow surgical access to the lesion. Those located below the VA are more likely to grow in such a way as to push the lower cranial nerves posteriorly and superiorly out of the surgical path. On the other hand, meningiomas above the VA displace the lower cranial nerves in an inconsistent manner, and these nerves need to be identified and protected during surgery. If the lesion is at either side of the VA, preserving the artery may be difficult, and leaving tumor surrounding the vessel may be the safest option if an arachnoid plane cannot be found between the tumor and the VA or its branches.[9]

Surgical Anatomy Pearl

Spinocranial meningiomas originate below the FM and displace the cranial nerves and the VA to the upper part of the tumor (as also happens with the tumors originating at the jugular foramen); anterior meningiomas displace the cranial nerves posterolaterally.[7]

■ Surgical Approaches

Safe surgical resection of symptomatic lesions is considered the ideal treatment of FM meningiomas. If surgery is contraindicated, radiosurgery is advisable.[10,11]

- The surgical approach is based on the anatomic location of the lesion, as well as the surgical corridor created by the lesion itself[12,13] (**Fig. 22.17**).
  - The midline posterior occipital craniotomy is used for posteriorly located FM meningiomas.[14] Removal of bony boundaries around the rim of the FM and posterior arch of the atlas facilitates visualization of the VA and provides access to more anteriorly based FM meningiomas. The advantages of this approach include good visualization of the VA, brainstem, and cranial nerves. The disadvantages are that the paravertebral muscles cannot be lateralized too much, and laterally positioned tumors are more likely to require neural retraction to be reached.
- Transcondylar approaches: Drilling some of the occipital condyle can widen the surgical access for FM lesions[9,15–21] (**Fig. 22.18**). Very rarely, resection of the adjacent portion of the superior articular facet of C1 and opening the hypoglossal canal or mastoidectomy may be required.[22]

> **Surgical Anatomy Pearl**
>
> Condylar resection of > 50% (with subsequent instability) requires occipitocervical fusion.

- Occipital condyle drilling is often unnecessary to achieve total resection of intradural FM tumors.[23] A transcondylar approach may be considered necessary to widen the surgical corridor, whenever required, but suboccipital craniotomy is usually good enough to perform a safe and total/subtotal resection, particularly if the suboccipital muscles have been adequately mobilized to enable bone removal from the lateral foramen magnum.
- Localized anterior lesions can be also approached by means of transoral approaches.[24,25]

> **Surgical Anatomy Pearls**
>
> - Most FM meningiomas tend to encase the lower cranial nerves, and may invade the hypoglossal canal and pars nervosa of the jugular foramen. It is fairly common to find CN XI and the cervical roots pushed back and stretched over the tumor. In these cases, do not resect the tumor en-bloc. Devascularize and then internally debulk the tumor to create a surgical corridor to improve and avoid retraction. Sharp dissection is often utilized in the confined space at the ventral aspect of these lesions to minimize manipulation and further compression of the medulla or brainstem.

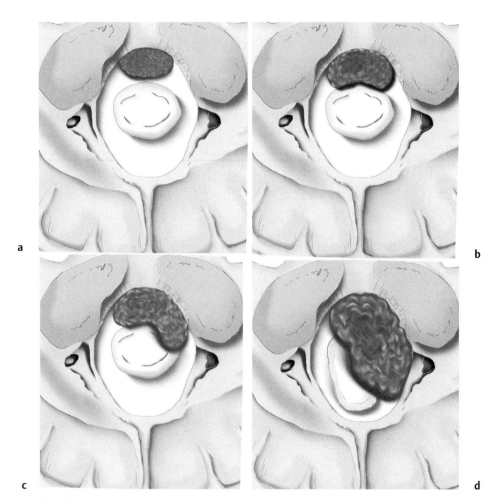

Fig. 22.17a–d Schema showing the growth of anterior and anterolateral foramen magnum meningiomas, with subsequent development of the surgical corridor, which is very narrow in the case of a purely anterior tumor **(a)** and very large when the tumor grows posterolaterally and displaces the brainstem **(d)**. If the surgical corridor is not large enough, a transcondylar approach may be required. (Adapted from Cusimano MD, Faress A, Chang Y, Luong W. Foramen magnum meningiomas. In: DeMonte F, McDermott MW, Al-Mefty O, eds. Al-Mefty's Meningiomas, 2nd ed. New York, Stuttgart: Thieme; 2011:297–309.)

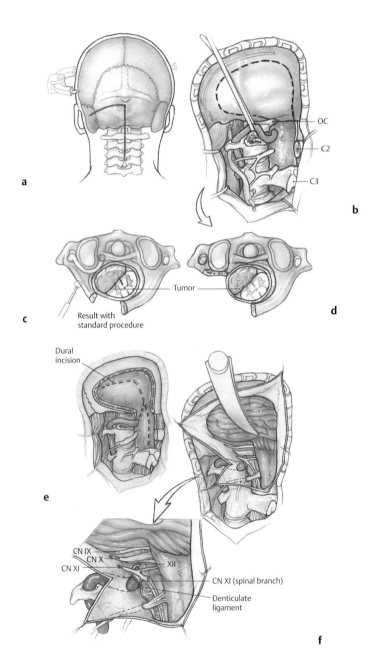

Fig. 22.18a–f Steps of the transcondylar approach for foramen magnum lesions. **(a)** Skin incision. **(b)** Craniotomy and vertebral artery (VA) exposure. **(c)** Partial and **(d)** extended laminectomy of C1 with partial occipital condylectomy. **(e)** Dural incision for **(f)** exposure of the foramen magnum/craniovertebral junction anatomic structures. CN, cranial nerve; OC, occipital condyle. (From George B. Foramen Magnum Tumors. In: Nader et al. (Eds.) Neurosurgery Tricks of the Trade. New York: Thieme; 2014:207.)

- Achieving dural removal after total excision of these lesions can be challenging, given the cranial nerves in the area. If cranial nerves such as CN XII are at risk, then it is often prudent to remove the tumor and coagulate the dural base. The tumor can be removed by working around and between the sensory roots of C1 and C2. The dentate ligament can be divided to access tumor anterior to it and the spinal cord.
- The arachnoid around the vertebral artery and the posterior inferior cerebellar artery (PICA) branch can be preserved and will protect the upper spinal cord and medulla during the dissection of the tumor. The arachnoid should stay with the patient whenever possible.

■ Outcome

- The surgery-related mortality rate is 0 to 13% (now most are under 5%), and the overall morbidity rate is 15 to 36%.[2,26-28]
- Similar data on the amount of resection of the tumor have been reported by using the suboccipital approach or more extended transcondylar approaches, with all the related variants.[7] Complete resection has been reported in the range of 63 to 100%,[3,19,29,30] with incomplete resection reported in 20% of patients.[7]
- Recurrences or remnants that grow over the follow-up may often be treated with radiosurgery.[31]
- The space lateral and sometimes anterior to the VA in the region of the jugular tubercle is a common location for residual tumor, so drilling the tubercle or accessing it with an angled endoscope may improve the outcome.
- An overall clinical improvement after surgery has been reported in the range 50 to 100%, with 15% of patients having worse clinical symptoms.[7]
- Poor prognostic factors are a low preoperative Karnofsky Performance Scale score, a progressive clinical course, lower cranial nerve involvement, VA encasement, anterior location, and quadriparesis.
- Complications after FM surgery include transient or permanent lower cranial nerve injuries (with possible subsequent aspiration pneumonia), CSF leak, meningitis, motor/sensory deficits, and vascular injury leading to stroke. Postoperative assessment of swallowing is important. Whenever required, early tracheostomy and percutaneous gastrostomy should be considered to avoid aspiration pneumonia and its sequelae.

■ 22.8 Cranial Base Rhizopathies

Cranial base rhizopathies entail symptomatic compression of posterior fossa cranial nerves, most commonly by vessels, causing the following (based on the compressed nerve):

1. **Trigeminal neuralgia** (also called tic douloureux): lancinating pain with referral to the territory of one or more branches of the trigeminal nerve
   - **Epidemiology**: incidence up to 27/100,000, more commonly afflicting the elderly.[1] Two to 6% of patients affected by multiple sclerosis have trigeminal neuralgia.[2,3] Bilateral trigeminal neuralgia is found in 18% of patients affected by multiple sclerosis, but very rarely in those without multiple sclerosis.[4]
   - **Pathophysiology:** secondary to vascular compression, posterior fossa tumor, demyelination, trauma, stroke, and herpes; it also can be idiopathic. The vascular compression of the trigeminal nerve at or near the root entry zone is the most common cause of trigeminal neuralgia,[5] but vascular compression may occur also in patients without trigeminal neuralgia.[6] High-resolution MRI may help in identifying neurovascular compression in trigeminal neuralgia, but this syndrome may also be unrelated to the compression itself.[7]
   - **Signs and symptoms:** May present with status trigeminus: rapid succession of tic-like spasms
     - Type I: classic presentation, usually called "typical trigeminal neuralgia": shooting, electrical-shock like, episodic pain lasting several seconds, often triggered by talking, chewing, shaving, brushing teeth, and walking in the wind. Responds well to carbamazepine initially. These patients are much better surgical candidates than type II patients because they have far better surgical outcomes in terms of pain relief.
     - Type II: idiopathic trigeminal facial pain: aching, throbbing, or burning for more than 50% of the time.[8] Rarely responds well to carbamazepine or to microvascular decompression.
     - These two types must be differentiated from other forms of trigeminal neuralgia (secondary to primary causes, such as tumors, or postherpetic, or associated with systemic diseases, such as fibromyalgia).[9]
   - **Treatment**
     - Generally treated with drugs (carbamazepine, oxcarbazepine, baclofen, gabapentin, phenytoin, or a combination of drugs), but 75% of patients may fail medical therapy or experience unbearable medication side effects and require a procedure.
     - Cases refractory to medical management may require percutaneous treatments (see below), radiosurgery (page 790), or microvascular decompression; a treatment algorithm is shown in **Fig. 22.19**.
     - Rarely, intradural retrogasserian trigeminal nerve section is indicated.
     - Microvascular decompression is the surgical gold standard.

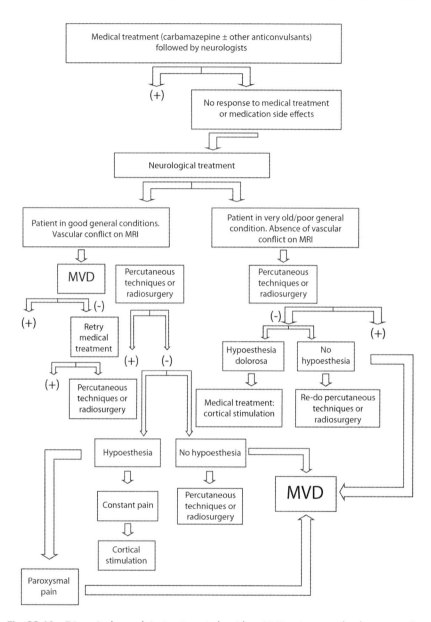

Fig. 22.19 Trigeminal neuralgia: treatment algorithm. MVD, microvascular decompression of the trigeminal nerve; +, successful treatment; −, unsuccessful treatment. (Adapted from Alvernia JE, Simon E, Sindou M. Percutaneous Lesioning: Procedures for Trigeminal Neuralgia. In: Nader R. et al. Neurosurgery Tricks of the Trade. New York: Thieme; 2014:617.)

- **Patterns**
    - The patterns of trigeminal neuralgia in decreasing likelihood are as follows: V_2 and V_3 together (42%), V_2 alone (20%), V_3 alone (17%), V_1 and V_2 together (14%), V_1 and V_2 and V_3 (5%), and V_1 alone (2%).[10,11]

2. Hemifacial spasm (HFS)

Abnormal clonic or tonic contractions of the facial muscles, initially starting in the orbicularis oculi and then spreading to all branches of the seventh cranial nerve.

- Caused by vascular compression of the root exit zone of the facial nerve, generally at the level of the supraolivary fossette.[12-15]
- Botulinum toxin injections may be used for temporary symptomatic treatment.[16]
- Microvascular decompression of the VII nerve is the gold standard and provides prolonged relief in up to 90% of patients.

3. Nervus intermedius neuralgia (geniculate neuralgia)

Sharp shooting pain in the ear, with occasional radiation to the posterior temple, mastoid, eye regions (in differential diagnosis with Ramsay Hunt syndrome type II, due to herpes zoster infection in the geniculate ganglion).

4. CN VIII vascular conflict

Positional vertigo and/or tinnitus.

5. Glossopharyngeal neuralgia

Sharp severe and intermittent pain in the throat or neck (pharyngeal type), or ear (tympanic type), or both, often triggered by swallowing, coughing, chewing, talking, yawning, or touching the earlobe. Sometimes associated with syncope and bradycardia. Peak onset occurs at 40 to 60 years of age. Almost 100 times less common than trigeminal neuralgia but can be effectively treated with microvascular decompression.

6. Bulbar compression by ectatic vertebral artery

Compression of the brainstem due to tortuous ectatic basilar/vertebral arteries, giving rise to progressive myelopathic features, low cranial nerve deficits, or systemic arterial hypertension. Few cases reported, with microvascular decompression of the brainstem proposed as treatment,[17] which is still controversial.

■ Radiological Investigations

Neuroimaging can rule out tumors, cysts, vascular lesions, or other causes giving rise to secondary neuralgias/spasms.

- CTA, MRA, and T2-weighted cisternography provide detailed information about the intracisternal structures at the CPA.[18-21] A 3D reconstructed balanced fast-field echo (BFEE) MRI fuses with 3D time-of-flight MRA and has been shown to have high sensitivity and specificity to detect compressions; however, they might not predict response.[7]

■ Neuromonitoring

- Intraoperative cranial nerves and BAEP neuromonitoring can be useful for reducing/avoiding cranial nerves deficits.[22-24]
- Electromyogram of the facial nerve in hemifacial spasm or the vocal cord in cases of glossopharyngeal decompression.
- Intraoperative monitoring of BAEP may reduce the risk of hearing loss in microvascular decompression (MVD).[25-27]

■ Microvascular Decompression

Microvascular decompression is recommended for patients who can no longer tolerate medications and can tolerate major surgery.

Surgical Position

The patient is placed in the lateral position or park-bench position, with the head secured in three- or four-point head holder.

❖ Surgical Steps

◈ Preoperative lumbar drainage may be useful, but in general opening of the cisterns during surgery provides enough brain relaxation.
◈ **Approach:** Retrosigmoid paracerebellar approach (see page 385).
◈ Perform craniotomy, with one or more bur holes, or craniectomy, exposing the posterior side of the sigmoid sinus and the inferior side of the transverse sinus. Avoid injury to the dural sinuses and beware of the mastoid emissary vein.
◈◈ Variation: The craniectomy can be round, oval, or isosceles triangle shaped.[28]
◈ Coagulate the mastoid emissary vein.
◈ Dura mater opening: Open the dura mater in a C-shaped fashion (or in other ways; see Chapter 14, **Fig. 14.23**, on page 389), medially to the sigmoid sinus and inferiorly to the lateral sinus.

◈ If no preoperative CSF lumbar drainage has been used, start the incision in the inferior segment of the C, to reach the lateral cerebellomedullary cistern or, if it is large, the cisterna magna. Open the cistern (with an arachnoid blade) and drain enough CSF to relax the cerebellum.

◈ After the durotomy, do not reflect the C-shaped dura. Leave it on the cerebellar surface, in order to avoid its drying.

◈ Make a T-shaped incision on the medial border of the dura, above the sigmoid sinus, and tack it up, making a gentle rotation of the sigmoid sinus. This maneuver opens more of the surgical angle into the CPA.

◈ Check the venous vascularization in the CPA and between the cerebellum and tentorium. Coagulation of some small bridging veins may be required, when strictly necessary for cerebellum retraction.

◈ Gently retract the cerebellum with suction. If the brain is still "tight," try draining more CSF or administering mannitol to help brain relaxation. In the event that retraction is deemed necessary, avoid retracting the cerebellum more than 1 cm from the petrous bone.[29]

◈ The surgical angle, and the position of the retractor, changes according to the target area: superiorly for exposing the root exit zone of the petrosal vein and the trigeminal nerve; in the middle for CN VII and VIII; inferiorly for access to the lateral cerebellomedullary cistern and exposure of the CNs IX to XI.

◈ In hemifacial spasm treatment, do gentle retraction of the flocculus. Excessive retraction causes deterioration of the brainstem evoked response.

◈◈ Variation: The surgical procedure is routine with the microscope, and angled endoscopes are very helpful for visualizing the distal aspects of nerves and the undersurface (anterior side) of the cranial nerves that are not easily visible with the microscope.

◈ Carefully dissect the arachnoid to access the cisterns and their contents.

◈ Do not move the vessel before a wide dissection of the entire length of the loop to its proximal and distal ends.[28]

◈ After identification of the target nerve, check the vessels, which may cause the compression.

◈ Always check for multiple areas of compression.
  • Typical causes of compression:
    ○ Trigeminal neuralgia: SCA or its branches (75%), AICA (10%), basilar artery or its branches, as sole cause of compression or in combination with a vein or multiple sites of compression.[30,31] In some cases, no compression can be found.
    ○ Hemifacial spasm: AICA, PICA, or small veins.
    ○ Glossopharyngeal neuralgia: PICA or VA.

◈ Dissect and mobilize carefully the compressive vessels from the nerves. Mobilization can be performed with microdissectors (e.g., Rhoton Nos. 5, 6, 7, 8, 9, or 10). The location of the compression is generally only on the root entry zone (63%), but is has been described also as only on the cisternal

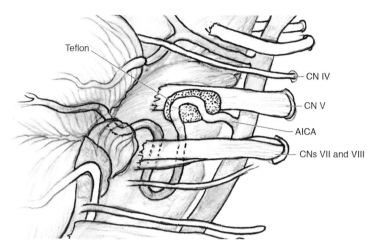

Fig. 22.20 Microvascular decompression for trigeminal neuralgia. In this example, the cause of the compression is the anterior inferior cerebellar artery (AICA), which can be separated from the trigeminal nerve with a piece of Teflon felt.

portion (4%), only on the petrous segment (1.5%), or combinations of these locations.[31]

◈ Insert one or more appropriately sized pieces of Teflon felt along the side of the compression to move the vessel off of the nerve (**Fig. 22.20**).

◈ Rarely is it necessary to tack up vessels using a fascial or other type of sling (e.g., Gore-Tex) or an anchoring stitch (e.g., 8-0 nylon) in the adventitia on the dura, to keep it away from the nerve.

◈◈ Variation: Reinforce the Teflon felt with a drop of fibrin glue, in order to avoid its migration.

■ Nervus Intermedius

❖ Surgical Steps

The nervus intermedius is formed by one or two fascicles between CNs VII and VIII. Explore not only the nervus intermedius but also the trigeminal nerve and glossopharyngeal nerves, which also supply the ear.

◈ Retract the facial nerve gently, visualize and cut the intermedius, if there is no vascular compression to resolve. Cutting the nerve seems well tolerated by patients, with no major complications and a success rate in relieving pain in up to 75%.[32–34]

◈◈ Variation: Section of the nervus petrosus major or geniculate ganglion.[35]

Complication

The sectioning of the nerve may cause tearing, but in general it is temporary and well tolerated by patients.[29]

■ Glossopharyngeal Nerve

In the microvascular treatment of glossopharyngeal neuralgia, a transcondylar approach has been suggested, to provide access to the lower cranial nerves, vertebral artery, and PICA,[36] but is rarely necessary.

❖ Surgical Steps

◈ If a vascular compression is found, use Teflon felt for decompression, or stitch the compressing vertebral artery to the dura in proximity of the jugular foramen.

◈◈ In the case of an absent clear vascular compression, section the glossopharyngeal nerve and the upper two fascicles of the vagus nerve.[37]

Complications

Temporary or permanent dysphagia and hoarseness.

■ Cranial Nerve VIII

It is very difficult to make the correct diagnosis, because positional vertigo and tinnitus can be found in several other diseases. The diagnosis should be made by a multidisciplinary team.

- A compression may be found on MRI or intraoperatively, from the brainstem to the AICA or PICA.
- In selected patients, the operation may have a success rate of up to 70%.[29]

❖ Surgical Steps

◈ The microvascular decompression techniques are performed in the same way as in the approaches for the other nerves.

◈◈ If there appears to be an AICA inside the IAC, the canal has to be drilled for adequate exposure and mobilization.

■ Closure in MVDs

Before closing the dura, the Valsalva maneuver may be indicated for checking venous oozing. Primary closure of the dura is generally possible; otherwise, reinforce it with pieces of muscle or fascia from the local flap, or fascia lata, or make a synthetic duraplasty. Fibrin glue may also be used.

> **Surgical Anatomy Pearl**
>
> Make sure to wax the mastoid air cells.

❖ Surgical Steps

◈ In the case of a craniotomy, reattach the bone flap with titanium microplates, or otherwise cover with titanium mesh or bone cement.

◈ Wax the bone edges on the sigmoidal side, in order to avoid CSF leakage via the mastoid cells.

◈ Closed-suction drainage is not recommended, so as not to cause CSF leakage.[38]

Postoperative Care

If there are no intraoperative complications and the patient is in good health, intensive care unit monitoring is not required. Patients are mobilized the day after surgery, and are discharged 1 to 4 days after surgery, if there are no complications.

Complications[31,39]

• Cerebellar contusion, hemorrhage: < 1%
• Injury to the dural sinuses
• Cranial nerve injuries: one of the most common is hearing loss,[40,41] occurring in 1% of cases in a recent series.[31]
  ○ Cranial nerve deficits may be managed by reducing the retraction of the cerebellum, and then the stretching the cranial nerves in the CPA, or by reducing the manipulation of the arteries (i.e., the labyrinthine artery, which, in the case of damage, may cause hearing loss). Direct trauma on the nerves may be caused by the instruments, or by coagulation heating, or by the illumination of the tip of the endoscope, if too high or too close; reduce excessive compression by the Teflon felt used for the MVD.
• Postoperative CSF leakage (generally treated by oversewing or spinal drainage): 3 to 7%
• Pseudomeningocele

- Wound infection
- Sensory loss: 5–10%
- Facial palsy: < 1%
- Hydrocephalus (requiring ventriculostomy): < 1%
- Hyponatremia: especially in those on carbamazepine preoperatively
- Chemical meningitis
- Teflon granuloma
- Death: 0.3–1%[2,42,43]

Outcomes of MVD

Trigeminal Neuralgia

About 90% of patients in whom a microvascular compression is found and treated obtain relief, usually starting immediately or within days of treatment.

- Good long-term control (pain free, off medication) was reported in 65 to 84% of cases[42,44]; 63% report having 20 years of pain relief.[42,44]
- In one series of 1,185 patients, recurrence of trigeminal neuralgia occurred in 23.8% of patients, especially in females, those with symptoms longer than 8 years, those who underwent decompression of a vein in surgery, and in those lacking immediate relief after surgery.[30]
- Recurrence within 2 years of surgery was seen in 16% (range 3–41%) of patients.[45]
- Patients in whom an arterial cause of compression was found and treated and who show recurrent symptoms within 2 years of surgery may be good candidates for reexploration. In many of these patients the Teflon will be found displaced, and remedying it can provide pain relief.
- Most series describe the following risk factors for recurrence: younger age, longer preoperative duration of symptoms, female gender, venous compression or involvement of more branches, and previous invasive procedures.[45–49] Although the venous compression on the nerve has been found as the most relevant cause of recurrence,[50] it seems that placing Teflon between the trigeminal nerve and the offending petrosal vein leads to a remission rate of 87%.[51]

Hemifacial Spasm

An analysis of 1,174 operations of MVD for hemifacial spasm found a success rate of 94.1%. Complications included transient hearing loss in 2.6%, permanent hearing loss in 1.1%, transient facial weakness in 7.6%, permanent facial weakness in 0.7%, CSF leakage in 0.25%, and cerebellar hemorrhage or infarction in 0.17%, with no mortality.[52]

Glossopharyngeal Neuralgia

Almost all the treated patients have shown immediate pain relief after surgery, with rare patients having recurring pain and requiring further surgery.[53,54]

Trigeminal Neuralgia: Other treatments

Radiosurgery

See page 790.

Percutaneous Trigeminal Rhizotomies

(1) Radiofrequency thermocoagulation; (2) percutaneous balloon compression; (3) glycerol rhizotomy.

All the percutaneous procedures require the placement of the needle into the foramen ovale.

❖ Surgical Steps

◈ *Needle placement:* The patient is placed in the supine position. In Hartel's technique, the entry point is 2.5 to 3 cm lateral to the oral commissure. The direction of the needle is toward one point, which is inferior to the pupil, and toward another one, which is 2 to 3 cm anterior to the external auditory canal, along the zygoma (**Figs. 22.21** and **Fig. 22.22a**).

- **General complications of the transovale placement of the needle:** dysesthesia, alterations in salivation, lacrimation, carotid cavernous fistula, aseptic meningitis, intracerebral hemorrhage or abscess, jaw

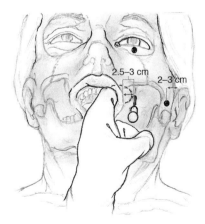

Fig. 22.21   Hartel's technique (see text).

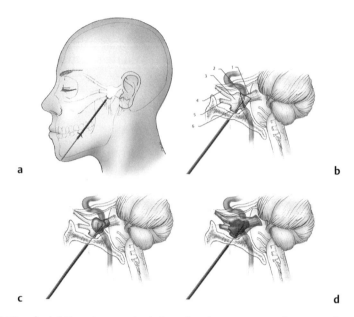

Fig. 22.22a–d **(a)** Percutaneous technique for the treatment of trigeminal neuralgia. **(b)** Glycerol injection. 1, motor branch of CN V; 2, plexus triangularis; 3, gasserian ganglion; 4, CN V$_1$; 5, CN V$_2$; 6, CN V$_3$. **(c)** Balloon compression. **(d)** Thermocoagulation. (From Alvernia JE, Simon E, Sindou M. Percutaneous Lesioning: Procedures for Trigeminal Neuralgia. In: Nader R. et al. Neurosurgery Tricks of the Trade. New York: Thieme; 2014:620.)

weakness, headache, diplopia, carotid artery puncture with bleeding, mild paresthesia/numbness, and herpes simplex perioralis. Very rarely, aseptic meningitis is a complication, occurring in about 2 of every 1,000 cases.

◈ Insert a gloved finger in the patient's mouth, laterally to the teeth, and insert the needle, or electrode, medial to the coronoid process toward a point 3 cm anterior to the external acoustic meatus and the medial aspect of the pupil. The introduction of the needle in the foramen ovale is marked by facial wince, which shows the contact with the mandibular nerve.

◈ Avoid advancing the cannula more than 8 mm beyond the clival line, in order to avoid abducens palsy, or penetration into the cavernous sinus, brainstem, or temporal lobe.[55]

◈ Check the position of the needle by intraoperative fluoroscopy or cisternography in the anteroposterior, lateral, and oblique anterolateral direction (head on to the foramen ovale). CSF should spill out of the needle.

◈ Twenty percent of patients may have a vasovagal response to the transo-vale needle penetration, especially in the balloon compression procedure.[56] The anesthetist should be aware of this possibility and should administer anticholinergic drugs at the first sign of bradycardia.[57]

1. Radiofrequency thermocoagulation (Fig. 22.22d)
- The patient is awake because his or her cooperation is critical during the stimulation phase.

❖ Surgical Steps

◈ Use straight or curved electrodes
◈ Check the position of the electrode by using a square-wave pulse (0.1 mS, 50 Hz), causing paresthesia. After stimulation, the patient can be sedated and the lesion treated with a thermocouple: 60°C for 60 seconds for V_1, 65°C for 65 seconds for V_2, and 70°C for 70 seconds for V_3.
◈ During the lesion procedure, monitor the corneal reflexes.
- **Outcome:** Initial pain relief up to 97.6%; 57.7% at 60 months and 42.2% at 180 months[58]; multiple treatments with thermocoagulation can increase these rates to 92% at 60 months and 97% at 180 months.
- **Complications:** high rate of masticatory weakness (up to 29%), dysesthesia, corneal numbness,[43] anesthesia dolorosa.

2. Percutaneous balloon compression (Fig. 22.22c)
Usually performed with the patient under general anesthesia. Patient is placed in the supine position, with the head on a neck roll (mild extension of the head).

❖ Surgical Steps

◈ Insert 14-gauge blunt cannula into the foramen ovale, according to Hartel's technique.
◈ Advance a No. 4 Fogarty catheter into Meckel's cave; based on the cave size, larger balloons may be required.
◈ Positioning the catheter in the center of the porous may affect all the divisions of the trigeminal nerve or sometimes more specifically the second division. A lateral placement usually has more effect on V_3, whereas a medial placement will affect V_1 most.
◈ Inflate the balloon with iohexol (pressure 1,000 to 1,200 mmHg) for 1 minute.
- **Outcome:** complete pain relief: up to 91% at 6 months and 69% at 3 years.[43]
  - Recurrence rate: 26% within an average of 18 months.[59]
  - In an analysis of 19 patients affected by multiple sclerosis, 95% of patients were pain free immediately after the procedure, with a 61%

recurrence rate after a median of 29 months; 53% of patients had temporary numbness, and one patient had severe numbness, weakness of masticator muscles, and impaired corneal reflex.[60] MVD in patients affected by multiple sclerosis is less satisfactory than in the idiopathic group[61]; balloon compression has the highest rate of initial pain-free response and duration of pain-free interval.[60] Repeated procedures are also associated with worse complications, such as carotid-cavernous fistula, subdural hematoma.

- **Advantage**: selective sparing of the small fibers for the corneal reflex; advantageous procedure in patients with ophthalmic-branch pain.[59]
- **Technique-related complication**: rupture and retention of the balloon. In the case of high pressure in the balloon, there will be higher rates of dysesthesia, severe numbness, and masseter weakness, and rarely anesthesia dolorosa.

3. Glycerol Rhizotomy (Fig. 22.22b)
Patient can be in deeper anesthesia or awake.

❖ Surgical Steps

◈ Insert a 20-gauge spinal needle into the foramen ovale, according to Hartel's technique.

◈ Check the position of the needle by X-ray and for CSF leaks caused by access into the subarachnoid cistern.

◈ After the insertion of the needle with the patient in the supine position, move the patient to the sitting position. Inject 0.2 to 0.5 mL of water-soluble contrast agent (e.g., iopamidol) to determine cistern volume and check the X-ray again for cisternography.

◈ Inject the cisternal volume with glycerol for lesioning of the involved division.

◈ Keep the patient flexed forward before and after the insertion of glycerol for several hours (at least 1 to 4 hours) to allow the glycerol to bathe the ganglion for as long as possible and to not let the glycerol flow out into the posterior fossa cisterns.

- **Complications:** dysesthesia, generally well tolerated, except anesthesia dolorosa, in 0.2 to 4% of patients, with severe and constant burning pain, refractory to all treatment.
- **Outcome:** immediate/early complete pain relief occurs in up to 90%[57], which can be long-lasting (11 years) in 75 to 85% of patients, 55% of whom may discontinue all the medications, but 22% still require some drugs.[62] There is the possibility of remaining pain free without medications: 61% after 1 year and 50% after 3 years.[63] The procedure can be performed again in some cases.

■ References

Boldfaced references are of particular importance.

22.1 Posterior Skull Base Surgery - Vestibular Schwannoma

1. Akalan N, Seçkin H, Kiliç C, Ozgen T. Benign extramedullary tumors in the foramen magnum region. Clin Neurol Neurosurg 1994;96:284–289
2. Arnautović KI, Al-Mefty O, Husain M. Ventral foramen magnum meningiomas. J Neurosurg 2000;92(1, Suppl):71–80
3. Couldwell WT, Fukushima T, Giannotta SL, Weiss MH. Petroclival meningiomas: surgical experience in 109 cases. J Neurosurg 1996;84:20–28
4. Little KM, Friedman AH, Sampson JH, Wanibuchi M, Fukushima T. Surgical management of petroclival meningiomas: defining resection goals based on risk of neurological morbidity and tumor recurrence rates in 137 patients. Neurosurgery 2005;56: 546–559, discussion 546–559
5. Natarajan SK, Sekhar LN, Schessel D, Morita A. Petroclival meningiomas: multimodality treatment and outcomes at long-term follow-up. Neurosurgery 2007;60:965–979, discussion 979–981
6. Woodruff JM, Selig AM, Crowley K, Allen PW. Schwannoma (neurilemoma) with malignant transformation. A rare, distinctive peripheral nerve tumor. Am J Surg Pathol 1994;18:882–895
7. Benson VS, Pirie K, Schüz J, Reeves GK, Beral V, Green J; Million Women Study Collaborators. Mobile phone use and risk of brain neoplasms and other cancers: prospective study. Int J Epidemiol 2013;42:792–802
8. Pettersson D, Mathiesen T, Prochazka M, et al. Long-term mobile phone use and acoustic neuroma risk. Epidemiology 2014;25:233–241
9. Koos WT, Matula C, Lang J. Color Atlas of Microneurosurgery of Acoustic Neurinomas. New York, Stuttgart: Georg Thieme Verlag; 2002
10. Khrais T, Romano G, Sanna M. Nerve origin of vestibular schwannoma: a prospective study. J Laryngol Otol 2008;122:128–131
11. Kondziolka D, Mousavi SH, Kano H, Flickinger JC, Lunsford LD. The newly diagnosed vestibular schwannoma: radiosurgery, resection, or observation? Neurosurg Focus 2012;33:E8
12. Al Sanosi A, Fagan PA, Biggs ND. Conservative management of acoustic neuroma. Skull Base 2006;16:95–100
13. Miyakoshi A, Kohno M, Nagata O, Sora S, Sato H. Hydrocephalus associated with vestibular schwannomas: perioperative changes in cerebrospinal fluid. Acta Neurochir (Wien) 2013;155:1271–1276
14. Harner SG, Laws ER Jr. Clinical findings in patients with acoustic neurinoma. Mayo Clin Proc 1983;58:721–728
15. Samii M, Matthies C. Management of 1000 vestibular schwannomas (acoustic neuromas): hearing function in 1000 tumor resections. Neurosurgery 1997;40: 248–260, discussion 260–262
16. Matthies C, Samii M. Management of vestibular schwannomas (acoustic neuromas): the value of neurophysiology for evaluation and prediction of auditory function in 420 cases. Neurosurgery 1997;40:919–929, discussion 929–930

17. Matthies C, Samii M, Krebs S. Management of vestibular schwannomas (acoustic neuromas): radiological features in 202 cases—their value for diagnosis and their predictive importance. Neurosurgery 1997;40:469–481, discussion 481–482

18. **Koos WT, Day JD, Matula C, Levy DI. Neurotopographic considerations in the microsurgical treatment of small acoustic neurinomas. J Neurosurg 1998;88:506–512**

19. Tos M, Drozdziewicz D, Thomsen J. Medial acoustic neuromas. A new clinical entity. Arch Otolaryngol Head Neck Surg 1992;118:127–133

20. Dunn IF, Bi WL, Erkmen K, et al. Medial acoustic neuromas: clinical and surgical implications. J Neurosurg 2014;120:1095–1104

21. Yamakami I, Kobayashi E, Iwadate Y, Saeki N, Yamaura A. Hypervascular vestibular schwannomas. Surg Neurol 2002;57:105–112

22. Sanna M, Sivalingam S, Russo A, Taibah A. Acoustic neuromas. Int Adv Otol 2011; 2:1–23

23. **Vachhrajani S, Fawaz C, Mathieu D, et al. Complications of Gamma Knife surgery: an early report from 2 Canadian centers. J Neurosurg 2008;109(Suppl): 2–7**

24. **Cusimano MD. Defining the optimal management for patients with large vestibular schwannomas. Can J Neurol Sci 2013;40:280–281**

25. Babu R, Sharma R, Bagley JH, Hatef J, Friedman AH, Adamson C. Vestibular schwannomas in the modern era: epidemiology, treatment trends, and disparities in management. J Neurosurg 2013;119:121–130

26. **Sekhar LN, Sarma S, Chanda A. Acoustic neuroma: Retrosigmoid and transpetrosal approaches. In: Sekhar LN, Fessler RG, eds. Atlas of Neurosurgical Techniques. New York, Stuttgart: Thieme; 2006:734–744**

27. **Sanna M, Mancini F, Russo A, Taibah A, Falcioni M, Di Trapani G. Atlas of Acoustic Neurinoma Microsurgery, 2nd ed. Stuttgart, New York: Thieme; 2011**

28. Abolfotoh M, Dunn IF, Al-Mefty O. Transmastoid retrosigmoid approach to the cerebellopontine angle: surgical technique. Neurosurgery 2013;73(1, Suppl Operative): ons16–ons23, discussion ons23

29. Cusimano MD, Sekhar L. Partial hypoglossal to facial nerve anastomosis for reinnervation of the paralyzed face in patients with lower cranial nerve palsies: technical note. Neurosurgery 1994;35:532–533, discussion 533–534

30. Day JD, Fukushima T, Giannotta SL. Microanatomical study of the extradural middle fossa approach to the petroclival and posterior cavernous sinus region: description of the rhomboid construct. Neurosurgery 1994;34:1009–1016, discussion 1016

31. House WF. Surgical exposure of the internal auditory canal and its contents through the middle, cranial fossa. Laryngoscope 1961;71:1363–1385

32. Brackmann DE, Fayad JN, Slattery WH III, et al. Early proactive management of vestibular schwannomas in neurofibromatosis type 2. Neurosurgery 2001;49:274–280, discussion 280–283

33. Neff BA, Welling DB. Current concepts in the evaluation and treatment of neurofibromatosis type II. Otolaryngol Clin North Am 2005;38:671–684, ix

34. **Samii M, Gerganov V, Samii A. Microsurgery management of vestibular schwannomas in neurofibromatosis type 2: indications and results. Prog Neurol Surg 2008;21:169–175**

35. Samii A, Lenarz M, Majdani O, Lim HH, Samii M, Lenarz T. Auditory midbrain implant: a combined approach for vestibular schwannoma surgery and device implantation. Otol Neurotol 2007;28:31–38
36. Maini S, Cohen MA, Hollow R, Briggs R. Update on long-term results with auditory brainstem implants in NF2 patients. Cochlear Implants Int 2009;10(Suppl 1):33–37
37. Sanna M, Di Lella F, Guida M, Merkus P. Auditory brainstem implants in NF2 patients: results and review of the literature. Otol Neurotol 2012;33:154–164
38. Mathieu D, Kondziolka D, Flickinger JC, et al. Stereotactic radiosurgery for vestibular schwannomas in patients with neurofibromatosis type 2: an analysis of tumor control, complications, and hearing preservation rates. Neurosurgery 2007;60:460–468, discussion 468–470
39. Subach BR, Kondziolka D, Lunsford LD, Bissonette DJ, Flickinger JC, Maitz AH. Stereotactic radiosurgery in the management of acoustic neuromas associated with neurofibromatosis Type 2. J Neurosurg 1999;90:815–822
40. Phi JH, Kim DG, Chung HT, Lee J, Paek SH, Jung HW. Radiosurgical treatment of vestibular schwannomas in patients with neurofibromatosis type 2: tumor control and hearing preservation. Cancer 2009;115:390–398
41. Baser ME, R Evans DG, Gutmann DH. Neurofibromatosis 2. Curr Opin Neurol 2003; 16:27–33
42. Ahmad RA, Sivalingam S, Topsakal V, Russo A, Taibah A, Sanna M. Rate of recurrent vestibular schwannoma after total removal via different surgical approaches. Ann Otol Rhinol Laryngol 2012;121:156–161
43. Ansari SF, Terry C, Cohen-Gadol AA. Surgery for vestibular schwannomas: a systematic review of complications by approach. Neurosurg Focus 2012;33:E14
44. Tatagiba M, Roser F, Schuhmann MU, Ebner FH. Vestibular schwannoma surgery via the retrosigmoid transmeatal approach. Acta Neurochir (Wien) 2014;156:421–425, discussion 425
45. Falcioni M, Fois P, Taibah A, Sanna M. Facial nerve function after vestibular schwannoma surgery. J Neurosurg 2011;115:820–826
46. Nonaka Y, Fukushima T, Watanabe K, et al. Contemporary surgical management of vestibular schwannomas: analysis of complications and lessons learned over the past decade. Neurosurgery 2013;72(2, Suppl Operative):ons103–ons115, discussion ons115
47. Sanna M, Taibah A, Russo A, Falcioni M, Agarwal M. Perioperative complications in acoustic neuroma (vestibular schwannoma) surgery. Otol Neurotol 2004;25:379–386
48. Mahboubi H, Ahmed OH, Yau AY, Ahmed YC, Djalilian HR. Complications of surgery for sporadic vestibular schwannoma. Otolaryngol Head Neck Surg 2014;150:275–281
49. Keiper GL Jr, Sherman JD, Tomsick TA, Tew JM Jr. Dural sinus thrombosis and pseudotumor cerebri: unexpected complications of suboccipital craniotomy and translabyrinthine craniectomy. J Neurosurg 1999;91:192–197
50. Slattery WH III, Francis S, House KC. Perioperative morbidity of acoustic neuroma surgery. Otol Neurotol 2001;22:895–902
51. Crocker M, Nesbitt A, Rich P, Bell B. Symptomatic venous sinus thrombosis following bone wax application to emissary veins. Br J Neurosurg 2008;22:798–800

22.2. Clival, Petroclival, and Petrous Meningiomas

1. Natarajan SK, Sekhar LN, Schessel D, Morita A. Petroclival meningiomas: multi-modality treatment and outcomes at long-term follow-up. Neurosurgery 2007; 60:965–979, discussion 979–981
2. Schaller B, Merlo A, Gratzl O, Probst R. Premeatal and retromeatal cerebellopontine angle meningioma. Two distinct clinical entities. Acta Neurochir (Wien) 1999; 141:465–471
3. Bassiouni H, Hunold A, Asgari S, Stolke D. Meningiomas of the posterior petrous bone: functional outcome after microsurgery. J Neurosurg 2004;100:1014–1024
4. Al-Mefty O. Operative Atlas of Meningiomas. Philadelphia: Lippincott-Raven; 1998
5. Samii MAM. Cerebellopontine angle meningioma (posterior pyramid meningiomas). In: Al-Mefty O, ed. Meningiomas. New York: Raven Press; 1991:503–515
6. Sekhar LN, Raso J, Schessel DA. The presigmoid petrosal approach. In: Sekhar LN, Oliveira ED, eds. Cranial Microsurgery: Approaches and Techniques. New York: Thieme; 1999:432–463
7. Li D, Hao SY, Wang L, et al. Surgical management and outcomes of petroclival meningiomas: a single-center case series of 259 patients. Acta Neurochir (Wien) 2013;155: 1367–1383
8. Nakamura M, Roser F, Dormiani M, Matthies C, Vorkapic P, Samii M. Facial and cochlear nerve function after surgery of cerebellopontine angle meningiomas. Neurosurgery 2005;57:77–90, discussion 77–90
9. Coopens JR, Couldwell WT. Clival and petroclival meningiomas. In: DeMonte F, McDermott MW, Al-Mefty O, eds. Al-Mefty's Meningiomas, 2nd ed. New York, Stuttgart: Thieme; 2011:270–282
10. Yamakami I, Higuchi Y, Horiguchi K, Saeki N. Treatment policy for petroclival meningioma based on tumor size: aiming radical removal in small tumors for obtaining cure without morbidity. Neurosurg Rev 2011;34:327–334, discussion 334–335
11. Sekhar LN, Jannetta PJ, Burkhart LE, Janosky JE. Meningiomas involving the clivus: a six-year experience with 41 patients. Neurosurgery 1990;27:764–781, discussion 781
12. Spetzler RF, Daspit CP, Pappas CT. The combined supra- and infratentorial approach for lesions of the petrous and clival regions: experience with 46 cases. J Neurosurg 1992;76:588–599
13. Bambakidis NC, Kakarla UK, Kim LJ, et al. Evolution of surgical approaches in the treatment of petroclival meningiomas: a retrospective review. Neurosurgery 2007;61(5, Suppl 2):202–209, discussion 209–211
14. Salas E, Sekhar LN, Ziyal IM, Caputy AJ, Wright DC. Variations of the extreme-lateral craniocervical approach: anatomical study and clinical analysis of 69 patients. J Neurosurg 1999;90(2, Suppl):206–219
15. Quiñones-Hinojosa A, Chang EF, Lawton MT. The extended retrosigmoid approach: an alternative to radical cranial base approaches for posterior fossa lesions. Neurosurgery 2006;58(4, Suppl 2):ONS-208–ONS-214, discussion ONS-214
16. Fraser JF, Nyquist GG, Moore N, Anand VK, Schwartz TH. Endoscopic endonasal minimal access approach to the clivus: case series and technical nuances. Neurosurgery 2010;67(3, Suppl Operative):ons150–ons158, discussion ons158

17. Fernandez-Miranda JC, Gardner PA, Rastelli MM Jr, et al. Endoscopic endonasal transcavernous posterior clinoidectomy with interdural pituitary transposition. J Neurosurg 2014;121:91–99

18. **Krisht AF. Transcavernous approach to diseases of the anterior upper third of the posterior fossa. Neurosurg Focus 2005;19:E2**

19. Kawase T, Toya S, Shiobara R, Mine T. Transpetrosal approach for aneurysms of the lower basilar artery. J Neurosurg 1985;63:857–861

20. **Bogaev C, Sekhar LN. Petroclival meningiomas. In: Sekhar LN, Fessler RG, eds. Atlas of Neurosurgical Techniques. New York: Thieme; 2006:695–710**

21. Sekhar LN, Schessel DA, Bucur SD, Raso JL, Wright DC. Partial labyrinthectomy petrous apicectomy approach to neoplastic and vascular lesions of the petroclival area. Neurosurgery 1999;44:537–550, discussion 550–552

22. Cass SP, Sekhar LN, Pomeranz S, Hirsch BE, Snyderman CH. Excision of petroclival tumors by a total petrosectomy approach. Am J Otol 1994;15:474–484

23. Kusumi M, Fukushima T, Mehta AI, et al. Tentorial detachment technique in the combined petrosal approach for petroclival meningiomas. J Neurosurg 2012;116:566–573

24. Hafez A, Nader R, Al-Mefty O. Preservation of the superior petrosal sinus during the petrosal approach. J Neurosurg 2011;114:1294–1298

25. Kusumi M, Fukushima T, Aliabadi H, et al. Microplate-bridge technique for watertight dural closures in the combined petrosal approach. Neurosurgery 2012;70(2, Suppl Operative):264–269

26. Couldwell WT, Fukushima T, Giannotta SL, Weiss MH. Petroclival meningiomas: surgical experience in 109 cases. J Neurosurg 1996;84:20–28

27. Goel A, Muzumdar D. Conventional posterior fossa approach for surgery on petroclival meningiomas: a report on an experience with 28 cases. Surg Neurol 2004;62:332–338, discussion 338–340

28. Little KM, Friedman AH, Sampson JH, Wanibuchi M, Fukushima T. Surgical management of petroclival meningiomas: defining resection goals based on risk of neurological morbidity and tumor recurrence rates in 137 patients. Neurosurgery 2005;56:546–559, discussion 546–559

29. Xu F, Karampelas I, Megerian CA, Selman WR, Bambakidis NC. Petroclival meningiomas: an update on surgical approaches, decision making, and treatment results. Neurosurg Focus 2013;35:E11

30. Bricolo AP, Turazzi S, Talacchi A, Cristofori L. Microsurgical removal of petroclival meningiomas: a report of 33 patients. Neurosurgery 1992;31:813–828, discussion 828

31. Almefty R, Dunn IF, Pravdenkova S, Abolfotoh M, Al-Mefty O. True petroclival meningiomas: results of surgical management. J Neurosurg 2014;120:40–51

32. **Coppens JR, Couldwell WT. Clival and petroclival meningiomas. In: De Monte F, McDermott MW, Al-Mefty O, eds. Al-Mefty's Meningiomas. New York, Stuttgart: Thieme; 2011:270–282**

33. **Samii M, Gerganov VM. Cerebellopontine angle meningiomas. In: DeMonte F, McDermott MW, Al-Mefty O, eds. Al-Mefty's Meningiomas, 2nd ed. New York, Stuttgart: Thieme; 2011:262–269**

34. Agarwal V, Babu R, Grier J, et al. Cerebellopontine angle meningiomas: postoperative outcomes in a modern cohort. Neurosurg Focus 2013;35:E10

35. Thomas NW, King TT. Meningiomas of the cerebellopontine angle. A report of 41 cases. Br J Neurosurg 1996;10:59–68
36. Voss NF, Vrionis FD, Heilman CB, Robertson JH. Meningiomas of the cerebellopontine angle. Surg Neurol 2000;53:439–446, discussion 446–447
37. Cho CW, Al-Mefty O. Combined petrosal approach to petroclival meningiomas. Neurosurgery 2002;51:708–716, discussion 716–718
38. Erkmen K, Pravdenkova S, Al-Mefty O. Surgical management of petroclival meningiomas: factors determining the choice of approach. Neurosurg Focus 2005;19:E7
39. Mathiesen T, Gerlich A, Kihlström L, Svensson M, Bagger-Sjöbäck D. Effects of using combined transpetrosal surgical approaches to treat petroclival meningiomas. Neurosurgery 2007;60:982–991, discussion 991–992

22.3. Epidermoid and Dermoid Tumors

1. Vellutini EA, de Oliveira MF, Ribeiro AP, Rotta JM. Malignant transformation of intracranial epidermoid cyst. Br J Neurosurg 2014;28:507–509
2. Abramson RC, Morawetz RB, Schlitt M. Multiple complications from an intracranial epidermoid cyst: case report and literature review. Neurosurgery 1989;24: 574–578
3. Szabó M, Majtényi C, Guseo A. Contribution to the background of Mollaret's meningitis. Acta Neuropathol 1983;59:115–118
4. Berger MS, Wilson CB. Epidermoid cysts of the posterior fossa. J Neurosurg 1985; 62:214–219
5. Peng Y, Yu L, Li Y, Fan J, Qiu M, Qi S. Pure endoscopic removal of epidermoid tumors of the cerebellopontine angle. Childs Nerv Syst 2014;30:1261–1267
6. Tuchman A, Platt A, Winer J, Pham M, Giannotta S, Zada G. Endoscopic-assisted resection of intracranial epidermoid tumors. World Neurosurg 2014;82:450–454
7. Safain MG, Dent WC, Heilman CB. An endoscopic assisted retrosigmoid approach to the cerebello-pontine angle for resection of an epidermoid cyst. Neurosurg Focus 2014;36(1, Suppl):1
8. **Schiefer TK, Link MJ. Epidermoids of the cerebellopontine angle: a 20-year experience. Surg Neurol 2008;70:584–590, discussion 590**
9. Gopalakrishnan CV, Ansari KA, Nair S, Menon G. Long term outcome in surgically treated posterior fossa epidermoids. Clin Neurol Neurosurg 2014;117:93–99

22.4. Chordoma and Chondrosarcoma

1. Eriksson B, Gunterberg B, Kindblom LG. Chordoma. A clinicopathologic and prognostic study of a Swedish national series. Acta Orthop Scand 1981;52:49–58
2. Unni KK. Dahlin's Bone Tumors: General Aspects and Data on 1187 Cases, 5th ed. Philadelphia: Lippincott-Raven; 1996
3. McMaster ML, Goldstein AM, Bromley CM, Ishibe N, Parry DM. Chordoma: incidence and survival patterns in the United States, 1973-1995. Cancer Causes Control 2001; 12:1–11
4. Smoll NR, Gautschi OP, Radovanovic I, Schaller K, Weber DC. Incidence and relative survival of chordomas: the standardized mortality ratio and the impact of chordomas on a population. Cancer 2013;119:2029–2037

5. Rostomily RC, Sekhar LN, Elahi F. Chordomas and chondrosarcomas. In: Sekhar LN, Fessler RG, eds. Atlas of Neurosurgical Techniques: Brain. New York, Stuttgart: Thieme; 2006:778–810

6. Cho YH, Kim JH, Khang SK, Lee JK, Kim CJ. Chordomas and chondrosarcomas of the skull base: comparative analysis of clinical results in 30 patients. Neurosurg Rev 2008;31:35–43, discussion 43

7. Diaz RJ, Cusimano MD. The biological basis for modern treatment of chordoma. J Neurooncol 2011;104:411–422

8. Pamir MN, Ozduman K. Tumor-biology and current treatment of skull-base chordomas. Adv Tech Stand Neurosurg 2008;33:35–129

9. Gagliardi F, Boari N, Riva P, Mortini P. Current therapeutic options and novel molecular markers in skull base chordomas. Neurosurg Rev 2012;35:1–13, discussion 13–14

10. Crockard HA, Cheeseman A, Steel T, et al. A multidisciplinary team approach to skull base chondrosarcomas. J Neurosurg 2001;95:184–189

11. Yeom KW, Lober RM, Mobley BC, et al. Diffusion-weighted MRI: distinction of skull base chordoma from chondrosarcoma. AJNR Am J Neuroradiol 2013;34:1056–1061, S1

12. Mehnert F, Beschorner R, Küker W, Hahn U, Nägele T. Retroclival ecchordosis physaliphora: MR imaging and review of the literature. AJNR Am J Neuroradiol 2004;25: 1851–1855

13. Colli B, Al-Mefty O. Chordomas of the craniocervical junction: follow-up review and prognostic factors. J Neurosurg 2001;95:933–943

14. Carpentier A, Blanquet A, George B. Suboccipital and cervical chordomas: radical resection with vertebral artery control. Neurosurg Focus 2001;10:E4

15. Carpentier A, Polivka M, Blanquet A, Lot G, George B. Suboccipital and cervical chordomas: the value of aggressive treatment at first presentation of the disease. J Neurosurg 2002;97:1070–1077

16. Harsh G. Chordomas and Chondrosarcomas of the Skull Base and Spine. New York, Stuttgart: Thieme; 2003

17. Boari N, Roberti F, Biglioli F, Caputy AJ, Mortini P. Quantification of clival and paraclival exposure in the Le Fort I transmaxillary transpterygoid approach: a microanatomical study. J Neurosurg 2010;113:1011–1018

18. Sekhar LN, Nanda A, Sen CN, Snyderman CN, Janecka IP. The extended frontal approach to tumors of the anterior, middle, and posterior skull base. J Neurosurg 1992; 76:198–206

19. Cass SP, Sekhar LN, Pomeranz S, Hirsch BE, Snyderman CH. Excision of petroclival tumors by a total petrosectomy approach. Am J Otol 1994;15:474–484

20. Sen CN, Sekhar LN. An extreme lateral approach to intradural lesions of the cervical spine and foramen magnum. Neurosurgery 1990;27:197–204

21. Benet A, Prevedello DM, Carrau RL, et al. Comparative analysis of the transcranial "far lateral" and endoscopic endonasal "far medial" approaches: surgical anatomy and clinical illustration. World Neurosurg 2014;81:385–396

22. Koutourousiou M, Gardner PA, Tormenti MJ, et al. Endoscopic endonasal approach for resection of cranial base chordomas: outcomes and learning curve. Neurosurgery 2012;71:614–624, discussion 624–625

23. Frank G, Sciarretta V, Calbucci F, Farneti G, Mazzatenta D, Pasquini E. The endoscopic transnasal transsphenoidal approach for the treatment of cranial base chordomas

and chondrosarcomas. Neurosurgery 2006;59(1, Suppl 1):ONS50–ONS57, discussion ONS50–ONS57

24. Fernandez-Miranda JC, Gardner PA, Rastelli MM Jr, et al. Endoscopic endonasal transcavernous posterior clinoidectomy with interdural pituitary transposition. J Neurosurg 2014;121:91–99

25. Forsyth PA, Cascino TL, Shaw EG, et al. Intracranial chordomas: a clinicopathological and prognostic study of 51 cases. J Neurosurg 1993;78:741–747

26. Evans HL, Ayala AG, Romsdahl MM. Prognostic factors in chondrosarcoma of bone: a clinicopathologic analysis with emphasis on histologic grading. Cancer 1977;40:818–831

27. Hasegawa T, Ishii D, Kida Y, Yoshimoto M, Koike J, Iizuka H. Gamma Knife surgery for skull base chordomas and chondrosarcomas. J Neurosurg 2007;107:752–757

28. Martin JJ, Niranjan A, Kondziolka D, Flickinger JC, Lozanne KA, Lunsford LD. Radiosurgery for chordomas and chondrosarcomas of the skull base. J Neurosurg 2007;107:758–764

29. Ito E, Saito K, Okada T, Nagatani T, Nagasaka T. Long-term control of clival chordoma with initial aggressive surgical resection and gamma knife radiosurgery for recurrence. Acta Neurochir (Wien) 2010;152:57–67, discussion 67

30. Ouyang T, Zhang N, Zhang Y, et al. Clinical characteristics, immunohistochemistry, and outcomes of 77 patients with skull base chordomas. World Neurosurg 2014;81:790–797

31. Chibbaro S, Cornelius JF, Froelich S, et al. Endoscopic endonasal approach in the management of skull base chordomas—clinical experience on a large series, technique, outcome, and pitfalls. Neurosurg Rev 2014;37:217–224, discussion 224–225

32. Tan NC, Naidoo Y, Oue S, et al. Endoscopic surgery of skull base chordomas. J Neurol Surg B Skull Base 2012;73:379–386

33. Fraser JF, Nyquist GG, Moore N, Anand VK, Schwartz TH. Endoscopic endonasal transclival resection of chordomas: operative technique, clinical outcome, and review of the literature. J Neurosurg 2010;112:1061–1069

34. Komotar RJ, Starke RM, Raper DM, Anand VK, Schwartz TH. The endoscope-assisted ventral approach compared with open microscope-assisted surgery for clival chordomas. World Neurosurg 2011;76:318–327, discussion 259–262

35. Gay E, Sekhar LN, Rubinstein E, et al. Chordomas and chondrosarcomas of the cranial base: results and follow-up of 60 patients. Neurosurgery 1995;36:887–896, discussion 896–897

36. Pamir MN, Kiliç T, Türe U, Ozek MM. Multimodality management of 26 skull-base chordomas with 4-year mean follow-up: experience at a single institution. Acta Neurochir (Wien) 2004;146:343–354, 354

37. Samii A, Gerganov VM, Herold C, et al. Chordomas of the skull base: surgical management and outcome. J Neurosurg 2007;107:319–324

38. Sekhar LN, Pranatartiharan R, Chanda A, Wright DC. Chordomas and chondrosarcomas of the skull base: results and complications of surgical management. Neurosurg Focus 2001;10:E2

39. Tzortzidis F, Elahi F, Wright D, Natarajan SK, Sekhar LN. Patient outcome at long-term follow-up after aggressive microsurgical resection of cranial base chordomas. Neurosurgery 2006;59:230–237, discussion 230–237

40. Diaz RJ, Maggacis N, Zhang S, Cusimano MD. Determinants of quality of life in patients with skull base chordoma. J Neurosurg 2014;120:528–537

22.5. Tentorial Meningiomas

1. Barrows HS, Harter DH. Tentorial Meningiomas. J Neurol Neurosurg Psychiatry 1962; 25:40–44
2. Bret P, Guyotat J, Madarassy G, Ricci AC, Signorelli F. Tentorial meningiomas. Report on twenty-seven cases. Acta Neurochir (Wien) 2000;142:513–526
3. MacCarty CS, Taylor WF. Intracranial meningiomas: experiences at the Mayo Clinic. Neurol Med Chir (Tokyo) 1979;19:569–574
4. Sekhar LN, Jannetta PJ, Maroon JC. Tentorial meningiomas: surgical management and results. Neurosurgery 1984;14:268–275
5. **Bassiouni H, Hunold A, Asgari S, Stolke D. Tentorial meningiomas: clinical results in 81 patients treated microsurgically. Neurosurgery 2004;55:108–116, discussion 116–118**
6. **Yasargil M. Meningiomas. In: Microneurosurgery of CNS Tumors, vol IVB. New York: Thieme; 1996:134–165**
7. Konovalov AN, Spallone A, Pitzkhelauri DI. Meningioma of the pineal region: a surgical series of 10 cases. J Neurosurg 1996;85:586–590
8. Okami N, Kawamata T, Hori T, Takakura K. Surgical treatment of falcotentorial meningioma. J Clin Neurosci 2001;8(Suppl 1):15–18
9. Raco A, Agrillo A, Ruggeri A, Gagliardi FM, Cantore G. Surgical options in the management of falcotentorial meningiomas: report of 13 cases. Surg Neurol 2004;61:157–164, discussion 164
10. **Bassiouni H, Asgari S. Tentorial meningiomas. In: DeMonte F, McDermott MW, Al-Mefty O, eds. Al-Mefty's Meningiomas, 2nd ed. New York, Stuttgart: Thieme; 2011:168–176**
11. Hashemi M, Schick U, Hassler W, Hefti M. Tentorial meningiomas with special aspect to the tentorial fold: management, surgical technique, and outcome. Acta Neurochir (Wien) 2010;152:827–834
12. Samii M, Carvalho GA, Tatagiba M, Matthies C, Vorkapic P. Meningiomas of the tentorial notch: surgical anatomy and management. J Neurosurg 1996;84:375–381
13. Asari S, Maeshiro T, Tomita S, et al. Meningiomas arising from the falcotentorial junction. Clinical features, neuroimaging studies, and surgical treatment. J Neurosurg 1995;82:726–738
14. Bassiouni H, Asgari S, König HJ, Stolke D. Meningiomas of the falcotentorial junction: selection of the surgical approach according to the tumor type. Surg Neurol 2008;69:339–349, discussion 349
15. **Harsh GR. Peritorcular meningiomas. In: DeMonte F, McDermott MW, Al-Mefty O, eds. Al-Mefty's Meningiomas, 2nd ed. New York, Stuttgart: Thieme; 2011:177–186**
16. Quiñones-Hinojosa A, Chang EF, Chaichana KL, McDermott MW. Surgical considerations in the management of falcotentorial meningiomas: advantages of the bilateral occipital transtentorial/transfalcine craniotomy for large tumors. Neurosurgery 2009; 64(5, Suppl 2):260–268, discussion 268

17. Gökalp HZ, Arasil E, Erdogan A, Egemen N, Deda H, Cerçi A. Tentorial meningiomas. Neurosurgery 1995;36:46–51, discussion 51
18. Guidetti B, Ciappetta P, Domenicucci M. Tentorial meningiomas: surgical experience with 61 cases and long-term results. J Neurosurg 1988;69:183–187
19. Sindou M, Hallacq P. Venous reconstruction in surgery of meningiomas invading the sagittal and transverse sinuses. Skull Base Surg 1998;8:57–64
20. Sindou MP, Alvernia JE. Results of attempted radical tumor removal and venous repair in 100 consecutive meningiomas involving the major dural sinuses. J Neurosurg 2006;105:514–525
21. Chen CM, Huang AP, Kuo LT, Tu YK. Contemporary surgical outcome for skull base meningiomas. Neurosurg Rev 2011;34:281–296, discussion 296
22. Colli BO, Assirati JA Jr, Deriggi DJ, Neder L, dos Santos AC, Carlotti CG Jr. Tentorial meningiomas: follow-up review. Neurosurg Rev 2008;31:421–430, discussion 430
23. Shukla D, Behari S, Jaiswal AK, Banerji D, Tyagi I, Jain VK. Tentorial meningiomas: operative nuances and perioperative management dilemmas. Acta Neurochir (Wien) 2009;151:1037–1051
24. Ciric I, Landau B. Tentorial and posterior cranial fossa meningiomas: operative results and long-term follow-up: experience with twenty-six cases. Surg Neurol 1993;39:530–537

22.6. Jugular Foramen Tumors

1. Brown JS. Glomus jugulare tumors revisited: a ten-year statistical follow-up of 231 cases. Laryngoscope 1985;95:284–288
2. Havekes B, van der Klaauw AA, Hoftijzer HC, et al. Reduced quality of life in patients with head-and-neck paragangliomas. Eur J Endocrinol 2008;158:247–253
3. Jansen JC, van den Berg R, Kuiper A, van der Mey AG, Zwinderman AH, Cornelisse CJ. Estimation of growth rate in patients with head and neck paragangliomas influences the treatment proposal. Cancer 2000;88:2811–2816
4. Caldemeyer KS, Mathews VP, Azzarelli B, Smith RR. The jugular foramen: a review of anatomy, masses, and imaging characteristics. Radiographics 1997;17:1123–1139
5. Jyung RW, LeClair EE, Bernat RA, et al. Expression of angiogenic growth factors in paragangliomas. Laryngoscope 2000;110:161–167
6. Gulya AJ. The glomus tumor and its biology. Laryngoscope 1993;103(11 Pt 2, Suppl 60):7–15
7. Vogl TJ, Bisdas S. Differential diagnosis of jugular foramen lesions. Skull Base 2009;19:3–16
8. Fisch U. Infratemporal fossa approach to tumours of the temporal bone and base of the skull. J Laryngol Otol 1978;92:949–967
9. Jenkins HA, Fisch U. Glomus tumors of the temporal region. Technique of surgical resection. Arch Otolaryngol 1981;107:209–214
10. Jackson CG, Glasscock ME III, Harris PF. Glomus Tumors. Diagnosis, classification, and management of large lesions. Arch Otolaryngol 1982;108:401–410
11. Graham MD, Larouere MJ, Kartush JM. Jugular foramen schwannomas: diagnosis and suggestions for surgical management. Skull Base Surg 1991;1:34–38

12. Song MH, Lee HY, Jeon JS, Lee JD, Lee HK, Lee WS. Jugular foramen schwannoma: analysis on its origin and location. Otol Neurotol 2008;29:387–391

13. **Brackmann DE, Fayad JN, Owens RM. Paragangliomas and schwannomas of the jugular foramen. In: Sekhar LN, Fessler RG, eds. Atlas of Neurosurgical Techniques: Brain. New York: Thieme; 2006:752–758**

14. Samii M, Babu RP, Tatagiba M, Sepehrnia A. Surgical treatment of jugular foramen schwannomas. J Neurosurg 1995;82:924–932

15. Arnautović KI, Al-Mefty O. Primary meningiomas of the jugular fossa. J Neurosurg 2002;97:12–20

16. Toyama C, Santiago Gebrim EM, Brito R, Bento RF. Primary jugular foramen meningioma. Otol Neurotol 2008;29:417–418

17. Roberti F, Sekhar LN, Kalavakonda C, Wright DC. Posterior fossa meningiomas: surgical experience in 161 cases. Surg Neurol 2001;56:8–20, discussion 20–21

18. Löwenheim H, Koerbel A, Ebner FH, Kumagami H, Ernemann U, Tatagiba M. Differentiating imaging findings in primary and secondary tumors of the jugular foramen. Neurosurg Rev 2006;29:1–11, discussion 12–13

19. Kwekkeboom DJ, van Urk H, Pauw BK, et al. Octreotide scintigraphy for the detection of paragangliomas. J Nucl Med 1993;34:873–878

20. **Liu JK, Gupta G, Christiano LD, Fukushima T. Surgery for jugular foramen tumors. In: Quinones-Hinojosa A, ed. Schmidek and Sweet's Operative Neurosurgical Techniques, 6th ed. Philadelphia: Elsevier; 2012:529–545**

21. Roche PH, Mercier P, Sameshima T, Fournier HD. Surgical anatomy of the jugular foramen. Adv Tech Stand Neurosurg 2008;33:233–263

22. **Choudhry OJ, Patel SK, Liu JK. Surgery versus radiosurgery for glomus jugulare tumors. In: Quinones-Hinojosa A, Raza SM, eds. Controversies in Neuro-Oncology: Best Evidence Medicine for Brain Tumor Surgery. New York: Thieme; 2014:469–479**

23. **Liu JK, Sameshima T, Gottfried ON, Couldwell WT, Fukushima T. The combined transmastoid retro- and infralabyrinthine transjugular transcondylar transtubercular high cervical approach for resection of glomus jugulare tumors. Neurosurgery 2006;59(1, Suppl 1):ONS115–ONS125, discussion ONS115–ONS125**

24. Ling PY, Mendelson ZS, Reddy RK, Jyung RW, Liu JK. Reconstruction after retrosigmoid approaches using autologous fat graft-assisted Medpor Titan cranioplasty: assessment of postoperative cerebrospinal fluid leaks and headaches in 60 cases. Acta Neurochir (Wien) 2014;156:1879–1888

25. Gottfried ON, Liu JK, Couldwell WT. Comparison of radiosurgery and conventional surgery for the treatment of glomus jugulare tumors. Neurosurg Focus 2004;17:E4

26. Sedney CL, Nonaka Y, Bulsara KR, Fukushima T. Microsurgical management of jugular foramen schwannomas. Neurosurgery 2013;72:42–46, discussion 46

27. Molony TB, Brackmann DE, Lo WW. Meningiomas of the jugular foramen. Otolaryngol Head Neck Surg 1992;106:128–136

28. Vrionis FD, Robertson JH, Gardner G, Heilman CB. Temporal bone meningiomas. Skull Base Surg 1999;9:127–139

29. Makek M, Franklin DJ, Zhao JC, Fisch U. Neural infiltration of glomus temporale tumors. Am J Otol 1990;11:1–5

30. Ramina R, Maniglia JJ, Fernandes YB, et al. Jugular foramen tumors: diagnosis and treatment. Neurosurg Focus 2004;17:E5
31. Green JD Jr, Brackmann DE, Nguyen CD, Arriaga MA, Telischi FF, De la Cruz A. Surgical management of previously untreated glomus jugulare tumors. Laryngoscope 1994;104(8 Pt 1):917–921

22.7. Foramen Magnum Tumors

1. **Bruneau M, Cornelius JF, George B. Antero-lateral approach to the V3 segment of the vertebral artery. Neurosurgery 2006;58(1, Suppl):ONS29–ONS35, discussion ONS29–ONS35**
2. Yasargil M, Mortara R, Curcic M. Meningiomas of basal posterior cranial fossa. In: Krayenbühl H, ed. Advances and Technical Standards in Neurosurgery. Vienna: Springer Verlag; 1980:1–115
3. Pamir MN, Ozduman K. Foramen magnum meningiomas. In: Pamir MN, Black PM, Fahlbusch R, eds. Meningiomas a Comprehensive Text. Philadelphia: WB Saunders; 2010:543–557
4. Akalan N, Seçkin H, Kiliç C, Ozgen T. Benign extramedullary tumors in the foramen magnum region. Clin Neurol Neurosurg 1994;96:284–289
5. **Arnautović KI, Al-Mefty O, Husain M. Ventral foramen magnum meningiomas. J Neurosurg 2000;92(1, Suppl):71–80**
6. Komotar RJ, Zacharia BE, McGovern RA, Sisti MB, Bruce JN, D'Ambrosio AL. Approaches to anterior and anterolateral foramen magnum lesions: a critical review. J Craniovertebr Junction Spine 2010;1:86–99
7. **Cusimano MD, Faress A, Chang Y, Luong W. Foramen magnum meningiomas. In: DeMonte F, McDermott MW, Al-Mefty O, eds. Al-Mefty's Meningiomas, 2nd ed. New York, Stuttgart: Thieme; 2011:297–309**
8. George B, Lot G, Velut S, Gelbert F, Mourier KL. [French language Society of Neurosurgery. 44th Annual Congress. Brussels, 8-12 June 1993. Tumors of the foramen magnum]. Neurochirurgie 1993;39(Suppl 1):1–89
9. **George B, Lot G, Boissonnet H. Meningioma of the foramen magnum: a series of 40 cases. Surg Neurol 1997;47:371–379**
10. **Nicolato A, Foroni R, Pellegrino M, et al. Gamma knife radiosurgery in meningiomas of the posterior fossa. Experience with 62 treated lesions. Minim Invasive Neurosurg 2001;44:211–217**
11. Bhatnagar AK, Gerszten PC, Ozhasaglu C, et al. CyberKnife Frameless Radiosurgery for the treatment of extracranial benign tumors. Technol Cancer Res Treat 2005;4:571–576
12. **Boulton MR, Cusimano MD. Foramen magnum meningiomas: concepts, classifications, and nuances. Neurosurg Focus 2003;14:e10**
13. **Suhardja A, Agur AM, Cusimano MD. Anatomical basis of approaches to foramen magnum and lower clival meningiomas: comparison of retrosigmoid and transcondylar approaches. Neurosurg Focus 2003;14:e9**
14. **Goel A, Desai K, Muzumdar D. Surgery on anterior foramen magnum meningiomas using a conventional posterior suboccipital approach: a report on an experience with 17 cases. Neurosurgery 2001;49:102–106, discussion 106–107**

15. George B, Dematons C, Cophignon J. Lateral approach to the anterior portion of the foramen magnum. Application to surgical removal of 14 benign tumors: technical note. Surg Neurol 1988;29:484–490

16. Babu RP, Sekhar LN, Wright DC. Extreme lateral transcondylar approach: technical improvements and lessons learned. J Neurosurg 1994;81:49–59

17. George B, Lot G. Anterolateral and posterolateral approaches to the foramen magnum: technical description and experience from 97 cases. Skull Base Surg 1995;5: 9–19

18. Salas E, Sekhar LN, Ziyal IM, Caputy AJ, Wright DC. Variations of the extreme-lateral craniocervical approach: anatomical study and clinical analysis of 69 patients. J Neurosurg 1999;90(2, Suppl):206–219

19. Gupta SK, Sharma BS, Khosla VK, Mathuria SN, Pathak A, Tewari MK. Far lateral approach for foramen magnum lesions. Neurol Med Chir (Tokyo) 2000;40:48–52, discussion 52–54

20. Wanebo JE, Chicoine MR. Quantitative analysis of the transcondylar approach to the foramen magnum. Neurosurgery 2001;49:934–941, discussion 941–943

21. Safavi-Abbasi S, de Oliveira JG, Deshmukh P, et al. The craniocaudal extension of posterolateral approaches and their combination: a quantitative anatomic and clinical analysis. Neurosurgery 2010;66(3, Suppl Operative):54–64

22. Sharma BS, Gupta SK, Khosla VK, et al. Midline and far lateral approaches to foramen magnum lesions. Neurol India 1999;47:268–271

23. Nanda A, Vincent DA, Vannemreddy PS, Baskaya MK, Chanda A. Far-lateral approach to intradural lesions of the foramen magnum without resection of the occipital condyle. J Neurosurg 2002;96:302–309

24. Miller E, Crockard HA. Transoral transclival removal of anteriorly placed meningiomas at the foramen magnum. Neurosurgery 1987;20:966–968

25. Crockard HA, Sen CN. The transoral approach for the management of intradural lesions at the craniovertebral junction: review of 7 cases. Neurosurgery 1991;28:88–97, discussion 97–98

26. Meyer FB, Ebersold MJ, Reese DF. Benign tumors of the foramen magnum. J Neurosurg 1984;61:136–142

27. Strang RD, al-Mefty O. Small skull base meningiomas. Surgical management. Clin Neurosurg 2001;48:320–339

28. Talacchi A, Biroli A, Soda C, Masotto B, Bricolo A. Surgical management of ventral and ventrolateral foramen magnum meningiomas: report on a 64-case series and review of the literature. Neurosurg Rev 2012;35:359–367, discussion 367–368

29. Samii M, Klekamp J, Carvalho G. Surgical results for meningiomas of the craniocervical junction. Neurosurgery 1996;39:1086–1094, discussion 1094–1095

30. Bassiouni H, Ntoukas V, Asgari S, Sandalcioglu EI, Stolke D, Seifert V. Foramen magnum meningiomas: clinical outcome after microsurgical resection via a posterolateral suboccipital retrocondylar approach. Neurosurgery 2006;59:1177–1185, discussion 1185–1187

31. Zenonos G, Kondziolka D, Flickinger JC, Gardner P, Lunsford LD. Gamma Knife surgery in the treatment paradigm for foramen magnum meningiomas. J Neurosurg 2012; 117:864–873

22.8. Cranial Base Rhizopathies

1. Hall GC, Carroll D, Parry D, McQuay HJ. Epidemiology and treatment of neuropathic pain: the UK primary care perspective. Pain 2006;122:156–162
2. **Sweet WH. The treatment of trigeminal neuralgia (tic douloureux). N Engl J Med 1986;315:174–177**
3. Putzki N, Pfriem A, Limmroth V, et al. Prevalence of migraine, tension-type headache and trigeminal neuralgia in multiple sclerosis. Eur J Neurol 2009;16:262–267
4. Brisman R. Bilateral trigeminal neuralgia. J Neurosurg 1987;67:44–48
5. **Jannetta PJ. Arterial compression of the trigeminal nerve at the pons in patients with trigeminal neuralgia. 1967. J Neurosurg 2007;107:216–219**
6. Miller JP, Acar F, Hamilton BE, Burchiel KJ. Radiographic evaluation of trigeminal neurovascular compression in patients with and without trigeminal neuralgia. J Neurosurg 2009;110:627–632
7. **Lee A, McCartney S, Burbidge C, Raslan AM, Burchiel KJ. Trigeminal neuralgia occurs and recurs in the absence of neurovascular compression. J Neurosurg 2014; 120:1048–1054**
8. **Eller JL, Raslan AM, Burchiel KJ. Trigeminal neuralgia: definition and classification. Neurosurg Focus 2005;18:E3**
9. Broggi G, Ferroli P, Franzini A, Galosi L. The role of surgery in the treatment of typical and atypical facial pain. Neurol Sci 2005;26(Suppl 2):s95–s100
10. van Loveren H, Tew JM Jr, Keller JT, Nurre MA. a 10-year experience in the treatment of trigeminal neuralgia. Comparison of percutaneous stereotaxic rhizotomy and posterior fossa exploration. J Neurosurg 1982;57:757–764
11. Taha JM, Tew JM Jr. Comparison of surgical treatments for trigeminal neuralgia: reevaluation of radiofrequency rhizotomy. Neurosurgery 1996;38:865–871
12. Campos-Benitez M, Kaufmann AM. Neurovascular compression findings in hemifacial spasm. J Neurosurg 2008;109:416–420
13. **Cohen-Gadol AA. Microvascular decompression surgery for trigeminal neuralgia and hemifacial spasm: naunces of the technique based on experiences with 100 patients and review of the literature. Clin Neurol Neurosurg 2011;113:844–853**
14. **Hitotsumatsu T, Matsushima T, Inoue T. Microvascular decompression for treatment of trigeminal neuralgia, hemifacial spasm, and glossopharyngeal neuralgia: three surgical approach variations: technical note. Neurosurgery 2003;53:1436–1441, discussion 1442–1443**
15. **Jannetta PJ, Abbasy M, Maroon JC, Ramos FM, Albin MS. Etiology and definitive microsurgical treatment of hemifacial spasm. Operative techniques and results in 47 patients. J Neurosurg 1977;47:321–328**
16. Naumann M, Albanese A, Heinen F, Molenaers G, Relja M. Safety and efficacy of botulinum toxin type A following long-term use. Eur J Neurol 2006;13(Suppl 4):35–40
17. Tomasello F, Alafaci C, Salpietro FM, Longo M. Bulbar compression by an ectatic vertebral artery: a novel neurovascular construct relieved by microsurgical decompression. Neurosurgery 2005;56(1, Suppl):117–124, discussion 117–124
18. Raslan AM, DeJesus R, Berk C, Zacest A, Anderson JC, Burchiel KJ. Sensitivity of high-resolution three-dimensional magnetic resonance angiography and three-dimensional

spoiled-gradient recalled imaging in the prediction of neurovascular compression in patients with hemifacial spasm. J Neurosurg 2009;111:733–736

19. Ryu H, Tanaka T, Yamamoto S, Uemura K, Takehara Y, Isoda H. Magnetic resonance cisternography used to determine precise topography of the facial nerve and three components of the eighth cranial nerve in the internal auditory canal and cerebello-pontine cistern. J Neurosurg 1999;90:624–634

20. Ohta M, Kobayashi M, Wakiya K, Takamizawa S, Niitsu M, Fujimaki T. Preoperative assessment of hemifacial spasm by the coronal heavily T2-weighted MR cisternography. Acta Neurochir (Wien) 2014;156:565–569

21. Kin T, Oyama H, Kamada K, Aoki S, Ohtomo K, Saito N. Prediction of surgical view of neurovascular decompression using interactive computer graphics. Neurosurgery 2009;65:121–128, discussion 128–129

22. Sindou M, Fobé JL, Ciriano D, Fischer C. [Intraoperative brainstem auditory evoked potential in the microvascular decompression of the 5th and 7th cranial nerves]. Rev Laryngol Otol Rhinol (Bord) 1990;111:427–431

23. Sindou M, Fobé JL, Ciriano D, Fischer C. Hearing prognosis and intraoperative guidance of brainstem auditory evoked potential in microvascular decompression. Laryngoscope 1992;102:678–682

24. Sindou MP. Microvascular decompression for primary hemifacial spasm. Importance of intraoperative neurophysiological monitoring. Acta Neurochir (Wien) 2005;147:1019–1026, discussion 1026

25. Hatayama T, Møller AR. Correlation between latency and amplitude of peak V in the brainstem auditory evoked potentials: intraoperative recordings in microvascular decompression operations. Acta Neurochir (Wien) 1998;140:681–687

26. Lee SH, Song DG, Kim S, Lee JH, Kang DG. Results of auditory brainstem response monitoring of microvascular decompression: a prospective study of 22 patients with hemifacial spasm. Laryngoscope 2009;119:1887–1892

27. Ying T, Thirumala P, Chang Y, Habeych M, Crammond D, Balzer J. Emprical factors associated with Brainstem auditory evoked potential monitoring during microvascular decompression for hemifacial spasm and its correlation to hearing loss. Acta Neurochir (Wien) 2014;156:571–575

28. **Jannetta PJ, McLaughlin MR, Casey KF. Technique of microvascular decompression. Technical note. Neurosurg Focus 2005;18:E5**

29. **Sekhar L, Stimac D, Elahi F. Microvascular decompression for cranial nerve compression syndromes. In: Sekhar LN, Fessler R, G., eds. Atlas of Neurosurgical Techniques: Brain. New York, Stuttgart: Thieme; 2006:860–869**

30. **Barker FG II, Jannetta PJ, Bissonette DJ, Larkins MV, Jho HD. The long-term outcome of microvascular decompression for trigeminal neuralgia. N Engl J Med 1996;334:1077–1083**

31. Jagannath PM, Venkataramana NK, Bansal A, Ravichandra M. Outcome of microvascular decompression for trigeminal neuralgia using autologous muscle graft: A five-year prospective study. Asian J Neurosurg 2012;7:125–130

32. Rowed DW. Chronic cluster headache managed by nervus intermedius section. Headache 1990;30:401–406

33. Rupa V, Saunders RL, Weider DJ. Geniculate neuralgia: the surgical management of primary otalgia. J Neurosurg 1991;75:505–511

34. Lovely TJ, Jannetta PJ. Surgical management of geniculate neuralgia. Am J Otol 1997; 18:512–517
35. Saers SJ, Han KS, de Ru JA. Microvascular decompression may be an effective treatment for nervus intermedius neuralgia. J Laryngol Otol 2011;125:520–522
36. Matsushima T, Goto Y, Natori Y, Matsukado K, Fukui M. Surgical treatment of glossopharyngeal neuralgia as vascular compression syndrome via transcondylar fossa (supracondylar transjugular tubercle) approach. Acta Neurochir (Wien) 2000;142: 1359–1363
37. Rey-Dios R, Cohen-Gadol AA. Current neurosurgical management of glossopharyngeal neuralgia and technical nuances for microvascular decompression surgery. Neurosurg Focus 2013;34:E8
38. Kim YH, Han JH, Kim CY, Oh CW. Closed-suction drainage and cerebrospinal fluid leakage following microvascular decompression : a retrospective comparison study. J Korean Neurosurg Soc 2013;54:112–117
39. Kalkanis SN, Eskandar EN, Carter BS, Barker FG II. Microvascular decompression surgery in the United States, 1996 to 2000: mortality rates, morbidity rates, and the effects of hospital and surgeon volumes. Neurosurgery 2003;52:1251–1261, discussion 1261–1262
40. Møller AR, Møller MB. Does intraoperative monitoring of auditory evoked potentials reduce incidence of hearing loss as a complication of microvascular decompression of cranial nerves? Neurosurgery 1989;24:257–263
41. **Samii M, Günther T, Iaconetta G, Muehling M, Vorkapic P, Samii A. Microvascular decompression to treat hemifacial spasm: long-term results for a consecutive series of 143 patients. Neurosurgery 2002;50:712–718, discussion 718–719**
42. Sarsam Z, Garcia-Fiñana M, Nurmikko TJ, Varma TR, Eldridge P. The long-term outcome of microvascular decompression for trigeminal neuralgia. Br J Neurosurg 2010; 24:18–25
43. Cheng JS, Lim DA, Chang EF, Barbaro NM. A review of percutaneous treatments for trigeminal neuralgia. Neurosurgery 2014;10(Suppl 1):25–33, discussion 33
44. Tronnier VM, Rasche D, Hamer J, Kienle AL, Kunze S. Treatment of idiopathic trigeminal neuralgia: comparison of long-term outcome after radiofrequency rhizotomy and microvascular decompression. Neurosurgery 2001;48:1261–1267, discussion 1267–1268
45. Sun T, Saito S, Nakai O, Ando T. Long-term results of microvascular decompression for trigeminal neuralgia with reference to probability of recurrence. Acta Neurochir (Wien) 1994;126:144–148
46. Rath SA, Klein HJ, Richter HP. Findings and long-term results of subsequent operations after failed microvascular decompression for trigeminal neuralgia. Neurosurgery 1996;39:933–938, discussion 938–940
47. Liao JJ, Cheng WC, Chang CN, et al. Reoperation for recurrent trigeminal neuralgia after microvascular decompression. Surg Neurol 1997;47:562–568, discussion 568–570
48. Lee SH, Levy EI, Scarrow AM, Kassam A, Jannetta PJ. Recurrent trigeminal neuralgia attributable to veins after microvascular decompression. Neurosurgery 2000;46:356–361, discussion 361–362

49. Sanchez-Mejia RO, Limbo M, Cheng JS, Camara J, Ward MM, Barbaro NM. Recurrent or refractory trigeminal neuralgia after microvascular decompression, radiofrequency ablation, or radiosurgery. Neurosurg Focus 2005;18:e12
50. Li ST, Wang X, Pan Q, et al. Studies on the operative outcomes and mechanisms of microvascular decompression in treating typical and atypical trigeminal neuralgia. Clin J Pain 2005;21:311–316
51. Li GW, Zhang WC, Yang M, Ma QF, Zhong WX. Clinical characteristics and surgical techniques of trigeminal neuralgia caused simply by venous compression. J Craniofac Surg 2014;25:481–484
52. Hyun SJ, Kong DS, Park K. Microvascular decompression for treating hemifacial spasm: lessons learned from a prospective study of 1,174 operations. Neurosurg Rev 2010; 33:325–334, discussion 334
53. **Ferroli P, Fioravanti A, Schiariti M, et al. Microvascular decompression for glossopharyngeal neuralgia: a long-term retrospective review of the Milan-Bologna experience in 31 consecutive cases. Acta Neurochir (Wien) 2009;151:1245–1250**
54. Kawashima M, Matsushima T, Inoue T, Mineta T, Masuoka J, Hirakawa N. Microvascular decompression for glossopharyngeal neuralgia through the transcondylar fossa (supracondylar transjugular tubercle) approach. Neurosurgery 2010;66(6, Suppl Operative):275–280, discussion 280
55. Janjua R, Taha J. Radiofrequency and glycerol rhizotomy for trigeminal neuralgia. In: Sekhar L, Fessler R, eds. Atlas of Neurosurgical Techniques: Brain. New York, Stuttgart: Thieme; 2006:870–875
56. Abdennebi B, Mahfouf L, Nedjahi T. Long-term results of percutaneous compression of the gasserian ganglion in trigeminal neuralgia (series of 200 patients). Stereotact Funct Neurosurg 1997;68(1-4 Pt 1):190–195
57. Kondziolka D, Lunsford LD. Percutaneous retrogasserian glycerol rhizotomy for trigeminal neuralgia: technique and expectations. Neurosurg Focus 2005;18:E7
58. Kanpolat Y, Savas A, Bekar A, Berk C. Percutaneous controlled radiofrequency trigeminal rhizotomy for the treatment of idiopathic trigeminal neuralgia: 25-year experience with 1,600 patients. Neurosurgery 2001;48:524–532, discussion 532–534
59. Brown JA, McDaniel MD, Weaver MT. Percutaneous trigeminal nerve compression for treatment of trigeminal neuralgia: results in 50 patients. Neurosurgery 1993;32:570–573
60. Mohammad-Mohammadi A, Recinos PF, Lee JH, Elson P, Barnett GH. Surgical outcomes of trigeminal neuralgia in patients with multiple sclerosis. Neurosurgery 2013; 73:941–950, discussion 950
61. **Broggi G, Ferroli P, Franzini A, et al. Operative findings and outcomes of microvascular decompression for trigeminal neuralgia in 35 patients affected by multiple sclerosis. Neurosurgery 2004;55:830–838, discussion 838–839**
62. Jho HD, Lunsford LD. Percutaneous retrogasserian glycerol rhizotomy. Current technique and results. Neurosurg Clin N Am 1997;8:63–74
63. **Pollock BE. Percutaneous retrogasserian glycerol rhizotomy for patients with idiopathic trigeminal neuralgia: a prospective analysis of factors related to pain relief. J Neurosurg 2005;102:223–228**

23 Extracranial Tumors Involving the Skull Base

Skull base tumors comprise a variety of different pathologies whose management requires a multidisciplinary approach. Although intracranial tumors may initially present to the neurosurgeon, extracranial tumors that involve the skull base warrant particular attention, given their distinct pathology, clinical presentation, and treatment. Many patients with these tumors initially present to the otolaryngologist–head and neck surgeon, and a thorough understanding of these pathologies is essential to provide comprehensive treatment of the skull base.

The traditional classification of intracranial skull base tumors is largely based on anatomic location (anterior, middle, posterior). In contrast, because skull base involvement with extracranial tumors occurs only in advanced disease or because of tumor growth through various skull base foramina, an appreciation of both tumor biology and anatomy is necessary in any classification scheme. One such system was developed by Irish et al[1] in 1994. It divides the skull base into three main regions, and groups together extracranial tumors that may have similarities in both clinical presentation and treatment approach (**Fig. 23.1**).

- **Region I**
    - Encompasses tumors that arise from the paranasal sinuses or anterior cranial fossa and can involve the orbit or other local structures
    - Also includes tumors that arise/extend to the clivus and foramen magnum, as many of the these tumors share a similar biology and are often resected via an anterior approach
    - Examples: See **Fig. 23.1**
- **Region II**
    - Tumors that involve the infratemporal and pterygopalatine fossa with extension into the middle cranial fossa and lateral skull base
- **Region III**
    - Tumors that arise from around the ear, parotid, and temporal bone and extend intracranially to involve the middle or posterior cranial fossa

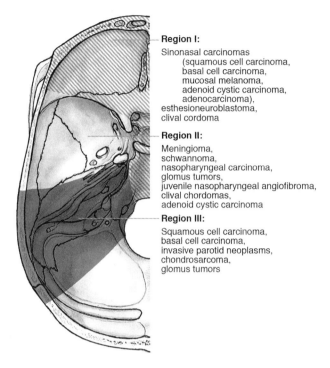

Region I:
Sinonasal carcinomas
    (squamous cell carcinoma,
     basal cell carcinoma,
     mucosal melanoma,
     adenoid cystic carcinoma,
     adenocarcinoma),
esthesioneuroblastoma,
clival cordoma

Region II:
Meningioma,
schwannoma,
nasopharyngeal carcinoma,
glomus tumors,
juvenile nasopharyngeal angiofibroma,
clival chordomas,
adenoid cystic carcinoma

Region III:
Squamous cell carcinoma,
basal cell carcinoma,
invasive parotid neoplasms,
chondrosarcoma,
glomus tumors

Fig. 23.1   Anatomic regions of the Irish et al[1] classification system with some examples of tumors.

■ Region I

Sinonasal Carcinoma[2–4]

Collectively, sinonasal carcinomas are rare, with an estimated incidence of 0.556 cases per 100,000 per year in the United States. They account for 3 to 5% of head and neck malignancies. Because of the anatomic location of the paranasal sinuses, these tumors often do not present until they are at an advanced stage with soft tissue, orbital, or skull base involvement. Although a variety of histological subtypes exist, the majority of these carcinomas arise from the maxillary sinus, nasal cavity, or ethmoid sinuses. Prognosis is generally poor, given the late stage at presentation.

Signs and Symptoms

- All sinonasal tumors can grow indolently with very few nonspecific local symptoms.

- Nasal obstruction, discharge, or epistaxis may be an initial clue to the presence of a malignancy.
- Most tumors present at an advanced stage with skull base or orbital involvement.
  - Symptoms may include epiphora (tearing), proptosis, diplopia, facial paresthesia, and headaches.

Staging

- Originally, a line connecting the medial canthus to the angle of the mandible was used to define the resectability of sinonasal malignancies. Tumors superior to this line were originally considered unresectable.[5]
- The American Joint Committee on Cancer (AJCC) has defined a tumor, lymph node, metastasis (TNM) staging system for tumors arising from the maxillary sinus, nasal cavity, or ethmoid sinus[6]:
  - TX: tumor cannot be assessed
  - T0: no evidence of tumor
  - Tis: carcinoma in situ
- Maxillary sinus **(Table 23.1)**
- Nasal cavity and/or ethmoid sinus **(Table 23.2)**
- Sinonasal carcinoma, lymph nodes involvement **(Table 23.3)**
- Distant metastasis
  - M0: no distant metastasis
  - M1: distant metastasis

Table 23.1   Sinonasal Carcinoma—Tumor, Lymph Node, Metastasis (TNM) System: Maxillary Sinus Invasion[6]

Stage	Description
T1	Tumor limited to maxillary sinus mucosa with no erosion or destruction of bone
T2	Tumor causing bone erosion or destruction including extension into hard palate and/or middle meatus, except extension to posterior wall of the maxillary sinus and pterygoid plates
T3	Tumor invades any of the following: bone of the posterior wall of the maxillary sinus, subcutaneous tissues, floor or medial wall of the orbit, pterygoid fossa, or the ethmoid sinuses
T4a	Moderately advanced local disease
	Tumor invades the anterior orbital contents, skin of the cheek, pterygoid plates, infratemporal fossa, cribriform plate, sphenoid or frontal sinuses
T4b	Very advanced local disease
	Tumor invades any of the following: dura, brain middle cranial fossa, cranial nerves (other than V_2), nasopharynx, or clivus

Table 23.2   Sinonasal Carcinoma—TNM System: Nasal Cavity and Ethmoid Sinus Invasion

Stage	Description
T1	Tumor restricted to any one sub-site, with or without bony invasion
T2	Tumor invading two sub-sites in a single region or extending to involve an adjacent region within the nasoethmoidal complex, with or without bony invasion
T3	Tumor extends to invade the medial wall or floor of the orbit, maxillary sinus, palate, or cribriform plate
T4a	Moderately advanced local disease
	Tumor invades any of the following: anterior orbital contents, skin of the nose or cheek, minimal extension to the anterior cranial fossa, pterygoid plates, sphenoid or frontal sinuses
T4b	Very advanced local disease
	Tumor invades any of the following: orbital apex, dura, brain, middle cranial fossa, cranial nerves (other than V_2), nasopharynx, or clivus

General Surgical Treatment Principles of Sinonasal Malignancies[7,8]

Because sinonasal malignancies often present at an advanced stage with skull base or orbital involvement, the gold standard for surgical excision has been the open craniofacial approach with bifrontal craniotomy and transfacial approach.

- With the advent and growth of endoscopic sinus surgery, early stage tumors (no skull base or orbital involvement) may be feasibly resected with a completely endonasal approach.
  - The tumor can initially be debulked in the sinonasal cavity, where it is not attached to the surrounding mucosa (i.e., filling an air-filled cavity).

Table 23.3   Regional Lymph Nodes: TNM System

Stage	Description
NX	Regional lymph nodes cannot be assessed
N0	No regional lymph node metastasis
N1	Metastasis in a single ipsilateral lymph node, ≤ 3 cm in greatest dimension
N2a	Metastasis in a single ipsilateral lymph node, > 3 cm but ≤ 6 cm in greatest dimension
N2b	Metastases in multiple ipsilateral lymph nodes, ≤ 6 cm in greatest dimension
N2c	Metastases in bilateral or contralateral lymph nodes, ≤ 6 cm in greatest dimension
N3	Metastasis in a lymph node, > 6 cm in greatest dimension

- ○ Once the tumor origin/attachment is identified with the endoscopic approach, it is then removed in an en-bloc fashion (typically in a submucoperiosteal plane) with adequate oncological mucosal margins.
- ○ Areas of bony attachment should either be resected where feasible or drilled down with a high-speed diamond drill bit.
- As experience has been gained with extended endoscopic approaches, selected advanced stage tumors have been treated successfully with endoscopic craniofacial resection (see page 464).
  - ○ The intranasal portion of the tumor is first debulked to provide visualization (again, no tissue planes are violated).
  - ○ The endoscopic transcribriform approach is often the standard corridor used to gain access to the anterior skull base (see page 424).
  - ○ The tumor attachment along the superior septum or skull base is left so that the entire skull base and cribriform plate can be mobilized in an en-bloc fashion.
  - ○ The bony medial orbital wall is often resected on the ipsilateral side of the tumor.
    - Control of the anterior and posterior ethmoidal arteries is necessary to devascularize the tumor and minimize bleeding and orbital complications.
  - ○ Once the skull base has been opened, the intracranial components of the tumor resection process proceed following oncological principles.
- Contraindications to the endoscopic craniofacial resection include brain parenchyma, intraorbital, cavernous sinus, or carotid artery involvement where complete resection is not surgically feasible.

Malignant Sinonasal Tumors of Epithelial Origin

Squamous Cell Carcinoma

Squamous cell carcinoma (SCC) is the most common sinonasal malignancy, with a peak incidence in the sixth to seventh decade of life.

- Maxillary sinus involvement is most common.
- Pathology (see also on page 156)
  - ○ Divided into keratinizing, nonkeratinizing or undifferentiated subtypes.
  - ○ 1 to 7% are seen in association with sinonasal inverted papilloma.
- **Treatment**
  - ○ Early-stage tumors T1 and T2 are effectively treated with single-modality treatment (surgery or radiotherapy).
    - Advanced tumors (T3 and T4) require a combined approach (surgery plus adjuvant radiation and/or chemotherapy).
- The 5-year survival ranges from 40 to 70%.

Adenoid Cystic Carcinoma[3,9]

- Adenoid cystic carcinoma (ACC) is the second most common sinonasal malignancy of epithelial origin and accounts for 10% of all non-SCC in the head and neck region.
- It commonly occurs in the maxillary sinus and nasal cavity.[10]
- There are three histological subtypes: cribriform, tubular, and solid (see on page 158).
- It is typically a slow-growing neoplasm, but recurrences can develop 10 to 20 years after the initial treatment.
- It has a propensity for perineural invasion with intracranial extension.
  - The most frequently involved cranial nerves are the maxillary and vidian nerves.
  - This one characteristic of ACC makes achieving negative surgical margins difficult and accounts for its poor long-term prognosis.
- Regional lymph node involvement ranges from 10 to 30%.[11] Distant hematogenous spread is more common, with an incidence of 40% (most likely to lung and bone).[12]
- **Treatment**
  - Surgical resection of tumors with negative surgical margins remains the gold standard of treatment.
    - Open or endoscopic approaches are used depending on the resectability of the tumor (the difficulty lies in achieving negative margins with perineural invasion).
  - Adjuvant postoperative radiation is often used to enhance local control.[13]
  - Systemic chemotherapy is not yet fully defined but can be considered for patients with recurrent, metastatic, or unresectable disease.[14]
  - The 5-year survival is 60 to 70%.[15]
  - The 10-year survival is 31%.

Adenocarcinoma[2,4,16,17]

- Adenocarcinoma is a malignancy arising from glandular cells in the sinonasal cavity, and it is the third most common sinonasal malignancy.
- There are two types: intestinal and nonintestinal (see also on page 157).
- Treatment involves complete surgical excision (open craniofacial or endoscopic) with possible adjuvant radiation (depending on margins and stage).
- Intestinal adenocarcinoma:
  - Similar to adenocarcinoma of the intestinal tract
  - Occupational risk factors: wood and leather dust exposure
  - Site of involvement: ethmoid sinus (40%), nasal cavity (20%), maxillary sinus (20%)
  - 5-year survival: 40 to 60%

- Nonintestinal adenocarcinoma:
  - Divided into low and high grade.
  - Low grade has a slower clinical presentation with a unilateral nasal mass.
  - High-grade tumors present with locally advanced symptoms of orbital, infratemporal fossa, or intracranial extension.
  - Low-grade tumors: 5-year survival is 85%.
  - High-grade tumors: 3-year survival is 20%.

Malignant Tumors of Nonepithelial Origin

Esthesioneuroblastoma (ENB)

Esthesioneuroblastoma is a rare malignant tumor of the nasal vault probably derived from the olfactory epithelium covering the superior third of the nasal septum, cribriform plate, and superior nasal conchae, although this is controversial.[18-21] It is also referred to as an olfactory placode tumor, esthesioneurocytoma, esthesioneuroepithelioma, esthesioneuroma, olfactory neuroblastoma, and olfactory neurogenic tumor.[19,21]

- Epidemiology and pathology (see also on page 161):
  - The histological findings suggest a classification system of four grades (Hyams's histopathological grades),[22] based on the cytoarchitecture of the tumor, the mitotic rate, the nuclear pleomorphism, the presence of rosettes, and necrosis. This classification is relevant to the prognosis, with grade I tumors having an excellent prognosis and grade IV being almost uniformly fatal.
  - The differential diagnoses includes sinonasal carcinoma, rhabdomyosarcoma, lymphoma, mucosal malignant melanoma, paraganglioma, meningioma, invasive pituitary adenoma, sarcoma, and chondrosarcoma.
- Esthesioneuroblastoma entails slow progression with aggressive clinical behavior, often involving and destroying the surrounding structures: ethmoid bone and cribriform plate, olfactory nerves, frontal sinus, sphenoid sinus, nasopharynx, anterior cranial fossa, orbits, nasal cavity, and antrum.

Surgical Anatomy Pearl

About 50 to 75% of esthesioneuroblastomas involve the anterior skull base.

- **Signs and symptoms**: The most typical presentation of esthesioneuroblastoma is unilateral nasal obstruction and epistaxis with or without olfactory impairment. Other possible findings[19,23-27] are headache, rhinitis/rhinorrhea, sinusitis, proptosis, diplopia, visual impairment, exophthalmia, facial pain, and excessive lacrimation. Nasal/facial masses may be visible or palpable. The involvement of the frontal lobes may give rise to frontal lobe symptoms or seizures.

Table 23.4   Esthesioneuroblastoma: TNM Staging System[30]

Stage	Description
T1	Nasal cavity or paranasal sinus involvement (excluding the sphenoid sinus)
T2	Like T1, but the sphenoid sinus is included, with extension/erosion of the cribriform plate
T3	Orbit/anterior skull base extension, without dural invasion
T4	Brain invasion
Cervical lymph-node metastasis No: N0; Yes: N1	*Metastases* No: M0; Yes: M1

- **Classification systems**
  - ◦ These tumors are classified according to tumor extension (Kadish and modified Kadish classifications).[28,29]
    - ▪ Stage A: tumor limited to the nasal cavity
    - ▪ Stage B: nasal cavity and paranasal sinuses
    - ▪ Stage C: tumor extension beyond the nasal cavity and paranasal sinuses
    - ▪ Stage D: cervical or distant metastases[29]
  - ◦ TNM staging system[30] (**Table 23.4**)
  - ◦ Hyams's histopathological grades are generally analyzed in two groups: grades I and II are typically grouped together, as are grades III and IV.[31]
- **Treatment:** Surgery followed by adjuvant radiotherapy is currently considered the gold standard for achieving the best prognosis, although there is controversy regarding the role of neoadjuvant/adjuvant chemotherapy.[31-34] Single-modality therapy (e.g., only surgery or only radiotherapy) may be considered in low-volume T1 disease.[31]
  - ◦ Chemotherapy can be considered in patients with advanced disease.[34-37]
  - ◦ Radiotherapy.
- **Surgical approaches:** The aim in surgical resection is to perform an en-bloc resection of the tumor. Because many tumors present at an advanced stage with intracranial involvement (Kadish stage C), the gold standard approach is the craniofacial resection (CFR). This can be performed via an external/transfacial or endonasal/endoscopic-assisted approach (see Chapters 15 and 16). The surgery involves removing the tumor along with the entire ipsilateral cribriform plate, crista galli, olfactory bulb, and dura.
- **Surgical complications**: There is an overall complication rate of 30 to 40%. Central nervous system (CNS) complications (cerebral haemorrhage, cerebral edema, meningitis, stroke, frontal syndrome, frontal abscess, cerebrospinal fluid [CSF] leak) occur at a rate of 19.2%, orbital complications occur at a rate of 1.3%, and wound infections occur at a rate of 14.6%.[33,35]

Table 23.5   Ten-Year Overall Survival and Disease-Specific Survival:
Kadish Classification

Kadish Stage	10-Year Overall Survival (%)	10-Year Disease-Specific Survival (%)
A	83.4	90
B	49	68.3
C	38.6	66.7
D	13.3	35.6

- **Outcome**: The overall 5-year survival rate is 62 to 83.4%, and the 10-year survival rate is 45 to 76.1%.[29-31,33-35,38-40] The local recurrence rate is 15 to 40%.[29,34,35,40,41] The regional recurrence rate is 15 to 20%.[29,30,35,42,43] An advanced Kadish stage (with intracranial and intraorbital involvement) has been found to be predictive of worse outcomes[39] **(Table 23.5)**.
  - A recent institutional review has suggested that Hyams's histological grading is also a significant predictor of outcome independent of Kadish stage (high-grade ENBs have worse overall survival and disease-free survival compared with low-grade ENBs).[34]

Mucosal Melanoma[4,44,45]

- Mucosal melanoma is a rare tumor arising from melanocytes either in the surface epithelium or the stroma (see also page 162).
- It most commonly arises de novo and not from a preexisting nevus or from skin metastases.
- It accounts for 0.1% of all sinonasal malignancies, with no gender-related differences.
- It is more commonly found in the nasal cavity, followed by the maxillary and ethmoid sinuses.
- Several histological subtypes have been described.
  - Various immunohistochemical stains are required to establish diagnosis and distinguish mucosal melanoma from other small blue-cell tumors.
- Mucosal melanoma is associated with a much poorer prognosis than other sinonasal malignancies involving the skull base, and it has a high risk of local recurrence.[46]
- **Treatment:** Traditionally, complete surgical excision of the tumor (either open craniofacial or endoscopic approaches) with negative margins was regarded as the gold standard of treatment.
  - Adjuvant postoperative radiotherapy has been used to enhance local disease control.[4]

- ○ A multicenter study demonstrated that the use of postoperative radiation is a key predictor of overall, disease-free, and recurrence-free survival (independent of negative surgical margins).[46]
- ○ Given the potential morbidity associated with either open or endoscopic craniofacial resections, the goals of surgery must be strongly considered and discussed in a multidisciplinary approach when the tumor invades the skull base or orbit.[47]
- ○ The role of systemic chemotherapy or immunotherapy is still not completely defined.
- ○ The 3-year overall, disease-free, and recurrence-free survival rates are 28.2%, 29.7%, 25.5%, respectively.[46]

Sinonasal Undifferentiated Carcinoma (SNUC)[2,45,48]

This is a rare, highly aggressive neuroendocrine tumor that typically presents with advanced disease.

- It has a broad age range, between the third and ninth decade of life, with a male predominance of 2–3:1.
- Clinically, symptoms progress rapidly (weeks to months) with local invasion of bone and surrounding structures.
- Histologically, differentiation between SNUC and olfactory neuroblastoma is important, given their vastly different clinical behavior and prognosis (see also page 159).
- Treatment consists of a multimodal approach that includes a combination of surgery (open craniofacial resection or endoscopic in carefully selected individuals) with adjuvant radiation and/or chemotherapy.
- Prognosis is poor, with a recent literature review demonstrating a 5-year survival of 6.25%, with a median overall survival of 12.7 months.[48]

Clival Chordoma

- See chordoma on page 165 (Pathology) and Chapter 22.4, page 585 (Treatment).

■ Region II[49,50]

Tumors of the infratemporal and pterygopalatine fossa not frequently originate primarily from these regions. Instead, these spaces are most often involved secondarily due to neoplastic processes from neighboring structures such as the paranasal sinuses and the nasopharynx. Moreover, because of the privileged anatomy of the infratemporal fossa and its close proximity to the middle cranial fossa and its various skull base foramina (review anatomy on page 35), malignant tumors that involve this region have multiple potential routes of spread to the cranial base.

Signs and Symptoms

- Clinically, primary tumors that occupy this region may not initially produce any significant symptoms because its location lateral to the nasal cavity and posterior to maxillary sinus.
- Advanced or neurogenic tumors may present with symptoms of pain or paresthesia along the maxillary or mandibular nerve distribution.
- Involvement of the pterygoid muscles may produce trismus.
- Extension through the inferior orbital fissure may produce orbital symptoms (e.g., diplopia, proptosis).

Tumors of the Infratemporal Fossa

Types

- **Primary**
  - Accounts for 25 to 30% of all tumors
  - Includes hemangioma, lipoma, hemangiopericytoma, meningioma, neurofibroma, osteosarcoma, schwannoma, rhabdomyosarcoma, fibrosarcoma, chondrosarcoma, lymphoma
- **Secondary**
  - Accounts for 70 to 75% of all tumors
  - Includes sinonasal carcinoma (e.g., squamous cell carcinoma, adenoid cystic carcinoma, adenocarcinoma), juvenile nasopharyngeal angiofibroma, nasopharyngeal carcinoma, glomus tumor

General Treatment Principles

- Most benign primary tumors of region II can be managed with a single modality if treatment is warranted (usually surgery).
- Malignant tumors of this region usually require multimodality therapy with surgery, radiation, and/or chemotherapy.

Surgical Approaches to the Infratemporal Fossa

- Traditionally, approaches to the infratemporal fossa have been performed via external approaches including the following:
  - Transfacial techniques: see Chapter 15.
  - Subtemporal/infratemporal approach with orbitozygomatic osteotomy: see frontotemporal-orbitozygomatic (FTOZ) approach (page 353).

○ More recently, expanded endoscopic techniques have been used to treat a variety of tumor pathologies in the pterygopalatine and infratemporal fossa.[51] This most often involves an extended trans-pterygoid approach: see Chapter 16, page 428.

Juvenile Nasopharyngeal Angiofibroma

- Juvenile nasopharyngeal angiofibroma (JNA) is a rare benign vascular tumor of the nasopharynx heavily skewed toward affecting males primarily during adolescence.
- It is believed that JNA accounts for 0.05 to 0.5% of head and neck tumors.
- The incidence is estimated to be 3.7 cases per million males in the age range of 10 to 24 years.[52]
- The median age is 15 years.

Etiology/Pathogenesis

- Juvenile nasopharyngeal angiofibroma is classically located in the nasopharynx, nasal cavity, sphenoid sinus, or pterygopalatine fossa.[53]
- The blood supply of JNA originates from the sphenopalatine artery and other end branches of the external carotid artery.
- In advanced disease, JNA can receive blood supply from the internal carotid artery system.
- Several staging systems (Andrews, Chandler, and Radkowski classifications) have been proposed based on extension of the tumor and the amount of intracranial extension.[54]
- Although JNA is a benign tumor, life-threatening complications can arise secondary to hemorrhage or intracranial extension.
- Its growth pattern is aggressive and can induce bone remodeling as it expands.
- Intracranial involvement has been reported to occur in 10 to 36% of cases, with the anterior and middle cranial fossa being the most common sites of invasion.[55]
- Four potential routes to the cranial cavity:
  ○ From the infratemporal fossa through the floor of the middle cranial fossa (most common)
  ○ From the pterygomaxillary fissure and infratemporal fossa into the superior and inferior orbital fissures
  ○ Through direct erosion of the sphenoid sinus into the region of the sella turcica and cavernous sinus
  ○ Along the ethmoid skull base and cribriform plate into the anterior cranial fossa

Pathology

See page 155.

Clinical Presentation

- Presenting symptoms include nasal obstruction, epistaxis, nasal discharge, pain, sinusitis, facial deformation, diplopia, hearing impairment, and otitis media[52]

Diagnosis

- Biopsy is not routinely performed due to the potential for severe epistaxis.
- On computed tomography (CT), the classic finding is the Holman-Miller sign with expansion of the pterygopalatine fossa and bulging of the posterior wall of the maxillary sinus.
- Computed tomography angiography (CTA) or angiography identifies the primary vessels that feed the tumor and enables preoperative embolization before surgical resection to minimize blood loss.[53]
- Magnetic resonance imaging (MRI) demonstrates the presence of soft tissue/intracranial extension.

Treatment

- Preoperative angiography + embolization of the feeding vessels of the external carotid artery system
- Surgery
  - Endoscopic transnasal approaches have been used successfully to treat JNA without intracranial extension.
    - Initially requires debulking of the intranasal portion of the tumor and isolating the main feeding vessel (often the sphenopalatine and maxillary artery)[54]
    - Commonly involves transpterygoid, and transsphenoidal approaches to fully resect the tumor; see Chapter 16
  - External transfacial approaches
    - Often reserved for JNA with intracranial involvement
    - Approaches include transpalatal, lateral rhinotomy, midfacial degloving, facial translocation; see external transfacial approaches (Chapter 15)
  - A recent systematic review did not find a statistically significant difference in the recurrence rates of JNA treated with endoscopic approaches and those treated with external approaches.[53]
    - One study suggests that open approaches should be reserved for tumors with significant intracranial involvement (e.g., internal carotid artery, cavernous sinus, optic nerve).[4]
- Radiotherapy
  - Can be used for unresectable tumors with intracranial extension or recurrences.

- ○ Tumor control has been found following a single course of 30 to 35 Gy.
- ○ Despite these results, it is still considered controversial to treat a benign neoplasm with potentially harmful radiotherapy. [55]

Outcome

- Recurrence rates range from 6 to 50%.[52,53]

Sinonasal Carcinoma

See discussion in Region I, above.

Nasopharyngeal Carcinoma

- Nasopharyngeal carcinoma (NPC) is a nonlymphomatous SCC arising from the epithelial lining of the nasopharynx.[56]

Epidemiology

- It is an uncommon disease in most countries (age-adjusted incidence < 1/100,000), but it occurs at a much higher frequency in southern China, northern Africa, and Alaska, especially among the Inuits of Alaska and the ethnic Chinese living in Guangdong.
- Reported incidence in Hong Kong (geographically adjacent to Guangdong province) is 20 to 30 per 100,000 men and 15 to 20 per 100,000 women. It is classified as World Health Organization (WHO) types II and III.
- In North America and Western Europe, NPC occurs sporadically and is primarily related to exposure to alcohol and tobacco. It is classified as WHO type I.[57]
  - ○ In North American populations and Mediterranean regions, the age distribution of NPC is bimodal, with peaks at 10 to 20 years and 40 to 60 years.

Etiology and Pathogenesis

- Epstein-Barr virus (EBV) is consistently detected in patients with NPC.[56] EBV-encoded RNA signal as detected by in-situ hybridization is present in nearly all tumor cells, and EBV can be detected from premalignant lesions, suggesting its role in the pathogenesis of the disease.
- There is a strong association with EBV infections as well as genetic factors such as human leukocyte antigen (HLA), suggesting that the interplay between environment and genetics is at the root of its pathogenesis.[57]

- Histologically classified by WHO into three groups: type I, keratinizing SCC; type II, nonkeratinizing SCC; type III, undifferentiated carcinoma (the most common form).[56]
- Children with NPC almost always have type III, which is more associated with locoregional spread and distant metastases.[58]

Pathology

See page 159.

Clinical Presentation[56,59]

- Nonspecific symptoms such as epistaxis, nasal obstruction, and nasal discharge may develop as the tumor enlarges in the posterior nasal space.
- Otologic symptoms such as unilateral serous otitis media/conductive hearing loss may be the initial presenting symptom as the tumor obstructs the eustachian tube.
- Cranial neuropathies (cranial nerves [CNs] V and VI) may develop as the tumor extends superiorly to involve the skull base, with symptoms of facial numbness and diplopia.
- Posterior triangle neck masses may indicate cervical metastases; this can be the initial presenting symptom.

Diagnosis

- If there is any suspicion of nasopharyngeal carcinoma, a thorough nasal-endoscopic exam is mandatory.
  - Particularly important in adult Asian patients who are presenting with a unilateral serous otitis media
- A definitive diagnosis is obtained with a biopsy.
- CT and MRI are again complementary modalities in determining the extent of the tumor.

Staging of Nasopharyngeal Carcinoma

See **Table 23.6**.

Treatment[56]

- External beam radiotherapy
  - Standard treatment for nasopharyngeal carcinoma.
  - Definitive radiotherapy alone in T1 tumors.

Table 23.6   Staging of Nasopharyngeal Carcinoma

Stage	Description
T stage	
T1	Tumor confined to nasopharynx, or tumor extends to oropharynx and/or nasal cavity without parapharyngeal extension
T2	Tumor with parapharyngeal extension
T3	Tumor involves bony structures of the skull base and/or paranasal sinuses
T4	Tumor with intracranial extension and/or involvement of cranial nerves, hypopharynx, orbit or with extension to the infratemporal/masticator space
N stage	
N0	No regional lymph node metastases
N1	Unilateral metastases in cervical lymph node ≤ 6 cm, above supraclavicular fossa, and/or unilateral or bilateral, retropharyngeal lymph nodes ≤ 6 cm
N2	Bilateral metastasis in cervical lymph nodes ≤ 6 cm, above supraclavicular fossa
N3	Metastases in a lymph node > 6 cm and/or to supraclavicular fossa
N3a	> 6 cm in dimension
N3b	Extension to the supraclavicular fossa

- ○ Used in combination with chemotherapy for T2–T4 tumors.
- ○ Prophylactic neck irradiation is undertaken given the high incidence of occult neck disease.
- Chemotherapy
  - ○ Studies have shown that concurrent chemotherapy alongside radiotherapy can improve both relapse-free survival and overall survival.[11] This approach is employed by most major centers for T2–T4 disease.
- Salvage therapy for residual/recurrent disease
  - ○ Re-irradiation
  - ○ Surgical resection
    - ▪ Primary NPC is generally not treated with surgery, given the complexity of the anatomy and the fact that the tumor is highly radiosensitive.
    - ▪ For residual/recurrent disease, nasopharyngectomy may be considered.
      - □ Infratemporal lateral approaches: see page 377.
      - □ Transfacial approaches: see Chapter 15.
      - □ More recently, endoscopic nasopharyngectomy has been described, which applies many of the extended endoscopic principles (transpterygoid, transclival)[60]; see Chapter 16.

Outcome[6]

- Overall 5-year survival rates:
  - Stage I: 70–80%
  - Stage II: 64%
  - Stage III: 62%
  - Stage IV: 38%

■ Region III

These are the rarest extracranial skull base neoplasms. Tumors can arise from the external auditory canal (EAC), middle ear, mastoid, or parotid gland. Because of their vastly different biology and treatment principles, we divide them into temporal bone and parotid neoplasms.

Temporal Bone Neoplasms

- Can involve primary neoplasms of the EAC, middle ear, mastoid, or secondary metastases to the temporal bone.
  - Note that primary neoplasms arising from the auricle (pinna) are considered separate from primary temporal bone neoplasms.
- Malignancies are extremely rare, with a reported incidence of 1 to 6 per million.[61,62]
- Accounts for 0.2% of head and neck tumors.
- Squamous cell carcinoma (SCC) is the most common malignancy in adults, followed by basal cell carcinoma, adenoid cystic carcinoma, and adenocarcinoma.[63]
- In pediatric patients, the most common diagnosis is rhabdomyosarcoma.[64]
- Given the rarity of temporal bone neoplasms reported in the literature, various histological subtypes are often grouped together when discussing management and treatment.
- As it relates to the skull base, temporal bone malignancies are the most relevant, and a general overview of the various histological subtypes and treatment paradigms will be discussed in this chapter.
- Differential diagnosis of temporal bone neoplasms: **Tables 23.7** and **23.8.**

Squamous Cell Carcinoma[65]

- Pathology: see page 160.
- Accounts for the majority of temporal bone malignancies.
- Most commonly arises from the skin of the external ear

Table 23.7   Benign Temporal Bone Neoplasms

Tissue	Neoplasm
Epithelial	Pleomorphic adenoma
	Ceruminous adenoma
	Papilloma
	Papillary adenoma
Mesenchymal	Lipoma
	Myxoma
	Hemangioma
	Schwannoma
	Neurofibroma
	Osteoma
	Chondroblastoma
Neuroendocrine	Paraganglioma
Other	Meningioma
	Teratoma

Table 23.8   Malignant Temporal Bone Neoplasms

Tissue	Neoplasm
Epithelial	Squamous cell carcinoma
	Basal cell carcinoma
	Ceruminal gland adenocarcinoma
	Adenoid cystic carcinoma
	Endolymphatic sac tumor
Mesenchymal	Rhabdomyosarcoma
	Osteosarcoma
	Chondrosarcoma
	Malignant schwannoma
Hematologic	Non-Hodgkin's lymphoma
	Plasmacytoma
Neuroendocrine	Neuroendocrine carcinoma
	Carcinoid
Other	Melanoma
	Langer's cell histiocytosis
	Metastases

- ○ Not associated with alcohol and tobacco use (unlike other head and neck SCCs)
  - ○ Associated with chronic inflammation or infection of the EAC
- Early lesions present as either a flat or raised lesion of the EAC or pinna.
- As the tumor grows, it can directly invade soft tissue and temporal bone or spread through perineural or lymphatic invasion.

Basal Cell Carcinoma[66]

- Pathology: Nonmelanocytic skin cancer arising from basal cells found in lower layer of epidermis.
- Commonly found in EAC and pinna.
- Presents as an ulcer with raised borders and telangiectasias.
- Actinic exposure is a risk factor.
- Previous studies have suggested a better prognosis than for SCC, although absolute numbers in any series are very small.

Adenoid Cystic Carcinoma[67]

- Pathology: see page 158
- Most common EAC malignancy of glandular origin
- Can also arise in the middle ear (secondary to glandular rests) or from an invasion from the parotid gland
- Most common symptom is intractable pain
- Propensity for perineural and intracranial involvement; difficult to achieve negative margins
- High risk of local recurrences and distant metastases
  - ○ 5-year overall survival: 75%
  - ○ 10-year overall survival: 60%

Ceruminous Carcinoma[68]

- Rare tumor with a peak incidence in the fifth decade of life
- Similar presentation to other EAC malignancies
- Arises from the ceruminous glands of the EAC
- Invasion of surrounding structures distinguishes this from ceruminous adenoma

Adenocarcinoma[69]

- Pathology: see page 158
- Rare tumor arising from the middle ear
- More common in females
- Peak incidence: fourth decade
- Aggressive bony invasion often on CT

Rhabdomyosarcoma[70]

- Malignant mesenchymal tumor primarily occurring in children
- Locally invasive and destructive
- Temporal bone involvement accounts for 7% of all head and neck rhabdomyosarcomas
- Median age of presentation is 4.5 years
- Can present as otorrhea, EAC mass, or hearing loss; frequently misdiagnosed as middle ear disease (otitis media)
- Treatment involves a combination of chemotherapy and radiation
  - 5-year disease-free survival: 81%

Endolymphatic Sac Tumors

- Rare slow-growing tumors arising from the endolymphatic sac or endolymphatic duct
- Typically locally aggressive, highly lytic into the temporal bone and mastoid process, with extension into the middle ear, posterior fossa, or cerebellopontine angle (CPA)
- Can cause massive destruction of the surrounding structures including the cochlea, vestibule, and internal auditory canal[71]
- Rare malignancy but associated with von Hippel–Lindau (VHL) disease in up to 16% of cases[19,71-74]
- Pathology: also known as adenocarcinoma of the endolymphatic sac
  - Papillary/glandular appearance with cuboidal epithelium that may resemble choroid plexus papilloma, especially given its vascular nature
  - Glandular areas may show secretions resembling a colloid (thyroid-like)
  - Immunohistochemistry: positive for cytokeratins and variable for glial fibrillary acid protein (GFAP)
- Slow-growing and invasive but not known to metastasize
- Sporadic cases appear to be more aggressive than ones associated with VHL.[75]

von Hippel-Lindau syndrome: Rare autosomal dominant genetic disease, with an incidence of 1 in 39,000 births, characterized by central nervous system and retinal hemangioblastoma, clear cell renal carcinomas, pheochromocytomas, pancreatic cysts, neuroendocrine tumors, cystoadenomas of the reproductive adnexal organs, and endolymphatic sac tumors. Patients are generally affected by headaches, ataxia, dizziness, unilateral hearing loss, visual loss, loss of spinal function, hypertension, or renal cell carcinoma.

- Generally hypervascular tumor
- Given the origin of the tumor, typically presents as progressive sensorineural hearing loss, tinnitus, and aural fullness before proceeding to cranial nerve dysfunction as it invades the posterior fossa and CPA
- Radiological findings:
  - CT: lytic lesion in region of endolymphatic sac
  - MRI: tumor is hyperintense on T1- and T2-weighted images with avid contrast enhancement.[76]
- Treatment involves radical surgical excision with radiotherapy reserved for unresectable tumors[77-79]
  - Surgical approaches: transmastoid/translabyrinthine, retrosigmoid, infratemporal, transcochlear
- Preoperative embolization is often suggested given the vascular nature of the tumor.[75,80]
- Overall survival is described from an aggregate of 40 patients published in the literature[81]:
  - 74%: no evidence of disease
  - 20%: alive with disease
  - 4%: died of disease
  - 2%: died of other cause

Temporal Bone Malignancies[69,82]

Clinical Symptoms

- Because malignancies of the temporal bone usually grow from the external ear canal inwards, symptoms often follow this clinical course.
- Early symptoms are nonspecific and can mimic common otologic diseases:
  - Pruritus
  - Otorrhea (discharge)
    - Present in 38 to 57% of patients
  - Conductive hearing loss
  - Pain
- Late symptoms reflect advanced disease.
  - Intractable pain (hallmark symptom of bone or dural invasion)
  - Facial paralysis
  - Sensorineural hearing loss
  - Vertigo
  - Tinnitus
  - Bloody otorrhea
- There can be a significant delay from onset of symptoms to diagnosis (4 months to 4 years).

Clinical Signs[83]

- Early lesions may be visible on the EAC as an ulcerated lesion or polyp of the ear canal.
  - However, up to 50% may not have any visible abnormality on otoscopy.
- Audiogram may demonstrated a conductive, sensorineural, or mixed hearing loss.
- Tumors of the EAC can spread through the fissures of Santorini (located in the bony ear canal) and invade the temporomandibular joint (TMJ), infratemporal fossa, or parotid gland.
  - Patients may have symptoms of trismus or present with a parotid mass.
- Advanced tumors that involve the mastoid and medial aspect of the temporal bone may present with cranial nerve deficits given the proximity of skull base foramina.
  - CNs VII, IX, X, and XI
- Occasionally, tumors may spread through the eustachian tube and present as a nasopharyngeal mass.

Investigations[84]

- Biopsy of the primary lesion with histopathological confirmation is the gold standard for diagnosis.
- The anatomy of the bony temporal bone and its close proximity to neurovascular structures requires both CT and MRI for assessing the size and extent of the primary tumor.
  - Search for possible involvement of the brain, dura, facial nerve, and internal carotid artery (ICA).
  - Search for extension into the parotid gland and soft tissues of the face.
  - Search for cervical node metastases.

Staging

- Given the rarity of temporal bone malignancies, there is no universally accepted staging system.
- The most commonly used staging system (for all malignancies) was originally developed for SCCs of the external auditory canal[85] **(Table 23.9)**.

General Surgical Treatment Principles[63,82,84]

- Although SCC is the most common temporal bone malignancy, other tumors behave in a similar fashion and have similar management approaches.
- In general, tumors of this region are treated by surgery, radiation, or a combination of both modalities.

Table 23.9   Staging of Temporal Bone Malignancies[85]

Stage	Description
T stage	
T1	Tumor limited to the external auditory canal without bony erosion or soft tissue extension
T2	Tumor with limited external auditory canal bony erosion (not full-thickness) or radiographic finding consistent with limited (< 0.5 cm) soft tissue involvement
T3	Tumor eroding osseous external auditory canal (full-thickness) with limited (< 0.5 cm) soft tissue involvement, or tumor involving the middle ear, mastoid
T4	Tumor eroding the cochlea, petrous apex, medial wall of the middle ear, carotid canal, jugular foramen, or dura, or with extensive (> 0.5 cm) soft tissue involvement, or evidence of facial paresis
N stage	
N0	No regional nodes
N1	Single ipsilateral regional node < 3 cm in size
N2a	Single ipsilateral node 3–6 cm in size
N2b	Multiple ipsilateral nodes
N2c	Bilateral or contralateral nodes
N3	Node > 6 cm
Overall stage	
I	T1N0
II	T2N0
III	T3N0
IV*	T4 N0, T1-T4 N+

*Any lymph node involvement automatically upstages tumor to stage IV.

- The role of chemotherapy has not yet been defined.
- Extent of surgery is dictated by the extent of the tumor and generally follows a lateral to medial extent.
- Four general procedures are described:
  - (1) Limited disease (confined to the EAC skin without bone or cartilage involvement). For select T1 lesions:
    - Local sleeve resection of skin with adequate margins (0.5 mm)
    - Can be combined with mastoidectomy
  - (2) Advanced disease:
    - Lateral temporal bone resection (LTBR) (for tumors confined to EAC without involvement of the middle ear or mastoid): for T1 and T2 lesions

- Removal of bony and cartilaginous EAC, tympanic membrane, malleus, and incus (medial limit is the incudostapedial joint)
- Preservation of the facial nerve along its vertical segment
- Requires a canal wall–up mastoidectomy with an extended facial recess opening
- Some centers combine LTBR with superficial parotidectomy
  - (3) Subtotal temporal bone resection (for tumors involving the middle ear and mastoid); for T3 and T4 lesions
    - Medial extension of the LTBR
    - Involves removal of the lateral temporal bone with preservation of the petrous apex and carotid artery
    - Requires identification of the internal auditory canal (IAC) and removal of the otic capsule
    - May require concurrent middle and posterior fossa craniotomies for exposure
    - Facial nerve is resected if involved with the tumor.
    - Superficial parotidectomy is often routinely performed.
  - (4) Total petrosectomy (for tumors involving the petrous apex); may be considered in select T4 lesions
    - Involves removal of the entire temporal bone with or without carotid artery sacrifice.
    - Combined with a subtemporal craniotomy to free the petrous apex.
    - Requires a medial dissection to expose the intrapetrous carotid artery.
    - Sigmoid sinus and jugular bulbs are also mobilized.
    - The ascending ramus, head, and coronoid process of the mandible are also removed.
    - A total parotidectomy is often incorporated in the resection.
    - Associated with significant morbidity.
  - Other surgical considerations depending on the extent of disease:
    - Concurrent parotidectomy (superficial or total)
      - Involvement is either through direct extension or from nodal metastases
      - Incidence of involvement ranges from 10 to 62% in EAC SCC tumors[86]
    - Concurrent neck dissection
      - Lymph node involvement is low, ranging from 10 to 36%.
      - Routine neck dissection is not often performed in the N0 neck (especially for T1 and T2 lesions).
      - Comprehensive neck dissection is performed for N+ neck.
    - Facial nerve sacrifice and reconstruction
    - Internal carotid artery sacrifice (whenever possible after preoperative balloon occlusion testing)

○ Finally, it is important to consider the surgical defect that will be created by these procedures, and multidisciplinary involvement with a head and neck reconstructive surgeon is mandatory (see Chapter 27).

Complications from Surgery

- Most common complication from temporal bone resection relates to intra-operative bleeding
  ○ Venous bleeding: sigmoid sinus, superior petrosal sinus, jugular bulb
  ○ Arterial bleeding: internal carotid artery
- Cranial nerve deficits
  ○ Facial nerve weakness (from retraction or secondary to nerve sacrifice and repair)
  ○ Hearing and balance disturbance from disturbance of otic capsule and labyrinth
  ○ Lower cranial nerves (CNs IX–XII)
    ▪ Because of their impact on airway protection and swallowing, patients may require a tracheotomy and a temporary feeding tube (see Chapter 8).
- CSF leak
- Wound infection

Postoperative Radiotherapy

- See Chapter 30.
- Adjuvant radiation is utilized in T1 and T2 lesions when there is evidence of bone or perineural invasion, a positive margin, or nodal metastases.
- Routinely used as adjuvant therapy in T3 and T4 lesions.

Role of Chemotherapy[87]

- Remains incompletely defined, but some studies have found a benefit for concurrent chemoradiation in advanced tumors

Outcomes

Because of the rarity of temporal bone malignancies, various tumor pathologies are often grouped together when reporting outcomes. SCC remains the most commonly reported malignancy.

- All temporal bone malignancies[63]:
  ○ 5-year overall survival of 62.3%
  ○ 5-year disease-specific survival of 70.4%
  ○ 5-year recurrence-free survival of 45.5%

- Squamous cell carcinoma:
  - 5-year overall survival of 63.2%
  - 5-year disease-specific survival of 67.7%
  - 5-year recurrence-free survival of 53.5%
  - Early-stage tumors have significantly better prognosis than late-stage tumors[84]:
    - T1: 48–100%
    - T2: 35–100%
    - T3: 17–100%
    - T4: 14.3–54%
  - Predictors of survival include advanced stage, middle ear invasion, mandible invasion, pathological bone invasion, pathological parotid invasion, performance of craniotomy, and need for facial nerve resection.[63]

Parotid Gland Neoplasms[79]

- Overall, incidence of salivary gland tumors varies from 0.4 to 13.5 per 100,000.[7]
  - Parotid gland tumors account for 60 to 75% of all salivary gland neoplasms
    - 80% benign: pleomorphic adenoma, Warthin's tumor, basal cell adenoma
    - 20% malignant: mucoepidermoid carcinoma (40–50% of this category), adenoid cystic carcinoma, adenocarcinoma, acinic cell carcinoma, SCC[80]
- Salivary gland malignancies account for 12% of oral and pharyngeal cancers, equivalent to ~ 0.3% of all cancers.
- Two thirds of patients diagnosed are ≥ 55 years of age, with an average age at diagnosis of 64 years.
- Parotid neoplasms with involvement of the skull base are indicative of a malignant process.

Pathology

- Pleomorphic adenoma:
  - Benign tumor composed of epithelial and myoepithelial elements
- Warthin's tumor (papillary cystadenoma lymphomatosum):
  - Benign tumor with double layer of epithelial cells in a lymphoid stroma
- Mucoepidermoid carcinoma:
  - Epithelial tumor that has various proportions of epidermoid and mucinous components with intermediate cells
    - Low grade: more mucinous components
    - High grade: more epithelial components
  - Grade is important in determining prognosis
- Adenoid cystic carcinoma:
  - See pathology on page 158

- Low grade typically has a cribriform or cylindromatous pattern
- High grade typically has a more solid pattern
- Adenocarcinoma:
  - See pathology on page 158
- Acinic cell carcinoma:
  - Some differentiation toward acinar cells
  - Variable patterns: solid, microcystic, papillary, follicular
- Squamous cell carcinoma
  - See pathology on page 160
  - Occurs from invasion of the parotid gland from overlying skin

Etiology/Pathogenesis

- Risk factors include exposure to ionizing radiation, medical radiation, or ultraviolet light; and full-mouth dental X-rays.
- A history of prior cancers, immunosuppression, and EBV infections has also been found to be associated with salivary gland cancers.[81]
- Patients with a history of benign salivary tumors (e.g., pleomorphic adenoma), which typically occur at a younger age, have a higher risk of developing malignant parotid carcinoma because these tumors can undergo malignant transformations in 3 to 10% of cases.

Clinical Symptoms[79,81]

- Chronic history of unilateral painless parotid swelling suggests a neoplastic process and is suspicious especially without signs of inflammation.
- Signs and symptoms suggestive of facial nerve involvement, such as paralytic ectropion, facial nerve palsy, rapid growth rate of the tumor, pain, and cervical adenopathy are indicative of a malignant rather than a benign tumor.
- Parapharyngeal fullness or palatal fullness, trismus, skin ulceration, and fistulas can present in advanced disease.

Diagnosis[79]

- Ultrasound has high sensitivity to detect lesions in the superficial lobe.
- CT and MRI are complementary and are used to delineate the location and extent of the tumor (e.g., superficial or deep lobe, skull base involvement), the presence of perineural invasion, as well as regional node involvement.
- Fine-needle aspiration (FNA) biopsy is performed to further refine the diagnosis.

Staging of Parotid Malignancy

See **Table 23.10.**

Table 23.10   Staging of Parotid Malignancy

Stage	Description
T stage	
T1	Tumor ≤ 2 cm without extraparenchymal extension
T2	Tumor > 2 cm but ≤ 4 cm without extraparenchymal extension
T3	Tumor > 4 cm and/or having extraparenchymal extension
T4a	Tumor invades the skin, mandible, ear canal, and/or facial nerve
T4b	Tumor invades the skull base and/or pterygoid plates and/or encases carotid artery
N stage	
N0	No regional nodes
N1	Single ipsilateral regional node < 3 cm in size
N2a	Single ipsilateral node 3–6 cm in size
N2b	Multiple ipsilateral nodes
N2c	Bilateral or contralateral nodes
N3	Node > 6 cm

Treatment Options[88]

- The mainstay of treatment for all parotid tumors (benign and malignant) involves surgery (e.g., parotidectomy).
  - The goal is to remove the tumor in an en-bloc fashion along with a margin of normal parotid gland while preserving the facial nerve where possible.
  - Superficial parotidectomy involves removing the entire superficial lobe of the parotid gland (i.e., superficial to the facial nerve).
  - Partial/limited parotidectomy is a subtotal superficial parotidectomy while still maintaining a cuff of normal tissue around the tumor. Often indicated for benign disease.
  - Total parotidectomy involves removing the entire parotid gland (superficial and deep to the facial nerve). Often indicated in malignant tumors involving both the superficial and deep lobes of the parotid gland.
  - Radical parotidectomy involves a total parotidectomy along with facial nerve sacrifice. Indicated for malignant tumors with facial nerve involvement.
    - Additional structures may be resected (e.g., temporal bone, mandible) depending on the extent of the tumor.
- Neck dissection
  - 16% of patients presenting with parotid gland carcinoma exhibit cervical lymph node metastases.
  - Neck dissection is indicated in patients with N+ disease.
  - Prophylactic neck dissection is considered in N0 disease in patients with high-grade tumors.

- Postoperative radiotherapy
  - Indications[89]:
    - T1 and T2 adenoid cystic carcinoma
    - T3 and T4 adenoid cystic carcinoma
    - T3 and T4 high-grade malignancies
    - Perineural invasion
    - Close or positive margins
    - Cervical node involvement
    - Lymphatic/vascular invasion
- Chemotherapy
  - Postoperative chemotherapy may be considered in patients with high-grade malignancies or with adverse features.
  - Chemotherapy alone is usually reserved for patients with unresectable disease (T4b).
- Outcomes/prognosis
  - Prognosis is strongly dependent on clinical stage, grade, and histology of the tumor.[90]
  - 5-year survival[89,90]:
    - Mucoepidermoid carcinoma low grade: 75–89%
    - Mucoepidermoid carcinoma high grade: 23–50%
    - Polymorphous low-grade adenocarcinoma: 95–100%
    - Adenoid cystic carcinoma: 35–70%
    - Acinic cell carcinoma: 75–96%

■ References

Boldfaced references are of particular importance.

1. Irish JC, Gullane PJ, Gentili F, et al. Tumors of the skull base: outcome and survival analysis of 77 cases. Head Neck 1994;16:3–10
2. Lund VJ, Stammberger H, Nicolai P, et al; European Rhinologic Society Advisory Board on Endoscopic Techniques in the Management of Nose, Paranasal Sinus and Skull Base Tumours. European position paper on endoscopic management of tumours of the nose, paranasal sinuses and skull base. Rhinol Suppl 2010;22: 1–143
3. Turner JH, Reh DD. Incidence and survival in patients with sinonasal cancer: a historical analysis of population-based data. Head Neck 2012;34:877–885
4. Haerle SK, Gullane PJ, Witterick IJ, Zweifel C, Gentili F. Sinonasal carcinomas: epidemiology, pathology, and management. Neurosurg Clin N Am 2013;24:39–49
5. Öhngren LG. Malignant tumours of maxillo-ethmoidal region: clinical study with special reference to treatment with electrosurgery and irradiation. Acta Otolaryngol 1933;Acta Otolaryngol Suppl. 1933;19:101–106
6. Edge SB, Byrd DR, Compton CC. Nasal cavity and paranasal sinuses. In: Edge SB, Byrd DR, Compton CC, eds. AJCC Cancer Staging Manual, 7th ed. New York: Springer; 2010:69–78

7. Snyderman CH, Carrau RL, Kassam AB, et al. **Endoscopic skull base surgery: principles of endonasal oncological surgery. J Surg Oncol 2008;97:658–664**

8. Eloy JA, Vivero RJ, Hoang K, et al. Comparison of transnasal endoscopic and open craniofacial resection for malignant tumors of the anterior skull base. Laryngoscope 2009;119:834–840

9. Dulguerov P, Jacobsen MS, Allal AS, Lehmann W, Calcaterra T. Nasal and paranasal sinus carcinoma: are we making progress? A series of 220 patients and a systematic review. Cancer 2001;92:3012–3029

10. Lupinetti AD, Roberts DB, Williams MD, et al. Sinonasal adenoid cystic carcinoma: the M. D. Anderson Cancer Center experience. Cancer 2007;110:2726–2731

11. Jones AS, Hamilton JW, Rowley H, Husband D, Helliwell TR. Adenoid cystic carcinoma of the head and neck. Clin Otolaryngol Allied Sci 1997;22:434–443

12. Spiro RH. Distant metastasis in adenoid cystic carcinoma of salivary origin. Am J Surg 1997;174:495–498

13. Naficy S, Disher MJ, Esclamado RM. Adenoid cystic carcinoma of the paranasal sinuses. Am J Rhinol 1999;13:311–314

14. Airoldi M, Pedani F, Succo G, et al. Phase II randomized trial comparing vinorelbine versus vinorelbine plus cisplatin in patients with recurrent salivary gland malignancies. Cancer 2001;91:541–547

15. **Howard DJ, Lund VJ, Wei WI. Craniofacial resection for tumors of the nasal cavity and paranasal sinuses: a 25-year experience. Head Neck 2006;28:867–873**

16. Kleinsasser O, Schroeder HG. Adenocarcinomas of the inner nose after exposure to wood dust. Morphological findings and relationships between histopathology and clinical behavior in 79 cases. Arch Otorhinolaryngol 1988;245:1–15

17. Bhayani MK, Yilmaz T, Sweeney A, et al. Sinonasal adenocarcinoma: a 16-year experience at a single institution. Head Neck 2014;36:1490–1496

18. Devaiah AK, Andreoli MT. Treatment of esthesioneuroblastoma: a 16-year meta-analysis of 361 patients. Laryngoscope 2009;119:1412–1416

19. Zhang M, Zhou L, Wang DH, Huang WT, Wang SY. Diagnosis and management of esthesioneuroblastoma. ORL J Otorhinolaryngol Relat Spec 2010;72:113–118

20. Kumar R, Ghoshal S, Khosla D, et al. Survival and failure outcomes in locally advanced esthesioneuroblastoma: a single centre experience of 15 patients. Eur Arch Otorhinolaryngol 2013;270:1897–1901

21. Modesto A, Blanchard P, Tao YG, et al. Multimodal treatment and long-term outcome of patients with esthesioneuroblastoma. Oral Oncol 2013;49:830–834

22. Hyams VJ. Tumors of the upper respiratory tract and ear. In: Hyams VJ, Batsakis JG, Michaels L, eds. Atlas of Tumor Pathology, 2nd ed. Washington, DC: Armed Forces Institute of Pathology; 1988:240–248

23. **Castelnuovo PG, Delù G, Sberze F, et al. Esthesioneuroblastoma: endonasal endoscopic treatment. Skull Base 2006;16:25–30**

24. Bisogno G, Soloni P, Conte M, et al. Esthesioneuroblastoma in pediatric and adolescent age. A report from the TREP project in cooperation with the Italian Neuroblastoma and Soft Tissue Sarcoma Committees. BMC Cancer 2012;12:117–240

25. El Kababri M, Habrand JL, Valteau-Couanet D, Gaspar N, Dufour C, Oberlin O. Esthesioneuroblastoma in children and adolescent: experience on 11 cases with literature review. J Pediatr Hematol Oncol 2014;36:91–95

26. Montava M, Verillaud B, Kania R, et al. Critical analysis of recurrences of esthesioneuroblastomas: can we prevent them? Eur Arch Otorhinolaryngol 2014;271:3215–
3222
27. Papacharalampous GX, Vlastarakos PV, Chrysovergis A, Saravakos PK, Kotsis GP, Davi-
lis DI. Olfactory neuroblastoma (esthesioneuroblastoma): towards minimally invasive surgery and multi-modality treatment strategies - an updated critical review of
the current literature. J BUON 2013;18:557–563
28. Kadish S, Goodman M, Wang CC. Olfactory neuroblastoma. A clinical analysis of 17
cases. Cancer 1976;37:1571–1576
29. Morita A, Ebersold MJ, Olsen KD, Foote RL, Lewis JE, Quast LM. Esthesioneuroblastoma: prognosis and management. Neurosurgery 1993;32:706–714, discussion 714–
715
30. Dulguerov P, Calcaterra T. Esthesioneuroblastoma: the UCLA experience 1970-1990.
Laryngoscope 1992;102:843–849
31. Dulguerov P, Allal AS, Calcaterra TC. Esthesioneuroblastoma: a meta-analysis and review. Lancet Oncol 2001;2:683–690
32. Kane AJ, Sughrue ME, Rutkowski MJ, et al. Posttreatment prognosis of patients with
esthesioneuroblastoma. J Neurosurg 2010;113:340–351
33. Patel SG, Singh B, Stambuk HE, et al. Craniofacial surgery for esthesioneuroblastoma:
report of an international collaborative study. J Neurol Surg B Skull Base 2012;73:208–
220
34. Bell D, Saade R, Roberts D, et al. Prognostic utility of Hyams histological grading and
Kadish-Morita staging systems for esthesioneuroblastoma outcomes. Head Neck
Pathol 2014
35. Eden BV, Debo RF, Larner JM, et al. Esthesioneuroblastoma. Long-term outcome
and patterns of failure—the University of Virginia experience. Cancer 1994;73:2556–
2562
36. McElroy EA Jr, Buckner JC, Lewis JE. Chemotherapy for advanced esthesioneuroblastoma: the Mayo Clinic experience. Neurosurgery 1998;42:1023–1027, discussion 1027–
1028
37. Bhattacharyya N, Thornton AF, Joseph MP, Goodman ML, Amrein PC. Successful treatment of esthesioneuroblastoma and neuroendocrine carcinoma with combined chemotherapy and proton radiation. Results in 9 cases. Arch Otolaryngol Head Neck Surg
1997;123:34–40
38. Irish J, Dasgupta R, Freeman J, et al. Outcome and analysis of the surgical management
of esthesioneuroblastoma. J Otolaryngol 1997;26:1–7
39. Jethanamest D, Morris LG, Sikora AG, Kutler DI. Esthesioneuroblastoma: a population-based analysis of survival and prognostic factors. Arch Otolaryngol Head Neck
Surg 2007;133:276–280
40. Rimmer J, Lund VJ, Beale T, Wei WI, Howard D. Olfactory neuroblastoma: a 35-year experience and suggested follow-up protocol. Laryngoscope 2014;124:1542–1549
41. Koka VN, Julieron M, Bourhis J, et al. Aesthesioneuroblastoma. J Laryngol Otol 1998;
112:628–633
42. Austin JR, Cebrun H, Kershisnik MM, et al. Olfactory neuroblastoma and neuroendocrine carcinoma of the anterior skull base: treatment results at the M.D. Anderson
Cancer Center. Skull Base Surg 1996;6:1–8

43. Broich G, Pagliari A, Ottaviani F. Esthesioneuroblastoma: a general review of the cases published since the discovery of the tumour in 1924. Anticancer Res 1997;17:2683–2706

44. Thompson LD, Wieneke JA, Miettinen M. Sinonasal tract and nasopharyngeal melanomas: a clinicopathologic study of 115 cases with a proposed staging system. Am J Surg Pathol 2003;27:594–611

45. Bridge JA, Bowen JM, Smith RB. The small round blue cell tumors of the sinonasal area. Head Neck Pathol 2010;4:84–93

46. Ganly I, Patel SG, Singh B, et al. Craniofacial resection for malignant melanoma of the skull base: report of an international collaborative study. Arch Otolaryngol Head Neck Surg 2006;132:73–78

47. Ledderose GJ, Leunig A. Surgical management of recurrent sinonasal mucosal melanoma: endoscopic or transfacial resection. Eur Arch Otorhinolaryngol 2014

48. Xu CC, Dziegielewski PT, McGaw WT, Seikaly H. Sinonasal undifferentiated carcinoma (SNUC): the Alberta experience and literature review. J Otolaryngol Head Neck Surg 2013;42:2–02

49. Tiwari R, Quak J, Egeler S, et al. Tumors of the infratemporal fossa. Skull Base Surg 2000;10:1–9

50. Hentschel SJ, Vora Y, Suki D, Hanna EY, DeMonte F. Malignant tumors of the anterolateral skull base. Neurosurgery 2010;66:102–112, discussion 112

51. Hosseini SM, Razfar A, Carrau RL, et al. Endonasal transpterygoid approach to the infratemporal fossa: correlation of endoscopic and multiplanar CT anatomy. Head Neck 2012;34:313–320

52. Glad H, Vainer B, Buchwald C, et al. Juvenile nasopharyngeal angiofibromas in Denmark 1981-2003: diagnosis, incidence, and treatment. Acta Otolaryngol 2007;127:292–299

53. Boghani Z, Husain Q, Kanumuri VV, et al. Juvenile nasopharyngeal angiofibroma: a systematic review and comparison of endoscopic, endoscopic-assisted, and open resection in 1047 cases. Laryngoscope 2013;123:859–869

54. Leong SC. A systematic review of surgical outcomes for advanced juvenile nasopharyngeal angiofibroma with intracranial involvement. Laryngoscope 2013;123:1125–1131

55. Lee JT, Chen P, Safa A, Juillard G, Calcaterra TC. The role of radiation in the treatment of advanced juvenile angiofibroma. Laryngoscope 2002;112(7 Pt 1):1213–1220

56. Wei WI, Sham JS. Nasopharyngeal carcinoma. Lancet 2005;365:2041–2054

57. Vokes EE, Liebowitz DN, Weichselbaum RR. Nasopharyngeal carcinoma. Lancet 1997;350:1087–1091

58. Ayan I, Kaytan E, Ayan N. Childhood nasopharyngeal carcinoma: from biology to treatment. Lancet Oncol 2003;4:13–21

59. Sham JS, Poon YF, Wei WI, Choy D. Nasopharyngeal carcinoma in young patients. Cancer 1990;65:2606–2610

60. Chen MY, Wen WP, Guo X, et al. Endoscopic nasopharyngectomy for locally recurrent nasopharyngeal carcinoma. Laryngoscope 2009;119:516–522

61. Prasad S, Janecka IP. Efficacy of surgical treatments for squamous cell carcinoma of the temporal bone: a literature review. Otolaryngol Head Neck Surg 1994;110:270–280

62. Madsen AR, Gundgaard MG, Hoff CM, et al. Cancer of the external auditory canal and middle ear in Denmark from 1992 to 2001. Head Neck 2008;30:1332–1338

63. Morris LG, Mehra S, Shah JP, Bilsky MH, Selesnick SH, Kraus DH. Predictors of survival and recurrence after temporal bone resection for cancer. Head Neck 2012;34:1231–1239

64. Wiatrak BJ, Pensak ML. Rhabdomyosarcoma of the ear and temporal bone. Laryngoscope 1989;99:1188–1192

65. Shih L, Crabtree JA. Carcinoma of the external auditory canal: an update. Laryngoscope 1990;100:1215–1218

66. **Chung SJ, Pensal ML. Tumors of the temporal bone. In: Jackler RK, Brackmann DE, eds. Neurotology, 2nd ed. Elsevier; 2005:1028–1036**

67. Leonetti JP, Marzo SJ, Agarwal N. Adenoid cystic carcinoma of the parotid gland with temporal bone invasion. Otol Neurotol 2008;29:545–548

68. Pulec JL. Glandular tumors of the external auditory canal. Laryngoscope 1977;87(10 Pt 1):1601–1612

69. **Curran AJ, Gullane PJ, Bance ML, Donald PJ. Temporal bone resection. In: Donald PJ, ed. Surgery of the Skull Base. Philadelphia: Lippincott-Raven; 1998:368–408**

70. Durve DV, Kanegaonkar RG, Albert D, Levitt G. Paediatric rhabdomyosarcoma of the ear and temporal bone. Clin Otolaryngol Allied Sci 2004;29:32–37

71. Friedman RA, Hoa M, Brackmann DE. Surgical management of endolymphatic sac tumors. J Neurol Surg B Skull Base 2013;74:12–19

72. Heffner DK. Low-grade adenocarcinoma of probable endolymphatic sac origin A clinicopathologic study of 20 cases. Cancer 1989;64:2292–2302

73. Lonser RR, Kim HJ, Butman JA, Vortmeyer AO, Choo DI, Oldfield EH. Tumors of the endolymphatic sac in von Hippel-Lindau disease. N Engl J Med 2004;350:2481–2486

74. Choo D, Shotland L, Mastroianni M, et al. Endolymphatic sac tumors in von Hippel-Lindau disease. J Neurosurg. 2004;100:480–487

75. Nevoux J, Nowak C, Vellin JF, et al. Management of endolymphatic sac tumors: sporadic cases and von hippel-lindau disease. Otol Neurotol 2014;35:899–904

76. Eze N, Huber A, Schuknecht B. De novo development and progression of endolymphatic sac tumour in von hippel-lindau disease: an observational study and literature review. J Neurol Surg B Skull Base 2013;74:259–265

77. Diaz RC, Amjad EH, Sargent EW, Larouere MJ, Shaia WT. Tumors and pseudotumors of the endolymphatic sac. Skull Base 2007;17:379–393

78. Poletti AM, Dubey SP, Barbo R, et al. Sporadic endolymphatic sac tumor: its clinical, radiological, and histological features, management, and follow-up. Head Neck 2013;35:1043–1047

79. Hou ZH, Huang DL, Han DY, Dai P, Young WY, Yang SM. Surgical treatment of endolymphatic sac tumor. Acta Otolaryngol 2012;132:329–336

80. Timmer FC, Neeskens LJ, van den Hoogen FJ, et al. Endolymphatic sac tumors: clinical outcome and management in a series of 9 cases. Otol Neurotol 2011;32:680–685

81. Diaz RC, Amjad EH, Sargent EW, Larouere MJ, Shaia WT. Tumors and pseudotumors of the endolymphatic sac. Skull Base 2007;17:379–393

82. Bacciu A, Clemente IA, Piccirillo E, Ferrari S, Sanna M. Guidelines for treating temporal bone carcinoma based on long-term outcomes. Otol Neurotol 2013;34:898–907

83. Prasad SC, D'Orazio F, Medina M, Bacciu A, Sanna M. State of the art in temporal bone malignancies. Curr Opin Otolaryngol Head Neck Surg 2014;22:154–165

84. Moody SA, Hirsch BE, Myers EN. Squamous cell carcinoma of the external auditory canal: an evaluation of a staging system. Am J Otol 2000;21:582–588

85. Zhang T, Li W, Dai C, Chi F, Wang S, Wang Z. Evidence-based surgical management of T1 or T2 temporal bone malignancies. Laryngoscope 2013;123:244–248

86. Sugimoto H, Ito M, Yoshida S, Hatano M, Yoshizaki T. Concurrent superselective intra-arterial chemotherapy and radiotherapy for late-stage squamous cell carcinoma of the temporal bone. Ann Otol Rhinol Laryngol 2011;120:372–376

87. Carlson ER, Webb DE. The diagnosis and management of parotid disease. Oral Maxillofac Surg Clin North Am 2013;25:31–48, v

88. Ho K, Lin H, Ann DK, Chu PG, Yen Y. An overview of the rare parotid gland cancer. Head Neck Oncol 2011;3:40–43

89. Guzzo M, Locati LD, Prott FJ, Gatta G, McGurk M, Licitra L. Major and minor salivary gland tumors. Crit Rev Oncol Hematol 2010;74:134–148

90. Guzzo M, Locati LD, Prott FJ, Gatta G, McGurk M, Licitra L. Major and minor salivary gland tumors. Crit Rev Oncol Hematol. 2010;74:134–148

24 Craniovertebral Junction

■ Anatomy

See Chapter 2.9, page 57.

■ Embryology

See Chapter 4, page 98.

■ Pathology

Table 24.1 summarizes the main pathologies of the craniovertebral junction (CVJ).[1]

■ Signs and Symptoms

- Pain is the most typical symptom in CVJ pathologies.
- Compressive myelopathy: weakness and clumsiness of the hands with or without spasticity of the extremities, sensory abnormalities.
- Classically, the sensory and/or motor findings start in the ipsilateral arm and then in the ipsilateral leg, followed by the contralateral leg and finally the contralateral arm.

Examination Pearl

To identify CN XI palsy, determine the presence of sternocleidomastoid and trapezius muscles atrophy. Note that slowly progressive pathologies provide time for the patient to compensate for shoulder movement by muscle groups innervated by nerves other than CN XI.

Table 24.1   Main Pathologies* of the Craniovertebral Junction

Developmental	• Malformations of the C0–C2 complex • Basilar invagination • Basilar impression in Paget's disease, osteogenesis imperfecta • Rheumatoid arthritis • Deformities related to hyperparathyroidism, arthropathies, osteomyelitis, tuberculosis, and other conditions • Chiari malformation
Neoplastic	• Meningioma, schwannoma, neurofibroma, arachnoid cyst • Benign primary osseous lesions: aneurysmal bone cyst, benign giant cell tumor, osteoblastoma, osteochondroma, osteoid osteoma, eosinophilic granuloma, solitary plasmacytoma, hemangioma • Malignant lesions: chordoma, myeloma, lymphoma, chondrosarcoma, osteosarcoma, Ewing's sarcoma, fibrosarcoma, hemangiopericytoma • Metastases • Central nervous systems tumors: astrocytomas, ependymomas
Traumatic	Fractures of the clivus, occipital condyles, odontoid, hangman's fracture, C2 vertebral body; atlanto-occipital dislocation; ligamentous disruptions
Vascular	Spinal arteriovenous malformations, vertebral artery (VA) and posterior inferior cerebellar artery (PICA) aneurysms, cavernous malformations of the cervicomedullary junction

*Congenital and acquired.

- Lower cranial nerve deficits, especially in CNs XI and XII.
- Internuclear ophthalmoplegia, downbeat nystagmus.
- Sleep apnea.
- Vertebrobasilar ischemia.

■ Surgical Approaches

The goals of surgery in the CVJ are (1) to decompress neurovascular structures; (2) to alleviate pain and stop the progression of neurologic deterioration; (3) to restore, whenever indicated, the stability of the junction; and (4) in the case of neoplastic disease, to resect the lesion as completely as possible and make a tissue diagnosis.

Table 24.2   Approaches to the Craniovertebral Junction

Anterior/anterolateral	• Transoral (± extensions/variants, e.g., ± transmaxillary, translabiomandibular, transpalatal, transglossal, etc.) • Transnasal endoscopic • Combined endoscopic transoral-transnasal • Retropharyngeal
Lateral/posterolateral	• Subtemporal with anterior petrosectomy • Posterior or extended transpetrosal • Retrosigmoidal • Far lateral transcondylar transtubercular
Posterior	• Suboccipital ± upper cervical laminectomy

- According to the nature and localization of the disease (e.g., ventral compression of the cervicomedullary junction caused by chordoma or dens displacement), the CVJ can be approached via anterior/anterolateral, lateral/posterolateral, and posterior approaches[1] (**Table 24.2**).

❖ Extended Endonasal Transclival Approaches to the CVJ

See Chapter 16, page 426.

❖ Transoral Odontoidectomy:

◈ The use of self-retaining retractors enables greater spreading of the space and better access to the clivus, the anterior arch of C1, and C2, and is highly recommended.

◈ Palpate the C1 tubercle to verify the midline and make a liner incision, cutting the median raphe of the posterior pharyngeal wall, the mucosa, pharyngeal muscles, and the anterior longitudinal ligaments in a single layer with a monopolar cautery.

◈ Using a drill and curettes, resect the required amount of bone to access the target space: the anterior arch of C1 and then the C2 body.

◈ Remove the joint capsule.

◈ Access the dens to remove it. Depending on the pathology, the dens may need to be cored out or simply transected at its base and pulled away from the cervicomedullary junction. Decompression of the cervicomedullary junction is achieved by removing all the bone components and soft tissue causing the compression.

◈ Irrigate the field with antibiotics, then suture the flap in a single layer.

◈ In the case of intradural access, use a dural patch (it is better to use biological tissues such as fascia lata) and use fibrin glue to assist in gaining a more watertight seal. A lumbar drain is recommended. Use a nasogastric tube in the postoperative period, with frequent inspection of the pharyngeal wall. Note that a large number of these incisions will spread apart simply because of the nature of the constrictors of the pharynx, which in their normal movements tend to pull the incision apart. Therefore, resting the swallowing mechanism by means of nasogastric tube or percutaneous gastrostomy will speed healing.

Occipitocervical Fusion

- Occipitocervical instability can be posttraumatic, iatrogenic, secondary to neoplastic diseases, or the result of basilar invagination. In such cases, occipitocervical fusion is required.[1,2]
- Contraindications to instrumented fusion are severe osteoporosis, osteolytic lesions in the region requiring fixation, or anomalously placed vertebral arteries, particularly in a patient who has a posterior circulation dependent on a single vertebral artery. Therefore, review the preoperative computed tomography angiography (CTA) carefully.
- After fusion is achieved, patients lose 30 to 60% of their neck mobility, and many patients find this quite limiting. Therefore be sure that a fusion is indicated before performing it.
- Several techniques have been described, such as occipital-C1 transarticular fusion, but the most often used technique, especially following skull base surgical approaches, is the occipitocervical fusion using an occipital plate connected with rods to the bilateral bicortical screws in the lateral masses of the lower cervical vertebrae (C3 down as far as C7 if required, but usually entailing only C3).
- The most relevant intracranial complication related to this technique is injury to the dural venous sinuses due to long transoccipital screws.

General Surgical Complications

- Cerebrospinal fluid (CSF) leakage and meningitis: above all in transoral intradural approaches
- Iatrogenic instability: managed by posterior fusion and, rarely, transoral bone graft, in a procedure using transoral approaches
- Vertebrobasilar injury
- Lower cranial nerve injury
- Cervicomedullary/cerebellum injury
- Infections

■ Basilar Invagination

Basilar invagination is an upward displacement of the odontoid process into the foramen magnum. It is not the same as platybasia, which is an abnormal obtuse angle between the anterior skull base and the clivus.

- Other findings related to basilar invagination include occipitalization of the atlas, vertebralization of the occiput, occipital condylar hypoplasia, atlas assimilation, aplasia/hypoplasia of the arches of the atlas, anomalies of the odontoid process, and fusion of the cervical vertebrae (as in Klippel-Feil syndrome).
- The tip of the odontoid generally lies below Chamberlain's line (in radiology, the line connecting the hard palate to the opisthion). In basilar invagination, the tip of the odontoid projects at least 2.5 to 3 mm above Chamberlain's line or more than 4.5 mm above McGregor's line (between the hard palate and occipital base, and used when the opisthion is not identifiable).

Treatment

Traction is applied if the basilar invagination can be reduced, followed by occipitocervical fusion, posterior fossa and upper cervical canal posterior decompression, and, if these fail, then transoral ventral decompression.

■ Chiari Malformations

Type I[4–10]

- Chiari malformation type I (CM-I) is the most common congenital malformation affecting the posterior fossa, named after the Austrian pathologist Hans Chiari, who in 1891 was the first to describe in detail and classify the different variations of the condition (although the Chiari type IV was described later by other investigators).[3]
- CM-I is associated with tonsillar herniation into the foramen magnum, small posterior cranial fossa, and altered CSF flow and tissue motion in the craniocervical junction.
- Presentation is usually in young and middle-aged adults. The most frequent presenting symptoms are cough-, laugh-, or sneeze-associated head pain.[4]
- Cerebellar tonsil descent below the foramen magnum > 5 mm is common.

Type II: Arnold-Chiari

- Caudal dislocation of inferior vermis, medulla, and fourth ventricle associated with lumbar or lumbosacral myelomeningocele. The cerebellar tonsils are dislocated at or below the foramen magnum.

- Often associated with hydrocephalus and very rarely with spina bifida occulta.
- Medullary kink is present in 55%.
- Presentation occurs in infancy, childhood, or adolescence. The more the severe the symptoms, the earlier the presentation. The usual presentation in infancy is with respiratory distress and hydrocephalus.
- Magnetic resonance imaging (MRI) can show a Z-bend deformity of the medulla, cerebellar peg, tectal fusion, enlarged massa intermedia, elongation of the medulla, low attachment of the tentorium, hydrocephalus, syringomyelia, trapped fourth ventricle, agenesis/dysgenesis of the corpus callosum, and cerebellomedullary compression.[11]
- If hydrocephalus is present, it should be first treated with a ventriculoperitoneal shunt.
- Suboccipital craniectomy with a cervical laminectomy and dural graft has been the treatment of choice. Obex plugging and tonsillar coagulation are now rarely performed.
- Upper cervical bone decompression with delamination of the outer layer of the dura has been reported as a safe and effective treatment for symptomatic Chiari type II malformation in neonates and young infants.[12]
- CM-II–related management guidelines are not well defined.
- Associated findings of syringomyelia, hydrocephalus, scoliosis, and symptomatic CM-II may be triggered by more than one underlying condition.
- Hydrocephalus is often involved in symptomatic CM-II and must always be considered first in any symptomatic patient. Intrinsic brainstem dysfunction cannot be treated surgically, and monitoring of vital functions is sometimes the only clinical means that can be offered to the patient. Knowledge of the complex background has led to improved follow-up programs for the affected children and has thus also improved long-term survival.[13]
- Respiratory arrest is the most typical cause of death. The rapidity of neurologic deterioration is an important prognostic factor.[11]

Type III

- Displacement of posterior fossa structures through an occipital and sometimes cervical encephalomeningocele. This is usually incompatible with life.[11]

Type IV

- Cerebellar hypoplasia without cerebellar herniation.

■ References

Boldfaced references are of particular importance.
1. **Bambakidis NC, Dickman CA, Spetzler RF, Sonntag VKH. Surgery of the Craniovertebral Junction, 2nd ed. New York, Stuttgart: Thieme; 2012**

2. Suchomel P, Choutka O. Reconstruction of Upper Cervical Spine and Craniovertebral Junction. New York: Springer; 2011
3. Massimi L, Peppucci E, Peraio S, Di Rocco C. History of Chiari type I malformation. Neurol Sci 2011;32(Suppl 3):S263–S265
4. **Chavez A, Roguski M, Killeen A, Heilman C, Hwang S. Comparison of operative and non-operative outcomes based on surgical selection criteria for patients with Chiari I malformations. J Clin Neurosci 2014;21:2201–2206**
5. Heiss JD, Suffredini G, Smith R, et al. Pathophysiology of persistent syringomyelia after decompressive craniocervical surgery. Clinical article. J Neurosurg Spine 2010; 13:729–742
6. **Clarke EC, Stoodley MA, Bilston LE. Changes in temporal flow characteristics of CSF in Chiari malformation Type I with and without syringomyelia: implications for theory of syrinx development. J Neurosurg 2013;118:1135–1140**
7. **Chotai S, Medhkour A. Surgical outcomes after posterior fossa decompression with and without duraplasty in Chiari malformation-I. Clin Neurol Neurosurg 2014;125:182–188**
8. Durham SR, Fjeld-Olenec K. Comparison of posterior fossa decompression with and without duraplasty for the surgical treatment of Chiari malformation Type I in pediatric patients: a meta-analysis. J Neurosurg Pediatr 2008;2:42–49
9. **Förander P, Sjåvik K, Solheim O, et al. The case for duraplasty in adults undergoing posterior fossa decompression for Chiari I malformation: a systematic review and meta-analysis of observational studies. Clin Neurol Neurosurg 2014; 125:58–64**
10. Royo-Salvador MB, Solé-Llenas J, Doménech JM, González-Adrio R. Results of the section of the filum terminale in 20 patients with syringomyelia, scoliosis and Chiari malformation. Acta Neurochir (Wien) 2005;147:515–523, discussion 523
11. Greenberg MS. Chiari malformation. In: Greenberg MS, ed. Handbook of Neurosurgery, 7th ed. New York: Thieme; 2010:233–240
12. Ogiwara H, Morota N. Surgical decompression without dural opening for symptomatic Chiari type II malformation in young infants. Childs Nerv Syst 2013;29:1563–1567
13. Messing-Jünger M, Röhrig A. Primary and secondary management of the Chiari II malformation in children with myelomeningocele. Childs Nerv Syst 2013;29:1553–1562

25 Skull Base Approaches in Cerebrovascular Surgery

Skull base approaches are commonly used in the treatment of cerebrovascular pathologies, such as intracranial aneurysms, arteriovenous malformations (AVMs), dural arteriovenous fistulas (dAVFs), and brainstem cavernous malformations (BCMs). Aneurysms that are most amenable for a skull base approach are aneurysms of the anterior circulation, (vertebro-)basilar artery aneurysms, and posterior circulation aneurysms.[1,2] In many cases, anterior communicating artery aneurysms or complex middle cerebral artery aneurysms can be treated best with a skull base approach by minimizing brain retraction and optimizing exposure and maneuverability.[3–6]

Due to the central location in the skull, BCMs are mostly treated by skull base approaches to ensure adequate exposure of the brainstem.

■ Anatomy

Review the cerebrovascular anatomy in Chapter 2, **Fig. 2.20**, page 65, as well as the classification systems of the segments of the internal carotid artery (ICA) and vertebral artery (VA) (**Fig. 2.21**, page 67).

■ Investigations and Imaging

- Digital subtraction angiography (DSA) and computed tomography angiography (CTA) are used to assess the angioarchitecture and projection of the aneurysm.
- Plain computed tomography (CT) with bone setting is used to delineate the anatomy of the skull base.
- Magnetic resonance imaging (MRI) is mandatory for BCMs to determine the optimal approach.
- Additionally, diffusion tensor imaging (DTI) can be helpful in determining the safest way to access the brainstem.[7]

Table 25.1   Skull Base Approaches to Cerebrovascular Pathology[8–10]

Approach	Pathology
Orbitozygomatic	AcomA, ICA, BCM, upper BA aneurysm, SCA aneurysm
Transcavernous	Retrosellar and upper BA aneurysm
Subtemporal with or without anterior petrosectomy	AICA aneurysm, retrosellar and upper BA aneurysm, PCA aneurysm
Presigmoid supra- or infratentorial	Middle BA aneurysm
Far lateral	BCM, PICA aneurysm, VB junction aneurysm
Retrosigmoid	BCM, PICA aneurysm

Abbreviations: AComA, anterior communicating artery; AICA, anterior inferior cerebellar artery; BA, basilar artery; BCM, brainstem cavernous malformations; ICA, internal carotid artery; PCA, posterior cerebral artery; PICA, posterior inferior cerebellar artery; SCA, superior cerebellar artery; VB, vertebrobasilar.

■ Treatment

Table 25.1 summarizes the potential skull base approaches for intracranial aneurysms and brainstem cavernous malformations.

■ Revascularization Techniques in Skull Base Surgery

Revascularization of intracranial arteries is sometimes necessary when the internal carotid artery (ICA) must be sacrificed. Reasons for occluding the ICA are the presence of an intracranial saccular, dissecting or blister aneurysms that cannot be secured by straightforward clipping or endovascular treatment, and skull base tumors that invade the arterial wall.[10–12]

- Cerebral revascularization surgery of the ICA is rarely indicated.
- A very selective approach with assessment of cerebrovascular reserve is advised to achieve the best outcome.
- Revascularization techniques include direct reconstruction, interposition graft or extracranial-intracranial (EC-IC) bypass.
- The most commonly used grafts are the saphenous vein and radial artery.

Indications

Most aneurysms of the ICA are treated by endovascular methods, such as coiling, balloon occlusion, or placement of a flow-diverting stent. If this treatment fails or is not feasible, or if the aneurysm cannot be clipped, intracranial revascularization surgery is indicated.

- The decision to occlude or resect the ICA for skull base tumors is controversial. In the era before the advent of stereotactic radiosurgery (SRS), it was performed in about 3% of cases.[13] Nowadays, remnants of skull base tumors can be treated by SRS, making complete tumor resection in most cases unnecessary. Therefore, revascularization surgery in skull base tumors is only indicated in very selective cases.[14]

Etiology/Pathophysiology

Sacrificing the ICA in skull base tumors is considered after evaluation of the following four aspects of the tumor: pathology, extent of infiltration, location,[12] and cerebrovascular reserve. The pathological diagnosis and the clinical behavior of the tumor are important factors to consider. Malignant tumors of the skull base where long-term control can only be achieved after complete surgical eradication, or "benign" skull base tumors with recurrent growth despite several treatment attempts may be indications to sacrifice the ICA.[12,15] The invasion of the vessel wall by the tumor, in contrast to encasement of the vessel, makes complete tumor resection impossible. In such cases, when complete surgical eradication is indicated and no additional therapy is possible, the ICA needs to be resected as well to achieve a complete tumor resection.

- A more rostral location of the tumor makes resection of the ICA more dangerous, due to the increased difficulty in approaching the artery and the presence of important branches and perforators.[12]

Clinical Presentation

Patients present with neurologic deficits related to the skull base/brain involvement, or intracranial (mostly subarachnoid) hemorrhage due to a ruptured aneurysm. Rarely, a patient can develop severe epistaxis due to rupture of a pseudoaneurysm of the ICA as a result of tumor invasion or radiation necrosis.[16]

Investigations and Imaging

The first step is to image the intracranial vessels and identify their relation with the surrounding structures to assess whether ICA sacrifice is necessary. Perform MRI/magnetic resonance angiography (MRA) and DSA. DSA is helpful in identifying the optimal site for arterial occlusion and bypass, examining the collateral circulation, and determining the size of the intended recipient and donor vessels. Additionally, a balloon test occlusion (BTO) can be helpful in

Table 25.2   Imaging Methods that Can Investigate Cerebral Blood Flow and Cerebral Vascular Reserve[19]

Digital subtraction angiography
Single photon emission computed tomography
Positron emission tomography
Arterial spin labeling magnetic resonance imaging
Blood oxygen level-dependent magnetic resonance imaging
Xenon computed tomography

assessing the stroke risk, although the 4 to 7% risk of (transient) complications and the 15% false-negative rate should be taken into account (see also page 301).[17,18] Assessment of cerebral vascular reserve during temporary ICA occlusion, which can be investigated by different studies **(Table 25.2)**, might be a good adjunctive to determine whether the patient can tolerate ICA sacrifice. When a bypass procedure is planned, a preoperative DSA of the extracranial arteries, a preoperative Doppler investigation of the saphenous vein, and the (modified) Allen's test to check the patency of the ulnar artery can be useful.

Treatment

There are different types of revascularization procedures, such as direct reconstruction by direct suture or patch (type 1), interposition grafting (type 2), EC-IC bypass (type 3), and direct intracranial revascularization (type 4).[20] The most common procedure in skull base aneurysms and tumors is the EC-IC bypass. There are different types of EC-IC bypass **(Table 25.3)**; each has benefits and drawbacks.

- The procedure of the EC-IC bypass using a graft, which is most commonly used for bypasses to the ICA, is discussed in detail below.

Preoperative

- When choosing the type of graft, consider the following factors: A saphenous vein is larger in diameter and can therefore provide a higher blood flow to the brain in comparison with the radial artery graft. On the other hand, the saphenous vein has lower long-term patency rates, a higher risk of kinking, and may cause a caliber mismatch with small intracranial arteries (< 2 mm). The drawbacks of the radial artery are its shorter length and its tendency to become spastic.[11]
- Patients are given acetylsalicylic acid preoperatively to reduce the risk of graft thrombosis.

Table 25.3   Types of Revascularization Procedures

Donor and Recipient Vessel	Interposition Graft	Type of Procedure*
Cervical to petrous ICA	Saphenous vein	2
Petrous to supraclinoid ICA	Saphenous vein	2
M1 to M2	Saphenous vein or radial artery	2
Cervical to supraclinoid ICA	Saphenous vein or radial artery	3
IMAX to supraclinoid ICA	Saphenous vein or radial artery	3
Cervical ICA to M1 or M2	Saphenous vein or radial artery	3
Cervical ICA to PCA or SCA	Saphenous vein or radial artery	3
IMAX to M1 or M2	Saphenous vein or radial artery	3
STA to M2 or M3	–	3
Cervical ICA to PCA	Saphenous vein or radial artery	3
STA to PCA or SCA	–	3
OA to PICA	–	3
Anastomosis between two adjacent cerebral arteries	–	4

Abbreviations: MCA, middle cerebral artery; M1, first branch of MCA; M2, second branch of MCA; IMAX, internal maxillary artery; STA, superior temporal artery; OC, occipital artery.
*See text.

Perioperative

- General[12]:
  - Normocapnea should be maintained: a partial pressure of carbon dioxide (PCO_2) of 35 to 40 mmHg.
  - Mannitol is administered if necessary for brain swelling.
  - Patients are allowed to become mildly hypothermic (34–36°C)
  - Electroencephalograph (EEG) monitoring is optional.
  - Deep sedation/burst suppression and elevation of the blood pressure by 20% from baseline is induced just before temporary occlusion of the intracranial artery.
- Surgical[10,11,15]:
- ◈ The necessary surgical sites are prepared: head, neck, lower arm or leg.
- ◈ The head is positioned in a radiolucent head holder.
- ◈ Graft harvesting is done following general surgical principles. A plastic surgeon (for radial artery harvest) or cardiothoracic surgeon (for saphenous vein harvest) can assist.
- ◈ The graft is marked proximally and distally, as well as on the superficial wall to identify whether the graft rotated during tunneling.

Surgical Pearl

Systemic heparinization is not advised when preoperative aspirin and mild hypothermia are used.

Surgical Anatomy Pearl

The internal maxillary artery (IMAX) can be used as an alternative donor vessel with the benefit of a shorter graft length and absence of a cervical incision.[21,22] A drawback is the more difficult exposure and technically challenging anastomosis to the IMAX.

◈ The graft is flushed and distended with heparinized saline (1,000 heparin units in 500 mL saline), and periadventitial tissue is sufficiently denuded at both ends for a length of 1 to 2 cm.

◈ The donor vessel—common carotid artery (CCA), internal carotid artery (ICA), or external carotid artery (ECA)—is exposed in the neck following general surgical principles.

◈ A craniotomy is performed. It is tailored to expose the recipient artery as well as the pathology that needs treatment.

◈ The recipient artery is exposed and occluded just distal to the pathology with a permanent clip, and the area of the arteriotomy is trapped by placing a second, temporary, clip.

◈ The graft is cut in a "fish-mouth" shape to optimize the diameter of the anastomosis.

◈ An arteriotomy of the recipient vessel is performed and flushed with heparinized saline.

◈ A end-to-side bypass is performed (with running or interrupted sutures) using 8-0 monofilament plastic sutures for an ICA anastomosis and 9-0 monofilament plastic sutures for middle cerebral artery (MCA) anastomosis

◈ After checking the patency of the bypass, a temporary clip is placed on the graft, close to the anastomosis, and the graft is flushed with heparinized saline.

◈ The temporary clip on the recipient artery is removed.

◈ With use of a chest tube, and with attention paid so as not to kink the vessel, the graft is tunneled in a preauricular-subzygomatic or retroauricular direction toward the cervical incision, unless the IMAX is used for the proximal anastomosis.

◈ The donor vessel is temporary clamped and an 8- to 10-mm arteriotomy is performed.

Surgical Pearl

With the excimer laser assisted nonocclusive anastomosis (ELANA) technique,[23] one can perform an intracranial anastomosis without temporary artery occlusion (see page 324). However, this technique can be applied only to ICA/proximal M1 vessels, and the practitioner needs training in the use of special laser equipment.

Surgical Pearl

Alternatively, tunneling is done through the submandibular-infratemporal route, which shortens the length of the bypass and eliminates the need for subcutaneous tunneling.[24]

◈ The graft is cut in a "fish-mouth" shape and in an appropriate length and is anastomosed to the cervical artery using 6-0 monofilament plastic sutures.

◈ After removal of the temporary clamps the patency of the bypass is tested by visual inspection, indocyanine green (ICG) videoangiography, flow measurement, intraoperative DSA, or a combination of these methods.

◈ Depending on the type of pathology, one can proceed with resection of the tumor or can plan additional surgery on another day.

◈ The wounds are closed after meticulous hemostasis, avoiding compression of the bypass.

Postoperative

Patients are continuously monitored in the first 24 to 48 hours after the surgery for normal to slightly elevated blood pressure. Patients are kept on acetylsalicylic acid for at least 6 months. A postoperative radiographic investigation of the intracranial vasculature (CTA, MRA, or DSA) is performed soon after surgery.

Complications

The most severe complication is occlusion of the graft, which can result in cerebral infarction. This is most often due to technical surgical errors, such as a poor anastomosis, kinking of the graft, or compression on it, but can also be a result of the underlying pathology.[12,20] Other possible complications of bypass surgery are listed in **Table 25.4**.

Table 25.4   Postoperative Complications After Bypass Surgery[12]

Complication	Possible Cause
Early postoperative infarct	Graft occlusion, arterial (graft) spasm, prolonged occlusion time, embolism, perforator occlusion
Late postoperative infarct	Graft thrombosis
Remote intraparenchymal hemorrhage	Hyperperfusion
Postoperative hematoma	Aspirin use, heparinization (if used), leakage from anastomosis
Graft infection	Most common in combination with malignant tumors and after radiation
Wound infection, meningitis	Long surgical exposure

694 Skull Base Surgery

Outcome

Patient selection and graft patency are the major factors that influence outcome. The graft patency is around 95%, when performed by an experienced surgical team.[12,20] The combined stroke rate in studies performed in the 1990s was 10 to 15%, and half of those patients had a favorable recovery.[13,20]

■ Dural Arteriovenous Fistulas

A dAVF is an arteriovenous shunt between a dural artery/arteries and a venous drainage channel, such as a leptomeningeal vein or dural sinus. DAVFs are most commonly supplied by branches of the ECA and ICA, meningeal branches of the vertebral artery, and occasionally by pial branches of the cerebral arteries.[25]

- They are named after the dural sinus into which they drain or their anatomic location, and are most commonly located at the transverse, sigmoid, and cavernous sinuses.[26]
- The fistulas that are considered for surgical treatment are most often located in the anterior fossa, or at the tentorial, petrosal, or superior sagittal sinus.[27,28]
- Classification systems must be taken into account when determining the timing of a surgical intervention, as each type of dAVF has a different natural history.
- Patients who present with intracranial hemorrhage are at high risk for early recurrent hemorrhage and need urgent treatment.
- The goal of treatment of dAVF is obliteration of the fistula or selective disconnection between the artery and cortical venous drainage, and can be achieved by endovascular treatment, surgery, radiosurgery, or a combination of these modalities.
- An endovascular approach is the mainstay of dAVF treatment, and surgical treatment is indicated in cases where endovascular treatment has failed or is not feasible, such as difficult access or when occlusion of the sinus is not desirable. Radiosurgery is considered in cases where other treatment options are too risky or have failed.

Epidemiology

Dural arteriovenous fistulas account for 10 to 15% of intracranial vascular malformations.[10,27] They typically occur at 40 to 70 years of age, and the male/female ratio depends on the type of fistula.[25] Borden type I fistulas **(Table 25.5)** are most often located at the cavernous and transverse/sigmoid junction and are more common in females. Anterior fossa and tentorial dAVFs, which tend to present more often as a Borden type II or III, are more common in males.[25,28]

Table 25.5   Dural Arteriovenous Fistula (dAVF) Classification Systems and Course of the Pathology

Type	Borden et al[29] Classification	Cognard et al[25] Classification	Course
I	Antegrade flow into dural sinus	Antegrade flow into dural sinus	Benign
II	Type I with retrograde flow into cortical vein		Aggressive
		Type I with reflux:	
IIa		• Retrograde into dural sinus	Benign
IIb		• Retrograde into cortical veins	Aggressive
IIc		• Retrograde into dural sinus and cortical veins	Aggressive
III	Exclusively retrograde flow into cortical vein	Exclusively drainage into cortical veins without venous ectasia	Aggressive
IV		Exclusively drainage into cortical veins with venous ectasia	Aggressive
V		Intracranial dAVF with drainage into medullary veins	Aggressive

The majority of dAVFs are believed to be acquired, but a specific event in the clinical history and syndromes associated with vascular fragility increase the risk for their development **(Table 25.6)**.

Etiology/Pathophysiology

The exact pathophysiological mechanism for the development of dAVFs is not completely understood. One theory is that the development of the fistula is triggered by sinus thrombosis, after which microscopic fistulas develop in the wall of the sinus influenced by angiogenic factors, such as vascular endothelial growth factor (VEGF). These fistulas expand afterward, owing to shear stress and the eventual recanalization of the thrombosed sinus.[35] In the end, the fistula

Table 25.6   Factors that Contribute to dAVF Formation

Specific event	
Previous trauma,[30] sinus infection,[25] cranial surgery,[31] sinus thrombosis,[32] meningitis,[33] hypercoagulable state[34]	
Syndrome[10]	
Ehlers-Danlos, fibromuscular dysplasia, neurofibromatosis type 1	

recruits new arterial feeding vessels with secondary venous hypertension, which can lead to leptomeningeal retrograde drainage.[36]

Clinical Presentation

The clinical presentation of dAVFs depends on the location and pattern of venous drainage, and is divided into nonhemorrhagic neurologic deficits and hemorrhagic presentation (**Table 25.7**).

The two most commonly used classification systems are those of Borden et al[29] and Cognard et al[25] (**Table 25.5**). The classification systems divide the fistulas into those with a benign course and those with an aggressive course. This depends mainly on the absence or presence or cortical venous drainage (CVD).

- Benign fistulas drain directly into a dural sinus and do not cause intracranial hemorrhage, although approximately 1% can transform into a more aggressive type and can subsequently cause hemorrhage.[28] Approximately 13% of benign fistulas resolve spontaneously.[37]
- Neurologic deficits in "aggressive" fistulas are a result of venous hypertension or intracranial hemorrhage. The annual hemorrhage risk is estimated to be 6 to 10%, with many factors increasing this risk, such as hemorrhagic presentation, isolated cortical drainage, and venous ectasia.[27–29,35,38,39] Patients who present with hemorrhage not uncommonly develop recurrent hemorrhage within days to weeks, so urgent treatment may be warranted.[25,38] "Aggressive" fistulas that are found incidentally without hemorrhage or neurologic deficits may have a more favorable course, with an annual hemorrhage rate of 1.5 to 2.0%.[28,35]

Table 25.7   Clinical Symptoms and Most Common Causes

Clinical Symptom	Most common Cause
Pulsatile tinnitus	Benign fistula
Ophthalmoplegia	
Proptosis	
Chemosis	Fistula at cavernous sinus
Retro-orbital pain	
Decreased visual acuity	
Headache	Benign fistula, venous hypertension, intracranial hemorrhage
Seizure	Venous hypertension, intracranial hemorrhage
Parkinsonism	Venous hypertension
Cerebellar symptoms	Venous hypertension, intracranial hemorrhage
Cognitive decline	Venous hypertension
Acute neurological deficit	Intracranial hemorrhage (parenchymal, subarachnoid, intraventricular, subdural)

Investigations and Imaging

The "gold standard" for imaging a dAVF is the DSA, because of its sensitivity and ability to delineate the exact arterial supply and venous drainage in order to classify the fistula. Other investigations, such as MRA and CTA or time-resolved imaging techniques, can be useful for identifying the anatomic location of the fistula, screening, and follow-up,[40] but are not sensitive enough to rule out the presence of a dAVF.[41] These techniques can be used as adjuncts by showing the anatomic location of dilated veins and venous pouches, the signs of venous hypertension and proptosis, and the bony relationships.[40]

Treatment

- Treatment of benign fistulas is not recommended, unless the symptoms, such as tinnitus, are intolerable for the patient. Carotid-cavernous fistulas may need treatment for proptosis, chemosis, increased intraocular pressure, and visual decline in the absence of retrograde cortical venous drainage.
- Patients who present with clinical symptoms related to venous hypertension or hemorrhage most often need direct admission, clinical stabilization (if necessary), and a plan for managing the fistula as soon as possible.
- The mainstay of treatment is endovascular therapy.[10,40,42] Surgical treatment is indicated in cases when endovascular treatment has failed or is not feasible, such as difficult access or when occlusion of a sinus is not desirable. Radiosurgery is considered in cases where other treatment options are not feasible or have failed.[43]
- Sometimes multiple procedures or a combination of treatments is the best way to obliterate the dAVF.

Endovascular Therapy[35,40]

- Complete elimination of the dAVF is usually necessary because incomplete treatment allows recruitment of new fistulous vessels and recurrence of symptoms.
- If complete elimination is not feasible or too risky, selective disconnection of the CVD can be considered.[44]
- Transarterial embolization can be done in the vast majority of fistulas, using coils or embolic agents, but seldom results in angiographic cure.
- Transvenous embolization is often the preferred approach and is aimed at preservation of normal venous drainage patterns. It can be advantageous for dAVFs with multiple arterial feeders (see also Chapter 12, page 298).

Surgery

- Fistulas that are most commonly amenable for surgical resection are located in the anterior fossa and tentorial, petrosal, or superior sagittal sinus.[40,42,45,46]

- General surgical recommendations:
  - ○ Coagulation of meningeal arteries and veins, occlusion of the draining dural sinus, resection of abnormal dura, skeletonization of the dural sinus, and selective disconnection of CVD are surgical options.[40,44]
  - ○ Proper exposure of the arterialized vein is necessary to check for complete obliteration of the fistula.
  - ○ ICG videoangiography, Doppler ultrasound, and intraoperative angiography can be helpful in the surgical strategy and to check if the fistula is obliterated.[47–49]

  > **Surgical Anatomy Pearl**
  >
  > Selective disconnection of CVD is the best surgical option for fistulas with isolated CVD or in cases where the draining sinus cannot be sacrified.[44,47]

- Surgical approaches in relation to the location of fistulas:
  - ○ Superior sagittal sinus fistula: tailored craniotomy and resection/incision of abnormal dura or falx or selective disconnection of CVD
  - ○ Anterior fossa fistula: unilateral or bifrontal craniotomy and resection/ incision of abnormal falx and anterior fossa dura or selective disconnection of CVD
  - ○ Cavernous sinus fistula: rarely necessary, pterional craniotomy and usually simple disconnection of CVD
  - ○ Petrosal sinus fistula: subtemporal or retrosigmoidal craniotomy and usually simple disconnection of CVD by clipping superior petrosal vein(s)[42]

  > **Surgical Anatomy Pearl**
  >
  > Bilateral exposure of the falx is advised in order not to miss a fistula on the opposite site of the falx.[42]

  - ○ Transverse-sigmoid junction fistula: combined supra- and infratentorial craniotomy with exposure and occlusion of the sinus; or skeletonization of the sinus with selective disconnection of CVD with a tailored (supra- or infratentorial) craniotomy
  - ○ Tentorial fistula: supra- or infratentorial craniotomy and resection of abnormal tentorium or selective disconnection of CVD

Radiosurgery

- General recommendations[43]:
  - ○ The latency period for occlusion of the fistula is a major disadvantage in the treatment of "aggressive" fistulas.
  - ○ The target is the arterial feeders, to induce diminished shunting and eventual obliteration.
  - ○ A radiation dose of 20 to 25 Gy can achieve an angiographic obliteration rate of 65 to 93%, with comparable percentages of clinical improvement,

although large series of cases have yet to be published with good long-term follow-up (see also Chapter 30, page 787).

Complications

Complications are either deficits that occur after hemorrhage of a conservatively treated dAVF or treatment related. The deficits that occur after hemorrhage are related to the location and the type of hemorrhage (parenchymal, subarachnoid, intraventricular, or subdural).

Treatment-related complications are either general or disease specific (**Table 25.8**). The overall rate of permanent complications after embolization is reported to be 4 to 8%, whereas surgery of Borden grade III fistulas caused complications in 8 to 17%.[28,35,40,44] The complication rate after radiosurgery is approximately 9%.[43]

Outcome

Even with a hemorrhagic presentation, patients can achieve an excellent outcome in 71% of cases.[45] Partially or untreated "aggressive" fistulas were associated with 45% mortality (nine of 20 patients) in one series.[39] The obliteration rate for the various treatment methods ranges from 71 to 88% for endovascular treatment to 96% for surgical treatment,[28,40] with a higher obliteration rate after combined treatments. More important, the rate of resolution of symptoms is higher because some treatments aim at selectively disconnecting the CVD instead of completely obliterating the fistula.[44]

Table 25.8   Most Common Complications per Treatment Modality

Treatment Modality	Complications
Embolization	Groin hematoma, radiation-induced injury, catheter entrapment, cranial nerve deficit, memory impairment, cerebral infarct, venous hypertension, vessel perforation with intracranial hemorrhage
Surgery	Significant blood loss, infection, postoperative hemorrhage, seizure, cranial nerve deficit, memory dysfunction, cerebral infarct
Radiosurgery	Hemorrhage during latency period, headache, nausea, malaise, radiation-induced injury, cranial nerve deficit

■ References

Boldfaced references are of particular importance.

1. Lawton MT, Spetzler RF. Surgical strategies for giant intracranial aneurysms. Acta Neurochir Suppl (Wien) 1999;72:141–156

2. **Gonzalez LF, Amin-Hanjani S, Bambakidis NC, Spetzler RF. Skull base approaches to the basilar artery. Neurosurg Focus 2005;19:E3**

3. Sekhar LN, Kalia KK, Yonas H, Wright DC, Ching H. Cranial base approaches to intracranial aneurysms in the subarachnoid space. Neurosurgery 1994;35:472–481, discussion 481–483

4. Andaluz N, Van Loveren HR, Keller JT, Zuccarello M. Anatomic and clinical study of the orbitopterional approach to anterior communicating artery aneurysms. Neurosurgery 2003;52:1140–1148, discussion 1148–1149

5. Andaluz N, Zuccarello M. Anterior communicating artery aneurysm surgery through the orbitopterional approach: long-term follow-up in a series of 75 consecutive patients. Skull Base 2008;18:265–274

6. Cunha AM, Aguiar GB, Carvalho FM, Simões EL, Pinto JR, Telles C. The orbitopterional approach for large and giant middle cerebral artery aneurysms: a report of two cases and literature review. Skull Base 2010;20:261–267

7. Ulrich NH, Kockro RA, Bellut D, et al. Brainstem cavernoma surgery with the support of pre- and postoperative diffusion tensor imaging: initial experiences and clinical course of 23 patients. Neurosurg Rev 2014;37:481–491, discussion 492

8. Figueiredo EG, Zabramski JM, Deshmukh P, Crawford NR, Spetzler RF, Preul MC. Comparative analysis of anterior petrosectomy and transcavernous approaches to retrosellar and upper clival basilar artery aneurysms. Neurosurgery 2006;58(1, Suppl): ONS13–ONS21, discussion ONS13–ONS21

9. **Abla AA, Turner JD, Mitha AP, Lekovic G, Spetzler RF. Surgical approaches to brainstem cavernous malformations. Neurosurg Focus 2010;29:E8**

10. Winn R. Neurological Surgery, 6th ed. Philadelphia: Elsevier; 2011

11. **Mura J, Rojas-Zalazar D, de Oliveira E. Revascularization for complex skull base tumors. Skull Base 2005;15:63–70**

12. Berg-Johnsen J, Helseth E, Langmoen IA. Cerebral revascularization for skull base tumors. World Neurosurg 2014;82:575–576

13. Lawton MT, Spetzler RF. Internal carotid artery sacrifice for radical resection of skull base tumors. Skull Base Surg 1996;6:119–123

14. Kalani MY, Kalb S, Martirosyan NL, et al. Cerebral revascularization and carotid artery resection at the skull base for treatment of advanced head and neck malignancies. J Neurosurg 2013;118:637–642

15. Abdulrauf SI. Extracranial-to-intracranial bypass using radial artery grafting for complex skull base tumors: technical note. Skull Base 2005;15:207–213

16. Chin SC, Jen YM, Chen CY, Som PM. Necrotic nasopharyngeal mucosa: an ominous MR sign of a carotid artery pseudoaneurysm. AJNR Am J Neuroradiol 2005;26:414–416

17. Tarr RW, Jungreis CA, Horton JA, et al. Complications of preoperative balloon test occlusion of the internal carotid arteries: experience in 300 cases. Skull Base Surg 1991;1:240–244

18. Origitano TC, al-Mefty O, Leonetti JP, DeMonte F, Reichman OH. Vascular considerations and complications in cranial base surgery. Neurosurgery 1994;35:351–362, discussion 362–363

19. Pandey P, Steinberg GK. Neurosurgical advances in the treatment of moyamoya disease. Stroke 2011;42:3304–3310

20. Sekhar LN, Bucur SD, Bank WO, Wright DC. Venous and arterial bypass grafts for difficult tumors, aneurysms, and occlusive vascular lesions: evolution of surgical treatment and improved graft results. Neurosurgery 1999;44:1207–1223, discussion 1223–1224

21. Abdulrauf SI, Sweeney JM, Mohan YS, Palejwala SK. Short segment internal maxillary artery to middle cerebral artery bypass: a novel technique for extracranial-to-intracranial bypass. Neurosurgery 2011;68:804–808, discussion 808–809

22. Nossek E, Costantino PD, Eisenberg M, et al. Internal maxillary artery-middle cerebral artery bypass: infratemporal approach for subcranial-intracranial (SC-IC) bypass. Neurosurgery 2014;75:87–95

23. Langer DJ, Van Der Zwan A, Vajkoczy P, Kivipelto L, Van Doormaal TP, Tulleken CA. Excimer laser-assisted nonocclusive anastomosis. An emerging technology for use in the creation of intracranial-intracranial and extracranial-intracranial cerebral bypass. Neurosurg Focus 2008;24:E6

24. Couldwell WT, Liu JK, Amini A, Kan P. Submandibular-infratemporal interpositional carotid artery bypass for cranial base tumors and giant aneurysms. Neurosurgery 2006;59(4, Suppl 2):ONS353–ONS359, discussion ONS359–ONS360

25. Cognard C, Gobin YP, Pierot L, et al. Cerebral dural arteriovenous fistulas: clinical and angiographic correlation with a revised classification of venous drainage. Radiology 1995;194:671–680

26. Kirsch M, Liebig T, Kühne D, Henkes H. Endovascular management of dural arteriovenous fistulas of the transverse and sigmoid sinus in 150 patients. Neuroradiology 2009;51:477–483

27. Söderman M, Pavic L, Edner G, Holmin S, Andersson T. Natural history of dural arteriovenous shunts. Stroke 2008;39:1735–1739

28. Gross BA, Dunn IF, Du R, Al-Mefty O. Petrosal approaches to brainstem cavernous malformations. Neurosurg Focus 2012;33:E10

29. Borden JA, Wu JK, Shucart WA. A proposed classification for spinal and cranial dural arteriovenous fistulous malformations and implications for treatment. J Neurosurg 1995;82:166–179

30. Dennery JM, Ignacio BS. Post-traumatic arteriovenous fistula between the external carotid arteries and the superior longitudinal sinus: report of a case. Can J Surg 1967;10:333–336

31. Sakaki T, Morimoto T, Nakase H, Kakizaki T, Nagata K. Dural arteriovenous fistula of the posterior fossa developing after surgical occlusion of the sigmoid sinus. Report of five cases. J Neurosurg 1996;84:113–118

32. Nishio A, Ohata K, Tsuchida K, et al. Dural arteriovenous fistula involving the superior sagittal sinus following sinus thrombosis—case report. Neurol Med Chir (Tokyo) 2002;42:217–220

33. Tsutsumi S, Yasumoto Y, Ito M, Oishi H, Arai H, Yoritaka A. Atypical dural arteriovenous fistula associated with meningitis. Neurol Med Chir (Tokyo) 2008;48:68–71

34. van Dijk JM, TerBrugge KG, Van der Meer FJ, Wallace MC, Rosendaal FR. Thrombophilic factors and the formation of dural arteriovenous fistulas. J Neurosurg 2007; 107:56–59

35. Hacein-Bey L, Konstas AA, Pile-Spellman J. Natural history, current concepts, classification, factors impacting endovascular therapy, and pathophysiology of cerebral and spinal dural arteriovenous fistulas. Clin Neurol Neurosurg 2014;121:64–75

36. Awad IA, Little JR, Akarawi WP, Ahl J. Intracranial dural arteriovenous malformations: factors predisposing to an aggressive neurological course. J Neurosurg 1990;72:839–850

37. Satomi J, van Dijk JM, Terbrugge KG, Willinsky RA, Wallace MC. Benign cranial dural arteriovenous fistulas: outcome of conservative management based on the natural history of the lesion. J Neurosurg 2002;97:767–770

38. Duffau H, Lopes M, Janosevic V, et al. Early rebleeding from intracranial dural arteriovenous fistulas: report of 20 cases and review of the literature. J Neurosurg 1999; 90:78–84

39. van Dijk JM, terBrugge KG, Willinsky RA, Wallace MC. Clinical course of cranial dural arteriovenous fistulas with long-term persistent cortical venous reflux. Stroke 2002;33:1233–1236

40. Gandhi D, Chen J, Pearl M, Huang J, Gemmete JJ, Kathuria S. Intracranial dural arteriovenous fistulas: classification, imaging findings, and treatment. AJNR Am J Neuroradiol 2012;33:1007–1013

41. Cohen SD, Goins JL, Butler SG, Morris PP, Browne JD. Dural arteriovenous fistula: diagnosis, treatment, and outcomes. Laryngoscope 2009;119:293–297

42. Macdonald RL. Neurosurgical Operative Atlas. New York: Thieme; 2009

43. Dalyai RT, Ghobrial G, Chalouhi N, et al. Radiosurgery for dural arterio-venous fistulas: a review. Clin Neurol Neurosurg 2013;115:512–516

44. van Dijk JM, TerBrugge KG, Willinsky RA, Wallace MC. Selective disconnection of cortical venous reflux as treatment for cranial dural arteriovenous fistulas. J Neurosurg 2004;101:31–35

45. Daniels DJ, Vellimana AK, Zipfel GJ, Lanzino G. Intracranial hemorrhage from dural arteriovenous fistulas: clinical features and outcome. Neurosurg Focus 2013;34:E15

46. Eftekhar B, Morgan MK. Surgical management of dural arteriovenous fistulas of the transverse-sigmoid sinus in 42 patients. J Clin Neurosci 2013;20:532–535

47. Youssef PP, Schuette AJ, Cawley CM, Barrow DL. Advances in surgical approaches to dural fistulas. Neurosurgery 2014;74(Suppl 1):S32–S41

48. Schuette AJ, Cawley CM, Barrow DL. Indocyanine green videoangiography in the management of dural arteriovenous fistulae. Neurosurgery 2010;67:658–662, discussion 662

49. Beynon C, Herweh C, Rohde S, Unterberg AW, Sakowitz OW. Intraoperative indocyanine green angiography for microsurgical treatment of a craniocervical dural arteriovenous fistula. Clin Neurol Neurosurg 2012;114:696–698

26 Dural Sinus Management

In skull base surgery, and especially in the posterior skull base approaches, it is of paramount importance to manage the dural sinuses, bridging veins (e.g., tentorial, petrosal), and the vein of Labbé.

Whenever possible, aim to preserve the sinuses and bridging veins, as occlusion may lead to a number of often unpredictable events, despite the use of pre- and intraoperative tests. A meningioma with a dominant sinus invasion may be best managed by subtotal-partial resection followed by radiotherapy of the intrasinus component; in rare situations and in expert hands, a total resection with venous reconstruction may be achievable.

- Preoperative magnetic resonance imaging (MRI), magnetic resonance venography (MRV), computed tomography venography (CTV), or cerebral angiogram are used to determine the involvement of the dural sinuses in the different pathologies (e.g., meningioma invasion of the sinus vs. compression of the wall), as well as the different anatomic variations of size and dominancy of the sinuses and the collateral drainage of the occluded sinuses.
- Preservation of the sinuses/veins is the main goal of surgery. Their reconstruction or their sacrifice are dependent on the existence of outflow collaterals, in order to avoid brain/cerebellum venous infarct and/or swelling.

Anatomic variations of the dural sinuses, vein of Labbé, and bridging veins should be studied in detail before deciding on the appropriate treatment (e.g., surgery vs. radiosurgery) and on the appropriate lateral approaches to the middle and posterior skull base (e.g., subtemporal/transpetrous approaches).

■ Anatomy of the Dural Sinuses and Vein of Labbé

Fig. 26.1 portrays the anatomy; also see page 33.

- In type 1 invasion (see **Fig. 26.2**), the lateral wall of the tumor may be peeled away, whereas reconstructive or nonreconstructive techniques have to be used for the other types.

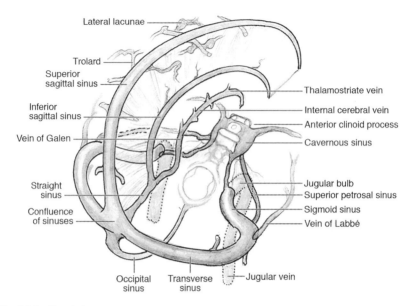

Fig. 26.1 Dural sinuses anatomy.

- In general, occlusion of one cavernous sinus, superior petrosal sinuses, and nondominant transverse and sigmoid sinuses is well tolerated by patients. Occlusion of the anterior third of the superior sagittal sinus is generally tolerated when the anterior cortical veins have collaterals; otherwise, there is still the risk of frontal lobe venous infarction/edema.
- Occlusion of a nondominant transverse sinus or a patent contralateral sinus is generally well tolerated by patients, but pseudotumor cerebri can develop, with subsequent headache and other symptoms related to raised intracranial pressure. There can be neuro-ophthalmological complications as well.[2]
- Iatrogenic cavernous sinus occlusion done intentionally by the skull base surgeon is usually well tolerated as long as the sinus is not overpacked. Overpacking can lead to cranial neuropathy, or internal carotid artery (or its branches) compression or occlusion.

❖ Intraoperative occlusion test[3–5]:

- There is uncontrolled evidence to support the use of intraoperative test occlusion.
- ◈ Insert a 20-gauge butterfly needle into the sinus for measuring the venous pressure (normally < 15 mmHg, but it is related to the position of the head).

Sinus Invasion Classification System[1] (Fig. 26.2)

Type 1: attachment to the outer layer of the sinus wall
Type 2: tumor fragment inside the lateral recess
Type 3: invasion of the lateral wall
Type 4: invasion of the lateral wall and roof
Type 5: complete sinus occlusion
Type 6: complete sinus occlusion with invasion of the contralateral wall

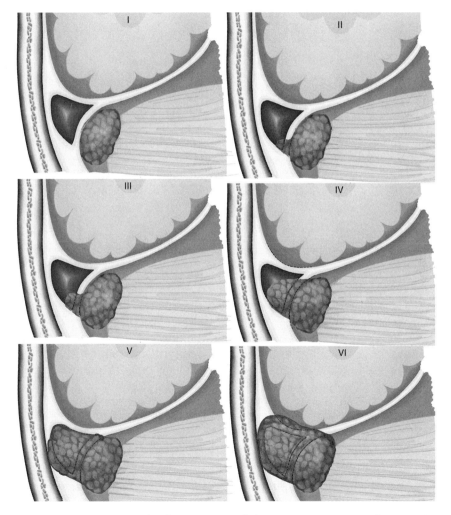

Fig. 26.2 Sinus invasions classification systems,[1] showing representations of a tumor invading the transverse sinus.

◈   By means of a pressure transducer, monitor the intrasinus pressure for at least 5 minutes before and after the application of a temporary clip (consider the risk of sinus wall injury by the application of the clip).
◈   Check for increasing pressure, cranial/cerebellar swelling, and changes in evoked potentials. In cases of swelling or pressure increases, the sinus cannot be sacrificed or it has to be reconstructed after sacrifice.

■ Reconstruction Techniques

- Small defects in the walls of the dural sinuses may be directly repaired by suturing with 5-0 or 6-0 Prolene, with or without a patch or graft.
- Application of hemostatic materials is also often successful, although efforts must be made to avoid migration of the material into the sinuses, causing thrombosis and potentially leading to pulmonary embolism. Fibrin-based sealants are the quickest solution for dural defects, although they may cause thrombosis.
- Local dura mater, temporal fascia, pericranium, and fascia lata or synthetic graft material can be used for patching.
- When defects are large and it is not possible to repair them by means of direct repair or sealants, graft reconstruction may be indicated.

■ Donors

Donors can be the saphenous vein (e.g., suture end-to-end), external jugular vein, radial artery (heparinized and sutured end-to-side[3]), or synthetic grafts (although they might entail a higher risk of thrombosis, irrespective of the use of anticoagulants[6]).

During grafting, temporary occlusion of the sinus may be achieved by using Surgicel, Surgifoam® (Ethicon, Bridgewater, NJ), balloons, or aneurysm clips, although endothelium damage should be avoided in order to lower the risk of thrombosis. As a result, plugging the lumen with Surgicel or leaving a residual tumor may be considered safer than a bypass.[6]

■ Examples of Bypasses

- Reconstruction of vein of Labbé by using a short saphenous vein bypass graft[7]
- Sinojugular bypass in case of occlusion of posterior third of the superior sagittal sinus, torcular, predominant lateral sinus, or internal jugular veins[8]

■ Medical Management After Surgery

After dural sinus/vein reconstruction, it may be necessary to use anticoagulation therapy to avoid graft thrombosis. One method involves intravenous heparin (2,000 units) during reconstruction, as well as subcutaneous heparin after surgery for 1 to 3 weeks, followed by aspirin 325 mg orally daily for 3 months.

• Endovascular thrombolysis is a therapeutic option in cases of dural sinus thrombosis with an intact dural sinus wall, although the immediate postoperative status may be a contraindication for thrombolysis. Hydrocephalus/pseudotumor cerebri can be treated with acetazolamide, dexamethasone, lumbar puncture, or a ventriculoperitoneal or lumboperitoneal shunt placement.

■ Outcomes

Outcomes are related to the primary cause of the dural occlusion. In one series of gross total resection of meningiomas invading the dural sinuses, sinus reconstruction was performed in 21 of 38 cases (13 cases by direct suture and eight by using a patch). Postoperatively, the sinus was patent in 52.4% of cases, and narrow but patent in 33.3% of cases.[9]

• Bypasses that develop thrombosis over time can still initially enable the brain venous system to achieve a gradual and slow compensatory venous outflow over time.[6]
• The patient who develops thrombosis of the sigmoid or transverse sinus after posterior fossa surgery should have a workup to look for sources of thrombophilia such as protein C deficiency or activated protein C (APC) resistance, and should be considered for a period of anticoagulation, although little evidence exists for the exact risk of pulmonary embolism in this situation.[10,11]

■ References

Boldfaced references are of particular importance.
1. **Sindou MP, Alvernia JE. Results of attempted radical tumor removal and venous repair in 100 consecutive meningiomas involving the major dural sinuses. J Neurosurg 2006;105:514–525**
2. Keiper GL Jr, Sherman JD, Tomsick TA, Tew JM Jr. Dural sinus thrombosis and pseudotumor cerebri: unexpected complications of suboccipital craniotomy and translabyrinthine craniectomy. J Neurosurg 1999;91:192–197
3. **Sekhar LN, Chanda A, Morita A. Cerebral veins and dural sinuses: Preservation and reconstruction. In: Sekhar LN, Fessler RG, eds. Atlas of Neurosurgical Techniques: Brain. New York, Stuttgart: Thieme; 2006:379–395**

4. Sekhar LN, Chanda A, Morita A. The preservation and reconstruction of cerebral veins and sinuses. J Clin Neurosci 2002;9:391–399

5. Schmid-Elsaesser R, Steiger HJ, Yousry T, Seelos KC, Reulen HJ. Radical resection of meningiomas and arteriovenous fistulas involving critical dural sinus segments: experience with intraoperative sinus pressure monitoring and elective sinus reconstruction in 10 patients. Neurosurgery 1997;41:1005–1016, discussion 1016–1018

6. Sindou MP, Alvernia JE. Surgical management of the cerebral venous sinuses. In: De Monte F, McDermott MW, Al-Mefty O, eds. Al-Mefty's Meningiomas, 2nd ed. New York, Stuttgart: Thieme; 2011:356–363

7. Morita A, Sekhar LN. Reconstruction of the vein of Labbé by using a short saphenous vein bypass graft. Technical note. J Neurosurg 1998;89:671–675

8. Sindou M, Auque J, Jouanneau E. Neurosurgery and the intracranial venous system. Acta Neurochir Suppl (Wien) 2005;94:167–175

9. Mantovani A, Di Maio S, Ferreira MJ, Sekhar LN. Management of meningiomas invading the major dural venous sinuses: operative technique, results, and potential benefit for higher grade tumors. World Neurosurg 2014;82:455–467

10. Ferro JM, Canhão P. Acute treatment of cerebral venous and dural sinus thrombosis. Curr Treat Options Neurol 2008;10:126–137

11. Ferro JM, Canhão P, Bousser MG, Stam J, Barinagarrementeria F, Stolz E; ISCVT Investigators. Cerebral venous thrombosis with nonhemorrhagic lesions: clinical correlates and prognosis. Cerebrovasc Dis 2010;29:440–445

27 Skull Base Reconstruction Techniques

Surgical resection of skull base tumors has improved because of our expanded ability to reconstruct cranial base defects. The basic principle of skull base reconstruction is the separation of the cranial contents from the sinonasal, orbital, or oral compartments. The treatment of cranial base tumors is most often multimodal, including radiation and chemotherapy; the principles, therefore, require the surgeon to consider the possibility and implications of adjuvant treatment, including delayed wound healing, infection, and resorption of non-vascularized tissues.

More recent advances in the endoscopic approach to the skull base have been paired with novel techniques in endoscopic reconstruction and may lead to an inside-out consideration of reconstruction rather than the traditional outside-in approach.

■ Classification of Skull Base Defects

The ideal classification system would categorize defects in a manner that would relate to a specific set of reconstructive approaches. Such a classification system has not yet been developed because of the anatomic complexity of the skull base and the complexity and variability of the defects. There needs to be a balance between making the system simple enough for effective communication among clinicians but complex enough to be useful as a defect-based decision-making tool.

There are several classification systems that categorize skull base defects. Irish and colleagues[1] classified tumors into skull base regions (I, II, and III) based on anatomic boundaries and tumor growth patterns (see Chapter 23, **Fig. 23.1**, page 647). This classification system is useful for describing the specific area of the skull base that requires reconstruction. A more sophisticated description of skull base defects has been developed, with the aim of comparing end results using different reconstructive techniques.[2] This classification takes into account the following anatomic components: (1) dura, (2) bone, (3) skin, (4) mucosa,

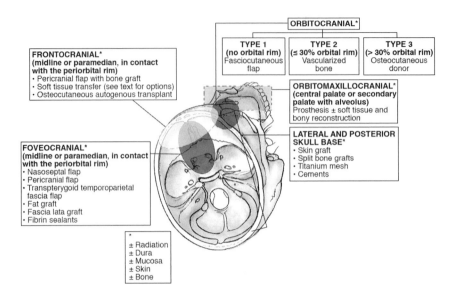

Fig. 27.1 Skull base reconstruction schema.

(5) cavity, (6) neurologic status, and (7) carotid artery. The classification system is very useful for describing the defect, determining the treatment plan, predicting potential postreconstructive complications, and counseling patients.

A classification system involving subdivisions of the anterior cranial fossa defects into compartments that direct the reconstructive algorithm is described here. In the anterior skull base, the regions are foveocranial, frontocranial, orbitocranial, and orbitomaxillocranial **(Fig. 27.1)**.

■ Anterior Defects: Foveocranial

Foveocranial defects are anterior cranial fossa defects that are in the median or paramedian location and that involve the ethmoid bone or the inner table of the frontal bone. They do not involve the orbit or the outer table of the frontal bone. Because the frontal and orbital rim bony structural supports remain intact, reconstruction of this defect is focused on separation of the cranial compartment from the nasal cavity with a watertight dural seal and use of vascularized tissue to prevent cerebrospinal fluid (CSF) leak and intracranial infectious complications. The foveocranial defect is well suited for endoscopic approaches to skull base lesions. Recent innovations with local pedicled flaps, such as the nasoseptal flap, have facilitated more extensive exposures and reliable reconstruction.

Nasoseptal Flap

- The vascularized pedicled nasoseptal flap significantly enhanced the reconstruction of skull base defects following both standard and extended endoscopic approaches to the skull base.[3–5]
- The risk of postoperative CSF leak with the nasoseptal flap is 5%, and is comparable to that with open reconstructive techniques.[4]

❖ Surgical Steps

- ◈ The pedicled nasoseptal flap utilizes blood supply from the posterior nasoseptal artery and is designed by making two parallel incisions, with the inferior one placed along the septum over the maxillary crest.
- ◈ When planning the flap, if the ipsilateral olfactory bulb is not involved in the resection, then the superior incision should be planned 1 cm below the most superior aspect of the septum in order to preserve the olfactory epithelium.
- ◈ See Chapter 16 for further details (page 420).

Pericranial Flap

- The pericranial flap is one of the most commonly used flaps in skull base surgery[6,7] (see Chapter 14, **Fig. 14.3**, page 342).
- For open skull base resections, the pericranial flap is the best option for supporting a dural closure and separating the cranial and nasal cavities for foveocranial defects.
- Studies utilizing injection data and blood vessel patterns show that the blood supply to pericranial flaps almost entirely depends on the deep branches and a variable component of the superficial branches of the supraorbital and the supratrochlear vessels.[6]
- The risk of CSF leak after reconstruction using this flap has been consistently reported to be approximately 5%.
- The flap is thin, pliable, and reported to be well vascularized even after regional irradiation.
- A minimally invasive endoscopic pericranial flap has been described for use in conjunction with an expanded endoscopic approach.[8] This approach uses an incision along the bicoronal line and the removal of bone in the region of the nasion to deliver the flap to the foveocranial defect.

❖ Surgical Steps

- ◈ Harvest of the pericranial flap begins near the bicoronal incision and involves elevation in the subgaleal plane down to the level of the supraorbital rims; in the supraorbital region, dissection is done so as to identify the supraorbital notch and free the supraorbital vascular bundle.

◈ If a foramen is present, a 4-mm osteotome can be used to preserve the neurovascular bundle and maintain the arterial supply to the flap.

◈ The pericranial flap is placed intracranially before the supraorbital bone is re-secured to enable coverage of the frontal bar.

Transpterygoid Temporoparietal Fascia Flap

• The temporoparietal fascial flap can be passed through a pterional bur hole to the foveocranial defect.

• This is an excellent alternative if a pericranial flap has already been harvested, particularly for patients who have had endoscopic surgery and have not had an incision crossing the territory of the superficial temporal artery.

❖ Surgical Steps

◈ The temporoparietal fascia flap is supplied by the superficial temporal artery and vein, and has been utilized extensively in head and neck reconstruction.

◈ The pedicle is located just deep to the bicoronal incision and can be injured during the opening of the skin.

◈ An elevation just deep to the hair follicles is performed and can result in skin loss overlying the donor site.

◈ The deep layer is harvested after the superficial layer and includes the pericranium above the temporal line and the superficial layer of temporal fascia below the temporal line.

◈ This site is most useful in revision cases; unfortunately, the bicoronal incision has frequently damaged the pedicle.

■ Anterior Defects: Frontocranial

Frontocranial defects involve the frontal bone and the anterior cranial fossa, but do not entail orbital exenteration. Frontocranial defects without orbital exenteration require attention to repair of the periorbita, prevention of transmission of the cerebral pulse to the globe, proper position and function of the lids, proper attachment of the canthi, and patency of the lacrimal system. Because of the projection of the frontal bone, reconstruction must be performed to avoid major deformity. To optimize the cosmetic result and adequately support the orbital contents, anterior frontal bone defects greater than 30% of the length of the orbital rim should be reconstructed with bone. There are two options:

nonvascularized calvarial bone grafts, which are most suited to the nonradiated patient, and vascularized bone transfers, which are appropriate for radiated or chemoradiated patients. The literature would suggest lower rates of surgical complications in radiated patients when a vascularized autogenous flap is utilized.[9]

Pericranial Flap with Bone Graft

- The pericranial flap with calvarial bone graft is the reconstruction of choice if the patient has not been previously irradiated.
- The split calvarial bone can be harvested from the inner table of the craniotomy bone flap.
- Some authors have reported excellent results using pericranium to wrap nonvascularized bone grafts when used in an irradiated field.[10] The use of calvarial bone graft in a radiated field can result in healing, but the associated complication rate is unacceptably high compared with the results of using vascularized tissue transplantation.

❖ Surgical Steps

- ◈ The pericranial flap harvest was described earlier in the chapter.
- ◈ Split calvarial bone grafts are harvested from the outer table of the cranium after raising a bicoronal skin flap and pericranial flap, or by harvesting the inner table of the craniotomy bone flap.
- ◈ When harvesting a cranial bone graft, care must be taken to avoid full-thickness bone cuts and dural injury.
- ◈ Troughs are cut around the calvarial bone graft with a fissure bur.
- ◈ Then an oscillating offset saw blade or a curved osteotome is used to undercut the graft in the cancellous space and to free it from the underlying inner table.
- ◈ After inset of the bone graft, the pericranium should be closely applied to the graft to separate it from contaminated fields.

Soft Tissue Transfer: Radial Forearm, Anterolateral Thigh, Rectus Abdominis, Latissimus Dorsi

- Soft tissue reconstruction of the frontocranial defect is a good alternative for patients with frontal bar defects 30% or less of the orbital rim diameter, particularly in a radiated field.
- In addition, if cosmesis is not a priority, then these donor sites can be used for frontal bar defects greater than 30% of the orbital rim diameter.

❖ Surgical Steps

- **Radial forearm:**
  - ◈ The radial forearm autogenous transplant is an excellent option for low-volume reconstructions if local tissue, such as the pericranial flap, is absent. This donor site is reliable, has a long vascular pedicle, provides thin pliable tissue, and has been shown to be effective for closing CSF leaks.[11]
  - ◈ Potential disadvantages of the radial forearm transplant over local flaps include a longer operative time and an additional, although low, risk of hand morbidity.

- **Anterolateral thigh:**
  - ◈ The anterolateral thigh autogenous transplant based on the lateral femoral circumflex artery is a good option when the volume of the defect is greater than the volume that the radial forearm donor site can obliterate.
  - ◈ This donor site also contains ample fascia, which can be used for dural repair. The fascia can remain vascularized for dural closure. The authors of a series of seven patients reconstructed with anterolateral thigh free tissue reported no CSF leaks or meningitis after a mean follow-up of 10 months.[12]
  - ◈ The donor site of the anterolateral thigh flap can be closed primarily. If a perforator-based harvest is chosen, the volume of the reconstruction is easier to control because there is no muscle in the transplant that will atrophy and result in volume loss.

- **Rectus abdominis:**
  - ◈ The rectus abdominis autogenous transplant is the historical donor site of first choice in skull base reconstruction.[13]
  - ◈ The vascular pedicle anatomy is long and reliable, with the ability to transfer large amounts of skin, fat, muscle, and fascia.
  - ◈ If long-term precise volume contouring is desired, then the donor site can be harvested as a perforator-based transplant so that muscle atrophy will not adversely affect the reconstructed contour.
  - ◈ When harvested as a myocutaneous skin paddle, the rectus has a tendency to become ptotic if the volume of the flap exceeds the volume of the defect.
  - ◈ The pale color of the donor site is a poor match for Caucasian patients.
  - ◈ The rectus donor site also places the patient at risk for ventral hernia, which has been reported as high as 43% in some series. The risk of hernia can be lowered, particularly when perforator-based harvests are performed and the fascia is preserved.

- **Latissimus dorsi:**
  - ◈ The latissimus dorsi autogenous transplant is useful as a myocutaneous donor site for defects of a medium to high surface area and for wounds that are poorly vascularized and require a long vascular pedicle.

◈ This transplant is useful for patients with multiple surgeries or a history of radiation, for patients for whom re-irradiation is planned, and for patients known to have osteoradionecrosis.

◈ For many patients the donor site is composed of a relatively thin muscle and cutaneous layers.

◈ The muscle can be positioned on the dural surface to help ensure a watertight seal, or on the bone to help prevent osteoradionecrosis.

◈ A myogenous or myocutaneous paddle can be used in large areas of the forehead and scalp.

Osteocutaneous Autogenous Transplant

Bony reconstruction improves cosmesis for patients with frontal bone defects involving the brow greater than 30% of the orbital rim diameter, although no published report has determined the exact size of the defect requiring vascularized bone. However, an approach and grading system has been reported.[14] Osteocutaneous free tissue transfer provides better wound healing, improved frontal contour, better frontal lobe protection, and fewer long-term complications. The high risk of resorption, extrusion, or osteoradionecrosis of free bone grafts when radiation is anticipated makes vascularized bone an optimal choice for reconstruction. The ultimate failure rate of free bone grafts in radiated fields has been reported in different series, and the risk of complications is unacceptably high.[15]

❖ Surgical Steps

◈ The two donor sites for this defect are the radial bone and the scapular tip.

◈ The radial forearm donor site is useful for a small-volume frontal bar with small-volume soft tissue defects.

◈ The second site, the thoracodorsal dorsal artery scapular tip, is better for a slightly larger volume of bone and for soft tissue defects. This donor site is discussed later in the chapter.

■ Anterior Defects: Orbitocranial

Orbitocranial defects can be divided into three types.[16] Type I defects include orbital exenteration with an intact rim. For these patients a soft tissue donor site, such as a fasciocutaneous forearm flap or an anterolateral thigh (ALT), rectus, or latissimus dorsi perforator based cutaneous flap, may be performed. Type II defects involve 30% or less of the bony orbital rim, with or without orbital exenteration. Vascularized bone can be used to restore the orbital rim when reconstructing this type of defect, particularly for the infraorbital rim or in cases where cosmesis is a priority. Type III defects involve greater than 30% of the bony orbital rim, with or without orbital exenteration, in addition to cheek skin or bony malar eminence. For these patients, an osteocutaneous subscapular artery system of donor paddles may be used in order to independently address the orbital and facial defects. Bone is important for orbital support, malar projection, and cosmesis in the appropriate patient. To clarify the classification system and distinguish these defects from frontocranial defects, type II and III defects involve the lateral, inferior, or medial orbital skeleton.

In orbitocranial defects with an orbital exenteration, the major decision is whether to leave the cavity open or closed. An open cavity may be lined with local soft tissue flaps that separate the intracranial space from the orbital and nasal cavities, and then a prosthesis can be used to reconstruct the aesthetic contour. Closed orbital reconstruction is an approach that uses autogenous transplantation to restore the volume of the orbit, maintain the skin in its normal location, and restore the bony architecture. The ultimate decision of open versus closed depends on the needs of the patient and the experience and preferences of the surgeon.

■ Techniques

Prosthesis for Orbitocranial Defect Types I, II and III with Orbital Exenteration

- The reconstructive priority is separation of the intracranial space, developing adequate bony fixation points for craniofacial implants, and keeping the soft tissue reconstruction to a minimum to improve prosthesis retention.
- To separate the intracranial space, there are several soft tissue options that include the temporalis muscle free flap (such as the temporoparietal fascia flap [TPFF]) or the radial forearm free flap (RFFF).

❖ Temporalis muscle:

◈ The temporalis muscle is supplied by the deep temporal arteries, which anastomose with the middle temporal artery as it arises from the superficial temporal artery at the level of the zygomatic arch.

◈ The muscle flap can be rotated into the orbit through a fenestration in the lateral orbital wall.

◈ The temporalis muscle fascia is sutured to the region of the medial canthal ligament to prevent retraction.

◈ The temporalis has a limited arc of rotation and limited length for reconstruction of medial dural defects.

◈ In addition, the harvest site develops a concavity that is not aesthetically pleasing.

❖ Temporoparietal fascia flap:

◈ The TPFF is a thin, pliable flap that has a reliable blood supply, enables a large degree of rotation, has minimal donor-site morbidity, and a large area available for harvest.

◈ Because of its dependable blood supply, the TPFF can be used to support calvarial bone grafting in patients who are not undergoing radiation and limited bone grafting for those who will undergo radiation.

❖ Radial forearm fasciocutaneous flap:

◈ The radial forearm autogenous transplant is useful in open orbit reconstruction to close dural defects or ethmoid defects when a pericranial flap is not available for closure.

◈ It is used for patients opting for an open cavity with a prosthesis because it leaves sufficient space for the placement of the prosthesis and can help provide a vascularized bed for craniofacial implants.

❖ Fasciocutaneous radial forearm and perforator-based fasciocutaneous autogenous transplant for type I orbital defects:

◈ The fasciocutaneous radial forearm autogenous transplant is well suited for type I orbital defects when the patient elects a closed reconstruction.

◈ In utilizing this donor site, it is important to ensure that there is adequate fat in the forearm for orbital volume restoration.

◈ A sunken orbital contour is considered a failure of closed orbital reconstruction. It is important to ensure that the fat is well vascularized so the volume of the reconstruction is maintained.

◈ Perforator-based rectus abdominis, anterolateral thigh, and latissimus dorsi can be used to perform closed orbital reconstruction. The descriptions of these flaps were presented above.
  • The amount of fat and the pedicle length can be tailored to the volume needs and available recipient vessels.
  • These flaps are useful for this defect because of the ample available volume and pedicle length.

❖ **Perforator-based fasciocutaneous autogenous transplant for type II and III with orbital exenteration:**

◈ When perforator-based soft tissue flaps, including the rectus abdominis, ALT, and latissimus dorsi are used for type II and III defects with orbital exenteration, a recognized trade-off takes place because the orbital and malar defect is not restored, and there may be flap ptosis that results in an overall loss of craniofacial contour.

◈ The clinician must decide whether to opt for soft tissue alone with a predictable degree of contour loss or to pursue osseous reconstruction of the craniofacial skeleton.

◈ Although utilizing soft tissue alone is faster, technically easier, and very reliable, it does result in significant secondary bone deformities.

❖ **Osteocutaneous radial forearm for type II orbital defects with orbital exenteration:**

◈ The osteocutaneous radial forearm autogenous transplant is a reliable option in patients with orbital exenteration defects involving 30% or less of the orbital rim.

◈ Orbital reconstruction requires consideration of the bone position relative to the skin paddle.

◈ This bone is well suited for use in orbital rim reconstruction and may be osteotomized once.

❖ **Osteocutaneous thoracodorsal artery scapular tip for type II and III orbital defects with or without orbital exenteration:**

◈ The thoracodorsal artery scapular tip (TDAST) autogenous transplant has become more widely used in orbital reconstruction.[17]

◈ Reconstructive advantages of the TDAST for orbital reconstruction include a long pedicle and the ability to meet the three-dimensional requirements of the orbit.

◈ In addition, the scapula tip can be used without osteotomy for reconstruction of the orbital rim or malar eminence in the presence or absence of a globe.

■ Anterior Defects: Orbitomaxillocranial

Orbitomaxillocranial defects involve the orbit, facial skin, and palate and may create a communication from the oral cavity to the intracranial space. In the majority of the cases, this defect type includes an orbital exenteration. In these cases, reconstruction of the contour of the orbit with bone is performed to improve the aesthetic result because reconstruction of the malar eminence and infraorbital rim reestablishes midface projection and contour. The principles of reconstructing this defect are separation of the cranial cavity from the nasal cavity, separation of the oral cavity from the nasal cavity, projection of the premaxilla, maintenance of oral competence, and reestablishment of the malar/orbital complex. Although soft tissue reconstruction without bone requires less operative time and may be associated with fewer complications, the use of vascularized bone can be preferred because of its superior reconstruction of the craniofacial contour. If prosthetics are used, the cranial compartment requires separate closure, and retention of the prosthesis must be part of the reconstructive plan.

Technique

❖ Prosthesis

◈ Prosthetics can provide a less technically demanding, noninvasive method of achieving oronasal separation, establishing maxillary dentition, and reestablishing the aesthetic contour of the face.

◈ The soft tissue reconstruction also needs to address dural closure and coverage of exposed bone to facilitate the placement of the prosthesis.

◈ A prosthesis functions best in a dry, well-epithelialized cavity. Retention of the prosthesis can be accomplished with glue, magnets between the maxillary prosthesis and the facial prosthesis, or bone-anchored craniofacial implants.

◈ In the case of orbitomaxillocranial defects with a large cranial component, free tissue transplantation could be used to separate the cranial cavity in combination with two separate prostheses: a large orbitofacial prosthesis to reduplicate the contour and appearance of the face, and a palatal prosthesis to provide oronasal separation. These two prostheses are connected to one another by a series of magnets.

◈ Another option for combining autogenous tissue transplantation with a prosthesis is to use the transplant for the cranial separation and the orbit/malar/facial reconstruction, and then use the prosthesis to reconstruct the infrastructure of the maxilla and to establish oronasal separation and a dental arch.

◈ Overall, the use of prostheses as the primary reconstructive approach to large orbitomaxillocranial defects is declining and is being replaced by autogenous free tissue transfer.

◈ Prostheses are still useful in combination with soft tissue and bony reconstruction, and retain their greatest use in (1) maxillary reconstruction for a secondary palate reconstruction to restore the dental arch, (2) orbital reconstruction, and (3) total nasal reconstruction.

❖ Soft Tissue Autogenous Transplant

- **Rectus abdominis:**
◈ The rectus abdominis autogenous transplant has been the most widely utilized flap for skull base defects involving the orbitomaxillary complex because of the anatomic consistency and length of the pedicle, its large volume, and the relative ease of harvest.[18]
◈ It can be used not only to provide dura protection and reinforcement but also to reconstruct the palate and nasal lining.
◈ If the external skin of the cheek is intact, the rectus abdominis can be harvested with a single skin island to close the palate.
◈ If the flap is thin, a second skin island may be used to restore the lateral nasal wall. A three-skin-island rectus abdominis template can be used to resurface an external cheek defect in addition to the palatal defect and nasal airway.
◈ A main disadvantage of soft tissue–only reconstructions without bony support is the expected loss of facial contour and eventual ptosis of the flap.

- **Anterolateral thigh:**
◈ The ALT donor site has been replacing the rectus abdominis donor site as the choice to reconstruct soft tissue defects in complex orbitomaxillary defects involving the cranial base because of its abundance of vascularized fat and availability of muscle.
◈ Like the rectus, the ALT has limitations with respect to establishing facial contour. It can also develop ptosis over time.

❖ Technique: Thoracodorsal Artery Scapular Tip

◈ The TDAST donor site is our reconstruction of choice for extensive orbito-maxillocranial defects.
◈ The soft tissue is adequate for the reconstruction of these large defects, as discussed previously in this chapter.
◈ The scapular tip bone contour matches the contour of the orbitomalar complex, facilitates re-projection of the midface, and prevents ptosis of the soft tissue component of this donor site.
◈ This donor site addresses the problems of flap ptosis, loss of facial contour, and the need for vascularized bone in a radiated field, and provides a long vascular pedicle.

■ Lateral Skull Base

Lateral skull base lesions involve the middle cranial fossa in combination with defects of the ear, lateral facial skin, lateral parotid, lateral temporal bone, and temporal mandibular joint. The principles of lateral skull base reconstruction are guided by the location and extent of the resection. They include appropriate dural support and coverage, cutaneous resurfacing, maintaining the appropriate facial contour, facial nerve reconstruction, reconstruction of the external auditory canal, and craniofacial implants for ear prosthesis.

Techniques
❖ Skin Grafts

◈ Skin grafts can effectively restore the epithelial covering of a lateral defect but result in noticeable contour deformity.

◈ When placed over bone, they require rotation of a vascular bed into the defect, most commonly the TPFF. The temporalis muscle donor site is infrequently used as vascular bed because of its limited arc of rotation and donor-site deformity.

◈ Wound vacuum-assisted closure systems (VACSs) may be helpful in securing a skin graft to a lateral defect.

◈ Skin grafts should not be used over an exposed facial nerve.

❖ Cervicofacial Rotational Flap

◈ The cervicofacial rotation flap is technically straightforward and is a good color match in the area of lateral skull base defects, but it does not effectively fill or fit into deeply contoured defects.

◈ Its reliability decreases when used to cover temporal bone defects, when the facial artery is divided, in radiated fields, and in smokers.

❖ Pedicled Flaps: Latissimus Dorsi, Trapezius, Pectoralis

• **Latissimus dorsi:**

◈ The latissimus dorsi flap is the best regional rotational flap for lateral temporal reconstruction.

◈ It is well vascularized and has sufficient pedicle length to reach this defect site.

◈ Because it is a musculocutaneous flap, it has a tendency to become ptotic, and is not useful for finesse recontouring.

◈ The patient positioning is more complex because the patient has to be placed in a semi-decubitus position.

• **Trapezius flap:**
◈ The trapezius flap has evolved with the development of perforator-based donor-site elevations.
◈ When first described, this donor site included harvest of the trapezius muscle and sacrifice of the accessory nerve.[19]
◈ Now the donor site can be harvested on a perforator from the transverse cervical artery located over the superior aspect of the deltoid.
◈ It has an adequate arc of rotation and is well vascularized.
◈ The flap may be utilized in conjunction with a neck dissection if the pedicle can be preserved in an oncologically sound manner.
◈ The use of perforator-based transverse cervical flaps is relatively new, and its reliability will have to be further evaluated.

• **Pectoralis flap:**
◈ The pectoralis flap has previously been shown to be a reliable flap in head and neck reconstruction.[20]
◈ However, it has limitations in lateral skull base reconstruction because of its inadequate length in reaching defects that involve the parietal or occipital scalp.

❖ Soft Tissue Free Flap

◈ A variety of donor sites can be used to resurface lateral temporal defects.
◈ These donor sites include the rectus abdominis, the latissimus dorsi, and the ALT.
◈ These donor sites have compartmentalized fat that is good for contour matching, is a good color match, and has ample nerve for nerve grafting.
◈ The rectus and the latissimus dorsi sites should not be elevated as musculocutaneous flaps because of the likelihood of ptosis and lack of contour matching.
◈ Perforator based elevations such as the ALT and the rectus provide better contour matching.

■ References

Boldfaced references are of particular importance.
1. Irish JC, Gullane PJ, Gentili F, et al. Tumors of the skull base: outcome and survival analysis of 77 cases. Head Neck 1994;16:3–10
2. Urken ML, Catalano PJ, Sen C, Post K, Futran N, Biller HF. Free tissue transfer for skull base reconstruction analysis of complications and a classification scheme for defining skull base defects. Arch Otolaryngol Head Neck Surg 1993;119:1318–1325

3. Hadad G, Bassagasteguy L, Carrau RL, et al. A novel reconstructive technique after endoscopic expanded endonasal approaches: vascular pedicle nasoseptal flap. Laryngoscope 2006;116:1882–1886

4. Zanation AM, Carrau RL, Snyderman CH, et al. Nasoseptal flap reconstruction of high flow intraoperative cerebral spinal fluid leaks during endoscopic skull base surgery. Am J Rhinol Allergy 2009;23:518–521

5. Kassam AB, Thomas A, Carrau RL, et al. Endoscopic reconstruction of the cranial base using a pedicled nasoseptal flap. Neurosurgery 2008;63(1, Suppl 1):ONS44–ONS52, discussion ONS52–ONS53

6. Wolfe SA. The utility of pericranial flaps. Ann Plast Surg 1978;1:147–153

7. Johns ME, Winn HR, McLean WC, Cantrell RW. Pericranial flap for the closure of defects of craniofacial resection. Laryngoscope 1981;91:952–959

8. Zanation AM, Snyderman CH, Carrau RL, Kassam AB, Gardner PA, Prevedello DM. Minimally invasive endoscopic pericranial flap: a new method for endonasal skull base reconstruction. Laryngoscope 2009;119:13–18

9. Chepeha DB, Wang SJ, Marentette LJ, Thompson BG, Prince ME, Teknos TN. Radial forearm free tissue transfer reduces complications in salvage skull base surgery. Otolaryngol Head Neck Surg 2004;131:958–963

10. Gil Z, Fliss DM. Pericranial wrapping of the frontal bone after anterior skull base tumor resection. Plast Reconstr Surg 2005;116:395–398, discussion 399

11. Burkey BB, Gerek M, Day T. Repair of the persistent cerebrospinal fluid leak with the radial forearm free fascial flap. Laryngoscope 1999;109:1003–1006

12. Chana JS, Chen H-C, Sharma R, Hao S-P, Tsai F-C. Use of the free vastus lateralis flap in skull base reconstruction. Plast Reconstr Surg 2003;111:568–574, discussion 575

13. Neligan PC, Mulholland S, Irish J, et al. Flap selection in cranial base reconstruction. Plast Reconstr Surg 1996;98:1159–1166, discussion 1167–1168

14. Moyer JS, Chepeha DB, Teknos TN. Contemporary skull base reconstruction. Curr Opin Otolaryngol Head Neck Surg 2004;12:294–299

15. Rodrigues M, O'malley BW Jr, Staecker H, Tamargo R. Extended pericranial flap and bone graft reconstruction in anterior skull base surgery. Otolaryngol Head Neck Surg 2004;131:69–76

16. Chepeha DB, Wang SJ, Marentette LJ, et al. Restoration of the orbital aesthetic subunit in complex midface defects. Laryngoscope 2004;114:1706–1713

17. Chepeha DB, Khariwala SS, Chanowski EJ, et al. Thoracodorsal artery scapular tip autogenous transplant: vascularized bone with a long pedicle and flexible soft tissue. Arch Otolaryngol Head Neck Surg 2010;136:958–964

18. Disa JJ, Pusic AL, Hidalgo DH, Cordeiro PG. Simplifying microvascular head and neck reconstruction: a rational approach to donor site selection. Ann Plast Surg 2001;47:385–389

19. Rosen HM. The extended trapezius musculocutaneous flap for cranio-orbital facial reconstruction. Plast Reconstr Surg 1985;75:318–327

20. Baek SM, Biller HF, Krespi YP, Lawson W. The pectoralis major myocutaneous island flap for reconstruction of the head and neck. Head Neck Surg 1979;1:293–300

28 Cranial Nerve Reconstruction

- Reconstruction of cranial nerves may be needed in cases of iatrogenic, tumor-related, or, rarely, traumatic cranial nerve damage.
- Common techniques: reanastomosis, grafting, partial transposition. Fine sutures (8-0, 9-0, or 10-0 monofilament depending on the sizes of the nerves) are used to appose the ends of the stumps with good fascicular pattern using standard anastomotic techniques. Fibrin glue can be used for stabilization of the anastomosis, although it might also be used alone for gluing the stumps.[1]
- General principles:
  - Excise the abnormal/damaged segment of the nerve.
  - Anastomose the healthy-appearing ends of the nerve.
  - In the case of a partial nerve anastomosis, only a segment of the nerve is utilized and the remainder is preserved.

■ Epineural Repair

❖ Technique

- ◈ Inspect the nerve for longitudinal blood vessels (for realigning the nerve).
- ◈ Use 8-0, 9-0, or 10-0 monofilament nylon sutures on a tapered needle for microsuturing the epineurium, making a tensionless end-to-end anastomosis.
- ◈ Do not produce tension or mismatch in the epineural repair.
- ◈ Use the minimal number of stitches to reapproximate the nerve, in order to avoid a foreign-body reaction, which may interrupt axon progression and regeneration. Avoid getting any foreign or epineural tissue into the growth space of the graft site (i.e., on the ends of the nerve).
- ◈◈ Variation: Cutting the stumps into a "fish-mouth" shape may increase the surface area usable for the anastomosis.[2]
- ◈ Reinforce the anastomosis with fibrin glue.

724

■ Nerve Graft

In the case of a large gap or tension be-tween the two parts of the nerve, use a graft, such as the sural nerve or the greater auricular nerve (in posterior fossa surgery, the latter may be obtained by using the same incision), or smaller nerves, such as the transverse cervical or supraclavicular nerves, or the supraorbital nerve.

Surgical Pearl

The sacrifice of these nerves is usu-ally not troublesome to the patient. Longer grafts have a lower chance of functional recovery.

Complications of Cranial Nerve Reconstructions

Complications include aberrant regeneration, misdirection of regenerating axons resulting in neuromas, foreign-body reaction at the site of the anastomosis, and synkinesis (which is normal at the beginning but can worsen over time).

■ Cranial Nerve VII Reconstruction

The goal of facial nerve reconstruction is the recovery of facial function, espe-cially after removal of large cerebellopontine angle (CPA) tumors, such as ves-tibular schwannomas, or following trauma. When the two nerve stumps are available, the primary end-to-end epineural anastomosis gives the best out-comes, although sometimes it cannot be done and an interposition graft has to be used (the greater auricular nerve has almost the same diameter as the facial nerve).

- In the case of a lack of the proximal stump of the nerve, or in the case of a lack of improvement 1 year after surgery, a **hypoglossal-facial anastomosis** might be performed.

❖ Technique

◈ Dissect the facial nerve at its exit from the stylomastoid foramen, by mak-ing an incision from the tip of the mastoid process downward to the ante-rior border of the sternocleidomastoid muscle.

◈◈ If it is difficult to find the nerve, drill the tip of the mastoid to identify the terminal mastoid segment of the facial nerve.

◈ Dissect the hypoglossal nerve, opening the carotid sheath between the ster-nocleidomastoid muscle and the posterior belly of the digastric muscle.

◈ After identification of the nerves, cut the facial nerve as close as possible to its foraminal emergence and the hypoglossal nerve as distal as possible, approximating the two nerves and performing an end-to-end tensionless anastomosis, by using 9-0 or 10-0 nylon sutures.

◈ The descending ramus can be anastomosed to the distal hypoglossal stump in order to minimize the hemitongue atrophy side effect.

Side Effects

Side effects include hemitongue atrophy, which is generally well tolerated by the patient, and dysarthria, which is usually transient for a few weeks.

◈◈ In patients who cannot tolerate speech impairment, a partial cranial nerve (CN) XII to CN VII anastomosis may be suggested, in which only a part of the hypoglossal nerve is used for the anastomosis, splitting it longitudinally, while the other part continues to serve the hypoglossal function.[3]

> **Surgical Anatomy Pearl**
>
> Check hypoglossal residual function by stimulating it at 1 mA.

- Upper eyelid gold implants can be used if the anastomosis fails or while the nerve recovers.
- It is debatable as to which technique gives the best results. In general, the longer the cable interposition grafts, the worse the ultimate outcome.
- Despite morbidities such as synkinesia, sural graft techniques may show better improvement in facial nerve function than a CN XII to CN VII anastomosis at 1- and 3-year follow-up after surgery.[4]
- In a successful facial nerve anastomosis, the typical recovery has the following trajectory[5]:
  - Six to 12 weeks after surgery: tingling/tightening in the face
  - 3 months: improvement in facial symmetry and muscle tone
  - 6 months: fine voluntary movement in the nasolabial fold, upper lip, lower eyelid
  - 9 months: increase of voluntary contractions, starting in the circumoral muscles followed by the circumorbicularis muscles
  - Nine to 18 months: maximal recovery, although some delayed recoveries are still possible

> **Surgical Anatomy Pearl**
>
> The temporalis branch (for the frontal muscle) as well as the mandibular branch are the two branches of the facial nerve less likely to recover.

- 90% of the cases with House-Brackmann (H-B, see **Table 8.2**, page 201) grade 6 palsy may have a fourth-degree palsy 1 year after surgery.
- The best recovery would be to a H-B grade 3.
- Physiotherapy with highly trained physiotherapists may be helpful in improving facial function.

■ Oculomotor Nerve Reconstructions

Experience with anastomoses of the intracavernous cranial nerves is limited to sporadic case reports or small case series. These are generally all done at the time of the primary surgery.

- **CN III:** The most feasible goals of the reconstruction of this nerve are the alleviation of ptosis[6] and prevention of synkinesis,[7] although occasionally full third nerve function returns. As an alternative to direct repair or graft of the injured nerve with sural nerve,[7,8] the trochlear nerve might be divided and anastomosed to the distal stump of the third nerve.[9,10]
- **CN IV:** used to maximize the chance for a full recovery of binocular vision.[6]
- ◈   Use a 10-0 nylon or fibrin glue for the epineural anastomosis.
- **CN VI:** also used to maximize the potential for a full recovery of binocular vision.[6]

Trochlear and abducens nerve anastomoses have a low potential for aberrant regeneration, because there are few fibers directed to a single muscle. However, for their size the anastomosis is technically challenging.

- In the case of failure of the anastomoses, or for patients with residual ophthalmoparesis due to cranial nerve dysfunction that has not recovered, prismatic glasses are prescribed or eye muscle surgery is performed some months after the operation for normal binocular vision. Other temporary options are injection of botulinum toxin into eye muscles. The neurosurgeon and the ophthalmologist or ocular plastic surgeon should collaborate closely (see Chapter 10).

■ Cranial Nerve V Reconstruction

This reconstruction is not often done. The potential indications are repair of the V_1 trigeminal branch for corneal sensation in order to avoid corneal keratitis (and potentially subsequent blindness).

■ References

Boldfaced reference is of particular importance.

1. **Bogaev CA, Sekhar LN. Cranial nerve and cranial base reconstruction. In: Sekhar LN, Fessler RG, eds. Atlas of Neurosurgical Techniques: Brain. Stuttgart, New York: Thieme; 2006:811–824**
2. Eby TL. Clinical experience in nerve grafting. Eur Arch Otorhinolaryngol 1994; December:S55–S56

3. Cusimano MD, Sekhar L. Partial hypoglossal to facial nerve anastomosis for reinnerva-tion of the paralyzed face in patients with lower cranial nerve palsies: technical note. Neurosurgery 1994;35:532–533, discussion 533–534

4. Wang Z, Zhang Z, Huang Q, Yang J, Wu H. Long-term facial nerve function following facial reanimation after translabyrinthine vestibular schwannoma surgery: A com-parison between sural grafting and VII-XII anastomosis. Exp Ther Med 2013;6:101–104

5. Spector JG, Lee P, Peterein J, Roufa D. Facial nerve regeneration through autologous nerve grafts: a clinical and experimental study. Laryngoscope 1991;101:537–554

6. Sekhar LN, Lanzino G, Sen CN, Pomonis S. Reconstruction of the third through sixth cranial nerves during cavernous sinus surgery. J Neurosurg 1992;76:935–943

7. Tariq F, Sekhar LN. Surgical management of nonvascular lesions around the oculomo-tor nerve and reconstruction of the oculomotor nerve. World Neurosurg 2014;81:693–694

8. Nonaka Y, Fukushima T, Friedman AH, Kolb LE, Bulsara KR. Surgical management of nonvascular lesions around the oculomotor nerve. World Neurosurg 2014;81:798–809

9. Frisén L, von Essen C, Roos A. Surgically created fourth-third cranial nerve commu-nication: temporary success in a child with bilateral third nerve hamartomas. Case report. J Neurosurg 1999;90:542–545

10. Lownie SP, Pinkoski C, Bursztyn LL, Nicolle DA. Eyelid and eye movements following fourth to third nerve anastomosis. J Neuroophthalmol 2013;33:66–68

III Postoperative and Surgery-Related Aspects

29 Postoperative Care and Complications Management

- Major complication rates in skull base surgery have been reported in the range of 10 to 50%.[1,2]
  - Infratentorial meningioma and craniopharyngioma are associated with higher rates of complications (medical and neurologic) than convexity lesions.[3]
  - For management of diabetes insipidus (DI), syndrome of inappropriate antidiuretic hormone (SIADH), and postoperative endocrine management, see Chapter 9.

■ Predictors of Complications for All Neurosurgical Cases[4]

- Emergency case
- Requirement of blood transfusion before surgery
- Presence of preexisting neurologic symptoms (altered mental status, paraplegia/paraparesis or quadriplegia/quadriparesis, prior stroke)
- Complex surgical approach and prolonged anesthetic treatment
- Preexisting comorbidities, especially cardiovascular and pulmonary diseases
- Alcohol use
- Chronic steroid use

> **Pearl**
>
> A team-oriented approach involving surgeons, anesthesiologists/intensivists, and other specialized health care providers is recommended to manage these challenging patients. The overall goal of this approach is prevention, early identification, and correct management of complications that can arise as a result of surgery.

■ Admission Considerations and Monitoring Strategies

- **The importance of patient handover (Table 29.1):** Appropriate care and monitoring of the postoperative neurosurgical patient requires accurate knowledge of
  - ◦ preoperative clinical status and comorbidities
  - ◦ intraoperative procedure
  - ◦ problems that may have occurred during surgery
  - ◦ anesthesia.
- **Admission considerations:** Immediate postoperative care and monitoring of patients after skull base surgery is traditionally provided in an intensive care unit (ICU) or in a high-dependency unit with advanced monitoring capability. However, in selected patients, ICU admission may not be necessary.[5] The required level and duration of monitoring after skull base surgery is determined by the following:
  1. Preoperative clinical status and comorbidities
  2. Characteristics of the surgical procedure
  3. Intraoperative events
  4. Specific needs in the immediate postoperative period

Pearl

Most of the major complications develop intraoperatively or in the immediate postoperative phase, with a very small number of postoperative neurosurgical patients requiring intensive monitoring beyond the first 6 to 24 hours, according to specific risk profiles. The majority of postoperative hematomas present with clinical signs of neurologic deterioration within 6 hours of surgery; therefore, an intensive but short postoperative monitoring period may be a cost-effective strategy in most neurosurgical patients.[5,6]

- **Monitoring strategies:** The goal of postoperative monitoring is to identify as soon as possible patients who are deteriorating after surgery. Any delay in identifying and treating these patients may severely affect the outcome.
- **Systemic monitoring:** Cardiovascular and respiratory monitoring is essential in patients undergoing skull base surgery **(Table 29.1)**.
- **Neuromonitoring (Table 29.1):** Routine assessment of level of consciousness and pupillary reactivity, and a neurologic examination focused on detection and monitoring of focal deficits are the cornerstones of early detection

Pearl

Both systemic monitoring and neuromonitoring strategies are essential. Early reestablishment of consciousness is ideal, to enable clinicians to administer a neurologic exam.

Table 29.1 Postoperative Considerations

STEP 1: The Patient Handover

1.A. Preoperative Data	1.B. Intraoperative Data	1.C. Immediate Postoperative Course
1.A.1. Neurosurgical data • Neurosurgical diagnosis • Neuroimaging results • Presurgical neurologic status (level of consciousness, presence of neurologic deficits, history of seizures) • Previous neurosurgical interventions **1.A.2. Preoperative clinical status** • Medical comorbidities (especially cardiovascular, respiratory, and neurohormonal diseases) • Preoperative medications • Relevant laboratory test results • Allergy • Mechanical DVT prophylaxis	**1.B.1. Neurosurgery** • Surgical goals and concerns • Patient surgical position • Surgical approach/technique • Duration of surgery • Intraoperative findings • Surgical issues and complications (e.g., brain swelling, brain ischemia, difficult hemostasis/intraoperative hemorrhage, temporary/permanent vascular occlusion, leaks, venous air embolism, nerve injury, rhabdomyolysis, etc.) **1.B.2. Anesthesia** • Airway management (technique used for intubation, level of difficulty, trauma to the airway/dental injury) • Type of anesthesia and analgesia used • Intravascular accesses available • Blood loss, transfusions, and fluid balance • Intraoperative laboratory values • Intraoperative complications/secondary brain insults (e.g., hypoxemia, hypercapnia, hypotension, hypertension, intraoperative seizures, etc.) • Hypothermia/hyperthermia • Neuropsychiatric complications (e.g., emergence delirium, agitation, somnolence, visual disturbance, etc.)	• Postoperative pain • Postoperative nausea and vomiting • Seizures • Respiratory complications (e.g., residual neuromuscular blockade, airway obstruction, laryngospasm, airway edema, compromised oxygen exchange) • Cardiovascular complications (e.g., hypotension, hypertension, arrhythmias)

(continued)

Table 29.1 *(continued)*

STEP 2: Postoperative Plan

2.A. General postoperative monitoring strategy

- Cardiovascular monitoring: continuous ECG and blood pressure (invasive or noninvasive)[a]
- In specific situations may consider central venous pressure[b] and other advanced hemodynamic monitoring strategies (e.g., pulmonary artery catheter, continuous arterial pulse-contours analysis devices, transpulmonary thermodilution technique)[c]
- Respiratory monitoring: pulse oximetry (SpO_2) and respiratory rate monitoring. Consider end-tidal carbon dioxide ($ETCO_2$).[d]
- Fluid balance assessment
- Temperature: peripheral temperature and/or core temperature
- Laboratory examination: blood gases, hematology (WBC, PLTs, Hgb), electrolytes, glucose, coagulation (INR, PTT). If indicated, consider lactate, cardiac markers (troponin) and CK (if rhabdomyolysis is suspected). In case of pituitary surgery, consider cortisol, thyroid hormones, LH, FSH, bioavailable testosterone, prolactin, free T_4, and IGF-1.

2.B. Neuromonitoring strategy

- Neurologic examination: level of consciousness (e.g., Glasgow Coma Scale, or FOUR score), pupillary reactivity, and comprehensive or focused neurologic examination (detection and monitoring of focal deficits, cranial nerves dysfunctions)
- Neurophysiology-based assessment (if indicated)
  - Intracranial pressure (ICP) and cerebral perfusion pressure (CPP) monitoring
  - Cerebral blood flow and oxygen delivery monitoring: cerebral blood flow devices, transcranial Doppler, jugular venous oximetry (SjO_2), near-infrared spectroscopy (NIRS), brain tissue oxygen partial pressure ($PbtO_2$)
  - Bioelectrical activity monitoring: electroencephalogram (EEG), evoked potentials
  - Cerebral metabolism monitoring: cerebral microdialysis
  - Biomarkers

2.C. Instructions for postoperative care

- General postoperative care (e.g., activity level allowed, position of the head of the bed, nutrition, goals and plan for airway management, if patient still intubated)
- Postoperative medications (e.g., need for antiseizure medications, antibiotics, steroids, analgesia, sedation, hyperosmolar agents, stress ulcer prophylaxis)
- Prevention of venous thromboembolism: mechanical prophylaxis (preferably with sequential intermittent pneumatic compression devices) versus pharmacological prophylaxis
- Instructions for management of drains and tubes (including EVDs), stitches, and monitors
- Instructions for postoperative follow-up imaging (e.g., CT or MRI, X-rays), if indicated/required

Abbreviations: CK, creatine kinase; CT, computed tomography; DVT, deep vein thrombosis; ECG, electrocardiogram; EVD, external ventricular drain; FSH, follicle-stimulating hormone; Hgb, hemoglobin; IGF-1, insulin-like growth factor-1; INR, international normalized ratio; LH, luteinizing hormone; MRI, magnetic resonance imaging; PLT, platelets; PTT, partial thromboplastin time; T_4, thyroxine; WBC, white blood count.

Source: Data from references 12, 14–17, and 78.

[a]Noninvasive blood pressure measurement may be sufficient in minor neurosurgical procedures, but continuous intra-arterial blood pressure measurement is essential when tight blood pressure control is required.

[b]The use of central venous pressure monitoring to assess fluid status and fluid responsiveness, despite still being widely diffused, has been recently challenged. A recent meta-analysis looking at its utility to predict fluid responsiveness concluded that there are no data to support this practice and recommends to abandon this approach in fluid resuscitation.[77]

[c]Advanced hemodynamic monitors are not routinely used in postoperatively neurosurgical patients, but they may be indicated in selected patients with severe cardiovascular complications or comorbidities.

[d]$ETCO_2$ should not be considered a reliable substitute for $PaCO_2$, especially in the presence of significant pulmonary disease (acute or preexistent).

of postoperative neurologic deterioration. Anything that interferes with the ability to perform this assessment should be avoided when possible. The assessment should be repeated at regular intervals (ideally every hour initially, if possible) and any time there are signs of change in clinical status (e.g., changes in respiratory pattern, blood pressure, increased intracranial pressure (ICP), if monitored).

○ Level of consciousness
  ▪ Glasgow Coma Scale (GCS)[7]: The best motor score response is considered the most important parameter.
  ▪ The FOUR (Full Outline of UnResponsiveness) score incorporates assessment of brainstem reflexes and ventilation pattern, and overcomes the failure to assess the verbal score in intubated patients[8] **(Table 29.2)**. The FOUR score has been shown to have a better ability to predict outcome than the GCS, but is more difficult to administer than the GCS and has not gained wide implementation.

Table 29.2   Full Outline of UnResponsiveness (FOUR) Score

Eye response	4 = Eyelids open or opened, tracking, or blinking to command
	3 = Eyelids open but not tracking
	2 = Eyelids closed but open to loud voice
	1 = Eyelids closed but open to pain
	0 = Eyelids remain closed with pain
Motor response	4 = Thumbs-up, fist, or peace sign
	3 = Localizing to pain
	2 = Flexion response to pain
	1 = Extension response to pain
	0 = No response to pain or generalized myoclonus status
Brainstem reflexes	4 = Pupil and corneal reflexes present
	3 = One pupil wide and fixed
	2 = Pupil or corneal reflexes absent
	1 = Pupil and corneal reflexes absent
	0 = Absent pupil, corneal, and cough reflex
Respiration	4 = Not intubated, regular breathing pattern
	3 = Not intubated, Cheyne-Stokes breathing pattern
	2 = Not intubated, irregular breathing
	1 = Intubated, breathes above ventilator rate
	0 = Breathes at ventilator rate or apnea

Source: From Wijdicks EFM, Bamlet WR, Maramattom BV, Manno EM, McClelland RL. Validation of a new coma scale: The FOUR score. Ann Neurol 2005;58:585–593. Copyright © 2005 American Neurological Association. Reprinted with permission.

○ Pupillary reactivity: Changes in the pupillary size and reactivity can provide important information on neurologic deterioration, presence of increased ICP, or herniation syndromes.[9] The automated pupillometer provides more accurate and sensitive measurements, although its clinical usefulness and reliability are still controversial.[10]

○ Neurologic examination: It is necessary to evaluate (1) persistence/worsening of previous deficits, (2) improvement of previous deficits after surgery, and (3) appearance of new neurologic findings.

Pearl

Challenge: differentiation between normal postoperative findings (often related to residual effects of general anesthesia) and symptoms/signs indicative of postoperative complications (e.g., intracranial hematoma, brain swelling).

- Common "normal" findings: transient headache; upturned Babinski reflex up to 2 hours postsurgery; depressed pupillary response, unilateral pupillary dilatation in awake patients, or eccentric pupil; dysarthria; asterixis; mild exacerbation of previous hemiparesis (normally lasting no more than 2 hours); unsustained clonus; and shivering unrelated to body temperature.[11–13]

- Concerning findings suggestive of postoperative complications: rapidly increasing headache (especially with associated vomiting), progressive drowsiness, seizures, new evolving hemiparesis, new or worsening paresthesias, vertigo, facial paresis, and pupillary changes in a fully awake patient.[12]

Pearl

Persistent weakness or bilateral ophthalmoplegia can be found after administration of nondepolarizing neuromuscular blockers. However, presence of ophthalmoplegia should always be investigated carefully before being attributed to neuromuscular blocking agents or emergence from anesthesia, given its association with basilar artery thrombosis.[12]

○ Neurophysiology-based assessment, consisting of advanced intracranial monitoring (e.g., ICP, cerebral blood flow and brain oxygen delivery, bioelectrical activity, cerebral metabolism), is recommended in patients with poor baseline neurologic status or requiring continuous sedation for concurrent nonneurologic complications. This form of assessment is rarely indicated for the elective, uncomplicated, skull base patient.[14–16]

Pearl

In case of significant changes in the neurologic status:

1. Immediate reassessment of patient clinical stability (ABC: airway, breathing, and circulation). If severely depressed level of consciousness (GCS ≤ 8, rapidly deteriorating
   level of consciousness, and uncontrolled seizures), early tracheal intubation is essential
   to protect the patient's airway (increased risk of aspiration, hypoxemia, and hypercar-
   bia). Close monitoring of gas exchange should be undertaken with the following goals:
   normal oxygenation (oxygen saturation > 94%, while avoiding hyperoxia), and normocarbia (partial pressure of carbon dioxide in arterial gas [$PaCO_2$] 35–45 mmHg). If signs
   of brain herniation are present or in the setting of increased ICP, hyperventilation
   should be instituted to acutely decrease ICP (goal $PaCO_2$: 28–32 mmHg). However,
   hyperventilation should never be instituted as a definitive treatment (risk of brain ischemia and rebound elevation of ICP), and normocarbia should be rapidly reinstituted
   as soon as other treatments to control ICP are in place.[17]
2. Urgent brain computed tomography (CT) scan ± intravenous contrast.

■ Blood Pressure Monitoring

Postoperative hypertension is relatively common in neurosurgical patients,
and it has been associated with a higher incidence of intracerebral hemorrhage,
ischemic stroke, worsening edema, and myocardial infarction.[18,19] Acute elevation of blood pressure can cause intracranial complications. Alternatively, it can
be a physiological response to maintain cerebral perfusion pressure in the presence of intracranial injury. Therefore, careful blood pressure monitoring and its
tight control are among the most important strategies in preventing complications in postoperative neurosurgical patients. Postoperative acute hypertension
can be attributed to different causes such as under-controlled pain, anxiety,
and preexisting arterial hypertension, or it can be a sentinel of a cerebrovascular event (e.g., intracerebral bleeding at operative site, subdural hematoma, or
epidural bleeding).

Management

- No absolute threshold can be recommended (the level to which elevated
  blood pressure should be lowered depends on several factors).
- The first step in the management of postoperative acute hypertension is the
  identification of the underlying problem (evaluate the patient for neurologic
  status changes, inadequate analgesia, bladder distention, shivering, etc.).
- If, after neurologic assessment, sufficient pain control, and exclusion of other
  reversible causes, the decision is made to control blood pressure with anti-

hypertensive drugs, a short-acting, titratable, intravenous agent should be administered to achieve the target blood pressure quickly, while minimizing the risk of cerebral hypoperfusion. Intravenous β-adrenergic antagonists (labetalol, metoprolol, esmolol) are an acceptable choice for treatment if there are no contraindications. With refractory hypertension or marked bradycardia, angiotensin-converting enzyme (ACE) inhibitors (e.g., enalapril) and vasodilators (e.g., hydralazine or calcium channel blockers) can be used. Nicardipine is considered the safest calcium channel blocker. Concerns regarding elevated ICP accompany the use of calcium channel blockers. Sodium nitroprusside and nitroglycerin increase ICP and lower cerebral blood flow, and should therefore be avoided in patients with reduced intracerebral compliance **(Table 29.3)**.[20,21] In patients with chronic hypertension, reinstitute the patient's previous oral antihypertensive medications early.[12]

Postoperative Hypotension

Postoperative hypotension following elective neurosurgery is uncommon (2–5%), and it has been associated with poorer outcome. Immediate resuscitation with fluid and possibly vasoactive agents should be instituted to avoid cerebral hypoperfusion. Transfusion therapy should also be considered. Causes of shock should be rapidly investigated and treated (hypovolemic, neurogenic, distributive, cardiogenic, and obstructive shock).

■ Prevention of Venous Thromboembolism

Neurosurgical patients are at high risk of developing venous thromboembolism (VTE).

- Pulmonary embolism has been reported in up to 5% of neurosurgical patients (mortality between 9% and 50%).[22]
- Estimated deep vein thrombosis (DVT) incidence ranges from 19 to 43% when standardized screening protocols are implemented.[23] In neurosurgical oncology, DVT has been shown to be the most common adverse event.[2] Meningiomas are associated with the highest postoperative rate of VTE events (the risk is three times higher than in patients with other brain tumors), especially skull base meningiomas.[24,25]
  - ○ Factors associated with increased risk of VTE in neurosurgical patients include cancer; advanced age; longer duration of surgery; prolonged immobilization (pre-, intra-, and postoperative); and the release of thromboplastin secondary to brain surgery.

Table 29.3 Intravenous Antihypertensive Agents in Postoperative Management of Neurosurgical Patients

Drug	Mechanism	Dose	Onset (min)	Duration of Action	Common Adverse Effects	Warnings
Labetalol	α_1, β_1, β_2 antagonist	Initial bolus dose: 5–20 mg IV push over 2 minutes; may administer 40–80 mg at 10 minutes intervals, up to 300 mg cumulative dose. Infusion: 0.5–2 mg/min	5–10	3–6 h	Bradycardia, nausea, vomiting, dizziness, bronchospasm, hypotension, liver injury	Asthma, COPD, LV failure, second or third AV block
Esmolol	β_1 antagonist	Initial bolus: 500 µg/kg. Infusion: 25–300 µg/kg/min. Titration: increase by 50 µg/kg/min every 4 min	1–2	10–30 min	Bradycardia, hypotension, nausea, bronchospasm	Asthma, COPD, LV failure, second or third AV block
Metoprolol	β_1 antagonist	1.25–5 mg (maximum total dose: 15 mg over a 10- to 15-minute period)	5–20	3–4 h (half-life)	Bradycardia, hypotension, dizziness, bronchospasm,	Asthma, COPD, LV failure, second or third AV block, pheochromocytoma
Nicardipine	L-type calcium channel blocker	Initial dose 5 mg/h, with titration by 2.5 mg/h every 15 min as needed; maximum dose 15 mg/h	5–10	30–240 min	Reflex tachycardia, headache, nausea, flushing	LV failure, severe aortic stenosis, cardiac ischemia

Drug	Class	Dose	Onset (min)	Duration	Side effects	Contraindications/comments
Enalaprilat	ACE inhibitor	0.625 mg bolus, followed by 0.625–5 mg every 6 hours	15–30	6–12 h	Hypotension, headache, cough	Acute MI, hypersensitivity, renal failure
Hydralazine	Direct arteriolar vasodilator	3–20 mg IV every 20–60 minutes as needed; Monitor blood pressure closely following IV administration; response may be delayed and unpredictable in some patients; titrate cautiously to response	5–20	1–4 h	Angina pectoris, flushing, orthostatic hypotension, palpitations, paradoxical hypertension, peripheral edema, dizziness, increased intracranial pressure (in patient with preexisting increased intracranial pressure), drug-induced lupus-like syndrome	Coronary artery disease, pulmonary hypertension, renal impairment, aortic dissection; Unpredictable blood pressure lowering effect

Abbreviations: ACE, angiotensin-converting enzyme; AV, atrioventricular; COPD, chronic obstructive pulmonary disease; IV, intravenous; LV, left ventricular; MI, myocardial infarction.
Source: Data from references 20 and 21.

Key Point

Longer duration of surgery, longer postoperative immobilization, and disease-specific morbidity (involvement of cranial nerves, pituitary stalk, or vascular structures) are contributing factors to the higher incidence of VTE events in skull base meningiomas. However, pharmacological VTE prophylaxis is frequently debated in neurosurgery because of the potential increased risk of intracranial bleeding (estimated baseline risk of intracranial hemorrhage [ICH] postcraniotomy: 1.1%, depending on patient- and procedure-specific factors[26]).

Management

Postoperative management of VTE prophylaxis is a balancing act between the risk of thrombotic events and the risk of intracerebral bleeding. Based on current evidence and available strategies,[23,27] the 2012 American College of Chest Physicians (ACCP) Guidelines[28] suggest risk stratification, with an individualized approach based on the risk of VTE (**Table 29.4**). In selected patients with specific risk of ICH (e.g., tumor type, intraoperative findings, and course of neurosurgical procedure), an even more individualized approach should be considered. As a general measure applicable to every group of patients, early mobilization of patients, if appropriate, should be instituted.

High Risk for Venous Thromboembolism Patients (Elective Craniotomy for Nonmalignant Disease)

Mechanical Techniques

The ACCP guidelines[28] suggest the use of **mechanical prophylaxis, preferably with sequential intermittent pneumatic compression (IPC) devices** (rather

Table 29.4   Venous Thromboembolism (VTE) Risk Stratification

Type of Patient	Risk Profile
Patient undergoing craniotomy for nonmalignant disease	High risk for VTE (~ 5%)
Patient undergoing craniotomy for malignant disease	Very high risk for VTE (≥ 10%)
Patient with traumatic brain injury	Very high risk for VTE (≥ 8–10%)

Source: Data from Gould MK, Garcia DA, Wren SM, et al; American College of Chest Physicians. Prevention of VTE in nonorthopedic surgical patients: Antithrombotic Therapy and Prevention of Thrombosis, 9th ed: American College of Chest Physicians Evidence-Based Clinical Practice Guidelines. Chest 2012;141(2, Suppl):e227S–e277S.

than no prophylaxis, grade 2C, or pharmacological VTE prophylaxis, also grade 2C).

- Risk reductions with IPC devices (versus no prophylaxis): 59% for asymptomatic DVT, and 63% for pulmonary embolism.
- IPC devices are favored over graduated compression stockings due to the increased risk of skin complications with elastic stockings.
- In cases of preexisting DVT or baseline immobility (potential presence of undiagnosed DVT), IPCs should not be used without ultrasonographic confirmation of the absence of DVT.
- IPC devices can be discontinued when the patient is able to ambulate at least 3 to 4 hours per day.

Pharmacological VTE prophylaxis with unfractionated heparin (UFH) or low molecular weight heparins (LMWH) at prophylactic doses is not recommended in high-risk neurosurgical patients

- In high-risk patients, the ACCP guidelines[28] consider pharmacological prophylaxis with LMWH more harmful than beneficial:
  - It is associated with a possible increase in the risk of death from any cause.
  - LMWH may prevent between eight and 36 VTE events/1,000 patients, but at a cost of four to 22 additional ICH events/1,000 patients.
- Low-dose UFH seems to have a more favorable trade-off, but the evidence is lacking.
- Therefore, the guidelines do not recommend UFH in high-risk neurosurgical patients.

Patients with Very High Risk for VTE (Elective Craniotomy for Malignant Disease)

- The use of IPC devices, low-dose UFH, or (possibly) LMWH seems to be associated with better outcome in very high-risk craniotomy patients as compared with no prophylaxis. However, when comparing LMWH with IPC devices, despite being associated with more nonfatal VTE events (6–26 more events/1,000 patients treated), IPC devices entail fewer episodes of nonfatal ICH (4–22 less events/1,000 patients treated)
- Adding pharmacological prophylaxis seems to prevent an additional 23 VTE events/1,000 patients treated, at the expense of 11 more ICH events/1,000 patients (considering 4.0% as the risk of symptomatic VTE in patients receiving IPC devices alone).
  - The current ACCP Guidelines[28] suggest a **combination strategy** in very high-risk patients, with the **addition of pharmacological prophylaxis to mechanical prophylaxis** once adequate hemostasis is established and the risk of bleeding decreases (grade 2C).

- **When should pharmacological prophylaxis be started?** No definitive answer exists and each case must be considered individually.
  - Surgical consideration of risk of bleeding is essential. Patients with significant pial invasion and dissection, large tumors, large exposures, and residual vascular lesions may be at higher risk of postoperative hemorrhage.
  - Most postoperative ICHs occur in the first 48 hours after craniotomy, whereas the vast majority of VTE events occurs in the first week or later. Therefore, the most favorable time for adding LMWH or low-dose UFH to IPC devices seems to be 24 to 48 hours after craniotomy, as long as adequate hemostasis has been achieved and the risk of bleeding is judged as not being excessively high.
  - A study shows that early use of subcutaneous low-dose UFH at either 24 or 48 hours was associated with a 43% reduction of lower extremity DVT without an increased incidence of ICHs.[29]

Patients with Traumatic Brain Injury (Very High Risk for VTE)

- The current ACCP Guidelines[28] suggest the use, as soon as possible, of mechanical prophylaxis (preferably with IPC) rather than no prophylaxis when not contraindicated by lower-extremity injury (grade 2C).
- If the risk of bleeding diminishes, most authors suggest adding pharmacological prophylaxis, ideally at 24 hours (but definitively within 48 hours).
- Inferior vena cava filters are not suggested for primary VTE prevention (grade 2C).

■ Stress Ulcer Prophylaxis

Critically ill patients are at risk of stress-related gastrointestinal mucosal damage, which can progress to ulceration and overt gastrointestinal (GI) bleeding. In the absence of adequate pharmacological prophylaxis, GI bleeding has been reported in 5 to 25% of critically ill patients, with an estimated incidence of clinically important GI bleeding varying between 0.1% and 4% in the most recent studies.[30-33]

Management

- Most neurosurgical postoperative patients, even if receiving corticosteroids, do not have high-risk profiles (**Table 29.5**) for GI bleeding and therefore should not receive stress ulcer prophylaxis.
- For patients at high-risk for GI complications, stress ulcer prophylaxis is currently considered the standard of care. The American Society of Health

Table 29.5   Risk Factors for Overt Gastrointestinal (GI) Bleeding

Major Risk Factors	Other Risk Factors*
• Mechanical ventilation ≥ 48 hours (odds ratio [OR] 15.6) • Coagulopathy (OR 4.3)	• Acute hepatic failure • Acute kidney injury • Nasogastric tube placement ≥ 5 days • History of alcohol abuse • Chronic renal failure • Positive for *Helicobacter pylori* • Severe head or spinal cord injury • Thermal injury (> 35% body surface area) • High-dose corticosteroids

Source: Data from references 30, 33, and 78.
*These factors are less strongly associated with significant GI bleeding.

System Pharmacists[34] recommends stress ulcer prophylaxis for patients with at least one major risk factor or at least two other risk factors **(Table 29.5)**.
• Suggested drugs are histamine-2 receptor antagonists (H2RAs) or proton pump inhibitors (PPIs). PPIs can significantly lower the risk of clinically important and overt gastrointestinal bleeding, without influencing ICU mortality or length of ICU stay **(Table 29.6)**. Optimal resuscitation and early enteral nutrition seem to be key factors in further preventing stress ulcer development.

There are some possible harms from pharmacological stress ulcer prophylaxis agents: H2RAs and PPIs have been associated with adverse drug events and increased medication costs, and they seem to enhance susceptibility to nosocomial pneumonia and *Clostridium difficile* infection.[33]

■ Anemia

Bleeding and anemia are among the most common complications following neurosurgical procedures,[3] and may require red blood cell (RBC) transfusion.

• Current evidence supports a restrictive RBC transfusion strategy (hemoglobin [Hb] threshold: ~ 70 g/L) in general critical care patients with normal brain function.[35,36] Moreover, in healthy subjects, brain hypoxia and dysfunction have been shown to manifest only when Hb is less than 60 to 70 g/L.
• Some physiological studies and observational data suggest that acute brain injury is exacerbated when Hb falls below 100 g/L.[37–39] In contrast, data on the effect of anemia in stable postoperative neurosurgical patients are very limited.[40]

Table 29.6 Pharmacological and Nonpharmacological Stress Ulcer Prophylaxis Agents

Agent	Mechanism	Evidence
Histamine 2 receptor antagonists (H2RAs)	H2RAs diminish gastric acid secretion by inhibiting the stimulation of the H^+-K^+- adenosine triphosphatase (ATPase) (H_2 receptors on the parietal cells).	Two meta-analyses comparing H2RAs to placebo found that they reduce the risk of clinically important bleeding; however no significant differences in length of intensive care unit stay or mortality were identified.[79,80]
Proton pump inhibitors (PPIs)	PPIs inhibit secretion of gastric acid by forming irreversible disulfide bonds with the H^+-K^+-ATPase pump. They can be administered enterally or intravenously; continuous intravenous infusion is more effective at controlling gastric pH.	In a recent meta-analysis, Alhazzani et al[31] found that PPIs were more effective than H2RAs at preventing clinically important and overt upper gastrointestinal bleeding (relative risk 0.36; 95% confidence interval [CI] 0.19–0.68; p = 0.002, and relative risk 0.35; 95% CI 0.21–0.59; p < 0.0001).
Sucralfate	Sucralfate, a basic aluminum salt, coats the gastric mucosa, forming a thin protective layer between the mucosa and the gastric acid in the lumen. It does not alter secretion of gastric acid or buffer acid.	Low level of evidence assessing the efficacy of sucralfate versus H2RAs.

Antacids	Antacids neutralize gastric acid and inactivate pepsin enzyme. They must be administered enterally at intervals of 1 to 2 hours and the dose depends on gastric pH (frequent monitoring and dose titration).	When compared with placebo, antacids did not seem to statistically reduce incidence of gastrointestinal bleeding.[79]
Prostanoids	Prostanoids (1) inhibit gastric acid secretion by reducing parietal cell production of cyclic adenosine monophosphate (cAMP) in response to histamine, and (2) enhance mucosal defense mechanisms (cytoprotective effect).	In a single randomized controlled trial involving critically ill patients and comparing antacid titration with fixed doses of a prostanoid agent (misoprostol), no statistically significant differences were identified.[81]
Enteral nutrition	Enteral nutrients buffer acid and may induce the secretion of cytoprotective prostaglandins and mucus, and increase mucosal blood flow. Moreover, the stress-triggered vagal stimulation seems to be blunted by enteral nutrition.	Small studies on critically ill patients and several animal studies suggest that enteral nutrition, especially if early, provides protection against stress gastropathy. However, these studies have many limitations (retrospective analyses, lack of randomization and adequate control groups) and therefore the level of evidence is currently very low.

- RBC transfusion has been shown to be an independent risk factor for adverse outcomes and complications in both general critical care[35,41] and neuro-critical care patients.[42,43]

> **Pearl**
>
> In brain-injured patients at high risk of secondary brain injury, the exact level at which anemia threatens tissue oxygenation and at which RBC transfusion is more beneficial than harmful is currently unknown (no level I evidence available).

Management

Existing guidelines recommend adhering to a restrictive transfusion strategy (70–80 g/L) in hospitalized, stable patients (strong recommendation; high-quality evidence), but little guidance is provided to clinicians for decision making in anemic patients with acute brain injury.[36,44] While waiting for more evidence-based data, a possible approach to anemia in postneurosurgical patients could be the one suggested in **Table 29.7**. In the presence of an actively bleeding patient, these recommendations are not valid, and the decision to transfuse should also consider the hemodynamic goals.

Table 29.7   Suggested Approach to Anemia in Brain-Injured Patients

Patient	Target Hemoglobin	Transfusion Threshold
Stable, hospitalized patients without evidence of cerebral ischemia or acute coronary syndrome	70–90 g/L	≤ 70 g/L Restrictive transfusion strategy
Patients with acute brain injury and evidence of cerebral ischemia (e.g., subarachnoid hemorrhage with delayed cerebral ischemia, acute ischemic stroke)	80–100 g/L	≤ 80 g/L Transfusion requirements should be influenced by illness severity, and patients' signs, symptoms, and comorbidities
Patients suffering from acute coronary syndrome	80–100 g/L	≤ 80 g/L

■ Postoperative Pain

Pain has been defined as an "unpleasant sensory and emotional experience associated with actual or potential tissue damage, or described in terms of such damage."[45] Pain is therefore a complex syndrome causing emotional and physical distress, significantly impacting patient recovery and general well-being.

- Perioperative pain management of patients undergoing craniotomy is challenging and controversial. Moderate to severe pain after craniotomy and its associated inadequate treatment is reported to occur in approximately 50% of patients. Neither strong evidence nor consensus on how to manage these patients is available.[46–48]
- Postoperative pain management in patients having craniotomy presents two key challenges[48]:
  ○ Overtreatment: Aggressive postoperative analgesia with opioids may result in an unintended risk of excessively sedating or causing nausea in patients, which could obfuscate the neurologic examination or interpretation of the patient's overall clinical status
  ○ Undertreatment: On the other hand, the fear of failing to detect in a timely fashion any change in mental status may lead to undertreatment of postoperative pain. Moreover, patients with altered neurologic status or neurologic deficits may not be able to effectively communicate their need for pain control. Inadequate analgesia may lead to agitation and hypertension, with increased risk of postoperative complications (e.g., intracranial bleeding).

Pain Assessment

Reproducible pain assessments and adequate monitoring of patients over time to determine the efficacy of treatment provided are key steps in pain management.[49]

- Patients may or may not be able to communicate their pain.
  ○ If the patient is able to communicate, self-report of pain is considered the "gold standard." Current guidelines suggest using a 0 to 10 visually enlarged horizontal numeric rating scale.[49]
  ○ When patients are unable to communicate, clinicians should use structured, reliable, and feasible tools to assess patients' pain. The Behavioral Pain Scale (BPS)[50,51] and the Critical Care Pain Observation Tool (CPOT)[52] can be used for monitoring postoperative patients unable to self-report, but only if motor function is intact and behavior is observable.

○ Vital signs are not reliable predictors of pain and therefore should not be used alone for pain assessment; however, changes in vital signs may be used as a cue to begin further assessment of pain.[49,53]

Management

Regional Analgesia

- **Preoperative and postoperative scalp block** can be considered as an adjunct for treating pain after craniotomies; however, the current evidence is poor and data are conflicting as to whether it eases pain and decreases the use of postoperative analgesia.[54]
- **Wound infiltration**
  ○ Intraoperative: often used to blunt systemic responses to craniotomy and to minimize bleeding with skin incision (epinephrine vasoconstrictive effect)
  ○ Postoperative: insufficient evidence available to support or discourage its use after craniotomy to improve postoperative analgesia[48]

Systemic analgesia

- **Opioids** represent the cornerstone drugs for managing moderate to severe postoperative pain.
  ○ Strategies:
    - Intermittent systemic administration (risk of oversedation followed by periods of inadequate analgesia); require upward titration of dose to effect
    - Patient-controlled analgesia (PCA)
  ○ Most commonly used opioids[48,49]:
    - **Fentanyl** (intravenous [IV] intermittent dosing: 0.35–0.5 µg/kg IV q 0.5–1 h; IV infusion rate: 0.7–10 µg/kg/h). Rapid onset of action (1–2 minutes) and short elimination half-life (2–4 hours) if used as intermittent bolus; if used as continuous infusion, significant context-sensitive half-life (200 minutes after 6-hour infusion; 300 minutes after 12-hour infusion; after 12 hours, and in case of end-organ dysfunction, the context-sensitive half-life increases unpredictably). Less hypotension than with morphine; accumulates with hepatic impairment.
    - **Hydromorphone** (IV intermittent dosing: 0.2–0.6 mg IV q 1–2 h or 0.5 mg IV every 3 hours; IV infusion rate: 0.5–3 mg/h; oral, immediate release: 2–4 mg every 4–6 hours as needed). Onset of action: 5–15 minutes. No active metabolites. It is a valid therapeutic option in patients tolerant to morphine/fentanyl. Risk of accumulation with hepatic (and

renal) impairment. Elderly/debilitated patients may require lower doses. Patients with prior opioid exposure may require higher initial doses.

- **Morphine** (IV intermittent dosing: 2–4 mg IV q 1–2 h or 4–8 mg IV every 3–4 hours; IV infusion rate: 2–30 mg/h; oral, immediate-release formulations: 10–30 mg every 4 hours as needed). Onset of action: 5–10 minutes; elimination half-life: 3–4 hours. It has 6- and 3-glucuronide active metabolites and accumulates with hepatic/renal impairment. Associated with histamine release. Patients with prior opioid exposure may require higher initial doses.
- **Remifentanil** (IV infusion rate: 0.025–0.2 µg/kg/min). Onset of action: 1–3 minutes; elimination half-life: 3–10 minutes. Does not accumulate in hepatic-renal failure. In cases of severe obesity (actual weight > 130% ideal body weight [IBW]), the IBW should be used instead of actual body weight.
  - ○ Adverse effects: nausea, vomiting, decreased gastrointestinal motility, pruritus, respiratory depression, and oversedation. Postoperative sedation in neurosurgical patients is a major concern because of the need for frequent neurologic examinations; however, excessive concern about oversedation may lead to inadequate analgesia in high-risk patients.[48]
- **Nonsteroidal anti-inflammatory drugs (NSAIDs)** achieve analgesia by central and peripheral inhibition of prostaglandin-mediated amplification of chemical and mechanical pain stimuli.
  - ○ Most commonly used NSAIDs[48,49]:
    - **Ketorolac** (30 mg IV/IM, then 15–30 mg IM/IV every 6 hours up to 5 days [maximum dose = 120 mg/day for 5 days]; for patients > 65 years of age or < 50 kg: 15 mg IV/IM every 6 hours [maximum dose = 60 mg/ day for 5 days]). Onset of action: 10 minutes; elimination half-life: 2.4–8.6 hours.
    - **Ibuprofen** (400–800 mg IV every 6 hours infused over > 30 minutes [maximum dose = 3.2 g/day]; 400 mg PO every 4 hours [maximum dose = 2.4 g/day]).
  - ○ Adverse effects: platelet dysfunction; peptic ulcer/gastrointestinal bleeding; nausea; renal dysfunction; hepatotoxicity (asymptomatic hepatitis, hepatocellular necrosis, fatal fulminant hepatitis); asthma; rash; cardiovascular events among patients receiving chronic cyclooxygenase-2 (COX-2) inhibitors. Platelet dysfunction, with the associated increased risk of bleeding, has limited the use of NSAIDs in the immediate postneurosurgery period, especially in patients at increased risk for bleeding (e.g., aneurysm repair, arteriovenous malformation resection, hematoma evacuations). Therefore, if possible, avoid NSAIDs in renal dysfunction, gastrointestinal bleeding, platelet abnormality, concomitant ACE inhibitor therapy, congestive heart failure, cirrhosis, asthma, and intracranial hemorrhage.

- **Acetaminophen (paracetamol)** alone does not seem to be sufficient to provide adequate analgesia for pain after craniotomy[46]; however, it definitely has a role as an opioid-sparing agent.
  - ○ Commonly used doses: PO/PR: 325–1,000 mg every 4–6 hours (maximum dose ≤ 4 g/day); IV: 650 mg IV every 4 hours to 1,000 mg IV every 6 hours (maximum dose ≤ 4 g/day).
  - ○ Adverse effects: the most severe and most common adverse effect is hepatotoxicity that can lead to severe liver failure.
- **Gabapentin** has been used, in addition to morphine PCA, for patients undergoing craniotomy and has been shown to be effective for prevention of acute postoperative pain.[55] However, its intrinsic sedative effects may offset the benefit of decreased opioid consumption.
  - ○ Starting dose = 100 mg PO t.i.d.; maintenance dose = 900–3,600 mg/day in three divided doses. Adjust dosing in renal failure patients.
  - ○ Adverse effects: ataxia; dizziness; somnolence; fatigue; movement disorders. Abrupt discontinuation is associated with drug withdrawal syndrome and seizures.

■ Postoperative Nausea and Vomiting

Postoperative nausea and vomiting (PONV) is the most common symptom in the immediate postoperative period. It is reported to be the most feared symptom by patients, even worse than the fear of potential surgical pain.[56]

- In postcraniotomy patients, avoidance of PONV is very important because of the potential risks caused by arterial hypertension and high intra-abdominal/intrathoracic pressures generated by retching or vomiting.[57]
- Risk factors: Neurosurgery is considered high-risk for PONV. Other risk factors include anesthesia with volatile anesthetics (e.g., sevoflurane, desflurane); opioid use; female gender; younger age; absence of a history of smoking (smokers have less PONV); prior PONV or motion sickness.[58,59]

Management

- Ideally, PONV should be prevented (prophylaxis), not just managed after its development (rescue therapy).
- The use of a throat/esophageal pack during transsphenoidal surgery, if placed correctly, can prevent the entry of blood into the stomach and potentially reduce PONV.
- Drug classes currently used for prophylaxis or rescue are serotonin-receptor antagonists, corticosteroids, phenothiazines, butyrophenones, antihistamine, anticholinergic, and neurokinin-receptor antagonists **(Table 29.8)**.[60]

- The rescue dose is lower than the dose needed for prophylaxis; patients who have failed to respond to one class of drugs as a prophylactic medication should be treated with another class as rescue antiemetic.[61]

■ Temperature Abnormalities

Both hypothermia and hyperthermia may have negative consequences in postoperative neurosurgical patients.

Hypothermia

Hypothermia affects drug metabolism (e.g., degradation of neuromuscular blocking agents) and decreases platelet function, with the potential impairment of hemostasis and an increased risk of postoperative bleeding.

- Hypothermia is very common in the postoperative setting, and it has been connected to several possible causes[62]: cold environment, infusion of room-temperature IV fluids, drug-induced vasodilatation, decreased basal metabolic rate, anesthetic-induced impairment of the hypothalamic thermostat, exposure of body cavities to room-temperature air, and ventilation with unwarmed gases.
- Ideally, all patients should be warmed to 36°C (96.8°F) within 15 minutes of their arrival from the operating room, and kept warm for the duration of their procedure.

Hyperthermia/Fever

Hyperthermia (temperature above 38°C or 100.4°F) is very common in the first few days after surgery, often caused by inflammatory response to surgery, and is self-limiting. However, elevated temperature is also common (present in up to 40% of cases) in brain-injured patients and has been independently associated with poor outcomes.

- Despite lack of evidence linking improved outcome with induced normothermia, there is general agreement that hyperthermia should be aggressively managed in this population, with the goal of maintaining normothermia (target core temperature below 37.5° to 38°C, considering that brain temperature is typically 0.5° to 0.8°C higher than core temperature).
- Many conditions are associated with postoperative fever, and a thorough differential diagnosis is essential. Historically, causes of postoperative fever have been classified as infectious or noninfectious. The timing of fever after surgery is also one of the most important factors to consider **(Table 29.9)**.[63]

Table 29.8 Drugs Commonly Used for Postoperative Nausea and Vomiting (PONV) Prophylaxis[60]

Drugs	Dose	Timing	Side Effects and Other Information
Ondansetron	4 mg IV	End of surgery	• Most commonly used agents for PONV
Dolasetron	12.5 mg IV	End of surgery	• No sedative side effects
Granisetron	0.35–1.5 mg IV	End of surgery	• Mechanism of action: suppress the initiation of nausea and vomiting by blocking serotonin peripherally at vagal afferents and centrally in the chemoreceptor trigger zone
Palonosetron	0.075 mg IV	End of surgery	• Adverse effects: headache; constipation; increased liver function tests; QT interval prolongation (dose-dependent effect of first-generation antagonists, including ondansetron, granisetron, and dolasetron; avoid in patients with congenital long-QT syndrome; use ECG monitoring in patients at risk of cardiac dysrhythmias, e.g., hypokalemia or hypomagnesemia, heart failure, bradyarrhythmias, and if concurrent administration of drugs that increase the risk of QT prolongation)
Dexamethasone	4–5 mg IV	At induction	• Prophylactic glucocorticoids (e.g., dexamethasone) are effective in reducing the incidence of PONV by approximately 50%
• Not useful for rescue therapy

Drug	Dose	Timing	Comments
Dimenhydrinate	1 mg/kg IV	–	• Not enough data available to establish optimal timing or its side-effect profile
Haloperidol	0.5–2 mg IM/IV	–	• At these doses, no sedation and cardiac arrhythmias reported; however, QT prolongation is described • No reports about optimal timing of administration
Prochlorperazine	5–10 mg IM/IV	End of surgery	• Adverse effects: akathisia; sedation; anticholinergic effects
Promethazine	6.25–25 mg IV	At induction	• Adverse effects: sedation; confusion; disorientation; extrapyramidal symptoms
Scopolamine	Transdermal patch	Prior evening or 4 hours before surgery	• Adverse effects: sedation; visual disturbances; dry mouth; dizziness; it should not be used in patients with narrow-angle glaucoma
Aprepitant	40 mg PO	3 hours before induction of anesthesia	• Mechanism of action: neurokinin is a naturally occurring proemetic substance; aprepitant is a neurokinin-receptor antagonist effective in prevent PONV • Because of cost consideration, reserved for patients in whom PONV would cause serious clinical problems • Not useful for rescue therapy

Table 29.9 Causes of Postoperative Fever

Immediate	Acute	Subacute	Delayed
Onset in the operating room or within hours after surgery	Onset within the first week after surgery	Onset within 1 to 4 weeks following surgery	Onset more than 1 month after surgery
Infectious • Infections present prior to surgery **Noninfectious** • Cerebral infarction • Hemorrhagic stroke (intracerebral and subarachnoid hemorrhage) • Hypothalamic dysfunction • Fat embolism • Medication reaction • Transfusion reaction • Trauma • Malignant hyperthermia • Hyperthyroidism • Hypoadrenalism • Neoplastic fever	**Infectious** • Nosocomial infections (e.g., surgical site infection; intravascular catheter infection; pneumonia—VAP and aspiration pneumonia; urinary tract infection) • Community-acquired infections **Noninfectious** • Cerebral infarction • Hemorrhagic stroke (intracerebral and subarachnoid hemorrhage) • Hypothalamic dysfunction • Trauma (especially brain injury) • Venous thromboembolic disease/thrombophlebitis • Myocardial infarction • Alcohol withdrawal • Acute gout • Pancreatitis • Hyperthyroidism • Hypoadrenalism • Neoplastic fever	**Infectious** • Nosocomial infections (e.g., surgical site infection; intravascular catheter infection; pneumonia – VAP and aspiration pneumonia; urinary tract infection; antibiotic-associated diarrhea; sinusitis; acalculous cholecystitis; foreign-body infection) **Noninfectious** • Febrile drug reactions (e.g., antibiotics, H_2-blockers, phenytoin, heparin) • Venous thromboembolic disease/thrombophlebitis • Neoplastic fever	**Infectious** (most common cause) • Nosocomial infections (e.g., surgical site infections due to more indolent microorganism, as coagulase negative staphylococci; intravascular catheter infection; pneumonia – VAP and aspiration pneumonia; urinary tract infection; antibiotic-associated diarrhea; sinusitis; acalculous cholecystitis; foreign-body infection; infective endocarditis) • Viral infections (e.g., CMV, hepatitis viruses; HIV) or parasitic infections (e.g., toxoplasmosis, babesiosis, malaria) from blood products • Neoplastic fever

Abbreviations: CMV, cytomegalovirus; HIV, human immunodeficiency virus; VAP, ventilator-assisted pneumonia.

Source: Data from Weed HG, Baddour LM. postoperative fever. *UpToDate Online.* http://www.uptodate.com/contents/postoperative-fever. Accessed September 15, 2014.

Management

- Discontinue any unnecessary treatment (including medications and catheters).
- Acetaminophen and nonpharmacological strategies (e.g., surface cooling devices) should be used to minimize patient discomfort and increased metabolic demand (risk of secondary brain injury).
- Clinical suspicion of a nosocomial infection should prompt immediate appropriate diagnostic workup and consideration of antimicrobial therapy. The decision to initiate antibiotic treatment in a patient with postoperative fever should take into consideration the probability of infectious origin of the fever and the patient's clinical stability. Critically ill patients with hemodynamic instability should be treated immediately with broad-spectrum antibiotics (with rapid de-escalation/narrowing once results of cultures are available; antimicrobial treatment beyond an empiric period of 48 hours should be reserved for patients in whom an infection has been identified).

■ Nosocomial Bacterial Meningitis

Postcraniotomy bacterial meningitis is a serious complication occurring in 0.8 to 1.5% of cases.[64,65] Factors that increase the risk of postcraniotomy bacterial meningitis are the presence of cerebrospinal fluid (CSF) leakage, a concomitant infection at the site of the incision, surgery duration of longer than 4 hours, and insertion of external ventricular drains (EVDs).[66] The rate of infection associated with EVD is approximately 8%, and increases linearly over time after insertion.[67]

- Classic symptoms and signs of meningitis (e.g., headache, photophobia, nuchal rigidity, and altered neurologic status) may be masked because of many confounding factors in postoperative patients (e.g., patient sedation, preexistent decreased level of consciousness, symptoms related to the primary brain injury, or presence of blood irritating the meninges). Fever and decreased level of consciousness are the most consistent clinical features of nosocomial meningitis.
- The diagnostic workup consists of the following:
  - Thorough history and neurologic/physical examination
  - Neuroimaging (CT or magnetic resonance imaging [MRI])
  - Immediate CSF analysis (cell counts, Gram stain, biochemical tests for glucose and protein, and aerobic and anaerobic cultures). Cultures are very specific but require prolonged incubation and results may be falsely negative in patients who have previously received antibiotics. Gram staining is also highly specific but not very sensitive, whereas cell counts have both low sensitivity and specificity in postoperative patients.[68,69] A simultaneous

blood glucose level is crucial for interpreting the CSF glucose and so should always be drawn concurrently with CSF analysis.
- ○ Blood, urine, and sputum cultures
- The most commonly isolated bacterial pathogens in nosocomial meningitis[66]:
  - ○ Facultative and aerobic gram-negative bacilli (including *Pseudomonas aeruginosa*) in cases of postneurosurgical infections, ventricular or lumbar catheters, and penetrating trauma
  - ○ *Staphylococcus aureus* in case of postneurosurgical infections, ventricular or lumbar catheters, and penetrating trauma
  - ○ Coagulase-negative staphylococci (especially *Staphylococcus epidermidis*) for postneurosurgical infections, ventricular or lumbar catheters, and penetrating trauma
  - ○ *Propionibacterium acnes* (ventricular or lumbar catheters)
  - ○ *Streptococcus pneumoniae, Haemophilus influenzae,* group A β-hemolytic streptococci for basilar skull fractures.

Management

- Immediate empirical antimicrobial therapy should be initiated for all patients who show signs of postoperative meningitis. A suggested empirical antimicrobial treatment for nosocomial bacterial meningitis includes vancomycin 15 mg/kg every 8 to 12 hours to maintain a serum vancomycin trough concentration of 15 to 20 µg/mL plus cefepime (2 g every 8 hours), ceftazidime (2 g every 8 hours), or meropenem (2 g every 8 hours) (suggested daily dosages in adults with normal renal and hepatic function).
- For treatment of infections caused by gram-negative bacilli in patients with severe allergy to β-lactams, aztreonam (2 g every 6 to 8 hours) or ciprofloxacin (400 mg every 8 to 12 hours) should be considered.
- In cases of skull base fractures, the recommended treatment includes vancomycin plus third-generation cephalosporin (e.g., ceftriaxone 2 g every 12 hours or cefotaxime 2 g every 8 to 12 hours).

Pearl

The choice of the specific agent should always be based on local antimicrobial susceptibility of aerobic gram-negative bacilli. An infectious disease consult is recommended to guide antibiotic treatment selection.

- In the event of negative CSF cultures after 72 hours, the need for antibiotic treatment should be reassessed and possibly discontinued. However, in cases of recent or concurrent antimicrobial therapy, continuation of treatment may still be appropriate despite negative culture results.[70]

■ Glucose Metabolism Disturbances

Hyperglycemia is common in postoperative neurosurgical patients, even in the absence of a previous history of diabetes mellitus.

- Many studies have shown that increased serum glucose is associated with an increased risk of poor outcome.[71,72] However, clear causality between hyperglycemia and poor outcome and, more interestingly, evidence of improved outcome with tight glycemic control have not clearly been shown.[28,73,74]
- Hypoglycemic episodes are more frequent, and increased mortality has been reported in ICU patients treated with tight glycemic control strategies.[75] Finally, recent microdialysis studies have demonstrated increased cerebral hypoglycemic events in patients treated with a tight glucose control strategy.[76]

Management

A less restrictive target has been suggested in patients with brain injury and in postoperative neurosurgical patients. Current guidelines, therefore, recommend glucose monitoring and avoidance of both hypoglycemia (< 70 mg/dL or < 3.9 mmol/L) and hyperglycemia (> 180 mg/dL or 10 mmol/L). Most authors agree on starting insulin infusion with serum glucose of more than 140 mg/dL (> 7.8 mmol/L), and the current consensus is moving toward a view that a more liberal approach to glycemic control is most appropriate.

■ References

Boldfaced references are of particular importance.

1. Manninen PH, Raman SK, Boyle K, el-Beheiry H. Early postoperative complications following neurosurgical procedures. Can J Anaesth 1999;46:7–14
2. **Wong JM, Panchmatia JR, Ziewacz JE, et al. Patterns in neurosurgical adverse events: intracranial neoplasm surgery. Neurosurg Focus 2012;33:E16**
3. Rolston JD, Han SJ, Lau CY, Berger MS, Parsa AT. Frequency and predictors of complications in neurological surgery: national trends from 2006 to 2011. J Neurosurg 2014;120:736–745
4. Beauregard CL, Friedman WA. Routine use of postoperative ICU care for elective craniotomy: a cost-benefit analysis. Surg Neurol 2003;60:483–489, 489
5. **Hanak BW, Walcott BP, Nahed BV, et al. Postoperative intensive care unit requirements after elective craniotomy. World Neurosurg 2014;81:165–172**
6. Taylor WA, Thomas NW, Wellings JA, Bell BA. Timing of postoperative intracranial hematoma development and implications for the best use of neurosurgical intensive care. J Neurosurg 1995;82:48–50
7. Teasdale G, Jennett B. Assessment of coma and impaired consciousness. A practical scale. Lancet 1974;2:81–84

8. Wijdicks EFM, Bamlet WR, Maramattom BV, Manno EM, McClelland RL. Validation of a new coma scale: The FOUR score. Ann Neurol 2005;58:585–593

9. Chesnut RM, Gautille T, Blunt BA, Klauber MR, Marshall LE. The localizing value of asymmetry in pupillary size in severe head injury: relation to lesion type and location. Neurosurgery 1994;34:840–845, discussion 845–846

10. Zafar SF, Suarez JI. Automated pupillometer for monitoring the critically ill patient: a critical appraisal. J Crit Care 2014;29:599–603

11. Rosenberg H, Clofine R, Bialik O. Neurologic changes during awakening from anesthesia. Anesthesiology 1981;54:125–130

12. **Ropper AH. Neurological and Neurosurgical Intensive Care. Philadelphia: Lippincott Williams & Wilkins; 2004**

13. **Lee K. The NeuroICU Book. New York: McGraw Hill Professional; 2012**

14. Oddo M, Villa F, Citerio G. Brain multimodality monitoring: an update. Curr Opin Crit Care 2012;18:111–118

15. **Stocchetti N, Le Roux P, Vespa P, et al. Clinical review: neuromonitoring—an update. Crit Care 2013;17:201**

16. Messerer M, Daniel RT, Oddo M. Neuromonitoring after major neurosurgical procedures. Minerva Anestesiol 2012;78:810–822

17. Seder DB, Riker RR, Jagoda A, Smith WS, Weingart SD. Emergency neurological life support: airway, ventilation, and sedation. Neurocrit Care 2012;17(Suppl 1):S4–S20

18. Rose DK, Cohen MM, DeBoer DP. Cardiovascular events in the postanesthesia care unit: contribution of risk factors. Anesthesiology 1996;84:772–781

19. Basali A, Mascha EJ, Kalfas I, Schubert A. Relation between perioperative hypertension and intracranial hemorrhage after craniotomy. Anesthesiology 2000;93:48–54

20. Marik PE, Rivera R. Hypertensive emergencies: an update. Curr Opin Crit Care 2011; 17:569–580

21. Rose JC, Mayer SA. Optimizing blood pressure in neurological emergencies. Neurocrit Care 2004;1:287–299

22. Hamilton MG, Hull RD, Pineo GF. Venous thromboembolism in neurosurgery and neurology patients: a review. Neurosurgery 1994;34:280–296, discussion 296

23. Iorio A, Agnelli G. Low-molecular-weight and unfractionated heparin for prevention of venous thromboembolism in neurosurgery: a meta-analysis. Arch Intern Med 2000;160:2327–2332

24. Cage TA, Lamborn KR, Ware ML, et al. Adjuvant enoxaparin therapy may decrease the incidence of postoperative thrombotic events though does not increase the incidence of postoperative intracranial hemorrhage in patients with meningiomas. J Neurooncol 2009;93:151–156

25. **Eisenring CV, Neidert MC, Sabanés Bové D, Held L, Sarnthein J, Krayenbühl N. Reduction of thromboembolic events in meningioma surgery: a cohort study of 724 consecutive patients. PLoS ONE 2013;8:e79170**

26. **Danish SF, Burnett MG, Ong JG, Sonnad SS, Maloney-Wilensky E, Stein SC. Prophylaxis for deep venous thrombosis in craniotomy patients: a decision analysis. Neurosurgery 2005;56:1286–1292, discussion 1292–1294**

27. Collen JF, Jackson JL, Shorr AF, Moores LK. Prevention of venous thromboembolism in neurosurgery: a metaanalysis. Chest 2008;134:237–249

28. Gould MK, Garcia DA, Wren SM, et al; American College of Chest Physicians. Prevention of VTE in nonorthopedic surgical patients: Antithrombotic Therapy and Prevention of Thrombosis, 9th ed: American College of Chest Physicians Evidence-Based Clinical Practice Guidelines. Chest 2012;141(2, Suppl):e227S–e277S

29. **Khaldi A, Helo N, Schneck MJ, Origitano TC. Venous thromboembolism: deep venous thrombosis and pulmonary embolism in a neurosurgical population. J Neurosurg 2011;114:40–46**

30. Cook DJ, Fuller HD, Guyatt GH, et al; Canadian Critical Care Trials Group. Risk factors for gastrointestinal bleeding in critically ill patients. N Engl J Med 1994;330:377–381

31. Alhazzani W, Alenezi F, Jaeschke RZ, Moayyedi P, Cook DJ. Proton pump inhibitors versus histamine 2 receptor antagonists for stress ulcer prophylaxis in critically ill patients: a systematic review and meta-analysis. Crit Care Med 2013;41:693–705

32. Mutlu GM, Mutlu EA, Factor P. GI complications in patients receiving mechanical ventilation. Chest 2001;119:1222–1241

33. Krag M, Perner A, Wetterslev J, Møller MH. Stress ulcer prophylaxis in the intensive care unit: is it indicated? A topical systematic review. Acta Anaesthesiol Scand 2013; 57:835–847

34. ASHP Therapeutic Guidelines on Stress Ulcer Prophylaxis. ASHP Therapeutic Guidelines on Stress Ulcer Prophylaxis. ASHP Commission on Therapeutics and approved by the ASHP Board of Directors on November 14, 1998. Am J Health Syst Pharm 1999; 56:347–379

35. Hébert PC, Wells G, Blajchman MA, et al. A multicenter, randomized, controlled clinical trial of transfusion requirements in critical care. Transfusion Requirements in Critical Care Investigators, Canadian Critical Care Trials Group. N Engl J Med 1999; 340:409–417

36. Retter A, Wyncoll D, Pearse R, et al; British Committee for Standards in Haematology. Guidelines on the management of anaemia and red cell transfusion in adult critically ill patients. Br J Haematol 2013;160:445–464

37. Naidech AM, Jovanovic B, Wartenberg KE, et al. Higher hemoglobin is associated with improved outcome after subarachnoid hemorrhage. Crit Care Med 2007;35:2383–2389

38. Naidech AM, Drescher J, Ault ML, Shaibani A, Batjer HH, Alberts MJ. Higher hemoglobin is associated with less cerebral infarction, poor outcome, and death after subarachnoid hemorrhage. Neurosurgery 2006;59:775–779, discussion 779–780

39. Oddo M, Milby A, Chen I, et al. Hemoglobin concentration and cerebral metabolism in patients with aneurysmal subarachnoid hemorrhage. Stroke 2009;40:1275–1281

40. LeRoux P. Haemoglobin management in acute brain injury. Curr Opin Crit Care 2013; 19:83–91

41. Marik PE, Corwin HL. Efficacy of red blood cell transfusion in the critically ill: a systematic review of the literature. Crit Care Med 2008;36:2667–2674

42. Festic E, Rabinstein AA, Freeman WD, et al. Blood transfusion is an important predictor of hospital mortality among patients with aneurysmal subarachnoid hemorrhage. Neurocrit Care 2013;18:209–215

43. Warner MA, O'Keeffe T, Bhavsar P, et al. Transfusions and long-term functional outcomes in traumatic brain injury. J Neurosurg 2010;113:539–546
44. Carson JL, Grossman BJ, Kleinman S, et al; Clinical Transfusion Medicine Committee of the AABB. Red blood cell transfusion: a clinical practice guideline from the AABB. Ann Intern Med 2012;157:49–58
45. International Association for the Study of Pain. *iasp-painorg.* http://www.iasp-pain.org/Education/Content.aspx?ItemNumber=1698&navItemNumber=576#Pain. Accessed July 25, 2014
46. Verchère E, Grenier B, Mesli A, Siao D, Sesay M, Maurette P. Postoperative pain management after supratentorial craniotomy. J Neurosurg Anesthesiol 2002;14:96–101
47. De Benedittis G, Lorenzetti A, Migliore M, Spagnoli D, Tiberio F, Villani RM. Postoperative pain in neurosurgery: a pilot study in brain surgery. Neurosurgery 1996;38:466–469, discussion 469–470
48. Lai LT, Ortiz-Cardona JR, Bendo AA. Perioperative pain management in the neurosurgical patient. Anesthesiol Clin 2012;30:347–367
49. Barr J, Fraser GL, Puntillo K, et al; American College of Critical Care Medicine. Clinical practice guidelines for the management of pain, agitation, and delirium in adult patients in the intensive care unit. Crit Care Med 2013;41:263–306
50. Payen JF, Bru O, Bosson JL, et al. Assessing pain in critically ill sedated patients by using a behavioral pain scale. Crit Care Med 2001;29:2258–2263
51. Chanques G, Payen J-F, Mercier G, et al. Assessing pain in non-intubated critically ill patients unable to self report: an adaptation of the Behavioral Pain Scale. Intensive Care Med 2009;35:2060–2067
52. Gélinas C, Fillion L, Puntillo KA, Viens C, Fortier M. Validation of the critical-care pain observation tool in adult patients. Am J Crit Care 2006;15:420–427
53. Hecht N, Spies C, Vajkoczy P. Routine intensive care unit-level care after elective craniotomy: time to rethink. World Neurosurg 2014;81:66–68
54. Bala I, Gupta B, Bhardwaj N, Ghai B, Khosla VK. Effect of scalp block on postoperative pain relief in craniotomy patients. Anaesth Intensive Care 2006;34:224–227
55. **Türe H, Sayin M, Karlikaya G, Bingol CA, Aykac B, Türe U. The analgesic effect of gabapentin as a prophylactic anticonvulsant drug on postcraniotomy pain: a prospective randomized study. Anesth Analg 2009;109:1625–1631**
56. Macario A, Weinger M, Carney S, Kim A. Which clinical anesthesia outcomes are important to avoid? The perspective of patients. Anesth Analg 1999;89:652–658
57. Eberhart LHJ, Morin AM, Kranke P, Missaghi NB, Durieux ME, Himmelseher S. Prevention and control of postoperative nausea and vomiting in post-craniotomy patients. Best Pract Res Clin Anaesthesiol 2007;21:575–593
58. Sinclair DR, Chung F, Mezei G. Can postoperative nausea and vomiting be predicted? Anesthesiology 1999;91:109–118
59. Gan TJ. Risk factors for postoperative nausea and vomiting. Anesth Analg 2006;102:1884–1898
60. Gan TJ, Meyer TA, Apfel CC, et al; Society for Ambulatory Anesthesia. Society for Ambulatory Anesthesia guidelines for the management of postoperative nausea and vomiting. Anesth Analg 2007;105:1615–1628
61. Habib AS, Reuveni J, Taguchi A, White WD, Gan TJ. A comparison of ondansetron with promethazine for treating postoperative nausea and vomiting in patients who re-

ceived prophylaxis with ondansetron: a retrospective database analysis. Anesth Analg 2007;104:548–551

62. Good KK, Verble JA, Secrest J, Norwood BR. Postoperative hypothermia—the chilling consequences. AORN J 2006;83:1054–1066, quiz 1067–1070

63. Weed HG, Baddour LM. postoperative fever. *UpToDate Online*. http://www.uptodate.com/contents/postoperative-fever. Accessed September 15, 2014

64. McClelland S III, Hall WA. Postoperative central nervous system infection: incidence and associated factors in 2111 neurosurgical procedures. Clin Infect Dis 2007;45:55–59

65. Korinek A-M, Baugnon T, Golmard J-L, van Effenterre R, Coriat P, Puybasset L. Risk factors for adult nosocomial meningitis after craniotomy: role of antibiotic prophylaxis. Neurosurgery 2006;59:126–133, discussion 126–133

66. van de Beek D, Drake JM, Tunkel AR. Nosocomial bacterial meningitis. N Engl J Med 2010;362:146–154

67. Lozier AP, Sciacca RR, Romagnoli MF, Connolly ES Jr. Ventriculostomy-related infections: a critical review of the literature. Neurosurgery 2008;62(Suppl 2):688–700

68. Schade RP, Schinkel J, Roelandse FWC, et al. Lack of value of routine analysis of cerebrospinal fluid for prediction and diagnosis of external drainage-related bacterial meningitis. J Neurosurg 2006;104:101–108

69. Mayhall CG, Archer NH, Lamb VA, et al. Ventriculostomy-related infections. A prospective epidemiologic study. N Engl J Med 1984;310:553–559

70. Infection in Neurosurgery Working Party of the British Society for Antimicrobial Chemotherapy. The management of neurosurgical patients with postoperative bacterial or aseptic meningitis or external ventricular drain-associated ventriculitis. Br J Neurosurg 2000;14:7–12

71. Krinsley JS. Association between hyperglycemia and increased hospital mortality in a heterogeneous population of critically ill patients. Mayo Clin Proc 2003;78:1471–1478

72. Lee S-H, Kim BJ, Bae H-J, et al. Effects of glucose level on early and long-term mortality after intracerebral haemorrhage: the Acute Brain Bleeding Analysis Study. Diabetologia 2010;53:429–434

73. Solheim O, Losvik OK. Tight glycemic control in the neuro-intensive care unit? Neurosurgery 2013;72:E694–E696

74. Finfer S, Chittock DR, Su SY-S, et al; NICE-SUGAR Study Investigators. Intensive versus conventional glucose control in critically ill patients. N Engl J Med 2009;360:1283–1297

75. Finfer S, Liu B, Chittock DR, et al; NICE-SUGAR Study Investigators. Hypoglycemia and risk of death in critically ill patients. N Engl J Med 2012;367:1108–1118

76. Oddo M, Schmidt JM, Carrera E, et al. Impact of tight glycemic control on cerebral glucose metabolism after severe brain injury: a microdialysis study. Crit Care Med 2008;36:3233–3238

77. Marik PE, Cavallazzi R. Does the central venous pressure predict fluid responsiveness? An updated meta-analysis and a plea for some common sense. Crit Care Med 2013;41:1774–1781

78. Ellison RT, Perez-Perez G, Welsh CH, et al; Federal Hyperimmune Immunoglobulin Therapy Study Group. Risk factors for upper gastrointestinal bleeding in intensive care unit patients: role of helicobacter pylori. Crit Care Med 1996;24:1974–1981

79. Cook DJ, Reeve BK, Guyatt GH, et al. Stress ulcer prophylaxis in critically ill patients. Resolving discordant meta-analyses. JAMA 1996;275:308–314
80. Marik PE, Vasu T, Hirani A, Pachinburavan M. Stress ulcer prophylaxis in the new millennium: a systematic review and meta-analysis. Crit Care Med 2010;38:2222–2228
81. Zinner MJ, Rypins EB, Martin LR, et al. Misoprostol versus antacid titration for preventing stress ulcers in postoperative surgical ICU patients. Ann Surg 1989;210:590–595

30 The Role of Radiation Therapy in Skull Base Pathologies

■ Introduction to Radiation Therapy

Background

- Radiation induces double-strand breaks within DNA to kill tumor cells.
- Normal tissues have a superior ability to repair radiation-induced DNA damage compared with tumor cells. This difference is exploited in therapeutic radiology.
- Radiation has been traditionally given in small daily fractions 5 days/week over several weeks.
  - This facilitates maximal normal tissue healing, and time for tumor reoxygenation and greater radiation sensitivity.
- Radiation therapy is usually delivered using a linear accelerator (LINAC) to deliver mega-voltage photons, which are particles without charge or mass.

Radiation Dose

- The unit of radiation is the gray (Gy) and 1 Gy is equal to 1 joule (J) of energy absorbed per kilogram of matter.
- Daily doses of radiation are usually in the range of 1.8 to 2.0 Gy.
- Total radiation doses depend on the tumor type and its histology, but the following are general principles:
  - 50 Gy/25 fractions (fx): used to sterilize microscopic malignant disease such as in the clinically negative neck at high risk for lymphatic nodal spread where few cells are likely harbored, or for the treatment of benign skull base tumors (e.g., glomus tumors, benign meningiomas, vestibular schwannomas)
  - 60 Gy/30 fx: used in the postoperative setting to control low-volume malignant microscopic residual disease within the postoperative bed, or for the treatment of high-grade skull base tumors such as atypical meningioma

- ○ 66 Gy/33 fx: used for close or positive malignant margins postoperatively as the tumor bulk is likely more significant than low-volume microscopic disease; thus, a higher dose is required
- ○ 70 Gy/35 fx (or 78 Gy/39 fx): used to control gross tumor with curative intent and for some radioresistant histologies that are considered "non-malignant" (e.g., chordoma)

Three-Dimensional Conformal Radiation Therapy (3D-CRT)

- Refers to radiation therapy that uses computed tomography (CT)-based planning.
- The tumor and structures that are critical to avoid irradiating, such as the brainstem or optic nerves, are contoured on axial CT images.
- Radiation therapy is planned, usually with two to six beams, with the goals of treating the tumor and avoiding critical structures.
  - ○ If a critical structure is adjacent to the tumor, it may be impossible to deliver the desired dose to the tumor without overdosing the critical structure. In this situation, either tumor underdosing or acceptance of the risk of treating to full dose is required, and typically tumor underdosing can be considered acceptable in order to avoid iatrogenic harm.
- The inability to shape the radiation beam to avoid critical normal structures (i.e., "modulate") is the major limitation of 3D-CRT.

Intensity-modulated Radiation Therapy (IMRT)

- A major advance that built upon the foundation of 3D-CRT.
- IMRT is the result of improvements in LINAC technology, treatment planning software, and the advent of multileaf collimators (beam-shaping devices that consist of leaves that move in and out of the field of irradiation to provide maximal exposure where tumor is visible and maximal sparing of eloquent normal structures where a critical structure is in the beam's eye view).
- Essentially it is now possible to shape the radiation around the critical structures to deliver higher doses at the tumor-critical structure interface, and minimize tumor underdosing **(Fig. 30.1)**.
- IMRT is the standard of care for treating complex tumors in the base of the skull (e.g., chordoma, meningioma) and the head and neck (e.g., nasopharynx and paranasal sinus), and it is now widely applied across tumor sites.

Image-Guided Radiation Therapy (IGRT)

- Incorporates three-dimensional imaging in the process of radiation delivery.
- Prior to each treatment delivery, an imaging study is performed to confirm alignment of the target volume prior to treatment delivery.

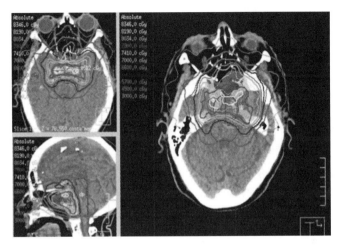

Fig. 30.1 Imaging of a postoperative clival chordoma patient treated with high-dose photon radiation using image-guided radiation therapy (IGRT) and intensity-modulated radiation therapy (IMRT) with a total dose of 78 Gy in 39 fractions.

- Imaging can consist of either orthogonal diagnostic quality X-rays that can render three-dimensional information, a limited volume CT scan with an on-board cone beam (CBCT), in-room CT (CT on rails), and, most recently, an integrated magnetic resonance imaging (MRI) (Viewray Inc., Cleveland, OH).
- IGRT increases the likelihood that treatment is delivered to the target volume, and allows for reduced margins applied for uncertainties beyond the target volume.

Stereotactic Radiation

- Stereotactic radiotherapy (SRT) is the precise delivery of focused irradiation to small targets using an advanced image-guidance delivery apparatus and patient immobilization systems.
- SRT is a resource-intensive treatment that requires specific equipment and practitioners with expertise in treatment planning.
- SRT requires prolonged treatment times on the unit, making it a specialized technique for selected applications.
- Submillimeter precision in therapy is mandated:
  - Fractionated stereotactic radiation therapy (FSRT): Conventionally fractionated radiation therapy is delivered with stereotactic precision to maximize dose at the tumor-critical structure interface and minimize normal tissue exposure.

- ○ Stereotactic body radiation therapy (SBRT): Stereotactic radiation therapy is delivered in a limited number of fractions, usually less than five, to an extracranial site.[1]
- ○ Stereotactic radiosurgery (SRS): Traditionally referred to as a treatment using stereotactic techniques, SRS entails delivering the entire dose of radiation in a single fraction.
- Fundamentally, the delivery of stereotactic radiation requires the following:
  - ○ Near-rigid or rigid immobilization devices
  - ○ IGRT
  - ○ IMRT
  - ○ Advanced radiation oncology delivery apparatus
  - ○ Rigorous quality assurance

Treatment Delivery Units

Stereotactic radiation apparatus can be categorized as follows:

- *LINAC-based stereotactic radiation*
  - ○ LINACs can be outfitted with subcentimeter width multileaf collimators leaves or stereotactic cones, image-guidance systems, and robotic couch tops.
  - ○ Together these features enable submillimeter motions in all six degrees of freedom, ensure precise patient positioning, deliver millimetric precision, and provide conformal dose distributions with steep gradients beyond the tumor edge to minimize normal tissue exposure.
  - ○ Given that these machines are capable of conventional 3D-CRT, IMRT, and stereotactic treatments, they are the most commonly used machines to deliver stereotactic radiation.
- *Stereotactic robotic radiosurgery*
  - ○ Stereotactic robotic radiosurgery refers to a dedicated LINAC system used to deliver SRS, FSRT, and SBRT.
  - ○ It consists of a miniaturized LINAC mounted onto a robotic arm that is able to move in all six degrees of freedom; for example, Cyberknife® (Accuray Inc., Sunnyvale, CA).
  - ○ The image-guidance system consists of a pair of orthogonal X-rays (i.e., stereoscopic X-ray) that can render three-dimensional information of the target location based on the imaging surrogate (a fiducial or bone in selected circumstances).
  - ○ The stereoscopic X-ray system has the advantage of being able to image the patient during treatment delivery in near-real time.
  - ○ The robotic arm also allows the LINAC to adjust for positioning inaccuracies and beam angles that are not possible using a conventional linear accelerator based system.

- ○ Treatment times tend to be much longer as a result of a limited number of beam paths and the fact that the dose contribution by the X-rays is greater than CT-based IGRT systems.
- **Gamma Knife**
  - ○ The Gamma Knife (GK; Elekta AB, Stockholm, Sweden) is the first dedicated brain SRS device and was invented by Lars Leksell.
  - ○ The most recent version is the Gamma Knife Perfexion® (Elekta AB).
  - ○ The system is based on cobalt sources, each emitting a beam of radiation that is collimated.
  - ○ A total of 192 beams are concentrated on a spot localized in three dimensions to deliver a single dose or "shot" of radiation with submillimeter precision.
  - ○ By applying several shots of radiation to cover the target, high doses in a single session are delivered with maximal sparing of the normal brain tissue as compared with other apparatuses.[2]
  - ○ GK has traditionally required the head to be immobilized using a stereotactic head frame; however, noninvasive head frames are now available, and they can be equipped with cone-beam CT image-guidance to enable performing IGRT. Ultimately these innovations permit the GK to deliver multiple fraction radiation therapy (such as FSRT) and expand this technology's scope beyond single-fraction SRS.
  - ○ GK has been used for lesions in the brain, skull base, eye, and occasionally upper cervical spine.
- **Charged particle therapy units**
  - ○ Charged particle therapy most commonly refers to proton therapy, although there are also carbon ion centers (in Europe and Asia).
  - ○ Protons and other charged particles, unlike photons, deposit the majority of their dose at a predictable depth, which is referred to as the Bragg peak.
  - ○ Very little dose is deposited beyond the Bragg peak, and this is the advantage of protons as compared with photon-based therapy.
  - ○ The Bragg peak has been exploited to treat tumors adjacent to critical structures such as the brainstem or optic structures; this is why charged particle therapy is often used for irradiation of skull base chordoma and chondrosarcoma.
  - ○ Charged particle therapy is also helpful in reducing low-dose deposition within normal tissues in pediatric patients, and it is postulated that the benefit will be a reduced risk of radiation-induced secondary malignancies.
  - ○ Treatments using protons or carbon ions are usually done with simple 3D-CRT plans, and require significant margins for uncertainty. As a result, the superiority of the technology as compared with modern linear accelerator systems able to deliver radiation with millimetric precision has been questioned.[3] As a result, some centers are now treating tumors that

were traditionally treated with proton therapy (such as chondrosarcoma and chordoma) with stereotactic LINAC-based techniques.

○ With new developments in proton delivery, such as intensity modulated proton therapy (IMPT) and the application of CBCT, the superiority of this technology may become evident once again.

○ Carbon ions have a greater relative biological effectiveness than photons or protons.[4]

○ With research and development, carbon ion therapy may be a highly useful technology for radioresistant tumor subtypes, but further study is needed to understand its application and implications.

■ Role of Radiation in Specific Pathologies of the Skull Base

Skull Base Meningioma

• The management of meningiomas depends on several factors: location, symptomatology, size, grade, and patient age.

• Observation may be reasonable for slow-growing lesions in asymptomatic patients.

• Late recurrences are common, and thus evaluation of therapeutic efficacy requires more than 5 years of follow-up.

• Reviews of nearly 1,200 patients have demonstrated > 90% rates of 5- to 10-year progression-free survival (PFS) for patients treated with SRS or external beam radiation therapy (EBRT) in recent years.[5]

• Both SRS and EBRT are reasonable options for treatment of meningioma. The ultimate choice should depend on available expertise, patient preferences, and tumor location in relationship to critical structures.

• Of note, for patients who decline, or are not good candidates for resection, definitive radiation has been used with excellent results. In a series of 189 patients with skull base meningioma treated to a median dose of 56.8 Gy, control rates were similar in patients who underwent primary EBRT (59 patients) and in those who underwent surgery followed by EBRT (130 patients).[6]

○ Toxicity in this series was low, with a 2.2% rate of grade 3 toxicity, consisting of reduced vision, a new visual field deficit, and trigeminal neuropathy.[6]

○ For large grade 1 meningiomas that are not amenable to gross total resection (GTR), it is still unknown whether subtotal resection followed by EBRT to residual disease or EBRT alone is preferred. It is unclear if the baseline pre-radiation tumor volume predicts local control.

- A fractionated dose of 54 Gy is recommended for grade 1 tumors, and 60 to 70 Gy for grade 2 or 3 tumors.
- For SRS, doses between 13 and 15 Gy are commonly used for grade 1 tumors. Grade 2 and 3 tumors typically are not treated with SRS.

Benign Meningioma

- Gross total resection (Simpson grade 1) for grade 1 (benign) meningioma is considered definitive treatment (see Chapter 18). A review of this approach demonstrated relapse rates at 5 years of 7 to 12%, which increase to 20 to 25% by 10 years.[5,7–9]
- Results of subtotal resection, even for benign tumors, are suboptimal. A review of over 3,500 patients reported recurrence rates greater than 35% at 5 years and 50% at 10 to 15 years of follow-up. The addition of postoperative radiation can yield PFS rates of over 90% at 10 years of follow-up.[10]

Atypical and Malignant Meningioma

- Grade 2 (atypical) meningioma has a seven- to eightfold increased risk of recurrence in the first 5 years of treatment following surgery alone, with recurrence rates of 38 to 62% and increasing to 81% at 8 years in one study.[7,11–14]
- Given the benefit of postoperative radiation for STR in benign tumors, the addition of radiation to atypical meningioma is relatively well accepted[10]; however, it is controversial as a routine practice following GTR of atypical meningiomas in non-eloquent observable areas of primary tumor.
  - A 108-patient study of atypical meningiomas that underwent GTR demonstrated a recurrence rate of 48% at 10 years. Eight of the patients received irradiation; none suffered a recurrence.[15]
  - A study of 45 patients who underwent GTR of atypical meningioma demonstrated local control in 92% of patients who underwent immediate irradiation versus 59% who underwent surgery alone.[16]
  - A systematic review, however, found that although adjuvant irradiation improved local control for atypical meningiomas, especially after subtotal resection, a statistically significant benefit of adjuvant irradiation after GTR could not be shown.[17]
  - Given the high recurrence rates for atypical tumors following resection alone, a suggested approach is to consider adjuvant irradiation in all patients, even those with GTR.
- Grade 3 (malignant) tumors are even more aggressive, with 5-year recurrence rates of 56 to 83% and a median survival of less than 2 years.[11,13,14]
- Given the poor outcomes with malignant meningioma, a reasonable approach is to offer all patients adjuvant irradiation.

Petroclival Meningioma

- A series of 168 patients with petroclival meningioma who underwent SRS to a median dose of 13 Gy has been reported.[18]
  - ○ SRS was used as the primary therapeutic modality in 97 patients, after STR in 32 patients, or for recurrent disease after GTR in 39 patients.
  - ○ With a median follow-up of 72 months, 10-year PFS was 86%.
  - ○ Twenty-six percent of patients had improvement in neurologic symptoms, 58% had stabilization of symptoms, 8% had clinical or neurologic deterioration, and 4% developed hydrocephalus requiring cerebrospinal fluid (CSF) diversion. SRS can provide durable control with acceptable rates of toxicity.

Sellar and Parasellar Meningioma

- A multi-institutional analysis, which included 763 patients treated to a median dose of 13 Gy, detailed the outcomes after SRS for sellar and parasellar meningiomas[19]:
  - ○ With a median follow-up of 67 months, the 10-year PFS rate was 82%.
  - ○ Functional improvements were seen in 34% of patients with preexisting deficits, in contrast to 9.6% of patients who had new or worsening cranial nerve deficits.
  - ○ Overall, 79.6% of patients had a favorable outcome, defined as tumor control with no new or worsened cranial nerve deficits. SRS provides excellent rates of local control with minimal morbidity.

Recurrent Meningioma

- Recurrent meningiomas should be managed aggressively.
- Rates of recurrence appear to be improved with surgery and irradiation, with one study reporting an 8-year PFS of 78% with combined therapy versus 11% with surgery alone.[20]
- There results were corroborated by another study demonstrating a 5-year PFS of 89% with combined therapy versus 30% with surgery alone. This study also demonstrated a 5-year overall survival (OS) benefit with the addition of radiation over surgery alone in the recurrent setting, 89% versus 43%, respectively.[21]

Cavernous Sinus Meningioma

- *Results of stereotactic radiosurgery*
  - ○ SRS has been used in tumors near the cavernous sinus with good results **(Table 30.1)**.

Table 30.1   Results of Therapy for Cavernous Sinus Meningiomas

Study	Technique	Patients	Follow-Up (Months)	Local Control	Toxicity
Lee et al[23]	SRS	115	89	93% at 10 years	12%
Slater et al[25]	FSRT	78	43	100%	Not detailed, but at least one trigeminal neuralgia and one transient ischemic attack
Castinetti et al[26]	Protons	72	74	96% at 5 years	12.5%

Abbreviations: FSRT, fractionated stereotactic radiation therapy; SRS, stereotactic radiosurgery.

○ Results from a 15-patient series of cavernous sinus meningioma treated with single-fraction SRS to a median marginal dose of 16 Gy were reported.[22]
  ▪ With a median follow-up of 89 months, the tumor control rate was 93% at 10 years.
  ▪ Permanent complications occurred in 12% of patients at a median of 23 months post-SRS and included trigeminal nerve dysfunction, ischemic stroke, diplopia, and hypopituitarism.
  ▪ The rate of complications was dependent on the size of the primary tumor: 3% for those ≤ 9.3 cc versus 21% for tumors ≥ 9.4 cc.
○ These results were similar to those from the University of Pittsburgh, in which 16 patients were treated with a dose of 13 Gy.
  ▪ The control rate was 93% at 10 years, and the crude rate of toxicity was 6.7%.
  ▪ The authors recommended SRS for cavernous sinus lesions < 3 cm in maximum diameter or < 15 cc in volume.[23]
• *Results of fractionated stereotactic radiation therapy*
  ○ Outcomes of fractionated stereotactic radiation in 222 meningioma patients, 78 of whom had cavernous sinus lesions were reported.[24]
  ○ The 10-year rate of local control was 86% overall, and 100% for cavernous sinus lesions.
  ○ Doses ranged from 50 to 55 Gy in 30 to 33 fractions.
  ○ The median tumor size was 12.0 cc in the 209 patients for whom data were available.

- *Results of proton therapy*
    - A review of 72 patients who were treated with 57 to 59 Gy using protons demonstrated a 5-year rate of local control of 96 to 99% in presumed grade 1 or biopsied lesions, and 50% in atypical tumors.[25]
    - Toxicities were considered acceptable at 12.5%, with adverse events consisting of hypopituitarism, optic nerve damage, and diplopia.

Pearls

- SRS is a reasonable option for cavernous sinus meningiomas up to 3 cm in size and at least 2 mm away from the optic nerves, chiasm, and optic tract.
- Larger tumors or those close to critical structures, such as the optic chiasm, may be better served by FSRT.
- Further study is needed to see if protons offer clinical advantages over IMRT and SRS.

Pituitary Adenoma

- Radiation therapy is generally used in four instances: incomplete resection, recurrent tumor, inoperable patient, and refractory secretory tumor.
- A limitation of radiation is that normalization of hormonal hypersecretion can take months to years, depending on the tumor type and radiation technique.
- Other considerations include tumor size and distance from the optic chiasm.
- The optimal SRS candidate has a tumor < 3 cm in maximal dimension that is at least 2 to 3 mm away from the optic apparatus.
- Recommended doses of radiation are as follows: 45–54Gy in 1.8–2.0 Gy daily fractions (regardless of secreting or nonsecreting status); 15 to 20 Gy for nonsecreting tumors undergoing single-fraction SRS; and 20 to 25 Gy for secreting tumors undergoing SRS.
- A review of results achieved with SRS demonstrated an overall 50% rate of control of secretion for hypersecreting tumors.[26]
- The rate of local control was 90% for nonsecreting tumors in a review of patients treated with SRS or FSRT.[27]

Results Specific to SRS

- Nonfunctioning tumors
    - Local control rates for nonfunctioning adenomas following single-fraction SRS range from 83 to 100%, with an average of 95.7%.[27]
    - Neurologic deficits are rare, with a range of 0 to 7.1%, with an average of 2.1%.[27]
    - Hypopituitarism ranges from 0 to 39%, with an average of 12%.[27]

- ○ The recommended SRS margin dose ranges from 12 to 18 Gy, and rates of < 12 Gy were shown to be inferior in at least one experience.[28]
- Cushing's disease
  - ○ Many adrenocorticotropic hormone (ACTH)-secreting pituitary adenomas demonstrate invasion into the dura or cavernous sinus, making surgical resection difficult.
  - ○ SRS is useful in patients with unresectable or persistent Cushing's disease following resection.
  - ○ Rates of remission after SRS range from 16.7% to 87%, with the majority of results demonstrating control rates of > 50%.[27]
  - ○ The average time to remission is 13 months following SRS (range 2–67 months).[29]
  - ○ Biochemical control rates range from 0 to 92%, with an average of 43.6%.[27]
  - ○ The mean time to endocrine remission appears longer than with Cushing's disease, and was found to be 27.6 months in a single institution experience of 136 patients.[30]
  - ○ Patients on octreotide in the perioperative period, were found to have a lower rate of biochemical control following SRS, at 11% versus 60% in patients not on such medications.[31]
- Prolactinoma
  - ○ Pharmacological therapy is the mainstay of treatment.
  - ○ Patients selected for radiation therapy are thus the subset of patients with the most recalcitrant disease. This may help explain why biochemical control rates are lower than with acromegaly and Cushing's disease.
  - ○ SRS has demonstrated biochemical remission rates ranging from 0 to 83%, with an average of 29.4%.[27]
  - ○ Patients on dopamine agonists at the time of SRS were found to have lower rates of biochemical control.[31,32]

Results of Fractionated Radiation Therapy

- EBRT in nonfunctioning tumors
  - ○ Doses of 45 to 54 Gy in 1.8- to 2-Gy daily fractions are typically used.
  - ○ The rate of local tumor control following conventional radiation is greater than 90% in most series.[27]
  - ○ A 24-patient series examining the results of proton therapy to 54 cobalt gray equivalents (CGEs) demonstrated 100% local control at a median follow-up of 47 months.[33]
  - ○ In a series of 63 patients who underwent FSRT, tumor control was 100% at a median follow-up of 82 months.[34]
- EBRT in Cushing's disease
  - ○ Remission rates of 0 to 84% have been reported, although the majority are within the 50 to 80% range.[35]

- ○ EBRT is associated with a longer time to endocrine remission in comparison with SRS for patients with Cushing's disease.
- ○ In a review of multiple series, SRS was associated with normalization of ACTH levels in a median of 7.5 to 33 months, whereas the median time with EBRT tend to be longer and ranged from 18 to 42 months.[35]
- EBRT in acromegaly
  - ○ EBRT results in remission rates ranging from 16 to 100% at 5 to 10 years, with 50 to 60% expected with modern techniques.[35]
  - ○ Overall time to remission appears longer as compared with SRS, with a mean time to remission of 6 to 10 years.[35]
  - ○ A series using proton therapy reported a 45% endocrine control rate in 11 patients with a median follow-up of 47 months.[33]
- EBRT in prolactinoma
  - ○ EBRT has demonstrated complete endocrine normalization with radiation alone in 25 to 50% of patients, and in conjunction with medical therapy to 80 to 100%.[35]
  - ○ The median time to response is quite variable, ranging from 1 to 10 years.[35]
- Toxicity of SRS
  - ○ Rates of hypopituitarism range from 20 to 40% following SRS, and the reported onset time ranges from 16 to 40 months in most reports; however, hypopituitarism has been reported at 100 months.[26]
  - ○ The second most common toxicity is related to cranial nerve toxicity, and is estimated to occur in 2% of patients or fewer.[27]
  - ○ Other rare side effects include ophthalmoplegia, transient ischemic attacks, temporal lobe epilepsy, transient hemiparesis, and memory loss.[26]
  - ○ The rate of second malignancy following Gamma Knife SRS is low, as one study examining 5,000 patients followed for more than 10 years demonstrated no increased risk of secondary malignancies.[36]
- Toxicity of EBRT
  - ○ Hypopituitarism is the most common side effect of pituitary irradiation.

Pearls

- Radiation therapy has a critical role in the management of pituitary tumors.
- The most common side effect is hypopituitarism.
- Both EBRT and SRS show excellent rates of local control for nonfunctioning tumors.
- SRS is preferable in secretory tumors due to faster rates of normalization of hormonal levels, potentially lower rates of hypopituitarism, and logistical ease.
  - ○ In patients undergoing SRS for secretory tumors, it is recommended to withhold hormonal therapy for 6 to 8 weeks prior to treatment.

- ○ The incidence varies widely depending on the study and length of follow-up, with reported values ranging from 28 to 57%.[37,38]
- ○ Other findings include a 1 to 3% risk of optic neuropathy.[37,39]
- ○ A 4% risk at 5 years of suffering a cerebrovascular accident, presumably from radiation-induced carotid stenosis, was seen in one study of patients treated with older techniques between 1962 and 1986.[40]
- ○ The risk of second malignancy following irradiation was found to be 2.4% at 20 years.[41]

Chordoma

- Maximal surgical resection is the mainstay of therapy.
- It is difficult to get a margin-negative complete resection due to the inherent proximity of multiple critical structures that can be functionally devastating to the patient if injured.
- Generally, GTR is achievable in < 50% of patients.[42,43]
- Even after GTR, recurrences are frequent as en-bloc excisions rarely possible.[44]
- Given the frequent rate of local recurrence, adjuvant radiation is usually recommended to patients.

Results of Conventional Photon Radiation Used in the Past

- Outcomes with conventional photon irradiation, particularly in cases of subtotal resection, are suboptimal.
- An older series of 48 chordoma patients (20 of which were skull base lesions) treated to a median dose of 50 Gy was reported.[45]
- Six of 13 patients (46%) with clival chordoma who were evaluated had no symptomatic response to radiation, and all 13 progressed.
- High rates of gross residual disease, limited imaging capacity with MRI, and the low doses of radiation delivered accounted for the poor outcomes.

Results of Proton Therapy and Stereotactic Radiation

- **Table 30.2** summarizes a systematic review regarding outcomes using different radiation modalities.[46]
- Outcomes for local control with postoperative photon radiation with doses of 50 to 60 Gy ranged from 23 to 47% with an average of 33.5%.
- Outcomes for proton therapy, using doses in the 70-CGE range, have demonstrated local control at 5 years in 46 to 73% and at 10 years in 54%.
- Outcomes with stereotactic radiation have demonstrated local control at 5 years in 32 to 72%, with an average of 56%.

Table 30.2   Results of Systematic Review of Radiation for Chordoma[47]

Technique	Local Control (Range)	Local Control (Average)	Time Point
Photon	23–47%	33.5%	5 years
Protons	46–73%	69.2%	5 years
		54%	10 years
Stereotactic radiation	32–72%	56%	5 years

Pearl

A caveat regarding the results of stereotactic radiation, either as SRS or FSRT:

- A selection bias exists in favor of these techniques. They are newer, are used for smaller lesions, and came into use predominantly at the same time as diagnostic MRI. Therefore, comparisons with historic data must be made with caution. Mature outcomes are required before conclusions can be drawn as to the superiority of any treatment modality.

Toxicity

- The 5-year risk of temporal lobe necrosis following proton therapy for skull base chordoma and chondrosarcoma was reported to be 13.2%; 80% of these patients had moderate to severe symptoms.[47]
- A separate experience of 58 patients with skull base chordoma or chondrosarcoma treated with protons reported grade 3 to 4 toxicities, as follows, in 7% of patients[48]:
  - Temporal lobe enhancement on MRI, seizures, severe hearing impairment, pituitary insufficiency, and hearing loss without the requirement for hearing aids.

Pearls

- Proton beam therapy appears to be more effective than 3D-CRT low-dose photon based therapy, due to the ability to deliver higher doses of radiation.
- Image-guided IMRT as a means for dose escalation has not been well studied. Whether this technology can yield outcomes similar to proton therapy is unclear, but preliminary data are promising and the concept is fundamentally sound.[3]
- SRS may have a role in small tumors or as a boost if proton/photon therapy is not available.

Table 30.3   Outcomes by Technique for Skull Base Chondrosarcomas

Study	Technique	Patients	Follow-Up (months)	Local Control
Iyer et al[51]	Proton/photon	200	65	98% at 10 years
Debus et al[52]	SRS	22	75	72% at 5 years 54% at 10 years
Dulguerov et al[53]	FSRT	8	19	100% at 5 years

Abbreviations: FSRT, fractionated stereotactic radiation therapy; SRS, stereotactic radiosurgery.

Chondrosarcoma

- Surgical resection of chondrosarcoma is the mainstay of therapy.
- Complete resection is difficult due to location and inherent proximity to critical organs at risk.
- Inadequate surgical margins are a risk factor for local recurrence.[49]
- Radiation therapy is advocated as an adjunctive therapy in nearly all cases of skull base chondrosarcoma (**Table 30.3**).
- High radiation doses of at least 65 Gy and often > 70 Gy are utilized for optimal results.

Results of Proton Therapy

- In the largest series of patients in the literature, 200 patients received a mixture of photon and proton therapy to a median dose of 72.1 CGE.[50]
- With a median follow-up of 65 months, local control at 10 years was 98% and overall survival at 10 years was 99%.

Results of SRS

- In a study of 22 patients treated with SRS, the median marginal dose was 15 Gy.[51]
- With a median follow-up of 75 months, the actuarial survival at 5 and 10 years was 70% and 56%, respectively. The rates of local control were 72% and 54% at 5 and 10 years, respectively. The median treated volume was 8 cc, emphasizing the potential bias given the small volumes typical of SRS series for this disease.

Results of FSRT

In an eight-patient series with a mean follow-up of 19 months, a FSRT total dose of 64.9 Gy yielded a 5-year local control rate of 50% and a 5-year survival of 82%.[52] Toxicity was similar to that for the chordoma (see above).

> **Pearls**
>
> - Adjuvant radiation therapy is typically recommended for all skull base chondrosarcomas (although in the setting of a GTR of a grade 1 chondrosarcoma, some have recommended observation).
> - Proton therapy, with its ability to deliver significantly higher doses of radiation, appears to be associated with the best outcomes.
> - Modern linear accelerators achieve similar results, but further research is ongoing.
> - Single-fraction SRS may be acceptable in selected cases, although high-dose FSRT is more commonly utilized.

Esthesioneuroblastoma (Olfactory Neuroblastoma)

Treatment Approaches

- A meta-analysis reported that surgery followed by radiation is the most common treatment approach (used in 44% of cases), whereas surgery with chemotherapy and radiation was used in the minority (13% of cases).[53]
- The best outcomes appeared to be in patients with surgery and radiation, yielding a 5-year survival of 65%, as compared with 48% for surgery alone and 37% for radiation alone, although only the latter difference was statistically significant.
- It is important to note that there have been no randomized trials; hence, these comparisons are subject to bias.
- A meta-analysis reporting patterns of failure data demonstrated local recurrence in 29%, regional recurrence in 16%, and distant metastases in 17%.[53]

Results with Radiation Alone

- Esthesioneuroblastomas are usually managed surgically.
- A small study examined local control results with radiation alone.[54]
  - Kadish A tumors (confined to the nasal cavity): 100% local control (6/6)
  - Kadish B tumors (involvement of paranasal sinuses): 58% local control (7/12)
  - Kadish C tumors (extension beyond nasal cavity and paranasal sinuses): 19% local control (7/37)
- It is thus thought that radiation alone may be acceptable treatment for Kadish A tumors, but not for more advanced disease. See on page 653 for the Kadish classification.

Benefit of Radiation Following Surgery

- In a study on 24 Kadish B or C patients, 92% of whom had negative margins, postoperative radiation was given in 46%.[55] Local recurrence was 71% in

Table 30.4   Results of Therapy for Esthesioneuroblastoma

Study	Patients	Treatment	Local Control	5-Uear LRFS	DFS
Herr et al[56]	14	Surgery alone	17%	29%	31% (5 years)
	12	Surgery +RT	71%	100%	87.5% (5 years)
Unger et al[57]	22	Surgery + RT ± chemotherapy	72.7% (crude)	NS	86% (4 years)

Abbreviations: NS, not stated; LRFS, local relapse–free survival; DFS, disease-free survival; RT, radiotherapy.

the surgery alone arm versus 17% in the postoperative radiation arm **(Table 30.4)**.

- Local relapse-free survival in patients receiving postoperative radiation was 100% at 5 years, which was significantly better that the survival in patients who had only surgery, which was 29% at 5 years. The 5-year disease-free survival was 87.5% with postoperative radiation versus 31% for surgery alone.

Elective Nodal Coverage

- Elective coverage of the neck nodes is controversial.
- In one study of patients who did not receive elective nodal irradiation, 26% (7/27) of patients developed regional nodal failure and less than 50% of these were salvaged.[55] Based on these data, elective irradiation to bilateral neck nodes has been recommended.

Results of Proton Therapy

- In one series, two patients with Kadish B and C tumors were treated using craniofacial resection followed by proton radiation to 66.5 CGE with or without chemotherapy.[56]
- With a mean follow-up of over 6 years, the 4-year disease-free survival and OS were 86% and 95%, respectively.
- There were six recurrences, and the recurrence rate in patients with positive margins was 56% (5/9).

Toxicity

- Toxicities in the above proton series were acceptable, with a single grade 4 toxicity of unilateral blindness.
- There were nine grade 3 toxicities, consisting of CSF leak (one patient), pneumocephalus (one), osteomyelitis (one), osteoradionecrosis (one), frontal sinus abscess (one), and sinocutaneous fistula (four).

Results of SRS

- A study reported results of 14 patients who underwent endoscopic resection and postoperative SRS.[57] With a median follow-up of 58 months, the initial control rate was 64%. Four patients were treated with additional SRS for failure, and one with salvage open surgery. The authors found toxicity to be acceptable.

Pearls

- Esthesioneuroblastomas are best managed with multimodal treatment with craniofacial resection followed by postoperative radiation.
- The majority of the data supports fractionated irradiation.
- The neck nodes can be electively treated, although this is controversial.
- Late recurrences are possible, and thus long-term follow-up is needed.
- Proton therapy may be of benefit.
- The role of SRS has yet to be defined.

Vestibular Schwannomas

- Radiation therapy is an attractive option for patients with vestibular schwannomas.
- It offers a noninvasive treatment with high rates of local control and low rates of facial nerve and trigeminal nerve toxicity.

Results of Stereotactic Radiosurgery

- Initial reports with SRS were based on single-fraction doses on the order of 16 Gy.
- Facial numbness and weakness rates on the order of 20 to 30% and hearing preservation rates of 50% have been reported.[58]
- Since then, the dose was reduced to marginal doses of 12 to 13 Gy and excellent results have been reported.[59,60]
- A study of 216 patients has demonstrated a 10-year actuarial local control rate of 98.3%.[60] Cranial nerve (CN) VII and V function was preserved in 100% and 95%, respectively. In 121 patients with serviceable hearing and > 3 years of follow-up, crude hearing preservation rates were 74%. The 10-year actuarial rate for preserving serviceable hearing was 44.5%, suggesting hearing results may decline over time. This study was limited by attrition of patients over the follow-up period.

Rare SRS-Related Toxicities

- The risk of hydrocephalus following vestibular schwannomas treatment is likely related to tumor volume and is in the range of 2 to 6%.[61,62]

- The risk of radiation-induced malignancy is quite low. A 440-patient experience with a median follow-up of 12.5 years had a single patient develop malignant transformation, for an overall incidence of 0.3%.[63]
- Delayed cyst formation was reported in one series to occur in 2.3% of patients. Of these patients, 30% required additional treatment with a craniotomy.[63]
- A dosimetric analysis of predictors of toxicity from 200 patients treated with SRS demonstrated treatment volume $\geq$ 5 cm^3 as the most significant predictor of toxicity.[62]

Results of Fractionated Stereotactic Radiation Therapy for Vestibular Schwannoma

- Typical dose regimens are 40 to 57.6 Gy in 1.8- to 2.0-Gy daily fractions.[64,65]
- Mature local tumor control has generally been excellent, in the 94 to 100% range.
- Trigeminal nerve and facial nerve preservation have been observed in approximately 95% of patients.

Results of Proton Therapy

- In a study including 31 patients treated to 54 to 60 Gy in 30 to 33 fractions, the results showed 100% local control and no CN V or VII injury.[66] Hearing preservation was achieved in only 31%.

Results of SRS Versus FSRT

- Two single institutions have retrospectively compared SRS and FSRT.
- In the University of Heidelberg experience, both techniques offered > 95% tumor control. The rates of CN V and VII dysfunction were 0% and 3%, respectively, for SRS doses of $\leq$ 13 Gy, and 5% and 2% for FSRT.[67]
- Rates of useful hearing preservation were similar (78%) if the dose of single-fraction SRS was limited to 13 Gy or less.
- The Thomas Jefferson University Hospital (Philadelphia, PA) group reports that local control and CN V and VII preservation rates were between 93 to 98%, with no significant difference between the groups.[68]
- However, hearing preservation was 81% in the FSRT group and 33% in the SRS group.
- Given the low rate of hearing preservation in the SRS arm, the short follow-up, and the lack of corroborating data, it is unclear if the rate of hearing preservation is higher with fractionated radiation therapy, and further study is needed.

Follow-Up

- A pattern of temporary enlargement followed by eventual shrinkage and long-term control has been described to occur in up to 41% of cases following single-fraction SRS.[69,70]

Pearls

- Local control appears to be equivalent among SRS, FSRT, and proton therapy **(Table 30.5)**.
- Further study is needed as to whether differences exist in terms of rates of serviceable hearing with either of these approaches and to determine long-term outcomes.

Juvenile Angiofibroma

- The most mature series on radiation in juvenile angiofibroma included 24 patients who were treated with the recommended dose of 36 Gy in 1.8-Gy daily fractions.[71] Findings from a median follow-up of 18 months were reported.
- About 90% of patients were locally controlled.
- A total dose of 30 Gy in 22 fractions was associated with a lower local control rate at 77%.

Toxicity

- Given the low doses used, complications are rare.
- There is a single reported case in the literature of a malignant transformation of a nasopharyngeal angiofibroma.[72]

Indications for Treatment

- Radiation should be used for recurrent or primary tumors that are not amenable surgical resection.

Results of SRS

- There are few reports of SRS as an adjunct to surgery.[73,74]
- Given the effectiveness and low toxicities observed with fractionated radiotherapy, the combination of surgery and SRS appears to offer little additional benefit.

Table 30.5   Results of Therapy for Vestibular Schwannoma

Study	Technique	Patients	Follow-Up	Local Control	Hearing Preservation	CN V Toxicity	CN VII Toxicity
Vachhrajani et al[61]	SRS	216	5.7 years (median)	98.3%	44.5% at 10 years	5%	0%
Combs et al[67]	Protons	31	2.9 years (mean)	100%	31%	0%	0%
Nakamura et al[69]	FSRT	56	2.2 years (mean)	97%	81%	7%	2%
	SRS	69	2.3 years (mean)	98%	33%	5%	2%

Abbreviations: CN, cranial nerve; FSRT, fractionated stereotactic radiation therapy; SRS, stereotactic radiosurgery.

Results of Proton Therapy

- There are no long-term data regarding the role of proton therapy for this disease.

Pearls

- Surgery is preferable given the young age of most patients, and concerns about secondary malignancy.
- If the tumor cannot be completely resected, then definitive radiation therapy remains a safe and effective option.
- Fractionated stereotactic radiation appears to be the most supported approach.
- Proton therapy and single fraction SRS require further study.

Hemangiopericytoma

Hemangiopericytoma (HPC) is a biologically aggressive tumor with a tendency for local and distant relapse. Surgical resection is the mainstay of treatment; however, GTR is possible in only slightly more than 50% of patients.[75,76]

Role of Radiation

- Analysis of national registry data has demonstrated a benefit in terms of cancer-specific survival and OS in a multivariate analysis for the addition of adjuvant irradiation.[77]
- Other studies have demonstrated a delay in recurrence but no overall survival benefit with adjuvant radiation.[76,78]

Results of Photon-Based Irradiation

- Mature outcomes of 39 patients with HPC (of whom 34 had intracranial disease) with a median follow-up of over 10 years have been reported.[79]
- The recurrence rate at 5 years was 46% and 92% at 15 years.
- 26% developed metastatic disease, at a median of 123 months posttreatment.
- Radiation increased the disease-free interval from 154 months to 254 months.
- Following GTR, the addition of radiation extended OS by 126 months ($p = 0.03$).

Results of SRS

- A series of SRS for recurrent or residual HPC included 20 patients with 29 lesions treated with a mean marginal dose of 15 Gy.[80]

- With a mean follow-up of 48 months, tumor control was 72% (21/29) and OS was 85.9% and 13.9% at 5 and 10 years, respectively.
- Lower grade and higher marginal dose appeared to be associated with improved PFS.

Results of Proton Therapy

- There are no data with proton therapy to guide its use in this tumor.

Pearls

- Hemangiopericytoma is an aggressive tumor with high rates of local recurrence, and a propensity for late failures and metastases.
- Given the high rates of local recurrence, radiation is typically recommended for all patients.
- FSRT or SRS are both reasonable approaches.
- The role of proton therapy has not been defined.

■ Skull Base Metastases

- Conventional EBRT is the mainstay of treatment for skull base metastases.
- A series of 43 patients with skull base metastases treated with conventional palliative radiation demonstrated symptomatic improvement in 86% of patients. For patients presenting with cranial nerve deficits, 16% had complete resolution, and 37% had partial improvement.[81]
- Timing of treatment is critical, as one study demonstrated an improvement in symptoms in 87% of patients who started radiation within 1 month of becoming symptomatic versus 25% if symptoms had been present for 3 months or longer.[82]

Results of SRS

- A series of 18 patients treated with SRS to a mean dose of 16.2 Gy and to a mean 50% isodose line demonstrated a 67% crude tumor control rate, and complete symptomatic resolution of cranial nerve deficits in 28% and partial resolution in 33%.[83]

Dural Arteriovenous Fistula (dAVF)

Surgical resection is the mainstay of therapy. SRS is used for dAVFs considered to have an unacceptably high risk associated with surgical excision or endovascular embolization, for patients who fail these traditional modalities, or for patients who require additional adjunctive therapy.

Results of SRS

- A review of outcomes with SRS to doses of 20 to 23 Gy demonstrated clinical improvement in 64 to 100%, with angiographic resolution in 65 to 93%.[84]
- Patients are still at risk for hemorrhage during the latency period—the period until complete angiographic obliteration of the lesion.
- This has in turn led some to recommend immediate post-SRS embolization.
- In a 23-patient series with this approach, 96% of patients had symptom resolution or improvement, and 65% of patients had total or near-total angiographic embolization. There were no intracerebral hemorrhages or documented radiation-related toxicities.[85]

Role of Photon and Proton-Based Therapy

- Currently there is no known role for fractionated radiotherapy in this disease.

Paraganglioma

- A 104-patient series of 121 paragangliomas treated with radiation with a median follow-up of 8.5 years demonstrated a 10-year local control rate of 94%.
  - Ninety-eight patients were treated with FSRT to a median dose of 45 Gy in 25 fractions, whereas the remaining six received SRS.[86]
- Complications were rare, with no severe complications. A 19% rate of mild to moderate complications was reported, which included headaches, hypopituitarism, cranial nerve XII palsy, mucositis, hearing loss, disequilibrium, and xerostomia, among others.
- Other published series demonstrated control rates of 80 to 100% with fractionated radiation and 75 to 100% with SRS.

Pearls

- Both SRS and FSRT offer high rates of local control for paraganglioma.
- Treatment is well tolerated, with low rates of toxicity.
- For well-selected smaller tumors, SRS is an option.

Sinonasal Undifferentiated Carcinoma (SNUC)

This is a rare aggressive tumor with very little data to guide management.

- An individual patient data meta-analysis of 167 cases with a mean and median follow-up of 23 months and 15 months, respectively, was recently reported.[87]
  - At last follow-up, 26% of patients were alive without evidence of disease, 21% were alive with disease, and 53% had died.
  - Surgery appeared to be the most important therapeutic modality.
  - Surgery with radiation with or without chemotherapy was associated with a significant gain in survival as compared to surgery alone (odds ratio [OR], 2.6; 95% confidence interval [CI], 0.82–7.87).

Role of Radiation Therapy

- A small series of 16 patients with a median follow-up of 14 months reported a benefit with radiation.[88]
  - Six patients received surgery alone, four patients had surgery followed by postoperative chemoradiation, and six patients had chemoradiation alone.
  - Overall survival was 30 months in the trimodality arm, 7 months in the surgery-alone arm, and 9 months in the nonoperative arm (non-significant).
  - The 2-year locoregional control was 78%, 37%, and 18% for the surgery plus chemoradiation arm, surgery-alone arm, and chemoradiation-alone arm, respectively.
    - A separate 18-patient review also supported a trimodality approach.[89]
      - The authors noted that a trimodality approach yielded 82% local control (LC) and 92% distant metastasis–free survival (DMFS), whereas surgery alone or definitive chemoradiation yielded 50% LC and 33% DMFS.
- Other published approaches include induction chemotherapy followed by chemoradiation,[90] and induction chemotherapy followed by radiation followed by craniofacial resection.[91] However, these tumors can be approached similarly to other head and neck sinus tumors, with surgical resection followed by adjuvant therapy.
- In the above series, long-term toxicities included 28% grade 1 xerostomia, 11% optic neuropathy/retinopathy, and 6% rates of orbital exenteration and grade 3 peripheral neuropathy.

Results of SRS and Proton Therapy

There are no data on the role of SRS in the treatment of SNUC. No reports regarding the benefit of proton therapy have been published.

Pearls

- SNUC is a rare aggressive tumor.
- There is a suggestion of benefit with aggressive trimodality therapy, which is the current recommendation.

Trigeminal Neuralgia

- SRS is often used for patients with medically refractory trigeminal neuralgia **(Table 30.6)**. There is no known role for fractionated photon or proton therapy.

Technique

- Deliver radiation to a point along the trigeminal nerve root entry zone at a dose of 70 to 90 Gy.
- With GK, a 4-mm shot is placed within the trigeminal nerve anterior to the junction of the pons.
- The largest series of 503 patients demonstrated an initial pain response of 89% at a median of 1 month; however, the response rate decreased to 41% at 5 years.[92]
- Eleven percent of patients developed or had worsened facial sensory dysfunction.
- Those who developed sensory loss along the trigeminal nerve had better pain control at 5 years (78%).

Table 30.6   Results of Therapy for Trigeminal Neuralgia

Study	Technique	Initial Pain Control	Late Pain Control	Sensory Toxicity
Smith et al[93]	Gamma Knife	89%	41% at 5 years (BNI I–IIIA)	11%
Villavicencio et al [94]	LINAC based	88.5% (good or excellent relief)	60% "excellent" at 3 years*	50%
Iannalfi et al[95]	Cyberknife	67%	50% at 2 years (completely off pain medications)	47%

Abbreviations: BNI: Barrow Neurological Institute score; LINAC, linear accelerator.
*Of patients with essential trigeminal neuralgia who had initial relief of symptoms, 60% continued to have "excellent" (complete pain relief, no medications) pain relief at 36 months.

Results of LINAC-Based SRS

- This modality is not performed as often as GK.
- In the largest series of 169 patients, 79% had significant pain relief and 19% of patients had recurrent pain at 13.5 months.[93]
- The rate of facial numbness varied based on the dose prescription and ranged from 35 to 50%.

Results of Cyberknife

- A multicenter study demonstrated favorable results with this apparatus and technique.[94]
- In 95 patients, the rate of "excellent" pain relief was 67%.
- Hypoesthesias occurred in 47% of patients.
- Sustained pain control was 50% at 2 years.
- The recommended dose was 78 Gy to a median length of nerve treated of 6 mm.

Pearls

- Gamma Knife has been the mainstream apparatus in the treatment of trigeminal neuralgia due to its unprecedented ability to deliver a single 4-mm dose of radiation to the trigeminal nerve.
- New technologies with high-accuracy dose delivery are becoming mainstream and will require further evaluation.
- Initial pain control rates are quite high but tend to decrease over time.
- There is no known role for fractionated stereotactic radiation therapy.

Craniopharyngioma

- Controversy exists about whether radical surgery with the goal of gross total resection is preferable to maximal safe resection followed by adjuvant irradiation for this tumor.
- Radiation therapy is generally used in cases of subtotal resection or at the time of recurrence.

Results of EBRT

- A review of results achieved with limited surgery followed by radiation demonstrated control rates of 77 to 100% at 10 years.[95]

Results of SRS

- A review of outcomes using Gamma Knife radiosurgery, largely as adjuvant treatment, demonstrated tumor control rates from 87 to 94%.[95]

Results of FSRT

- A review of outcomes with FSRT demonstrated a tumor control rate of 93% at a median follow-up of 67 months.[96]

Results of Cyberknife

- A review of outcomes with Cyberknife radiosurgery demonstrated local control rates of 85 to 91% at 2 to 3 years of follow-up.[95]

Results of Proton Therapy

- A review of results with proton therapy demonstrated a crude rate of local control of 93% in one series, and a 10-year actuarial control rate of 85% in another.[95]

Toxicity of Treatment

- With modern radiation techniques and standard doses, the incidence of visual deterioration ranges from 0 to 2.5%.[95]
- New or worsening pituitary deficits are seen in 20 to 60% of patients at 5 to 10 years following treatment.[96]
- Other rare complications include radionecrosis, cognitive deficits, epilepsy, cerebrovascular accidents, and secondary tumors.

Pearls

- Radiation therapy is used either in cases of subtotal resection or in cases of recurrence after initial resection.
- Control rates appear to be excellent regardless of the radiation modality chosen.

■ References

Boldfaced references are of particular importance.
1. Sahgal A, Roberge D, Schellenberg D, et al; The Canadian Association of Radiation Oncology-Stereotactic Body Radiotherapy Task Force. The Canadian Association

of Radiation Oncology scope of practice guidelines for lung, liver and spine stereotactic body radiotherapy. Clin Oncol (R Coll Radiol) 2012;24:629–639

2. Ma L, Petti P, Wang B, et al. Apparatus dependence of normal brain tissue dose in
stereotactic radiosurgery for multiple brain metastases. J Neurosurg 2011;114:1580–
1584

3. **Combs SE, Laperriere N, Brada M. Clinical controversies: proton radiation therapy
for brain and skull base tumors. Semin Radiat Oncol 2013;23:120–126**

4. **Combs SE, Kessel KA, Herfarth K, et al. Treatment of pediatric patients and young
adults with particle therapy at the Heidelberg Ion Therapy Center (HIT): establishment of workflow and initial clinical data. Radiat Oncol 2012;7:170**

5. Rogers L, Mehta M. Role of radiation therapy in treating intracranial meningiomas.
Neurosurg Focus 2007;23:E4

6. Debus J, Wuendrich M, Pirzkall A, et al. High efficacy of fractionated stereotactic radiotherapy of large base-of-skull meningiomas: long-term results. J Clin Oncol 2001;
19:3547–3553

7. Condra KS, Buatti JM, Mendenhall WM, Friedman WA, Marcus RB Jr, Rhoton AL. Benign meningiomas: primary treatment selection affects survival. Int J Radiat Oncol
Biol Phys 1997;39:427–436

8. Mirimanoff RO, Dosoretz DE, Linggood RM, Ojemann RG, Martuza RL. Meningioma:
analysis of recurrence and progression following neurosurgical resection. J Neurosurg
1985;62:18–24

9. Stafford SL, Perry A, Suman VJ, et al. Primarily resected meningiomas: outcome and
prognostic factors in 581 Mayo Clinic patients, 1978 through 1988. Mayo Clin Proc
1998;73:936–942

10. **Gondi V, Tome WA, Mehta MP. Fractionated radiotherapy for intracranial meningiomas. J Neurooncol 2010;99:349–356**

11. Perry A, Scheithauer BW, Stafford SL, Lohse CM, Wollan PC. "Malignancy" in meningiomas: a clinicopathologic study of 116 patients, with grading implications. Cancer
1999;85:2046–2056

12. Perry A, Stafford SL, Scheithauer BW, Suman VJ, Lohse CM. Meningioma grading: an
analysis of histologic parameters. Am J Surg Pathol 1997;21:1455–1465

13. Hug EB, Devries A, Thornton AF, et al. Management of atypical and malignant meningiomas: role of high-dose, 3D-conformal radiation therapy. J Neurooncol 2000;48:
151–160

14. Jääskeläinen J, Haltia M, Servo A. Atypical and anaplastic meningiomas: radiology,
surgery, radiotherapy, and outcome. Surg Neurol 1986;25:233–242

15 Aghi MK, Carter BS, Cosgrove GR, et al. Long-term recurrence rates of atypical meningiomas after gross total resection with or without postoperative adjuvant radiation.
Neurosurgery 2009;64:56–60, discussion 60

16. Komotar RJ, Iorgulescu JB, Raper DM, et al. The role of radiotherapy following gross-
total resection of atypical meningiomas. J Neurosurg 2012;117:679–686

17. Kaur G, Sayegh ET, Larson A, et al. Adjuvant radiotherapy for atypical and malignant
meningiomas: a systematic review. Neuro-oncol 2014;16:628–636

18. Flannery TJ, Kano H, Lunsford LD, et al. Long-term control of petroclival meningiomas
through radiosurgery. J Neurosurg 2010;112:957–964

19. Sheehan JP, Starke RM, Kano H, et al. Gamma Knife radiosurgery for sellar and parasellar meningiomas: a multicenter study. J Neurosurg 2014;120:1268–1277
20. Miralbell R, Linggood RM, de la Monte S, Convery K, Munzenrider JE, Mirimanoff RO. The role of radiotherapy in the treatment of subtotally resected benign meningiomas. J Neurooncol 1992;13:157–164
21. Taylor BW Jr, Marcus RB Jr, Friedman WA, Ballinger WE Jr, Million RR. The meningioma controversy: postoperative radiation therapy. Int J Radiat Oncol Biol Phys 1988; 15:299–304
22. Pollock BE, Stafford SL, Link MJ, Garces YI, Foote RL. Single-fraction radiosurgery of benign cavernous sinus meningiomas. J Neurosurg 2013;119:675–682
23. Lee JY, Niranjan A, McInerney J, Kondziolka D, Flickinger JC, Lunsford LD. Stereotactic radiosurgery providing long-term tumor control of cavernous sinus meningiomas. J Neurosurg 2002;97:65–72
24. Soldà F, Wharram B, De Ieso PB, Bonner J, Ashley S, Brada M. Long-term efficacy of fractionated radiotherapy for benign meningiomas. Radiother Oncol 2013;109:330–334
25. Slater JD, Loredo LN, Chung A, et al. Fractionated proton radiotherapy for benign cavernous sinus meningiomas. Int J Radiat Oncol Biol Phys 2012;83:e633–e637
26. Castinetti F, Régis J, Dufour H, Brue T. Role of stereotactic radiosurgery in the management of pituitary adenomas. Nat Rev Endocrinol 2010;6:214–223
27. **Sheehan JP, Xu Z, Lobo MJ. External beam radiation therapy and stereotactic radiosurgery for pituitary adenomas. Neurosurg Clin N Am 2012;23:571–586**
28. Mingione V, Yen CP, Vance ML, et al. Gamma surgery in the treatment of nonsecretory pituitary macroadenoma. J Neurosurg 2006;104:876–883
29. Jagannathan J, Sheehan JP, Pouratian N, Laws ER, Steiner L, Vance ML. Gamma Knife surgery for Cushing's disease. J Neurosurg 2007;106:980–987
30. Lee CC, Vance ML, Xu Z, et al. Stereotactic radiosurgery for acromegaly. J Clin Endocrinol Metab 2014;99:1273–1281
31. Landolt AM, Haller D, Lomax N, et al. Octreotide may act as a radioprotective agent in acromegaly. J Clin Endocrinol Metab 2000;85:1287–1289
32. Pouratian N, Sheehan J, Jagannathan J, Laws ER Jr, Steiner L, Vance ML. Gamma knife radiosurgery for medically and surgically refractory prolactinomas. Neurosurgery 2006;59:255–266, discussion 255–266
33. Ronson BB, Schulte RW, Han KP, Loredo LN, Slater JM, Slater JD. Fractionated proton beam irradiation of pituitary adenomas. Int J Radiat Oncol Biol Phys 2006;64:425–434
34. Colin P, Jovenin N, Delemer B, et al. Treatment of pituitary adenomas by fractionated stereotactic radiotherapy: a prospective study of 110 patients. Int J Radiat Oncol Biol Phys 2005;62:333–341
35. Loeffler JS, Shih HA. Radiation therapy in the management of pituitary adenomas. J Clin Endocrinol Metab 2011;96:1992–2003
36. Rowe J, Grainger A, Walton L, Silcocks P, Radatz M, Kemeny A. Risk of malignancy after gamma knife stereotactic radiosurgery. Neurosurgery 2007;60:60–65, discussion 65–66
37. Erridge SC, Conkey DS, Stockton D, et al. Radiotherapy for pituitary adenomas: long-term efficacy and toxicity. Radiother Oncol 2009;93:597–601

38. Estrada J, Boronat M, Mielgo M, et al. The long-term outcome of pituitary irradiation after unsuccessful transsphenoidal surgery in Cushing's disease. N Engl J Med 1997; 336:172–177

39. Brada M, Rajan B, Traish D, et al. The long-term efficacy of conservative surgery and radiotherapy in the control of pituitary adenomas. Clin Endocrinol (Oxf) 1993;38: 571–578

40. Brada M, Burchell L, Ashley S, Traish D. The incidence of cerebrovascular accidents in patients with pituitary adenoma. Int J Radiat Oncol Biol Phys 1999;45:693–698

41. Minniti G, Traish D, Ashley S, Gonsalves A, Brada M. Risk of second brain tumor after conservative surgery and radiotherapy for pituitary adenoma: update after an additional 10 years. J Clin Endocrinol Metab 2005;90:800–804

42. Gay E, Sekhar LN, Rubinstein E, et al. Chordomas and chondrosarcomas of the cranial base: results and follow-up of 60 patients. Neurosurgery 1995;36:887–896, discussion 896–897

43. Forsyth PA, Cascino TL, Shaw EG, et al. Intracranial chordomas: a clinicopathological and prognostic study of 51 cases. J Neurosurg 1993;78:741–747

44. Tzortzidis F, Elahi F, Wright D, Natarajan SK, Sekhar LN. Patient outcome at long-term follow-up after aggressive microsurgical resection of cranial base chordomas. Neurosurgery 2006;59:230–237, discussion 230–237

45. Catton C, O'Sullivan B, Bell R, et al. Chordoma: long-term follow-up after radical photon irradiation. Radiother Oncol 1996;41:67–72

46. Amichetti M, Cianchetti M, Amelio D, Enrici RM, Minniti G. Proton therapy in chordoma of the base of the skull: a systematic review. Neurosurg Rev 2009;32:403–416

47. Santoni R, Liebsch N, Finkelstein DM, et al. Temporal lobe (TL) damage following surgery and high-dose photon and proton irradiation in 96 patients affected by chordomas and chondrosarcomas of the base of the skull. Int J Radiat Oncol Biol Phys 1998; 41:59–68

48. Hug EB, Loredo LN, Slater JD, et al. Proton radiation therapy for chordomas and chondrosarcomas of the skull base. J Neurosurg 1999;91:432–439

49. Fiorenza F, Abudu A, Grimer RJ, et al. Risk factors for survival and local control in chondrosarcoma of bone. J Bone Joint Surg Br 2002;84:93–99

50. Rosenberg AE, Nielsen GP, Keel SB, et al. Chondrosarcoma of the base of the skull: a clinicopathologic study of 200 cases with emphasis on its distinction from chordoma. Am J Surg Pathol 1999;23:1370–1378

51. **Iyer A, Kano H, Kondziolka D, et al. Stereotactic radiosurgery for intracranial chondrosarcoma. J Neurooncol 2012;108:535–542**

52. Debus J, Schulz-Ertner D, Schad L, et al. Stereotactic fractionated radiotherapy for chordomas and chondrosarcomas of the skull base. Int J Radiat Oncol Biol Phys 2000; 47:591–596

53. **Dulguerov P, Allal AS, Calcaterra TC. Esthesioneuroblastoma: a meta-analysis and review. Lancet Oncol 2001;2:683–690**

54. Benfari G, Fusconi M, Ciofalo A, et al. Radiotherapy alone for local tumour control in esthesioneuroblastoma. Acta Otorhinolaryngol Ital 2008;28:292–297

55. Demiroz C, Gutfeld O, Aboziada M, Brown D, Marentette LJ, Eisbruch A. Esthesioneuroblastoma: is there a need for elective neck treatment? Int J Radiat Oncol Biol Phys 2011;81:e255–e261

56. Herr MW, Sethi RK, Meier JC, et al. Esthesioneuroblastoma: an update on the Massachusetts Eye and Ear Infirmary and Massachusetts General Hospital experience with craniofacial resection, proton beam radiation, and chemotherapy. J Neurol Surg B Skull Base 2014;75:58–64

57. Unger F, Haselsberger K, Walch C, Stammberger H, Papaefthymiou G. Combined endoscopic surgery and radiosurgery as treatment modality for olfactory neuroblastoma (esthesioneuroblastoma). Acta Neurochir (Wien) 2005;147:595–601, discussion 601–602

58. Kondziolka D, Lunsford LD, McLaughlin MR, Flickinger JC. Long-term outcomes after radiosurgery for acoustic neuromas. N Engl J Med 1998;339:1426–1433

59. Sun S, Liu A. Long-term follow-up studies of Gamma Knife surgery with a low margin dose for vestibular schwannoma. J Neurosurg 2012;117(Suppl):57–62

60. Chopra R, Kondziolka D, Niranjan A, Lunsford LD, Flickinger JC. Long-term follow-up of acoustic schwannoma radiosurgery with marginal tumor doses of 12 to 13 Gy. Int J Radiat Oncol Biol Phys 2007;68:845–851

61. Vachhrajani S, Fawaz C, Mathieu D, et al. Complications of Gamma Knife surgery: an early report from 2 Canadian centers. J Neurosurg 2008;109(Suppl):2–7

62. Hayhurst C, Monsalves E, Bernstein M, et al. Predicting nonauditory adverse radiation effects following radiosurgery for vestibular schwannoma: a volume and dosimetric analysis. Int J Radiat Oncol Biol Phys 2012;82:2041–2046

63. Hasegawa T, Kida Y, Kato T, Iizuka H, Kuramitsu S, Yamamoto T. Long-term safety and efficacy of stereotactic radiosurgery for vestibular schwannomas: evaluation of 440 patients more than 10 years after treatment with Gamma Knife surgery. J Neurosurg 2013;118:557–565

64. Selch MT, Pedroso A, Lee SP, et al. Stereotactic radiotherapy for the treatment of acoustic neuromas. J Neurosurg 2004;101(Suppl 3):362–372

65. Fuss M, Debus J, Lohr F, et al. Conventionally fractionated stereotactic radiotherapy (FSRT) for acoustic neuromas. Int J Radiat Oncol Biol Phys 2000;48:1381–1387

66. Bush DA, McAllister CJ, Loredo LN, Johnson WD, Slater JM, Slater JD. Fractionated proton beam radiotherapy for acoustic neuroma. Neurosurgery 2002;50:270–273, discussion 273–275

67. Combs SE, Welzel T, Schulz-Ertner D, Huber PE, Debus J. Differences in clinical results after LINAC-based single-dose radiosurgery versus fractionated stereotactic radiotherapy for patients with vestibular schwannomas. Int J Radiat Oncol Biol Phys 2010;76:193–200

68. Andrews DW, Suarez O, Goldman HW, et al. Stereotactic radiosurgery and fractionated stereotactic radiotherapy for the treatment of acoustic schwannomas: comparative observations of 125 patients treated at one institution. Int J Radiat Oncol Biol Phys 2001;50:1265–1278

69. Nakamura H, Jokura H, Takahashi K, Boku N, Akabane A, Yoshimoto T. Serial follow-up MR imaging after gamma knife radiosurgery for vestibular schwannoma. AJNR Am J Neuroradiol 2000;21:1540–1546

70. Murphy ES, Suh JH. Radiotherapy for vestibular schwannomas: a critical review. Int J Radiat Oncol Biol Phys 2011;79:985–997

71. Amdur RJ, Yeung AR, Fitzgerald BM, Mancuso AA, Werning JW, Mendenhall WM. Radiotherapy for juvenile nasopharyngeal angiofibroma. Pract Radiat Oncol 2011;1:271–278

72. Makek MS, Andrews JC, Fisch U. Malignant transformation of a nasopharyngeal angiofibroma. Laryngoscope 1989;99(10 Pt 1):1088–1092
73. López F, Suárez V, Costales M, Suárez C, Llorente JL. Treatment of juvenile angiofibromas: 18-year experience of a single tertiary centre in Spain. Rhinology 2012;50:95–103
74. Dare AO, Gibbons KJ, Proulx GM, Fenstermaker RA. Resection followed by radiosurgery for advanced juvenile nasopharyngeal angiofibroma: report of two cases. Neurosurgery 2003;52:1207–1211, discussion 1211
75. Ghia AJ, Chang EL, Allen PK, et al. Intracranial hemangiopericytoma: patterns of failure and the role of radiation therapy. Neurosurgery 2013;73:624–630, discussion 630–631
76. Rutkowski MJ, Jian BJ, Bloch O, et al. Intracranial hemangiopericytoma: clinical experience and treatment considerations in a modern series of 40 adult patients. Cancer 2012;118:1628–1636
77. Ghia AJ, Allen PK, Mahajan A, Penas-Prado M, McCutcheon IE, Brown PD. Intracranial hemangiopericytoma and the role of radiation therapy: a population based analysis. Neurosurgery 2013;72:203–209
78. Melone AG, D'Elia A, Santoro F, et al. Intracranial hemangiopericytoma—our experience in 30 years: a series of 43 cases and review of the literature. World Neurosurg 2014;81:556–562
79. Schiariti M, Goetz P, El-Maghraby H, Tailor J, Kitchen N. Hemangiopericytoma: long-term outcome revisited. Clinical article. J Neurosurg 2011;114:747–755
80. Kano H, Niranjan A, Kondziolka D, Flickinger JC, Lunsford LD. Adjuvant stereotactic radiosurgery after resection of intracranial hemangiopericytomas. Int J Radiat Oncol Biol Phys 2008;72:1333–1339
81. Greenberg HS, Deck MD, Vikram B, Chu FC, Posner JB. Metastasis to the base of the skull: clinical findings in 43 patients. Neurology 1981;31:530–537
82. Vikram B, Chu FC. Radiation therapy for metastases to the base of the skull. Radiology 1979;130:465–468
83. Iwai Y, Yamanaka K. Gamma Knife radiosurgery for skull base metastasis and invasion. Stereotact Funct Neurosurg 1999;72(Suppl 1):81–87
84. **Dalyai RT, Ghobrial G, Chalouhi N, et al. Radiosurgery for dural arterio-venous fistulas: a review. Clin Neurol Neurosurg 2013;115:512–516**
85. Friedman JA, Pollock BE, Nichols DA, Gorman DA, Foote RL, Stafford SL. Results of combined stereotactic radiosurgery and transarterial embolization for dural arteriovenous fistulas of the transverse and sigmoid sinuses. J Neurosurg 2001;94:886–891
86. Hinerman RW, Amdur RJ, Morris CG, Kirwan J, Mendenhall WM. Definitive radiotherapy in the management of paragangliomas arising in the head and neck: a 35-year experience. Head Neck 2008;30:1431–1438
87. Reiersen DA, Pahilan ME, Devaiah AK. Meta-analysis of treatment outcomes for sinonasal undifferentiated carcinoma. Otolaryngol Head Neck Surg 2012;147:7–14
88. Yoshida E, Aouad R, Fragoso R, et al. Improved clinical outcomes with multi-modality therapy for sinonasal undifferentiated carcinoma of the head and neck. Am J Otolaryngol 2013;34:658–663
89. Mourad WF, Hauerstock D, Shourbaji RA, et al. Trimodality management of sinonasal undifferentiated carcinoma and review of the literature. Am J Clin Oncol 2013;36:584–588

90. Rischin D, Porceddu S, Peters L, Martin J, Corry J, Weih L. Promising results with chemoradiation in patients with sinonasal undifferentiated carcinoma. Head Neck 2004;26:435–441

91. Musy PY, Reibel JF, Levine PA. Sinonasal undifferentiated carcinoma: the search for a better outcome. Laryngoscope 2002;112(8 Pt 1):1450–1455

92. Kondziolka D, Zorro O, Lobato-Polo J, et al. Gamma Knife stereotactic radiosurgery for idiopathic trigeminal neuralgia. J Neurosurg 2010;112:758–765

93. Smith ZA, Gorgulho AA, Bezrukiy N, et al. Dedicated linear accelerator radiosurgery for trigeminal neuralgia: a single-center experience in 179 patients with varied dose prescriptions and treatment plans. Int J Radiat Oncol Biol Phys 2011;81:225–231

94. Villavicencio AT, Lim M, Burneikiene S, et al. Cyberknife radiosurgery for trigeminal neuralgia treatment: a preliminary multicenter experience. Neurosurgery 2008;62: 647–655, discussion 647–655

95. Iannalfi A, Fragkandrea I, Brock J, Saran F. Radiotherapy in craniopharyngiomas. Clin Oncol (R Coll Radiol) 2013;25:654–667

96. Minniti G, Esposito V, Amichetti M, Enrici RM. The role of fractionated radiotherapy and radiosurgery in the management of patients with craniopharyngioma. Neurosurg Rev 2009;32:125–132, discussion 132

31 Chemotherapy of Skull Base Malignancies

Chemotherapy involves the use of synthetic or natural molecules for the purposes of blocking tumor cell functions required for cell division or maintenance of cell viability.

- The hallmark traits of cancer that serve as targets of cancer therapy[1] are resistance to cell death, angiogenesis, replicative immortality, sustained proliferation signaling, evasion of growth suppressors, activation of migration or invasion, alteration of energy metabolism, and evasion of immune response.
- The development of chemotherapeutics for skull base malignancies has focused on the adaptation of cytotoxic agents that have been shown to induce significant tumor cell death or tumor growth inhibition in preclinical models of solid malignancy.
- Given the rare nature of skull base malignancy and the diverse pathology, large clinical trials evaluating the use of chemotherapeutic agents are infrequent. Current chemotherapeutic strategies for selected tumors have relied on case series or phase II studies with comparison to historical or contemporaneous control groups.

■ Indications

The use of chemotherapy for the management of skull base malignancy is dependent on the histological diagnosis.[2] Chemotherapy may be administered prior to surgery or radiation, following surgery, or in the palliative setting for primary or recurrent tumors where surgical or radiation options are absent or limited.

Chemotherapy in combination with radiation may be considered as the primary treatment paradigm for moderately to poorly differentiated neuroendocrine carcinomas, lymphoma, Ewing's sarcoma, rhabdomyosarcoma, and malignant peripheral nerve sheath tumors of the skull base.[2]

- Induction chemotherapy for reduction of tumor burden prior to surgical resection should be considered for patients with squamous cell carcinoma[3–5] and sinonasal undifferentiated carcinoma.[6,7]

- The addition of chemotherapy to standard radiation treatment in nasopharyngeal carcinoma provides a 20% overall survival advantage at 2 to 4 years over treatment not involving chemotherapy.[8]
- Squamous cell cancer of the head and neck is treated with induction chemotherapy using the TPF regimen, which consists of docetaxel, cisplatin, and 5-fluorouracil.[4,9] This regimen may be combined with concurrent radiation in the event of temporal bone tumors.[10]
- Concurrent chemotherapy with postoperative radiation is employed for esthesioneuroblastoma patients at high risk of recurrence. Neoadjuvant chemotherapy can be considered for advanced cases of esthesioneuroblastoma.[11]
- Nonresectable malignant skull base tumors may be treated with a regimen of radiation therapy and concomitant cisplatin or mitomycin C plus adjuvant cisplatin and vinblastine.[12]
- Chemotherapy for salivary gland carcinomas has not been shown to have a survival effect and is reserved for cases in which the tumor is causing severe symptoms or showing rapid progression.[13]
- Effective chemotherapy regimens for chordoma, meningioma, or chondrosarcoma have not been described to date. Biological therapies for these tumors are currently under investigation. **Fig. 31.1** shows the current treatment indications for chemotherapy in the management of malignant skull base tumors.

■ Mechanism of Action

Cytotoxic chemotherapeutic agents act by inducing DNA damage or impairing DNA synthesis, which initiates cell death pathways in cells that are in the midst of an active cell cycle. DNA damage may be induced directly (doxorubicin [Adriamycin], cyclophosphamide, etoposide, ifosfamide, cisplatin) or indirectly by interfering with mitosis (vincristine, taxanes). Antimetabolites such as methotrexate and hydroxyurea block production of DNA precursors required for DNA synthesis. These agents do not discriminate between proliferating normal cells and tumor cells, which explains side effects involving proliferative tissues of the hematopoietic system, skin, and gastrointestinal tract.

Cytotoxic Agents

- Mitotic inhibitors: vincristine, vinblastine, paclitaxel, docetaxel
- Antimetabolites: methotrexate, 5-fluorouracil, hydroxyurea
- Anthracycline: doxorubicin (Adriamycin)
- DNA-damaging: cyclophosphamide, ifosfamide, cisplatin, mitomycin-C
- Topoisomerase inhibitor: etoposide

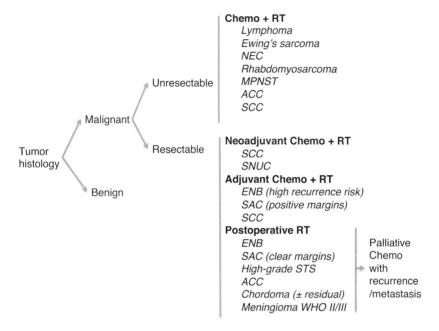

Fig. 31.1 Current treatment indications for chemotherapy in the management of malignant skull base tumors. ENB, esthesioneuroblastoma; SCC, squamous cell carcinoma; ACC, adenoid cystic carcinoma; SAC, sinonasal adenocarcinoma; SNUC, sinonasal undifferentiated carcinoma; NEC, neuroendocrine carcinoma; MPNST, malignant peripheral nerve sheath tumor; RT, radiation therapy; STS, soft tissue sarcoma; WHO, World Health Organization.[8,12–26]

Biological Agents

* Epidermal growth factor inhibitors: e.g., gefitinib
   ◦ Side effects: rash, diarrhea, corneal keratopathy, anemia, fatigue
* Vascular endothelial growth factor inhibitors: e.g., Bevacizumab
   ◦ Side effects: impaired wound healing, elevated liver enzymes, proteinuria, hypertension, hemorrhage, thromboembolism

Biological Therapies

Targeted biological therapies are in development for neoplasms that have shown poor response to cytotoxic chemotherapy in the past. These include meningioma, chordoma, chondrosarcoma, and neurofibromatosis type 2 (NF2)–associated vestibular schwannoma. These therapies take advantage of an understanding of the molecular mechanisms underlying tumor cell growth, survival, and migration pathways, and attempt to interfere with these pathways to arrest tumor growth, induce cell death, or block migration and invasion. **Table 31.1** shows

Table 31.1 Experimental Biological Therapies for Skull Base Tumors

Tumor	Biological Targeted Therapy	Mechanism of Action	Investigational Status
Chordoma	Imatinib mesylate	Tyrosine kinase inhibitor targeting plate-let-derived PDGFRB, BCR-ABL, and KIT	Case series[27,28]
	Cetuximab, gefitinib, lapatinib	EGFR inhibitor	Case series, phase II[29]
	CDDO-ME	STAT 3 inhibitor; blocks chordoma cell growth	Preclinical[30]
	Rapamycin	mTOR inhibitor	Case report[31]
Meningioma	Bevacizumab	VEGF is a soluble ligand that binds VEGFR, inducing cellular signals involved in angiogenesis. Bevacizumab is a monoclonal antibody with affinity for VEGF. By binding VEGF, it prevents VEGF binding to VEGFR, blocking downstream signaling pathways that promote angiogenesis.	Case series[32-35]
	Somatostatin analogues (Sandostatin, pasireotide)	Somatostatin inhibits meningioma growth in vitro. Meningioma cells express somatosta-tin receptors.	Preclinical, case series.[36] phase II [37,38]
	Erlotinib, gefitinib	Inhibitor of EGFR, which is overexpressed by meningioma cells	Single-arm phase II[39]
	Interferon-α	Signals blockade of DNA synthesis	Preclinical,[40] case series[41]
Chondrosarcoma	Zoledronic acid	Inhibits cell proliferation and increases cell death	Preclinical,[42] case report[43]
	Recombinant human apoptosis ligand-2/tumor necrosis factor–related apoptosis-inducing ligand (dulanermin)	Activates the extrinsic cell-death pathway, which is independent of p53	Phase I[44,45]

	Melphalan: quaternary ammonium conjugate	Localizes the effects of melphalan (DNA alkylating agent) to sites of aggrecan deposition due to interaction between proteoglycans and quaternary ammonium	Preclinical[46]
	PI3K and MEK inhibitors	PI3K and MEK activation is involved in integrin mediated signaling of chondrosarcoma cell migration	Preclinical[47]
	PPAR-γ agonist	PPAR-γ activation suppresses chondrosarcoma cell proliferation and induces apoptosis	Preclinical[48]
Ewing's sarcoma	IGF-1R antibodies	IGF-1R has been implicated in the proliferation, metastasis, and resistance of sarcoma	Phase I[49–51]
Osteosarcoma	Bisphosphonates	Inhibits cell proliferation and increases cell death; inhibits angiogenesis and osteolysis	Preclinical[52,53]
	MET inhibitors	Inhibits MET receptor, which is overexpressed in OS and responsible for tumor progression	Preclinical[54]
	Bevacizumab	Inhibits VEGF, which is overexpressed in OS	Preclincial[55]
Esthesioneuroblastoma	Sunitinib mesylate	Multikinase inhibitor (PDGFR, VEGFR, KIT)	Case report[56]
Paraganglioma	Lactate dehydrogenase inhibitor (oxamate)	SDH mutant tumors are dependent on glycolysis and are therefore limited in NAD+ regeneration. Pyruvate is converted to lactate by lactate dehydrogenase, which generates NAD+ from NADH	Preclinical[57]

(continued)

Table 31.1 (continued)

Tumor	Biological Targeted Therapy	Mechanism of Action	Investigational Status
Vestibular schwannoma	Bevacizumab	Inhibits VEGF, which is overexpressed in VS	Case series[58,59]
	PTC299	Blocks VEGF synthesis	Phase II[60]
	Trastuzumab	ERBB2 inhibitor	Preclinical[61]
	Erlotinib	EGFR tyrosine kinase inhibitor	Preclinical, case series[62]
	Lapatinib	Dual inhibitor of EGFR and HER2	Preclinical, phase 0[63]
	PAK inhibitor (IPA-3)	Merlin acts as a tumor suppressor in its active form. PAK phosphorylation of Merlin is required for maintenance in the inactive state. Inhibition of PAK allows maintenance of Merlin in the active state	Preclinical[64,65]

Abbreviations: EGFR, epidermal growth factor receptor; ERBB2/HER2, v-Erb-B2 avian erythroblastic leukemia viral oncogene homologue 2; PAK, p21 activated kinase; MET, hepatocyte growth factor receptor; VEGF, vascular endothelial growth factor; VEGFR, vascular endothelial growth factor receptor; pRB, retinoblastoma protein; PI3K, phosphoinositide 3 kinase; MEK, mitogen-activated protein kinase/extracellular signal-regulated kinase kinase; PPAR-γ, peroxisome proliferator-activated receptor gamma; KIT, V-Kit Hardy-Zuckerman feline sarcoma viral oncogene homologue 4; IGF-1R, insulin-like growth factor-1 receptor; CDDO-ME, 1,2-cyano-3,12-dioxo-oleana-1,9 (11)-dien-28-oic acid-methyl ester; BCR-ABL, breakpoint cluster and Abelson tyrosine kinase oncogene; mTOR, mammalian target of rapamycin; OS, osteosarcoma; NAD, nicotinamide adenine dinucleotide; NADH, reduced nicotinamide adenine dinucleotide; PDGFRβ, platelet-derived growth factor receptor-β; SDH, succinate dehydrogenase; STAT3, signal transducer and activator of transcription 3; VS, vestibular schwannoma.

the current experimental biological therapies for various types of skull base neoplasms.

■ References

Boldfaced references are of particular importance.

1. Hanahan D, Weinberg RA. Hallmarks of cancer: the next generation. Cell 2011; 144:646–674

2. Demonte F. Management considerations for malignant tumors of the skull base. Neurosurg Clin N Am 2013;24:1–10

3. Posner MR, Hershock DM, Blajman CR, et al; TAX 324 Study Group. Cisplatin and fluorouracil alone or with docetaxel in head and neck cancer. N Engl J Med 2007; 357:1705–1715

4. Vermorken JB, Remenar E, van Herpen C, et al; EORTC 24971/TAX 323 Study Group. Cisplatin, fluorouracil, and docetaxel in unresectable head and neck cancer. N Engl J Med 2007;357:1695–1704

5. Hanna EY, Cardenas AD, DeMonte F, et al. Induction chemotherapy for advanced squamous cell carcinoma of the paranasal sinuses. Arch Otolaryngol Head Neck Surg 2011;137:78–81

6. Diaz EM Jr, Kies MS. Chemotherapy for skull base cancers. Otolaryngol Clin North Am 2001;34:1079–1085, viii

7. Righi PD, Francis F, Aron BS, Weitzner S, Wilson KM, Gluckman J. Sinonasal undifferentiated carcinoma: a 10-year experience. Am J Otolaryngol 1996;17:167–171

8. Huncharek M, Kupelnick B. Combined chemoradiation versus radiation therapy alone in locally advanced nasopharyngeal carcinoma: results of a meta-analysis of 1,528 patients from six randomized trials. Am J Clin Oncol 2002;25:219–223

9. Posner M, Vermorken JB. Induction therapy in the modern era of combined-modality therapy for locally advanced head and neck cancer. Semin Oncol 2008;35:221–228

10. Shiga K, Ogawa T, Maki A, Amano M, Kobayashi T. Concomitant chemoradiotherapy as a standard treatment for squamous cell carcinoma of the temporal bone. Skull Base 2011;21:153–158

11. Ow TJ, Bell D, Kupferman ME, Demonte F, Hanna EY. Esthesioneuroblastoma. Neurosurg Clin N Am 2013;24:51–65

12. Harrison LB, Pfister DG, Kraus D, et al. Management of unresectable malignant tumors at the skull base using concomitant chemotherapy and radiotherapy with accelerated fractionation. Skull Base Surg 1994;4:127–131

13. Laurie SA, Licitra L. Systemic therapy in the palliative management of advanced salivary gland cancers. J Clin Oncol 2006;24:2673–2678

14. Austin JR, Cebrun H, Kershisnik MM, et al. Olfactory neuroblastoma and neuroendocrine carcinoma of the anterior skull base: treatment results at the M.D. Anderson cancer center. Skull Base Surg 1996;6:1–8

15. Kim WT, Nam J, Ki YK, et al. Neoadjuvant intra-arterial chemotherapy combined with radiotherapy and surgery in patients with advanced maxillary sinus cancer. Radiat Oncol J 2013;31:118–124

16. Rossi A, Molinari R, Boracchi P, et al. Adjuvant chemotherapy with vincristine, cyclophosphamide, and doxorubicin after radiotherapy in local-regional nasopharyngeal

cancer: results of a 4-year multicenter randomized study. J Clin Oncol 1988;6:1401–1410

17. Bhayani MK, Yilmaz T, Sweeney A, et al. Sinonasal adenocarcinoma: A 16-year experience at a single institution. Head Neck 2013

18. Baujat B, Audry H, Bourhis J, et al; MAC-NPC Collaborative Group. Chemotherapy as an adjunct to radiotherapy in locally advanced nasopharyngeal carcinoma. Cochrane Database Syst Rev 2006;4:CD004329

19. Zhang X, Ma K, Wang J, Wu W, Ma L, Huang D. A prospective evaluation of the combined helical tomotherapy and chemotherapy in pediatric patients with unresectable rhabdomyosarcoma of the temporal bone. Cell Biochem Biophys 2014;70:103–108

20. DeMonte F. Soft tissue sarcomas of the skull base: time for a new paradigm. Cancer 2007;110:939–940

21. Robbins KT, Ferlito A, Silver CE, et al. Contemporary management of sinonasal cancer. Head Neck 2011;33:1352–1365

22. Finnegan V, Parsons JT, Greene BD, Sharma V. Neoadjuvant chemotherapy followed by concurrent hyperfractionated radiation therapy and sensitizing chemotherapy for locally advanced (T3-T4) oropharyngeal squamous cell carcinoma. Head Neck 2009;31:167–174

23. Bradley PJ. Adenoid cystic carcinoma of the head and neck: a review. Curr Opin Otolaryngol Head Neck Surg 2004;12:127–132

24. Adeberg S, Hartmann C, Welzel T, et al. Long-term outcome after radiotherapy in patients with atypical and malignant meningiomas—clinical results in 85 patients treated in a single institution leading to optimized guidelines for early radiation therapy. Int J Radiat Oncol Biol Phys 2012;83:859–864

25. Haddad RI, Posner MR, Busse PM, et al. Chemoradiotherapy for adenoid cystic carcinoma: preliminary results of an organ sparing approach. Am J Clin Oncol 2006;29:153–157

26. Harrison LB, Pfister DG, Fass DE, et al. Concomitant chemotherapy-radiation therapy followed by hyperfractionated radiation therapy for advanced unresectable head and neck cancer. Int J Radiat Oncol Biol Phys 1991;21:703–708

27. Casali PG, Messina A, Stacchiotti S, et al. Imatinib mesylate in chordoma. Cancer 2004;101:2086–2097

28. Ferraresi V, Nuzzo C, Zoccali C, et al. Chordoma: clinical characteristics, management and prognosis of a case series of 25 patients. BMC Cancer 2010;10:22

29. Stacchiotti S, Tamborini E, Lo Vullo S, et al. Phase II study on lapatinib in advanced EGFR-positive chordoma. Ann Oncol 2013;24:1931–1936

30. Yang C, Hornicek FJ, Wood KB, et al. Blockage of Stat3 with CDDO-Me inhibits tumor cell growth in chordoma. Spine 2010;35:1668–1675

31. Ricci-Vitiani L, Runci D, D'Alessandris QG, et al. Chemotherapy of skull base chordoma tailored on responsiveness of patient-derived tumor cells to rapamycin. Neoplasia 2013;15:773–782

32. Wilson TJ, Heth JA. Regression of a meningioma during paclitaxel and bevacizumab therapy for breast cancer. J Clin Neurosci 2012;19:468–469

33. Puchner MJ, Hans VH, Harati A, Lohmann F, Glas M, Herrlinger U. Bevacizumab-induced regression of anaplastic meningioma. Ann Oncol 2010;21:2445–2446

34. Goutagny S, Raymond E, Sterkers O, Colombani JM, Kalamarides M. Radiographic regression of cranial meningioma in a NF2 patient treated by bevacizumab. Ann Oncol 2011;22:990–991
35. Lou E, Sumrall AL, Turner S, et al. Bevacizumab therapy for adults with recurrent/progressive meningioma: a retrospective series. J Neurooncol 2012;109:63–70
36. Schulz C, Mathieu R, Kunz U, Mauer UM. Treatment of unresectable skull base meningiomas with somatostatin analogs. Neurosurg Focus 2011;30:E11
37. **Chamberlain MC, Glantz MJ, Fadul CE. Recurrent meningioma: salvage therapy with long-acting somatostatin analogue. Neurology 2007;69:969–973**
38. **Chamberlain MC. The role of chemotherapy and targeted therapy in the treatment of intracranial meningioma. Curr Opin Oncol 2012;24:666–671**
39. Norden AD, Raizer JJ, Abrey LE, et al. Phase II trials of erlotinib or gefitinib in patients with recurrent meningioma. J Neurooncol 2010;96:211–217
40. Koper JW, Zwarthoff EC, Hagemeijer A, et al. Inhibition of the growth of cultured human meningioma cells by recombinant interferon-alpha. Eur J Cancer 1991;27:416–419
41. Kaba SE, DeMonte F, Bruner JM, et al. The treatment of recurrent unresectable and malignant meningiomas with interferon alpha-2B. Neurosurgery 1997;40:271–275
42. Gouin F, Ory B, Rédini F, Heymann D. Zoledronic acid slows down rat primary chondrosarcoma development, recurrent tumor progression after intralesional curettage and increases overall survival. Int J Cancer 2006;119:980–984
43. Montella L, Addeo R, Faiola V, et al. Zoledronic acid in metastatic chondrosarcoma and advanced sacrum chordoma: two case reports. J Exp Clin Cancer Res 2009;28:7
44. Herbst RS, Eckhardt SG, Kurzrock R, et al. Phase I dose-escalation study of recombinant human Apo2L/TRAIL, a dual proapoptotic receptor agonist, in patients with advanced cancer. J Clin Oncol 2010;28:2839–2846
45. Subbiah V, Brown RE, Buryanek J, et al. Targeting the apoptotic pathway in chondrosarcoma using recombinant human Apo2L/TRAIL (dulanermin), a dual proapoptotic receptor (DR4/DR5) agonist. Mol Cancer Ther 2012;11:2541–2546
46. Peyrode C, Weber V, David E, et al. Quaternary ammonium-melphalan conjugate for anticancer therapy of chondrosarcoma: in vitro and in vivo preclinical studies. Invest New Drugs 2012;30:1782–1790
47. Bloch O, Parsa AT. Skull base chondrosarcoma: evidence-based treatment paradigms. Neurosurg Clin N Am 2013;24:89–96
48. Nishida K, Furumatsu T, Takada I, et al. Inhibition of human chondrosarcoma cell growth via apoptosis by peroxisome proliferator-activated receptor-gamma. Br J Cancer 2002;86:1303–1309
49. Kurzrock R, Patnaik A, Aisner J, et al. A phase I study of weekly R1507, a human monoclonal antibody insulin-like growth factor-I receptor antagonist, in patients with advanced solid tumors. Clin Cancer Res 2010;16:2458–2465
50. Tolcher AW, Sarantopoulos J, Patnaik A, et al. Phase I, pharmacokinetic, and pharmacodynamic study of AMG 479, a fully human monoclonal antibody to insulin-like growth factor receptor 1. J Clin Oncol 2009;27:5800–5807
51. Olmos D, Postel-Vinay S, Molife LR, et al. Safety, pharmacokinetics, and preliminary activity of the anti-IGF-1R antibody figitumumab (CP-751,871) in patients with sar-

coma and Ewing's sarcoma: a phase 1 expansion cohort study. Lancet Oncol 2010; 11:129–135

52. Ohba T, Cates JM, Cole HA, et al. Pleiotropic effects of bisphosphonates on osteosarcoma. Bone 2014;63:110–120

53. Ohba T, Cole HA, Cates JM, et al. Bisphosphonates inhibit osteosarcoma-mediated osteolysis via attenuation of tumor expression of MCP-1 and RANKL. J Bone Miner Res 2014;29:1431–1445

54. Sampson ER, Martin BA, Morris AE, et al. The orally bioavailable met inhibitor PF-2341066 inhibits osteosarcoma growth and osteolysis/matrix production in a xenograft model. J Bone Miner Res 2011;26:1283–1294

55. Scharf VF, Farese JP, Coomer AR, et al. Effect of bevacizumab on angiogenesis and growth of canine osteosarcoma cells xenografted in athymic mice. Am J Vet Res 2013; 74:771–778

56. Preusser M, Hutterer M, Sohm M, et al. Disease stabilization of progressive olfactory neuroblastoma (esthesioneuroblastoma) under treatment with sunitinib mesylate. J Neurooncol 2010;97:305–308

57. Bancos I, Bida JP, Tian D, et al. High-throughput screening for growth inhibitors using a yeast model of familial paraganglioma. PLoS ONE 2013;8:e56827

58. Plotkin SR, Stemmer-Rachamimov AO, Barker FG II, et al. Hearing improvement after bevacizumab in patients with neurofibromatosis type 2. N Engl J Med 2009;361: 358–367

59. Mautner VF, Nguyen R, Kutta H, et al. Bevacizumab induces regression of vestibular schwannomas in patients with neurofibromatosis type 2. Neuro-oncol 2010;12: 14–18

60. Terry AR, Plotkin SR. Chemotherapy: present and future. Otolaryngol Clin North Am 2012;45:471–486, x

61. Clark JJ, Provenzano M, Diggelmann HR, Xu N, Hansen SS, Hansen MR. The ErbB inhibitors trastuzumab and erlotinib inhibit growth of vestibular schwannoma xenografts in nude mice: a preliminary study. Otol Neurotol 2008;29:846–853

62. Plotkin SR, Halpin C, McKenna MJ, Loeffler JS, Batchelor TT, Barker FG II. Erlotinib for progressive vestibular schwannoma in neurofibromatosis 2 patients. Otol Neurotol 2010;31:1135–1143

63. Ammoun S, Cunliffe CH, Allen JC, et al. ErbB/HER receptor activation and preclinical efficacy of lapatinib in vestibular schwannoma. Neuro-oncol 2010;12:834–843

64. Yi C, Wilker EW, Yaffe MB, Stemmer-Rachamimov A, Kissil JL. Validation of the p21-activated kinases as targets for inhibition in neurofibromatosis type 2. Cancer Res 2008;68:7932–7937

65. Licciulli S, Maksimoska J, Zhou C, et al. FRAX597, a small molecule inhibitor of the p21-activated kinases, inhibits tumorigenesis of neurofibromatosis type 2 (NF2)-associated Schwannomas. J Biol Chem 2013;288:29105–29114

32 Cerebrospinal Fluid Fistula in Skull Base Surgery

Cerebrospinal fluid (CSF) leak, or CSF fistula, is the direct passage of CSF from the subarachnoid space to lower pressure areas, often the upper respiratory tract or skin. It manifests most commonly as either CSF rhinorrhea or otorrhea, or as a leakage directly through a surgical incision.[1–3]

- A CSF leak may be classified according to its location or to the known or presumed cause.[4] Clinical communication regarding CSF rhinorrhea should include the site as well as the presumed cause.[4]

■ Classification

By Location

- Clivus (rare)
- Temporal bones: from the posterior or middle fossa, via mastoid air cells, eustachian tube, or petrous apex through an extensive lateral pneumatization of the sphenoid sinus. In the pediatric population, three usual routes of fistula are the facial canal, the petromastoid canal, and Hyrtl's fissure.[5]
- Anterior fossa: through the cribriform plate, ethmoid, sphenoid, or frontal bones
- Persistence of lateral craniopharyngeal canal or Sternberg canal[6,7]: results from incomplete fusion of the greater wing of the sphenoid bone with the basisphenoid, causing a weak region of the skull base
- Along the path of the internal carotid artery[5]
- Percutaneously
- Rosenmüller's fossa (pharyngeal recess): from Meckel's cave through the medial part of the sphenoid bone in the nasopharynx[8]
- Unknown

By Cause

- Traumatic
  - ○ Surgical (iatrogenic): planned or unplanned (acute and delayed)—10%[9]
  - ○ Nonsurgical: penetrating or nonpenetrating (acute and delayed)—80–90%[9]
- Nontraumatic
- High-pressure leak: tumor, hydrocephalus, idiopathic intracranial hypertension
  - ○ Normal pressure leak: congenital (Gorham-Stout disease, dehiscence of the footplate of the stapes, Mondini dysplasia; see Box 32.1), tumors, bone necrosis following chemotherapy or radiotherapy, arachnoid granulations, infection (osteomyelitis), empty sella—10%[9]
  - ○ Primary spontaneous rhinorrhea (PSR)—3–4%[9]

Pearl

Tumors can either cause high-pressure leak (because of obstruction or edema following treatment) or normal pressure leak (because of a direct effect on the skull base from the tumor and/or treatment).[4]

- **Pseudo-CSF rhinorrhea**: a surgical complication that mimics CSF rhinorrhea.[10] It has been described in patients who underwent mobilization or resection of the ipsilateral petrous or cavernous sinus segments of the internal carotid artery (ICA), presenting with ipsilateral rhinorrhea, typically exacerbated by exertion, an increase in room temperature, or feeling an intense emotion. In such patients, lacrimation is typically absent ipsilaterally to rhinorrhea, and β_2-transferrin testing is negative. The pathophysiological explanation for this nasal hypersecretion is probably related to the parasympathomimetic state caused by the surgical interruption of the sympathetic innervation of the nasal cavity during surgery.[10]

■ Diagnosis

The diagnosis of a suspected CSF leak has two end points:

1. To demonstrate the presence of CSF
2. To identify the precise site of the leak

Appearance

- CSF is generally clear and colorless ("crystal-clear water").
- When it is blood tinged, allowing it to drip onto linen will leave a ring of blood with a larger concentric ring of clear fluid (ring sign or halo sign).[5]

- Patients with CSF leaks may complain of a salty taste or even a sweet taste because CSF contains two-thirds the glucose content of blood.
- CSF leak may be induced by a Valsalva maneuver, compression of the neck veins, or a change in position because the sphenoid and frontal sinuses may act as reservoirs.[11]

Biochemical Analyses

- β_2-transferrin: a carbohydrate-free (desialated) isoform of transferrin that is almost exclusively found in the CSF. It is not present in blood, nasal mucus, tears, or mucosal discharge. It has been reported to have a sensitivity of nearly 100% and a specificity of about 95%.[12,13] False-positive and false-negative results can occur in patients with chronic liver disease, inborn errors of glycoprotein metabolism, or genetic variants of transferrin.[11] It is detected using protein electrophoresis.[14]
- Beta-trace protein: another CSF marker that is reported to have high predictive value.[11]
- Glucostix test: a traditional method for detection of the presence of CSF. It is not recommended as a confirmatory test due to its lack of specificity and sensitivity.[13] Normal CSF glucose is > 30 mg%, whereas secretions are < 5 mg%.[5] Interpretation of the results is confounded by various factors such as contamination from glucose-containing fluid (tears, nasal mucus, blood in nasal mucus) or relatively low CSF glucose levels (meningitis).

Fluorescein Nasal Endoscopic Evaluation

When the biochemical examination of a fluid sample, nasal endoscopy, or imaging techniques give positive results that confirm and identify the leak, then surgical repair of the dural lesion is indicated.[15] When these preliminary tests are unable to identify the leak, the fluorescein test follows in order to locate and to confirm or exclude a CSF leak.[16] When the fistula is evident, the nasal endoscopic approach is successful in treating the fistula—also without the use of intrathecal fluorescein.

- Fluorescein can be administered suboccipitally into the cisterna magna (rarely used) or through a lumbar injection.
- It should be administered in a 5% concentration up to 1 mL (50 mg) of total dose. Fluorescein should be mixed with previously withdrawn CSF (ideal quantity of 9 mL) and slowly injected into the lumbar subarachnoid space.[16,17]
- Applying a blue filter on the light source and a yellow filter on the endoscope lens is a useful technique to enhance fluorescein in very low flow fistulas. Fluorescein appears greenish.
- Rare complications including seizures, grand mal epilepsy, opisthotonos, and peripheral nerve palsy have been reported for doses > 100 mg.[16]

Radiological Investigations

- Plain X-rays: generally ineffective. They can demonstrate indirect signs such as fractures and pneumoencephalos, but they are rarely helpful in localization of the fistula.
- High-resolution computed tomography (CT): useful screening examination for the initial workup of CSF rhinorrhea or otorrhea. The study should include thin coronal cuts and can be performed with or without intravenous contrast. CT offers superb bony detail and can reveal bone defects and opacification of sinuses or air cells. The site of the leak is usually associated with abnormal enhancement of the brain.[5,11]
- Magnetic resonance imaging (MRI): reserved for characterizing underlying pathology (e.g., inflammatory tissue, meningoencephalocele, or tumor). MRI can demonstrate brain herniation into the ethmoid, sphenoid, or frontal sinuses.[13]
- Radionuclide cisternography: an old test that does not provide precise anatomic localization of CSF leaks but is very sensitive to small leaks. It requires that nasal pledgets be placed in the nasal cavity adjacent to each foramina before the test.
- CT or MR cisternography: With active leaks, cisternography demonstrates movement of contrast through the defect in 85% of the cases.[11] It is considered the procedure of choice when a patient is leaking clinically. If the patient is not leaking, there is no point in giving intrathecal contrast, as the test is almost always negative in the absence of active CSF leak.

■ Treatment

- Antibiotics: The role of antibiotic prophylaxis in patients with CSF leaks has been studied extensively, yet remains controversial.[18] Some reports suggest that the use of antibiotic therapy in patients with a CSF leak may increase the risk of meningitis, rather than decrease it, via eradication of commensal organisms and colonization of pathogenic flora (that may be antibiotic resistant).[19]
- Acetazolamide: a carbonic anhydrase inhibitor and a sulfonamide derivative. Following an initial dose of acetazolamide, more than 99% of brain carbonic anhydrase activity is inhibited, thus decreasing CSF production by as much as 48%. Early acetazolamide administration as part of the conservative measures in patients with skull base fractures can be useful in preventing CSF leakage and shortening the duration of leakage in patients who already have either otorrhea or rhinorrhea. However, no decrease in the incidence of meningitis or in the number of patients needing surgical intervention to ter-

minate the leakage have been demonstrated. Therefore, the drug is considered to be of limited value.[1]

- ○ Dosage: 25 mg/kg/day by mouth to be continued for 48 hours after cessation of the leakage.[1]

Traumatic Cerebrospinal Fluid Leak

A CSF leak is a complication in 2% of all patients who have sustained a head injury and in 12 to 30% of all cases of basilar skull base fractures. Fractures involving the frontal or ethmoidal sinuses and longitudinal temporal bone fractures are most commonly associated with CSF leakage.[18] Although penetrating head trauma is an obvious cause of CSF leak, most traumatic CSF leaks occur as a result of blunt trauma.

Most traumatic CSF leaks resolve spontaneously, with the majority resolving within the first 24 to 48 hours. The mechanism of CSF leak cessation is thought to involve blood products, inflammatory adhesions, or herniation of brain at the site of the dural breach and associated skull fracture. However, persistent fistulas do occur, particularly in patients with fractures involving the anterior cranial fossa. The rate of spontaneous cessation of traumatic CSF leaks has been reported to be 53 to 95%.[18,20] CSF leaks associated with temporal bone fractures have historically been thought to have a higher propensity to cease spontaneously.[21] Delayed CSF leaks occur at an average time interval of 13 days and a range of up to 30 days.[18]

- Some authors have suggested that lumbar drainage may be a safe and effective treatment in patients with traumatic CSF leakage, but it entails the risk of cerebral transtentorial herniation, which must be assessed.[22]
- Traditionally, anterior fossa CSF leaks are approached intracranially via a bifrontal craniotomy for both intradural and extradural approaches (see Chapter 14). After the craniotomy is performed, loose bone fragments are removed. The dural tear is identified and closed primarily, whenever possible. Modest resection of herniated brain tissue may be required. When the dural tear is extensive, an autologous graft, such as fascia lata or pericranium, is preferable to nonautologous material, given the contaminated nature of the field. Frequently, fibrin glue is used as a sealant, although its true efficacy in preventing CSF fistulas is unproven.[18]
- The endoscopic endonasal approach has largely replaced the traditional open craniotomy approaches as the primary mode of repair due to its minimal invasiveness and to the optimal results obtained (≥ 90% success in sealing the dural defect after the first endoscopic intervention and ≥ 97% success after the second endoscopic attempt).[16] These outcomes have reduced the indications for conservative treatment, thus limiting the use of CSF drainage for acute posttraumatic fistulas. To optimize the endoscopic approach, the fol-

lowing steps must be taken preoperatively: define precisely the site and size of the fistula; determine the presence of multiple fistulas; and adequately prepare the area surrounding the gap in order to guarantee good adhesion of the graft.[16]

- For defects of the middle cranial fossa, an intracranial approach via a temporal craniotomy and primary dural closure, or an extracranial approach via a mastoidectomy, can be used. The extracranial approach offers the advantage of enabling extensive packing of the middle ear with fat and cartilage, but it may be contraindicated if hearing is to be preserved.[18]

Iatrogenic Cerebrospinal Fluid Leak

An iatrogenic CSF leak can occur in pituitary and posterior fossa surgery.

- **Anterior skull base surgery**: There has been a rapid evolution in the surgical approach to many anterior skull base pathologies. The endoscopic route is now a preferred option in many surgical centers when managing both benign and malignant disease. The majority of small defects (< 1 cm) in the skull base are reliably repaired using multilayered free grafts, with success rates surpassing 90% and minimal differences among the methods or material used.[23]
  - Multilayer free graft reconstruction can be tailored according to the CSF leak grading systems, such as the one in **Table 32.1**.[24] Similar algorithms for skull base reconstruction have also been proposed by other authors.[25]
  - Collagen seems to be effective as a dural substitute because it provides scaffolding for fibroblast ingrowth and stimulates the coagulation cascade and platelet aggregation.[24] Tissue glues do not stop CSF leaks, but they can help prevent migration of the repair construct.[26]
  - For larger skull base defects (> 3 cm), materials used for free graft repairs have included cadaveric pericardium, acellular dermis, fascia lata, and titanium mesh.[23]
  - With multilayer reconstruction, the estimated postoperative CSF leak rate is considered to be less than 5% for traditional transsphenoidal surgery (< 1-cm defects) and around 15.6% for the extended surgery (> 3-cm defects).
  - A nasoseptal flap has been proposed to reconstruct large dural defects.[27] Subsequently, other intranasal and regional vascular flaps were described and made available for skull base reconstruction. Options for skull base reconstructions includes avascular grafts, nasoseptal pedicled flaps, turbinate flaps, and novel endoscopic regional flaps[28] (**Table 32.2**). See also Chapter 16.
  - A systematic review of the literature showed that vascular flaps decrease the CSF leak rate in large skull base defects from 15.6% to 6.7%.[23] Although

Table 32.1   Example of a Cerebrospinal Fluid (CSF) Leak Grading System in Endonasal Transsphenoidal Surgery

Grade	Description	Repair Method
0	Absence of CSF leak, confirmed by Valsalva maneuver	Collagen sponge
1	Small "weeping" leak, confirmed by Valsalva maneuver, without an obvious, or with only a small, diaphragmatic defect	1. Collagen sponge (intrasellar fat graft if large dead space present after tumor removal) 2. Titanium mesh buttress (intrasellar, extradural) 3. Second-layer collagen sponge over mesh 4. Tissue glue to hold repair in position
2	Moderate CSF leak with obvious diaphragmatic defect	1. Intrasellar fat graft 2. Collagen sponge over sellar dura 3. Titanium mesh buttress (intrasellar, extradural) 4. Additional fat in sphenoid sinus 5. Tissue glue to hold repair in position
3	Large CSF leak, typically created as part of an extended transsphenoidal approach trough in the supradiaphragmatic or clival dura for tumor access	1. Intrasellar fat graft 2. Collagen sponge over sellar dura 3. Titanium mesh buttress (intrasellar, extradural) 4. Additional fat in sphenoid sinus 5. Tissue glue to hold repair in position 6. Lumbar CSF diversion for 48 hours

Source: Adapted from Esposito F, Dusick JR, Fatemi N, Kelly DF. Graded repair of cranial base defects and cerebrospinal fluid leaks in transsphenoidal surgery. Neurosurgery 2007;60(4, Suppl 2):295–303, discussion 303–304. Reprinted with permission.

the current literature suggests that skull base repair with vascularized tissue is associated with a lower rate of CSF leak compared with free tissue graft,[27,29] this study was limited by its search strategy. Selected trials included subjects of any age, with any comorbidity, and of varied duration of follow-up.[23]

Lateral Skull Base Surgery

A CSF leak may occur following lateral skull base craniotomies for the excision of cerebellopontine angle (CPA) neoplasms or microvascular decompression (MVD). CSF leakage can occur in lateral skull base surgery, regardless of the approach used.[30] In these cases, CSF leakage can present as leakage through the

Table 32.2   Flaps Used for Dural Defect Repairs

Location	Vascular Tissue Flap	Pedicle
Intranasal vascular tissue flaps	Nasoseptal flap	Posterior nasoseptal from sphenopalatine artery
	Inferior turbinate flap	Inferior turbinate artery
	Middle turbinate flap	Middle turbinate artery
Regional vascular tissue flaps	Pericranial flap	Supraorbital and supratrochlear artery
	Temporoparietal fascia flap	Superficial temporal artery
	Palatal flap	Greater palatine artery

Source: Adapted from Patel MR, Stadler ME, Snyderman CH, et al. How to choose? Endoscopic skull base reconstructive options and limitations. Skull Base 2010;20:397–404. Reprinted with permission.

surgical wound or by the presence of rhinorrhea or otorrhea, as the CSF escapes into the eustachian tube to the nasopharynx and nasal cavity or from the mastoid cavity to the middle ear and external auditory canal, respectively.[31]

- The CSF leak rates for the translabyrinthine (TL), suboccipital (SO), and middle fossa (MF) approaches have been found to be 12%, 12%, and 13%, respectively, with no significant difference in leak rates between the approaches.[32] However, combined approaches have a significantly higher leak rate when compared with singular approaches.[32] A wound leak is the most common CSF leak presentation following the TL approach (54%), but rhinorrhea is the most common CSF leak presentation following the SO (68%) and MF (70%) approaches. This can be explained by the meticulous obliteration of the eustachian tube and middle ear space with fat and muscle grafts during the TL approach. Also, routine MF and SO approaches require only bone waxing of the air cells and occasional use of muscle graft in the internal auditory canal (IAC). If an air cell tract persists at the end of the IAC or into the mastoid, then CSF has an unobstructed path into the middle ear space and the eustachian tube, resulting in rhinorrhea.[32]
- Conservative treatment includes any combination of acetazolamide, elevation of the head of the bed, oversewing the wound, bed rest, or placement of a lumbar drain. Surgical treatment includes reexploration of the wound, mastoid obliteration, eustachian tube obliteration, or shunt placement.[32] It is imperative to be more aggressive with CSF rhinorrhea when initial conservative management fails due to the decreased success when treating rhinorrhea conservatively after initial failure.[32]
- Shunting should be considered as the primary treatment when the diagnosis of hydrocephalus has been established.[33]

- In cases of persistent or recurrent CSF leak, a subtotal petrosectomy can be considered. This is accomplished by converting the mastoid and petrous elements of the temporal bone into a single cavity while the ossicles and bony external canal are sacrificed. The likelihood of subsequent ascending infection is diminished by occluding the eustachian tube, blind sacking the external meatus, and obliterating the temporal bone cavity. This procedure results in a conductive deafness. Other techniques may be considered if the hearing on the opposite side is also compromised.[34] For persistent leaks, consideration should be given to the fact that the patient may in fact have increased intracranial pressure, and the leak is a manifestation of hydrocephalus. In this case, once the leak is stopped, typically with a lumbar drain at minimum, a ventriculoperitoneal shunt should be considered.

Primary Spontaneous Rhinorrhea

This is the term used for rhinorrhea without an identifiable cause.[4,35] A careful history, combined with endoscopic, radiological, and surgical examination will commonly result in the identification of a probable cause of the leak.[36]

- Primary spontaneous rhinorrhea often occurs in middle aged or older women, with a body mass index (BMI) > 30 in most patient series.[37]
- The so-called focal atrophy theory proposes that atrophy of the normal content of the cribriform plate or sella turcica results in reduced bone tissue bulk through which arachnoidal pouches exert a local erosive effect. However, this theory lacks anatomic studies to support it.[35]
- The arachnoid granulation theory, which is supported by anatomic studies, proposed that skull base arachnoid granulations are not covered by endothelium but by an extension of the dura. This creates a closed system of CSF within the arachnoid granulation that transmits pulsations through its capsule to cause destruction of the surrounding bone.[38]
- Primary spontaneous rhinorrhea may be due to an elevated intracranial pressure (ICP) and is a rare symptom of idiopathic intracranial hypertension (IIH).[37] As with PSR, IIH is a diagnosis of exclusion. High ICP is the most important sign in the diagnosis of IIH. Normal ICP values registered in PSR might be due to the fact that rhinorrhea may reduce the ICP due to CSF leakage. In one study, pressures obtained after repair of the skull base and resolution of the leakage were indeed significantly higher.[37]
- Conservative management has little effect on PSR and may increase the risk of meningitis; thus, surgery should be performed as soon as the condition is diagnosed. Even though conservative treatment is sometimes effective, ICP could again become elevated, and the already weakened skull base may be destroyed again, thereby causing a recurrence. PSR is an indication for surgery and should be followed by postoperative control of high ICP.[37]

■ Complications

The significance of a persistent CSF fistula is not the leak itself but its sequelae: posture-related headache, pneumocephalus, and, most significantly, bacterial meningitis. CSF rhinorrhea and otorrhea are independent predictors of post-traumatic meningitis.[39] Additionally, they may lead to a significantly increased cost of hospitalization.[39] CSF leaks have been associated with about a 10% risk of developing meningitis per year.[13]

- Overall, between 7% and 30% of all patients with posttraumatic CSF leakage develop meningitis, and this rate increases as the duration of CSF leakage increases.[40,41] *Streptococcus pneumoniae* is by far the most common pathogen.[42]

> **Pearl**
>
> Meningitis does not aid in the spontaneous resolution of the CSF rhinorrhea. Thus, surgical intervention, whenever required, should not be delayed.[43]

> **Box 32.1**   Congenital Conditions Causing Normal Pressure Leak
>
> - **Gorham-Stout disease:** a rare disease characterized by nonmalignant intraosseous proliferation of hemangiomatous or lymphangiomatous tissue that causes massive osteolysis. It is nonhereditary with no gender-related predilection. It predominantly affects patients younger than 40 years of age. Pelvic and shoulder regions are most frequently affected. The skull is among the least common locations of involvement.[44]
> - **Cochlear dysplasias:** associated with a defect in the stapes footplate. It can cause a CSF leak. Mondini dysplasia is a rare malformation of the inner ear commonly associated with loss of hearing and vestibular function. Children with Mondini dysplasia are predisposed to developing a spontaneous CSF leak and recurrent meningitis.[45,46]

■ References

Boldfaced references are of particular importance.

1. Abrishamkar S, Khalighinejad N, Moein P. Analysing the effect of early acetazolamide administration on patients with a high risk of permanent cerebrospinal fluid leakage. Acta Med Iran 2013;51:467–471
2. Brandt MT, Jenkins WS, Fattahi TT, Haug RH. Cerebrospinal fluid: implications in oral and maxillofacial surgery. J Oral Maxillofac Surg 2002;60:1049–1056
3. Mokri B. Spontaneous cerebrospinal fluid leaks: from intracranial hypotension to cerebrospinal fluid hypovolemia—evolution of a concept. Mayo Clin Proc 1999;74:1113–1123
4. Har-El G. What is "spontaneous" cerebrospinal fluid rhinorrhea? Classification of cerebrospinal fluid leaks. Ann Otol Rhinol Laryngol 1999;108:323–326
5. Greenberg MS. Handbook of Neurosurgery. New York: Thieme; 2010

6. Rossi Izquierdo M, Martín Martín C, Labella Caballero T. [Association between cerebrospinal fluid leakage and persistence of Sternberg's canal: coincidence or cause?]. Acta Otorrinolaringol Esp 2012;63:144–146 (English Edition)

7. Bendersky DC, Landriel FA, Ajler PM, Hem SM, Carrizo AG. Sternberg's canal as a cause of encephalocele within the lateral recess of the sphenoid sinus: a report of two cases. Surg Neurol Int 2011;2:171

8. Jaffe B, Welch K, Strand R, Treves S. Cerebrospinal fluid rhinorrhea via the fossa of Rosenmuller. Laryngoscope 1976;86:903–907

9. Iffenecker C, Benoudiba F, Parker F, et al. [The place of MRI in the study of cerebrospinal fluid fistulas]. J Radiol 1999;80:37–43

10. Cusimano MD, Sekhar LN. Pseudo-cerebrospinal fluid rhinorrhea. J Neurosurg 1994; 80:26–30

11. **Han Z-L, He D-S, Mao Z-G, Wang H-J. Cerebrospinal fluid rhinorrhea following trans-sphenoidal pituitary macroadenoma surgery: experience from 592 patients. Clin Neurol Neurosurg 2008;110:570–579**

12. Irjala K, Suonpää J, Laurent B. Identification of CSF leakage by immunofixation. Arch Otolaryngol 1979;105:447–448

13. Abuabara A. Cerebrospinal fluid rhinorrhoea: diagnosis and management. Med Oral Patol Oral Cir Bucal 2007;12:E397–E400

14. McCudden CR, Senior BA, Hainsworth S, et al. Evaluation of high resolution gel b(2)-transferrin for detection of cerebrospinal fluid leak. Clin Chem Lab Med 2013; 51:311–315

15. **Locatelli D, Rampa F, Acchiardi I, Bignami M, De Bernardi F, Castelnuovo P. Endoscopic endonasal approaches for repair of cerebrospinal fluid leaks: nine-year experience. Neurosurgery 2006; 58(4, Suppl 2)ONS-246–ONS-256, ONS-256–ONS-257**

16. **Felisati G, Bianchi A, Lozza P, Portaleone S. Italian multicentre study on intrathecal fluorescein for craniosinusal fistulae. Acta Otorhinolaryngol Ital 2008;28: 159–163**

17. Wolf G, Greistorfer K, Stammberger H. [Endoscopic detection of cerebrospinal fluid fistulas with a fluorescence technique. Report of experiences with over 925 cases]. Laryngorhinootologie 1997;76:588–594

18. Friedman JA, Ebersold MJ, Quast LM. Persistent posttraumatic cerebrospinal fluid leakage. Neurosurg Focus 2000;9:e1

19. Yilmazlar S, Arslan E, Kocaeli H, et al. Cerebrospinal fluid leakage complicating skull base fractures: analysis of 81 cases. Neurosurg Rev 2006;29:64–71

20. Brodie HA, Thompson TC. Management of complications from 820 temporal bone fractures. Am J Otol 1997;18:188–197

21. Brodie HA. Prophylactic antibiotics for posttraumatic cerebrospinal fluid fistulae. A meta-analysis. Arch Otolaryngol Head Neck Surg 1997;123:749–752

22. Shapiro SA, Scully T. Closed continuous drainage of cerebrospinal fluid via a lumbar subarachnoid catheter for treatment or prevention of cranial/spinal cerebrospinal fluid fistula. Neurosurgery 1992;30:241–245

23. **Harvey RJ, Parmar P, Sacks R, Zanation AM. Endoscopic skull base reconstruction of large dural defects: a systematic review of published evidence. Laryngoscope 2012;122:452–459**

24. Esposito F, Dusick JR, Fatemi N, Kelly DF. Graded repair of cranial base defects and cerebrospinal fluid leaks in transsphenoidal surgery. Neurosurgery 2007;60(4, Suppl 2):295–303, discussion 303–304

25. Tabaee A, Anand VK, Brown SM, Lin JW, Schwartz TH. Algorithm for reconstruction after endoscopic pituitary and skull base surgery. Laryngoscope 2007;117: 1133–1137

26. Kumar A, Maartens NF, Kaye AH. Evaluation of the use of BioGlue in neurosurgical procedures. J Clin Neurosci 2003;10:661–664

27. Hadad G, Bassagasteguy L, Carrau RL, et al. A novel reconstructive technique after endoscopic expanded endonasal approaches: vascular pedicle nasoseptal flap. Laryngoscope 2006;116:1882–1886

28. Patel MR, Stadler ME, Snyderman CH, et al. How to choose? Endoscopic skull base reconstructive options and limitations. Skull Base 2010;20:397–404

29. Zanation AM, Snyderman CH, Carrau RL, Kassam AB, Gardner PA, Prevedello DM. Minimally invasive endoscopic pericranial flap: a new method for endonasal skull base reconstruction. Laryngoscope 2009;119:13–18

30. Hardy DG, Macfarlane R, Moffat DA. Wound closure after acoustic neuroma surgery. Br J Neurosurg 1993;7:171–174

31. Netto AA, Colafêmina JF, Centeno RS. Dural defect repair in translabyrinthine acoustic neuroma surgery and its implications in cerebrospinal fluid leak occurrence. J Neurol Surg B Skull Base 2012;73:327–330

32. Mangus BD, Rivas A, Yoo MJ, et al. Management of cerebrospinal fluid leaks after vestibular schwannoma surgery. Otol Neurotol 2011;32:1525–1529

33. Spetzler RF, Wilson CB. Management of recurrent CSF rhinorrhea of the middle and posterior fossa. J Neurosurg 1978;49:393–397

34. Hamilton JW, Foy PM, Lesser TH. Subtotal petrosectomy in the treatment of cerebrospinal fluid fistulae of the lateral skull base. Br J Neurosurg 1997;11:496–500

35. Ommaya AK, Di Chiro G, Baldwin M, Pennybacker JB. Non-traumatic cerebrospinal fluid rhinorrhoea. J Neurol Neurosurg Psychiatry 1968;31:214–225

36. Hubbard JL, McDonald TJ, Pearson BW, Laws ER Jr. Spontaneous cerebrospinal fluid rhinorrhea: evolving concepts in diagnosis and surgical management based on the Mayo Clinic experience from 1970 through 1981. Neurosurgery 1985;16:314–321

37. Yang Z, Wang B, Wang C, Liu P. Primary spontaneous cerebrospinal fluid rhinorrhea: a symptom of idiopathic intracranial hypertension? J Neurosurg 2011;115: 165–170

38. Gacek RR. Arachnoid granulation cerebrospinal fluid otorrhea. Ann Otol Rhinol Laryngol 1990;99:854–862

39. Sonig A, Thakur JD, Chittiboina P, Khan IS, Nanda A. Is posttraumatic cerebrospinal fluid fistula a predictor of posttraumatic meningitis? A US Nationwide Inpatient Sample database study. Neurosurg Focus 2012;32:E4

40. Choi D, Spann R. Traumatic cerebrospinal fluid leakage: risk factors and the use of prophylactic antibiotics. Br J Neurosurg 1996;10:571–575

41. MacGee EE, Cauthen JC, Brackett CE. Meningitis following acute traumatic cerebrospinal fluid fistula. J Neurosurg 1970;33:312–316

42. Kaufman BA, Tunkel AR, Pryor JC, Dacey RG Jr. Meningitis in the neurosurgical patient. Infect Dis Clin North Am 1990;4:677–701

43. Malik TH, Bruce IA, Kelly G, Ramsden RT, Saeed SR. Does meningitis stop CSF rhinorrhea following lateral skull base surgery? Skull Base 2007;17:235–238
44. Lo C-P, Chen C-Y, Chin S-C, Juan C-J, Hsueh C-J, Chen A. Disappearing calvarium in Gorham disease: MR imaging characteristics with pathologic correlation. AJNR Am J Neuroradiol 2004;25:415–418
45. Kaftan H, Adamaszek M, Hosemann W. [Mondini dysplasia: traumatic cerebrospinal fluid otorrhea with meningitis]. HNO 2006;54:624–627
46. Syal R, Tyagi I, Goyal A. Cerebrospinal fluid otorhinorrhea due to cochlear dysplasias. Int J Pediatr Otorhinolaryngol 2005;69:983–988

33 Skull Base Infections

With the introduction and use of antibiotics over the past century, infections of the skull base have become rare, especially in the Western countries.[1] These serious conditions occur most often in predisposed patient populations, including diabetic, elderly, or immunocompromised individuals,[2-11] making their management difficult **(Table 33.1)**.

The most common skull base infections, according to location, are illustrated in **Fig. 33.1**.

■ Infections of the Anterior Skull Base

- Osteomyelitis with, or without, bony erosion and destruction
- Mass lesions, e.g., subperiosteal abscesses or fungal masses
- Basal meningitis
- Cerebritis

Extension from Paranasal Sinus Infections

Pathophysiology

Sinusitis affects an estimated 16% of the adult population in the United States.[12] Intracranial complications of paranasal sinusitis include subdural empyema, brain abscess, meningitis, subperiosteal abscess, and osteomyelitis of the anterior skull base.[13-15] Infection spreads in susceptible individuals to the anterior cranial base and orbit through either direct extension (from the nose, ethmoid, sphenoid, or frontal air sinuses) or retrograde thrombophlebitis.[13] Although bacterial and viral infections are more common in sinusitis, they are usually noninvasive and thus are infrequently associated with a skull base infection.[12] The only exception is posttraumatic sinusitis with pyocele formation, ultimately leading to subperiosteal abscess, brain abscess, osteomyelitis, and bony destruction.[13,14] This condition is most commonly seen in frontal sinus penetrating injuries. Fungal infections tend to be more invasive. Invasive fungal sinusitis most

Table 33.1   Precipitating Factors of the Most Common Skull Base Infections, and Patients Affected[2–11]

General	Diabetes
	Old age
	Trauma
	Surgery
	Immunocompromised
	CNS infections causing basal arachnoiditis (e.g., cysticercosis)

Specific
- Paranasal sinus infection   Pediatrics and young adults
- Orbital infections   Pediatrics
- Osteomyelitis   Trauma, surgery
- Malignant otitis externa   Old age, DM
- Mastoiditis   Pediatrics, immunocompromised
- Fungal infections   DM, AIDS, immunocompromised
- Odontoid infections   Old age, immunocompromised
- Apical petrositis   Middle ear infections

Abbreviations: AIDS, acquired immunodeficiency syndrome; CNS, central nervous system; DM, diabetes mellitus.

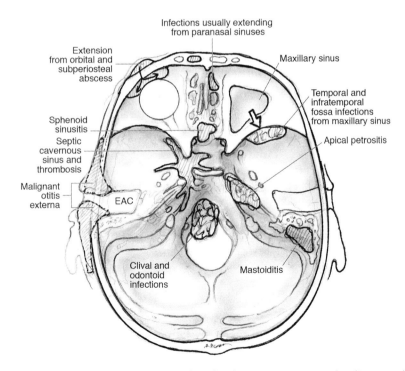

Fig. 33.1   Common skull base infections based on location. EAC, external auditory canal.

commonly starts in the nose or paranasal sinuses, then extends to the orbit, with the destruction of the cribriform plate or orbital apex, and to the cranial base, causing mass effect on intracranial structures.[2] The most common pathogens for invasive fungal sinusitis are *Mucoraceae* (mucormycosis) followed by *Aspergillus*[2] (**Table 33.2**). Mortality from invasive fungal sinusitis in immunocompromised patients is 50 to 90%.

Clinical Presentation and Sequelae

Presentation often occurs in childhood or young adulthood, and the condition is usually precipitated by trauma, diabetes mellitus (DM), or immunocompromised states, such as corticosteroids therapy, malignancies, burns, AIDS, or renal failure.[16] Fever and other constitutional manifestations are usually absent in fungal and chronic sinus infections. The most common presentations are as follows[2,11-16]:

- History of trauma or recurrent sinusitis.
- Local pain, swelling, and redness over the affected sinus. Frontal sinusitis can cause a Pott's puffy tumor, which is swelling and edema over the eyebrow due to subperiosteal abscess formation, and is usually associated with frontal bone osteomyelitis.[17] This was originally described with a tuberculous subperiosteal abscess.
- Focal neurologic manifestations or symptoms of increased intracranial pressure from intracranial mass effect (e.g., fungal mass).
- Mass lesions from mucormycosis can extend to involve the temporal and infratemporal fossae.
- Ophthalmoplegia, proptosis, or blindness from extension to the orbit or cavernous sinus thrombosis (see **Box 33.1**).
- Other intracranial complications of paranasal sinusitis include basal meningitis, cavernous sinus thrombosis, subdural empyema, and brain abscess. Approximately half of subdural empyema and parenchymal brain abscesses are caused by paranasal sinusitis.

Workup[12,18]

- Laboratory:
  - Leukocytosis is nonspecific, but may denote acute infection, with elevated erythrocyte sedimentation rate (ESR) and C-reactive protein (CRP) (nonspecific and elevated in many inflammatory and infectious conditions).
  - Neutropenia can occur with fungal infections.
  - Culture and sensitivity analysis of the sinus aspiration.
  - Blood cultures are usually sterile. Cerebrospinal fluid (CSF) cultures may be indicated in selected patients, but, because of the potential presence of mass effects, should be considered only after imaging is completed.

Box 33.1.   Cavernous Sinus Thrombosis[21–25]

Septic cavernous sinus thrombosis is a serious complication of acute sinusitis and orbital and midface infections in an otherwise healthy individual. Infection usually spreads directly through the valveless ophthalmic veins. In the pre-antibiotic era, mortality was almost 100%, but with antimicrobial agents it is now less than 30%.

The clinical presentation is usually acute, and includes the following:

1. Retro-orbital pain is usually the first sign. It is followed by periorbital edema and ecchymosis.
2. Ophthalmoplegia (abducens nerve is affected first).
3. Exophthalmos.
4. Increased intraocular pressure.
5. Sluggish papillary responses and decreased visual acuity.
6. Extension to the contralateral eye is suggestive.
7. Meningeal signs.
8. Subarachnoid hemorrhage or carotid occlusion can occur with fungal infections.

Imaging studies include CT and MRI with contrast, supplemented by magnetic resonance venography (MRV), magnetic resonance angiography (MRA) and diffusion-weighted magnetic resonance imaging (DW-MRI). Common findings with imaging are as follows:

1. Filling defects within the cavernous sinus with contrast injection indicating thrombi
2. Widening of the cavernous sinus evident by its walls turning convex instead of concave
3. Absence of flow signals and restricted diffusion, especially in superior ophthalmic veins
4. Dilation of cavernous sinus tributaries

- Polymerase chain reaction (PCR) for detection of circulating DNA from mucorales.[19,20]
- Imaging: computed tomography (CT) and magnetic resonance imaging (MRI) of the brain, orbit, and paranasal sinuses
  - Opacification of the paranasal sinuses or air–fluid level
  - Mucosal thickening or enhancement within the sinus
  - Orbital cellulitis (see below)
  - CT to assess bony destruction within the anterior cranial base and its extent
  - Herniation of the brain through cranial base defects, into orbits or ethmoid
  - Subperiosteal abscess, subdural empyema, or intracranial mass lesions
  - Cavernous sinus thrombosis (see **Box 33.1**)
- D-dimer testing
  - A recent study suggested that D-dimer testing may be useful in diagnosing cavernous sinus thrombosis.[24]

Extension from Orbital Cellulitis

Pathophysiology

Orbital cellulitis is an orbital infection commonly seen in the pediatric age group following (1) direct spread from ethmoid, maxillary, or sphenoid sinusitis; (2) traumatic inoculation; or (3) hematogenous spread from nasopharyngeal pathogens.[7,15,26] The usual causative organisms are *Streptococcus pneumoniae, Haemophilus influenzae,* and *Moraxella catarrhalis,* as well as others[7] **(Table 33.2)**. Orbital cellulitis can be associated with subperiosteal abscess formation and osteomyelitis. Infection can spread through the roof of the orbit to the anterior base, causing anterior skull base osteomyelitis and bony destruction.[27] Septic thrombosis of the ophthalmic veins can result in cavernous sinus thrombosis.[7,28]

Clinical Presentation and Sequelae[7,27,28]

Presentation usually occurs in childhood, or, less commonly, young adulthood, and usually consists of one or more of the following:

- Fever, headache, and malaise
- Orbital pain, swelling, and ecchymosis
- Ophthalmoplegia and proptosis from cavernous sinus thrombosis, subperiosteal abscess, or rarely herniation of the brain through the osteomyelitic orbital roof
- Enophthalmos, if the roof of the maxillary sinus (floor of the orbit) is destroyed
- Progression to blindness

Workup[7,21,29]

- Laboratory
  - Complete blood count may reveal leukocytosis, with elevated ESR and CRP.
  - Blood cultures reveals an organism in 30 to 60% of the cases.
  - CSF cultures are usually negative, but may show pleocytosis.
  - Cultures and sensitivity analysis of aspirate from the affected sinus or percutaneously from the orbital subperiosteal abscess.
- Imaging: CT and MRI of the brain, orbit and paranasal sinuses. Intracranial and paranasal sinuses as described above for paranasal sinusitis; orbital findings include the following:
  - Edema of the orbital contents (best seen on T2) and proptosis
  - Differentiation among subperiosteal abscess, orbital abscess, and cellulitis
  - Thrombosis of the superior ophthalmic veins: engorged superior ophthalmic vein (best seen on T2 coronal to differentiate from rectus muscle); DW-MRI shows restricted diffusion within the vessel[22,23]

Table 33.2 Empiric Antimicrobial Therapy for Some of the Most Common Skull Base Infections

Type of Infection	Common Organism	First Line	Second Line (If Not Resolving or Intracranial Complications)
Fungal infections (mucormycosis or aspergillosis)[2,31,32,49]	Mucoraceae (mucormycosis) Aspergillus	Lipid formulation of amphotericin B infusion (5 mg/kg/d) + caspofungin[51] for 3 weeks then oral posaconazole (800 mg/d divided in 3 doses) prophylaxis for life Note: Amphotericin B deoxycholate has higher renal toxicity than lipid formulations	Escalate amphotericin B dose to 7.5–10 mg/kg/d + consider GM-CSF (250 µg/m²/d) + hyperbaric oxygen therapy
Anterior skull base, bacterial infections from paranasal sinusitis or orbital cellulitis[10–13,22,23]	Streptococcus pneumoniae, Haemophilus influenzae, and Moraxella catarrhalis Others include Staphylococcus aureus, Streptococcus pyogenes, and anaerobic bacteria of the upper respiratory tract	For sinusitis or orbital cellulitis: cefuroxime IV (150 mg/kg/d divided into 3 doses every 8 h) + metronidazole IV (30 mg/kg/d divided into 2 doses every 12 h) if evidence of anaerobic infection; switch to oral antibiotics once clinical improvement occurs, for 3 weeks	Advanced-generation cephalosporins such as cefotaxime or ceftriaxone (150 and 100 mg/kg/d divided into 8- and 12-h doses, respectively) + vancomycin (60 mg/kg/d divided into doses every 6 h) if CSF pleocytosis; continue treatment for 10 days, then oral treatment for 2 to 4 weeks
Mastoiditis and its complications (apical petrositis or skull base osteomyelitis)[1,4,9,52]	Pseudomonas aeruginosa, Streptococcus pneumoniae, Haemophilus influenzae, and group A streptococci	• For simple mastoiditis in children less than 2 years: amoxicillin–clavulanate (Augmentin ES, GlaxoSmithKline), at a daily dose of 90 mg of amoxicillin/kg combined with 6.4 mg of clavulanate/kg twice daily for 10 days • Over 2 years of age: ceftriaxone IV 1 g/d for 2 weeks	Nonresolving or development of complications: ceftriaxone IV 2–4 g/d for 2 weeks followed by 4 weeks of oral therapy + consider adding vancomycin if intracranial complications occur

Abbreviations: CSF, cerebrospinal fluid; GM-CSF, granulocyte macrophage colony-stimulating factor.
Note: These treatments are to be used initially until the results of culture and sensitivity testing are received. Treatment is then changed according to the results.

■ Infections of the Middle and Posterior Skull Base

Sphenoid Sinusitis

Pathophysiology

Isolated sphenoid sinus infections are the rarest form of paranasal sinus infections and account for roughly 2.5% of all sinus infections. Commonly, sphenoidal sinus infections follow initial infections of another group of paranasal sinuses.[30] As with other paranasal sinuses, the infection could be viral, bacterial, or fungal (**Table 33.2**). More than 60% of cases of isolated sphenoid sinusitis, especially the invasive type, are fungal. *Aspergillus* is the most common species.[31] Invasive fungal sinusitis usually occurs in immunocompromised individuals, although case reports of isolated and invasive disease in immunocompetent patients have been described.[32] Due to close proximity of the sphenoid sinus to the cavernous sinus, invasive fungal sinusitis can spread to the cavernous sinus through afferent communicating veins or directly through osteomyelitis of the sphenoid bone or bony defects within the sphenoid sinus walls.[30]

Classically, *Aspergillus* hyphae proliferate within the sinus. Necrosis and deposition of calcium crystals follows with mucopurulent discharge.[30,31] Some authors refer to the fungal mass inside the sphenoid as a "fungal ball or a mycetoma."[31]

Clinical Presentation and Sequelae[30–33]

The most common presentations of isolated sphenoid sinusitis are headache, retro-orbital pain, and purulent rhinorrhea. Constitutional manifestations are rarely present. Sphenoid sinusitis produces very few localizing symptoms, and thus is difficult to diagnose by routine clinical and radiological examination. Consequently, sphenoid sinusitis is frequently misdiagnosed on presentation; patients are referred initially to clinicians other than otolaryngologists, and the condition is suspected only after the development of complications.

Possible sequelae of the disease include the following:

- Osteomyelitis and destruction of the sphenoid bone
- Extension to other paranasal sinuses
- Extension to the orbit
- Cavernous sinus thrombosis, infection, or compression by mucocele or fungal balls (also with eventual invasion of the internal carotid artery [ICA] by *Aspergillus*)
- Meningitis and brain abscess

- Extension to a pneumatized anterior clinoid through the optic strut, eventually compressing the optic nerve[33]

Workup[30,31]

Workup and imaging findings for sphenoid sinus infections are similar to those of other paranasal sinus infections described above. Fungal sinusitis, however, have some pathognomonic features:

- Laboratory
  - Culture or pathology the sphenoid sinus contents during endoscopic sinus surgery (ESS) can reveal the fungal hyphae.
  - Blood: elevated ESR and CRP, sometimes with neutropenia and eosinophilia. Culture is often negative.
- Imaging
  - CT usually shows central hyperdense areas of calcification (calcium crystals) and areas of bone destruction, if invasive.
  - MRI can assess intracranial and intraorbital complications, such as cavernous sinus thrombosis, meningitis, and others. Of particular note, fungal elements are typically hypodense on T2-weighted images.

Sphenoid Wing, Temporal, and Infratemporal Fossa Infections

- Usually an extension of mucormycosis or maxillary sinus infections.

Mastoiditis

Pathophysiology

Acute mastoiditis is a serious complication of acute otitis media (AOM). It is more common in the pediatric age group, as most patients are younger than 4 years of age.[4] AOM extends through the aditus to the mastoid antrum into mastoid air cells, and inflammation of mastoid epithelium blocks adequate drainage, facilitating the propagation of the infection.[3] There are two stages for the disease: stage 1, which is mastoiditis with periostitis, and stage 2, termed acute coalescent mastoiditis. The most common organisms causing the infection are *Pseudomonas aeruginosa, Streptococcus pneumoniae, Haemophilus influenzae,* and group A *Streptococcus.*[34] With progression, especially in immunocompromised individuals, the disease could extend to the surrounding areas of the cranial base with development of malignant otitis externa, also known as skull base osteomyelitis[35] (see **Box 33.2**).

Box 33.2.   Malignant Otitis Externa (Skull Base Osteomyelitis)[35,37,38]

A serious osteomyelitis of the temporal bone and skull base usually follows otitis externa, or less commonly otitis media, in elderly patients. One of the hallmarks of this progression is granulation tissue in the bone–cartilage junction of the external auditory canal. With the exception of a few case reports, the causative organism is *Pseudomonas* and the condition is usually facilitated by impaired host immunity. There is usually a history of otitis externa or acute otitis media with the following superimposed:

- Severe otalgia and ear discharge, not responding to medical treatment.
- Severe headache.
- Cranial nerve deficits due to secretion of neurotoxins or the compressive effect of the destructive process through the relevant foramina. The facial nerve is usually the first nerve affected, followed by lower cranial nerve palsies in advanced cases.
- Late osteomyelitis can spread to other skull base locations, such as the sphenoid bone or infratemporal fossa.
- Central nervous system (CNS) complications (see Mastoiditis. above).

    In addition to the clinical picture, diagnosis can be made by any of the following:

- Pathological examination of granulation tissue in the external auditory canal.
- CT scan of the petrous bone and skull base in order to assess the extent of disease and bone destruction.
- MRI of the brain is useful for detecting intracranial complications.
- CT bone scan and gallium scans are positive with skull base osteomyelitis. Gallium scan assesses mainly soft tissue disease. Both can also be used to monitor the response to treatment.

Clinical Presentation and Sequelae

The disease can present with the following[3,4,36]:

- Fever or other constitutional manifestations
- Pain, swelling, erythema, and tenderness over the mastoid prominence
- Anteroinferior displacement of the auricle
- Otitis media (middle ear effusion with erythema of the tympanic membrane), which occurs in almost all cases of ear discharge
- Hearing loss and otalgia
- Postauricular fistula
- Apical petrositis (Gradenigo's syndrome) (see **Box 33.3**)

With progressive AOM, the following complications can occur in 15 to 55% of cases[3,4]:

- Malignant otitis externa, especially in patients with diabetes mellitus and other immunocompromised states
- Permanent hearing loss
- Labyrinthitis

Box 33.3.   Gradenigo's Syndrome (Apical Petrositis)[9,38]

This syndrome is a complication of acute mastoiditis. The condition is characterized by a triad of suppurative otitis media, pain in the distribution of the trigeminal nerve, and abducent palsy. The trigeminal ganglion and abducens nerve are separated from the bony petrous apex by only a fold of dura mater, hence their vulnerability to the inflammatory process. Involvement of the sixth nerve is due to extension of the inflammatory process under the petroclinoid ligament through Dorello's canal.

Possible associations and sequelae include the following:

- Meningitis
- Intracranial abscess
- Spread to skull base and involvement of cranial nerves IX, X, and XI (Vernet's syndrome, see page 184)
- Prevertebral/parapharyngeal abscess
- Spread to the sympathetic plexus around the carotid sheath

Computed tomography of the petrous bone may not be helpful in assessing the petrous apex because air cells only extend to the petrous apex in 30% of individuals. Thus, relying on opacification and obliteration of air cells in the petrous bone is not accurate in diagnosing this condition. Bony destruction, however, is easily demonstrated. An MRI of the brain may show the inflammatory process and associated intracranial complications. A radioisotope bone scan shows increased uptake at the petrous apex.

Historically, this condition has been managed with aggressive surgical intervention; however, the advent of modern antibiotics facilitates conservative treatment in most cases.

- Bezold's abscess (in the sternocleidomastoid muscle)
- Zygomatic arch abscess
- Facial palsy
- Sigmoid or lateral sinus thrombosis
- CNS complications: meningitis, brain abscess, subdural empyema, or otitic hydrocephalus

Workup[3,4,34]

Diagnosis can usually be made clinically and by otoscopy of the tympanic membrane. Further workup is done for suspected complications:

- Culture and sensitivity analysis of the discharge, which can also be obtained by tympanocentesis
- CT scan of temporal bone: shows opacification of the mastoid with obliteration of air paces
- Audiogram for hearing loss
- MRI of the brain to evaluate CNS complications

Basal Arachnoiditis and Meningitis

Pathophysiology

Infections of the basal meninges (basilar meningitis) can occur with almost any CNS infection.[39] The most common organisms vary by age, immunocompetence of the host, and the prevalence of organisms in the host's environment. In general, the most common ones are *Tuberculosis, Cryptococcosis, Aspergillosis, Candidiasis, Listeria,* and *Echinococcosis.*[40] It is worth noting that the organisms and pathophysiology cited here are related only to basilar meningitis (and not the general broad entity of meningitis, where pneumococci are the most common organisms). Spread of infection to the basal meninges can occur with immune-deficient states, through direct spread from a primary intracranial abscess or via hematogenous spread from a distant focus, as in tuberculosis (Rich focus: rupture of an infected parameningeal tubercle). The inflammatory process may then extend to involve much of the skull base, with adhesive arachnoiditis involving the cranial nerves and blocking CSF pathways, resulting in an increase in intracranial pressure.[41–45] Basal arachnoiditis can also occur, but rarely, from extension of a spinal subarachnoid source.[45]

Clinical Presentation and Sequelae

The clinical picture of basilar meningitis is classically a triad of headache, focal neurologic deficit, and altered mental status, with nuchal rigidity and other meningeal irritation signs on examination.[39,43,46,47] Fever is sometimes absent because most cases are subacute or chronic. Prior surgery or trauma with CSF leak may precede the development of basal meningitis.

Possible complications are as follows[39–47]:

- Communicating hydrocephalus
- Visual deficits: from adhesive arachnoiditis extending to the optic nerve, compression by nodules, or increased CSF pressure within the subarachnoid space
- Other cranial neuropathies
- Seeding of infection in the spinal subarachnoid space causing myelopathy or radiculopathies
- Associated neurologic deficits resulting from the primary intracranial lesion (e.g., *Echinococcosis* or *Cysticercosis* cyst)

Workup

Identifying the etiology and offending pathogen is the most important step in the management of these cases. **Table 33.3** lists the CSF workup required for the most common pathogens causing basal meningitis. Elevated ESR and CRP in

Table 33.3   Cerebrospinal Fluid (CSF) Workup and Findings for Different Infections Causing Basal Arachnoiditis and Meningitis

Infection	CSF Analysis	CSF Specific Tests
Tuberculosis[40,41,47]	• Lymphocytosis • Elevated protein • Low glucose	• Mycobacterial antigen and antibody by ELISA • PCR for detection of mycobacterial DNA • Culture with Ziehl-Neelsen stain and mycobacterial growth indication tube • Xpert MTB/RIF assay is a new technique for detection of mycobacterial DNA and resistance to rifampicin
Cryptococcosis[43,46]	• Lymphocytosis • Elevated protein • Low glucose • Sometimes acellular CSF in AIDS patients with only an increase in opening pressure	• Culture of *Cryptococcus neoformans* • Cryptococcal antigen titer (CRAG); higher titers in AIDS than in non-AIDS patients.
Fungal[45,50] (*Aspergillus* and *Candida*)	• Neutropenia	• CSF culture and biopsy may reveal fungal hyphae • CSF galactomannan (GM) • PCR assays for DNA detection

Abbreviations: AIDS: acquired immunodeficiency syndrome; ELISA, enzyme-linked immunosorbent assay; PCR, polymerase chain reaction.

blood samples is common; however, blood cultures may not be specific or may be sterile.[39–41,48]

• Radiological findings[39,43,47]: In addition to an intracranial mass or abscess from the primary infection, basal meningitis can be demonstrated by the following:
  ○ CT scan showing meningeal and sometimes gyral enhancement after contrast administration. Enhancement is also found in the basal subarachnoid cisterns and around the brainstem. Hydrocephalus is a common finding.
  ○ Brain MRI with contrast may show the same findings as CT, but in addition can show diffuse thickening and enhancement of affected cranial nerves, and meningeal nodules. Fungal meningoencephalitis characteristically may show dilated perivascular spaces, usually in the basal ganglia (so-called soap-bubble lesions).

- Diffusion MRI studies have been used recently to differentiate fungal from bacterial CNS lesions. Fungal lesions seems to have higher average apparent diffusion coefficient (ADC) values, indicating less average restricted diffusion, when compared with bacterial lesions.[49]

■ Treatment

- Medical treatment
  - *Antibiotic treatment:* This is the mainstay of treatment for most skull base infections, if surgical treatment is not indicated. Depending on the condition (**Table 33.2**), empiric treatment is started promptly, and then treatment is modified according to the results of the culture and sensitivity test.
  - *Corticosteroids:* These should be used with caution as they could exacerbate the infections in immunocompromised patients in addition to their usual side effects. They may also decrease the penetration of antibiotics into abscesses.
  - *Antiepileptic drugs:* reserved for cases with intracranial masses or if seizures develop.
- Surgical treatment
  - *General indications* (these are only general guidelines, not absolute indications; treatment should be tailored to the patient's specific medical condition based on the clinician's judgment):
    - Intracranial mass lesions causing neurologic compromise, such as abscesses or fungal masses
    - Decompression of neural foramina if causing cranial neuropathies
    - No response to medical treatment
    - Culture and biopsy of lesions if diagnosis cannot be made by other methods
    - CSF diversion procedures for hydrocephalus or increased intracranial pressure
    - Debridement of osteomyelitic bone + reconstruction for cosmetic purposes (e.g., frontal bone osteomyelitis)
  - *General guidelines:*
    - If possible, stop antibiotic therapy 24 to 48 hours before surgery to avoid negative cultures.
    - Most acute sinus-related infections are treated medically with antibiotics and topical nasal treatments (e.g., saline sprays, corticosteroid sprays, short-term decongestants). Endoscopic sinus surgery is generally reserved for patients with complicated acute sinusitis not responding to medical treatment (e.g., orbital subperiosteal abscess).

For invasive fungal sinusitis localized to the sinuses, endoscopic sinus surgery is indicated to debride all necrotic sinonasal tissue until healthy bleeding mucosa is encountered (in addition to continued medical therapy with systemic antifungal agents).

- Osteomyelitis of the skull base and the cranial vault is generally treated with long-term antibiotics. If infected, bone needs to be surgically debrided; reconstruction is generally performed as a secondary procedure.
- Bleeding from bone may be profuse. Control with bone wax and always have blood products available.
- Meticulous closure and sealing of the skull base with free fascia lata or pericranial flaps, fat and sealant materials
- In cases where CSF diversion is required, external ventricular drains (EVDs) are preferred over ventriculoperitoneal (VP) shunts when CNS infections are present. They can also be used for intrathecal administration of antibiotics. Once CSF is clear and the condition is stable, the EVD can be replaced with VP shunts.
- Continue antibiotic treatment for 2 to 4 weeks following surgery.

■ References

Boldfaced references are of particular importance.

1. Tarantino V, D'Agostino R, Taborelli G, Melagrana A, Porcu A, Stura M. Acute mastoiditis: a 10 year retrospective study. Int J Pediatr Otorhinolaryngol 2002;66:143–148
2. Javadi M, Mohammadi S. Fungal infection of the sinus and anterior skull base. Med J Islam Repub Iran 2008;22:137–140
3. Harker LA. Cranial and intracranial complications of acute and chronic otitis media. In: Snow JB, ed. Ballenger's Otorhinolaryngology Head and Neck Surgery. Hamilton, Ontario: BC Decker; 2003:294–316
4. **Rea P, Gragam J. Acute otitis media in children. In: Gleeson M, Browning GG, Burton MJ, et al, ed. Scott-Brown's Otorhinolaryngology, Head and Neck Surgery. Birmingham, UK: Hodder Arnold; 2008:912–927**
5. Haridas A, Walsh DC, Mowle DH. Polymicrobial osteomyelitis of the odontoid process with epidural abscess: case report and review of literature. Skull Base 2003;13:107–111
6. Thiagarajan BS. Sphenoidal fungal sinusitis with intracranial extension. An interesting case report. Online J Otolaryngol 2013;3:29–33
7. Wald ER. Periorbital and orbital infections. Pediatr Rev 2004;25:312–320
8. Chang PC, Fischbein NJ, Holliday RA. Central skull base osteomyelitis in patients without otitis externa: imaging findings. AJNR Am J Neuroradiol 2003;24:1310–1316
9. Kantas I, Papadopoulou A, Balatsouras DG, Aspris A, Marangos N. Therapeutic approach to Gradenigo's syndrome: a case report. J Med Case Reports 2010;4:151

10. Rosenfeld RM, Andes D, Bhattacharyya N, et al. Clinical practice guideline: adult sinusitis. Otolaryngol Head Neck Surg 2007;137(3, Suppl):S1–S31
11. Abzug MJ. Acute sinusitis in children: do antibiotics have any role? J Infect 2014; 68(Suppl 1):S33–S37
12. Leung RS, Katial R. The diagnosis and management of acute and chronic sinusitis. Prim Care 2008;35:11–24, v–vi
13. Osei-Yeboah C, Neequaye J, Bulley H, Darkwa A. Osteomyelitis of the frontal bone. Ghana Med J 2007;41:88–90
14. Gupta S, Goyal R, Shahi M. Frontal sinus mucopyelocele with intracranial and intra-orbital extension. Nepal J Ophthalmol 2011;3:91–92
15. Sajid T, Kazmi HS, Shah SA, et al. Complications of nose and paranasal sinus disease. J Ayub Med Coll Abbottabad 2011;23:56–59
16. Finn DG. Mucormycosis of the paranasal sinuses. Ear Nose Throat J 1988;67:813, 816–818, 821–822
17. Aínsa Laguna D, Pons Morales S, Muñoz Tormo-Figueres A, Vega Senra MI, Otero Reigada MC. [Pott's puffy tumor: a rare complication of frontal sinusitis]. An Pediatr (Barc) 2014;80:317–320
18. Nancy F. Crum-Cianflone. Mucormycosis. Drugs Dis. 2013. http://emedicine.medscape.com/article/222551-overview
19. Millon L, Larosa F, Lepiller Q, et al. Quantitative polymerase chain reaction detection of circulating DNA in serum for early diagnosis of mucormycosis in immunocompromised patients. Clin Infect Dis 2013;56:e95–e101
20. Bernal-Martínez L, Buitrago MJ, Castelli MV, Rodriguez-Tudela JL, Cuenca-Estrella M. Development of a single tube multiplex real-time PCR to detect the most clinically relevant Mucormycetes species. Clin Microbiol Infect 2013;19:E1–E7
21. Herrmann BW, Forsen JW Jr. Simultaneous intracranial and orbital complications of acute rhinosinusitis in children. Int J Pediatr Otorhinolaryngol 2004;68:619–625
22. Pendharkar HS, Gupta AK, Bodhey N, Nair M. Diffusion restriction in thrombosed superior ophthalmic veins: two cases of diverse etiology and literature review. J Radiol Case Rep 2011;5:8–16
23. Cumurcu T, Demirel S, Keser S, et al. Superior ophthalmic vein thrombosis developed after orbital cellulitis. Semin Ophthalmol 2013;28:58–60
24. Misra UK, Kalita J, Bansal V. D-dimer is useful in the diagnosis of cortical venous sinus thrombosis. Neurol India 2009;57:50–54
25. Ito E, Saito K, Nagatani T, Teranishi M, Aimi Y, Wakabayashi T. Cavernous sinus thrombophlebitis caused by porphyromonas gingivalis with abscess formation extending to the orbital cavity. Case report. Neurol Med Chir (Tokyo) 2009;49:370–373
26. Allan K, Atkinson H, Agada F. Posterior orbital cellulitis: case report and literature review. J Laryngol Otol 2013;127:1148–1151
27. Soon VT. Pediatric subperiosteal orbital abscess secondary to acute sinusitis: a 5-year review. Am J Otolaryngol 2011;32:62–68
28. Saetang S, Preechawai P, Hirunpat S. Retrograde cavernous sinus thrombosis and orbital cellulitis secondary to meningitis in immunocompetence child. J Med Assoc Thai 2012;95:1485–1488
29. Bedwell J, Bauman NM. Management of pediatric orbital cellulitis and abscess. Curr Opin Otolaryngol Head Neck Surg 2011;19:467–473

30. Komatsu H, Matsumoto F, Kasai M, Kurano K, Sasaki D, Ikeda K. Cavernous sinus thrombosis caused by contralateral sphenoid sinusitis: a case report. Head Face Med 2013;9:9
31. Pagella F, Pusateri A, Matti E, et al. Sphenoid sinus fungus ball: our experience. Am J Rhinol Allergy 2011;25:276–280
32. Lee TJ, Huang SF, Huang CC, Chen YL. Isolated sphenoid sinus aspergillosis: report of two cases. Chang Gung Med J 2002;25:464–468
33. Kwon SH, Kim SH, Yoon JH. Anterior clinoid mucocele coexisting with sphenoid sinus mucocele. Auris Nasus Larynx 2009;36:598–600
34. Stähelin-Massik J, Podvinec M, Jakscha J, et al. Mastoiditis in children: a prospective, observational study comparing clinical presentation, microbiology, computed tomography, surgical findings and histology. Eur J Pediatr 2008;167:541–548
35. Handzel O, Halperin D. Necrotizing (malignant) external otitis. Am Fam Physician 2003;68:309–312
36. Courson AM, Vikram HR, Barrs DM. What are the criteria for terminating treatment for necrotizing (malignant) otitis externa? Laryngoscope 2014;124:361–362
37. Soheilipour S, Meidani M, Derakhshandi H, Etemadifar M. Necrotizing external otitis: a case series. B-ENT 2013;9:61–66
38. Colpaert C, Van Rompaey V, Vanderveken O, et al. Intracranial complications of acute otitis media and Gradenigo's syndrome. B-ENT 2013;9:151–156
39. Shahlaie K, Hawk MW, Hu BR, Theis JH, Kim KD. Parasitic central nervous system infections: echinococcus and schistosoma. Rev Neurol Dis 2005;2:176–185
40. Nhu NT, Heemskerk D, Thu DA, et al. Evaluation of GeneXpert MTB/RIF for diagnosis of tuberculous meningitis. J Clin Microbiol 2014;52:226–233
41. Ou Q, Liu X, Cheng X. An iTRAQ approach to quantitative proteome analysis of cerebrospinal fluid from patients with tuberculous meningitis. Biosci Trends 2013;7:186–192
42. Garg RK, Paliwal V, Malhotra HS. Tuberculous optochiasmatic arachnoiditis: a devastating form of tuberculous meningitis. Expert Rev Anti Infect Ther 2011;9:719–729
43. Nakae Y, Kudo Y, Yamamoto R, Johkura K. Pseudo-subarachnoid hemorrhage in cryptococcal meningitis: MRI findings and pathological study. Neurol Sci 2013;34:2227–2229
44. Horta-Baas G, Guerrero-Soto O, Barile-Fabris L. Central nervous system infection by Listeria monocytogenes in patients with systemic lupus erythematosus: analysis of 26 cases, including the report of a new case. Reumatol Clínica (English Ed.) 2013;9:340–347
45. Vivek V, Kavar B, Hogg M, Eisen DP, Butzkueven H. Aspergillus arachnoiditis post intrathecal baclofen pump insertion. J Clin Neurosci 2013;20:1159–1160
46. de Vedia L, Arechavala A, Calderón MI, et al. Relevance of intracranial hypertension control in the management of Cryptococcus neoformans meningitis related to AIDS. Infection 2013;41:1073–1077
47. Sher K, Firdaus, Abbasi A, Bullo N, Kumar S. Stages of tuberculous meningitis: a clinicoradiologic analysis. J Coll Physicians Surg Pak 2013;23:405–408
48. Mohindra S, Savardekar A, Gupta R, Tripathi M, Rane S. Varied types of intracranial hydatid cysts: radiological features and management techniques. Acta Neurochir (Wien) 2012;154:165–172

49. Lin DJ, Sacks A, Shen J, Lee TC. Neurocandidiasis: a case report and consideration of the causes of restricted diffusion. J Radiol Case Rep 2013;7:1–5

50. Reinwald M, Buchheidt D, Hummel M, et al. Diagnostic performance of an Aspergillus-specific nested PCR assay in cerebrospinal fluid samples of immunocompromised patients for detection of central nervous system aspergillosis. PLoS ONE 2013;8:e56706

51. Reed C, Bryant R, Ibrahim AS, et al. Combination polyene-caspofungin treatment of rhino-orbital-cerebral mucormycosis. Clin Infect Dis 2008;47:364–371

52. Hoberman A, Paradise JL, Rockette HE, et al. Treatment of acute otitis media in children under 2 years of age. N Engl J Med 2011;364:105–115

34 Skull Base Traumatology

- Skull base fractures (SBFs) occur in 3.5 to 24% of head injuries.[1]
- SBFs can cause death or coma. They may be associated with immediate or delayed complications, such as cerebrospinal fluid (CSF) leakage, possible meningitis, and neurovascular damage (injury of arteries, dural sinuses, and/or cranial nerves).[2,3]

■ Causes

The causes of SBFs vary depending on the severity of the injury. Although sports and recreation activities account for large numbers of head injuries, these injuries are rarely severe enough to lead to a SBF. The most common mechanisms of head injury are motor vehicle accidents (which account for 40% in both the adults and children), followed by falls, direct trauma by falling/penetrating objects, and assaults.[1,4] In the pediatric population, SBFs are caused by falls from heights (32%), falls on the ground (10%), falls related to sports (3%), and episodes of violence (8%)[4] (for the pediatric skull base traumatology, see page 876).

- Skull base fractures are among the most difficult fractures to evaluate and manage.
- They are an epiphenomenon in polytrauma patients, occurring alongside other body trauma with or without neurologic deficits.

Pearl

In skull base fractures or penetrating injuries, always investigate for other fractures (midface, cranial vault, spine), brain injury, neurovascular injury, and neurologic deficits, and assess the general clinical and neurologic status (more than just using the Glasgow Coma Scale [GCS]).

- Patients with SBF require prompt multidisciplinary assessment and management, often involving a neurologist, an ophthalmologist, an otorhinolaryngologist, and/or maxillofacial, plastic, and trauma surgeons.
- Anatomic location of SBFs: 70% involve the anterior skull base, 5% the middle skull base, 5% the posterior skull base, and 20% the central midline skull base.

■ Typical Signs of Skull Base Fractures

- Battle's sign (postauricular ecchymosis)
- Raccoon's eyes or panda's eyes (periorbital ecchymosis). This is an indicator that is not always associated with SBFs. It occurs in 42% of cases, of which 53% have been found to occur in the petrous bone/middle skull base. Periorbital ecchymosis has been associated with several further findings, such as intracranial hemorrhage, cranial nerve injury, soft tissue injury with or without fracture, and convexity fracture. Surgical intervention is required in 22% of patients with periorbital ecchymosis.[5]
- CSF rhinorrhea/otorrhea/orbitorrhea or leak from the traumatic wound
- Hemotympanum with or without laceration of the external auditory canal
- Cranial nerve injuries

■ Imaging

Computed tomography (CT) is the imaging gold standard for the detection of SBFs, and several classification systems are CT-based. To overcome the limits of low-resolution single slices to detect fractures, high-resolution CT (1-mm slice thickness) is often required with solid and transparent three-dimensional (3D) volume-rendering reconstructions[6–9] or curved maximum intensity projection (cMIP) reconstructions to improve fracture detection.[9,10]

- A step-by-step analysis of the axial and multiplanar reconstructions of the skull base is critical to avoid missing fractures and clinically relevant neurologic findings.[11] Frontobasilar fractures require special attention to assess the integrity of the nasofrontal ducts or nasofrontal outflow tracts, and the involvement of the cribriform plate, posterior wall of the frontal sinus, optic canal, sella turcica, and orbit walls and contents.
- CT angiography (CTA) or digital subtraction angiography (DSA) should be performed in cases of SBF with possible vascular injury (laceration, thrombosis, dissection, pseudoaneurysm[12]).

- On CT imaging, determine the involvement of the exocranial structures of the skull base: lateral and medial pterygoid processes, styloid process of the temporal bone, tip of the mastoid, and occipital condylar processes.
- Have a high index of suspicion for vascular, neural, or dural injuries in any patient with SBFs.
- The involvement of specific regions of the skull base already suggests the possible neurovascular involvement of the anatomically contiguous structures:
  - Petrous portion of the internal carotid artery (ICA) and facial nerve in petrous bone fractures
  - Dissection of the vertebral artery in craniovertebral trauma
  - Injury of the intracavernous ICA, carotid-cavernous fistula in sellar/parasellar fractures
  - Laceration of the middle meningeal artery in middle fossa/temporal squama fractures
  - Venous dural sinuses injuries in cranial vault/skull base fractures
- Whenever feasible, magnetic resonance imaging (MRI) is helpful for the detection of traumatic involvement of soft tissues (brain, orbit contents) and dural defects.

■ Classification Systems

Classification systems of SBFs should consider radiological, anatomic, and clinical information related to clinical decision making.

- Anatomy-based classification systems offer a general framework including the specific complications related to the site of the SBFs.
- The involvement of the skull base must also be investigated in facial fractures. For example, Le Fort II and III fractures are associated with an increased risk of blunt injury to the carotid arteries,[14] and Le Fort III may have skull base involvement (**Table 34.1**).
- Fractures of the petrous bone can cause facial palsy, deafness, and CSF leakage with otorrhea or paradoxical (oto)rhinorrhea (see Chapter 32). Fractures of the posterior fossa may lacerate the major venous sinuses and affect craniocervical stability.[3]

Pearl

- A classification system should be logically structured, accurate, comprehensive, and systematic, and should provide information regarding the severity of the injury and recommendations regarding therapeutic options.[13]

Table 34.1   Le Fort Fracture Types

Type and Definition	Fracture Pattern	Signs and Symptoms
I: horizontal/transverse	Fracture line above the apices of the upper teeth, crossing the pterygoid plate and the maxilla, then entering into the maxillary sinus	Ecchymosis, swelling, teeth mobility
II: pyramidal	Pyramidal pattern involving the medial orbital walls, inferior orbital rim, nasofrontal suture, pterygoid plates	Face deformity with midface mobility, cranial nerve V_2 anesthesia/paresthesia
III: transverse, craniofacial dislocation	Zygomatic arches, zygomaticofrontal and nasofrontal sutures, pterygoid plates, orbital floors	Separation of the frontozygomatic suture, eyeball deviation, often associated with other injuries in polytrauma

Clinical- and Radiology-Based Classification Systems of the Skull Base Fractures

In a 48-patient study, high-resolution thin-section CT scan enabled the classification of fractures into four major types[15]:

- I: cribriform
- II: frontoethmoidal
- III: lateral frontal
- IV: complex (combination of the other three types)

The major finding of this study was that there is a trend of increased infection rate related to (1) prolonged duration of rhinorrhea, (2) large size of fracture displacement, and (3) proximity of the fracture to the midline (to the cribriform plate).

- Cranial and facial injuries in high-velocity injury events can be classified[16] as frontal, basal, or combined, as well as central, lateral, or combined. Moreover, fractures can be classified as unilateral or bilateral, as well as pure or impure, depending on the absence (pure) or presence (impure) of midfacial fractures. The most common injuries are the combined frontobasal type (30% of cases), with CSF leak occurring more commonly in impure types of frontobasal fractures.[16]
- Frontobasal and midface fractures involving the skull base are classified into the following three types, based on the fracture pattern, location, involvement of the midface, and related complications[14]:
  - Type I: isolated linear cranial base fractures
  - Type II: vertical-linear fracture of the skull vault (frontal bone) in combination with a SBF
  - Type III: comminuted fracture of the frontolateral skull vault and orbital roof in association with a linear SBF
- In this classification system, in which 290 patients were analyzed, type III patients had the highest rate of complications (CSF leaks and infections), followed by type II.[17]
- Radioanatomic and clinical findings (rhinorrhea, periorbital hematoma, and pneumocephalus) have been analyzed in two studies of the Arbeitsgemeinschaft für Osteosynthesefragen: Association for the Study of Internal Fixation (AO), to develop a hierarchical classification system in which the score stratifies patients' risk of complications and suggests a treatment approach.[18,19] The classification system defined three fracture types (A, B, C), three groups (1, 2, 3), and three subgroups (1.1, 1.2, 1.3) with increasing severity from A1.1 (lowest severity) to C3.3 (highest). The operative cases had significantly higher severity scores than the nonoperative ones. More severe fracture grades were significantly associated with the occurrence of pneumocephalus and rhinorrhea, and with the treatment approach. A correlation among the se-

verity of the fracture, the number of posttraumatic functional limitations, the need for bone grafting or duraplasty, and facial asymmetry was observed. The proposed classification system enables standardized documentation of midfacial and craniofacial fractures, including those not precisely defined by other schemas, as well as the relationship among the severity of the fracture, the posttraumatic functional limitations, and the need for different therapeutic strategies. The classification, although limited by the fact that it is roughly regional, also has been found to be of reliable utility in arriving at a prognosis, demonstrating that almost 87.5% of patients who died had sustained group 3 fractures involving the skull base.[18]

- The most recent AO proposed classification system also has a hierarchical system: levels 1 and 2 define the anatomic localizers (region of the head, cranial vault, and skull base involvement), whereas level 3 describes the fracture morphology in an array of modules specific for anatomic regions and subregions.[20,21] According to this model, the skull base is divided into two lateral compartments and a central compartment, from the frontal sinuses to the foramen magnum (see Chapter 2, **Fig. 2.3b**, page 12), and the types of fractures can be classified by means of classifier software.[22]

- Based on their morphology, fractures are defined as single or multiple, crossing one or more bones, displaced or nondisplaced, depressed or not depressed, and involving or not involving the paranasal sinuses. Radiologically, it is important to correlate the presence of fractures with other findings, such as the presence of pneumocephalus or intracranial mass lesions (epidural, subdural, subarachnoid, intraventricular, or intraparenchymal hematoma, brain contusions, foreign bodies).

■ Anterior Skull Base Fractures

Craniofacial fractures may involve the anterior skull base, which includes the posterior wall of the frontal sinus, the ethmoid cells, the cribriform-ethmoid junction, and the orbits.

Head injury with frontobasal involvement is generally associated with facial fractures (87% of patients), as well as hematomas (epidural/subdural or subarachnoid) or otobasal fractures (15%).[23]

Signs typically associated with these fractures are CSF rhinorrhea with (3%) or without (37%) meningitis, hyposmia/anosmia (91%), and raccoon's eyes (21%).[23]

Frontal Sinus Involvement

A three-grade classification system exists for frontobasal fractures involving the frontal sinus[24] **(Fig. 34.1)**:

- Type A: The anterior wall of the frontal sinus is fractured.
- Type B: Both anterior and posterior walls are fractured.
- Type C: The frontobasal fracture does not involve the frontal sinus.

Patients in type B generally present with pneumocephalus, CSF rhinorrhea, and displaced fractures, and they often require surgery. Type A patients generally require surgery only for cosmetic reasons. Type C patients generally do not require surgery for their fracture.[24]

The complication rate in patients undergoing surgery of the frontal sinus (see below) is up to 10%, and should be considered before proceeding with surgery.[25–27] Moreover, the presence of an obstructed outflow tract must be considered as well, because it might be treated by stenting of the duct.[28]

Fractures of the anterior wall may undergo reconstruction by using bony fragments and titanium mesh.[29]

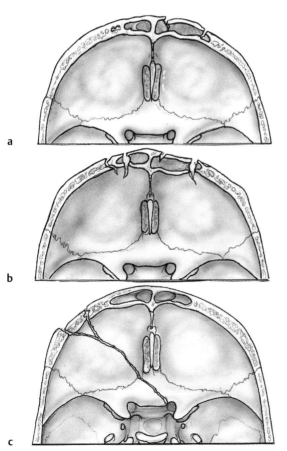

a

b

c

Fig. 34.1a–c Frontobasal fractures. **(a)** Type A: anterior wall of the frontal sinus involvement. **(b)** Type B: anterior and posterior walls fractured. **(c)** Type C: frontobasal fracture not involving the frontal sinus.[24]

Cranialization of the Frontal Sinus

The so-called cranialization of the frontal sinus is a technique used to resect sinus muco-sal tissue from the frontal sinus and separate the nasal cavity from the cranial fossa. Al-though this can almost always be effectively accomplished without resorting to removal of the posterior table of the frontal sinus, the procedure to do so is still in use. In cases with a comminuted fracture of the posterior table, the main reason to remove it is to avoid the development of sequestra.

In general, a coronal scalp incision approach is used for the cranialization procedure (see Chapter 14, **Fig. 14.3**, page 342).

- Using an extradural dissection, expose the posterior table of the frontal sinus and the anterior skull base. The ethmoidal arteries should be identified as they exit the bone, and they are later coagulated and cut.
- Remove the posterior wall of the sinus by means of rongeurs or drills. A drill should be used to smooth the contour of the remaining bone.
- Strip out the sinus mucosa, and use a fine high-speed drill to remove any remnant of the mucosa. One can entirely exenterate the mucosa or, rarely, invert it, pushing it inferiorly in order to obstruct the outflow tract. The tract can be plugged also with fragments of bone or fascia.
- Cover the frontal sinus and the anterior skull base with the pericranial flap.
- To close the bone flap, use miniscrews, mini-plates, titanium meshes, or cement, depending on the size of the defect. Avoid strangulating the pericranial flap across too tight a gap in the bone or across a too posteriorly placed craniotomy cut.

Surgical Pearl

To make a "watertight" compart-mentalization, the pericranial flap has to be intact. If some holes are present, repair it with sutures.

Ocular/Orbital Involvement

Patients with major trauma and facial injuries have a high risk of vision-threat-ening injury. Patients with orbital fractures, SBFs, eyelid lacerations, or superfi-cial eye injuries should be assessed by an ophthalmologist as part of the early management of their trauma to determine whether an ocular injury is pres-ent.[30] Documentation of visual acuity and the pupillary responses including searching for a Marcus Gunn pupil are important in all patients with trauma. (See Chapter 10).

- Nondisplaced orbital fractures do not require surgical treatment.[31]
- Superiorly displaced fractures (isolated blowup) may be associated with neurologic deficits (including brain contusion, CSF leakage, and hematoma), whereas inferiorly displaced fractures (isolated blow-in) result in ophthal-mic injury (including proptosis, hematoma, blindness, globe rupture, and ophthalmoparesis).[31,32] Only 10% of patients with orbital fracture require surgical repair (orbital roof and dural defect repair).[33]

- Orbital roof fracture may also be associated with supraorbital rim or frontal sinus involvement.
- Surgical treatment of orbital fractures may require a coronal bifrontal approach, optic nerve decompression, repair of the orbital roof, cranialization of the frontal sinus, open reduction and internal fixation, external orbital frame, or restoration of the internal orbital volume (see Chapters 20 and 27).[34]

> **Pearl**
>
> Patients who have complete loss of vision at the time of injury should be investigated for optic nerve transection with CT or MRI as appropriate.

■ Temporal Bone Fractures

Temporal bone fractures are most commonly caused by motor vehicle accidents, followed by assaults and falls,[35] and account for 14 to 22% of all skull fractures. They are more common in men than in women.[36,37]

- Typical signs and symptoms: sensorineural hearing loss, conductive hearing loss, perilymphatic fistula, cerebrovascular injury, CSF leak (otorrhea), and facial nerve paralysis.[38]
- High-resolution CT is fundamental for identification of temporal bone fractures.

> **Radiology Pearl**
>
> Recognize normal anatomy and avoid misinterpreting the sutures (tympanomastoid, tympanosquamous, petrosquamosal, petrotympanic sutures) as fractures.[39,40] Temporal bone fractures caused by gunshot wounds are frequently complex, and CT scan may be limited by metallic streak artifacts.

- Classically, petrous temporal bone fractures have been classified as longitudinal, transverse, or mixed.
- The most common associated injury is to the facial nerve in its geniculate or proximal tympanic segment.
- A careful search for various types of ossicular dislocations should be performed in patients with temporal bone fractures, because this may result in conductive hearing loss. Otoscopic examination is recommended.
- The site of CSF otorrhea resulting from temporal bone fractures can usually be identified on plain high-resolution temporal bone images, but intrathecal contrast can be used to definitively identify the source in leaks that persist longer than 72 hours (see Chapter 32).

- Petrous bone fractures generally require a high-energy mechanism, and are present in 3.4% of patients with head injury, often associated with other skull fractures and with an overall mortality rate of 17%.

> **Pearl**
>
> Subdural bleeding is often associated with petrous bone fractures.[41]

- Pediatric patients have different proportions of facial nerve injury and types of hearing loss in comparison with adults.[42]
- Temporal bone fractures can be also defined as otic capsule violating and otic capsule sparing. However, this classification system has not been shown to be significantly better than the traditional systems in predicting the chances of sustaining hearing loss, facial nerve injury, or CSF leak.[43]
- Another system classifies the fractures based on the involvement of one or more of the four anatomic components of the temporal bone (i.e., the squamous, tympanic, mastoid, and petrous parts) to provide a clinically useful association with the clinical symptoms.[44]
- Isolated fractures of the styloid process are rare, but may be associated with facial trauma or may be iatrogenic.[45] The clinical presentation is similar to Eagle's syndrome[46,47] with stylalgia: cervical, oropharyngeal, and craniofacial pain associated with an elongated styloid process (see also Chapter 7, page 184).

Treatment

Generally, fractures of the temporal bone do not require surgery, except in the following cases: facial nerve entrapment with progressing paresis over time, subdural hematoma with mass-effect on the underlying brain, encephaloceles, and persisting CSF leakage. Lumbar drainage or dural repair grafting may be required in cases of persistent CSF leakage. Prior to lumbar drain insertion, the risk of inducing brain herniation must be considered.[48]

■ Clivus Fractures

Isolated fractures of the clivus are rare, with an overall incidence of less than 0.5% in head trauma patients.[49,50] They are typically the result of high-velocity trauma and are often associated with fatal mechanisms.[51,52] Static loading forces produce typical traumatic diastasis in the clivus.[53]

Types

Clivus fractures can be transverse (intersecting both petrous ridges), longitudinal (between the clivus and the dorsum sellae), or oblique (extending form one of the petrous ridges into the clivus)[49,50] **(Fig. 34.2)**.

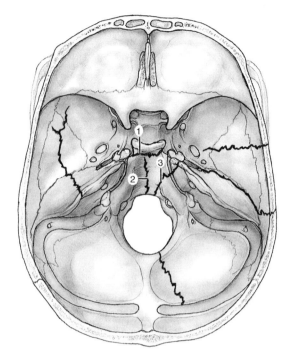

Fig. 34.2 Examples of middle and posterior skull base fractures. The numbers point to the different kind of fractures of the clivus: 1, transverse; 2, longitudinal; 3, oblique.

- Fractures of the clivus are frequently associated with a high rate of complications and neurologic sequelae, including a 24% mortality rate, and 46% neurologic and vascular complication rate.[49] Cases of traumatic basilar artery occlusion with locked-in syndrome, basilar artery entrapment (particularly in the longitudinal fractures), brainstem dysfunction, posterior fossa epidural hematoma, and subarachnoid bleeding have been described following clivus fracture.
- Clivus fractures may be associated with CSF rhinorrhea or otorrhea, and cranial nerve (CN) palsy (most commonly CNs III, V, and VII, as well as CN VI for the anatomic position of Dorello's canal). CN VI palsy is often associated with transverse fractures, whereas longitudinal fractures are associated mainly with CN VII palsy.[51,54]
- Clivus fracture with retroclival hematoma extending downward to

> **Pearl**
>
> Occipital–C1 dislocation requires occipitocervical fusion. Fractures without associated ligamentous or other injury on MRI may be managed conservatively.

the foramen magnum may be caused by a hyperextension injury with tectorial membrane damage, requiring the use of a rigid collar fixation.[49]

In patients with clivus fractures, radiological assessment of occipitocervical ligamentous lesions as well as C0-C1 dislocation should be performed.

■ Occipital Condyle Fractures

Occipital condyle fractures are unusual but not rare findings, with an overall incidence estimated at 1 to 4% of trauma patients.[55-58] Even more rarely, bilateral occipital condyles fractures may occur.

Types

- The most used classification system for occipital condyle fractures is the one proposed by Anderson and Montesano[59]:
  - Type I: Comminuted impaction fracture, generally resulting from axial loading (stable)
  - Type II: Condylar fracture with extension into the skull base (stable)
  - Type III: Avulsion-type fractures at the insertion of the alar ligament (unstable)

An alternative is that proposed by Tuli et al[60]:

Type	Description	Anderson and Montesano's Type
I	Undisplaced and stable	I and II
IIA	Displaced fracture with stability at the occiput-C1 junction	III
IIB	Displaced fracture with craniocervical junction instability	III

Signs and Symptoms

Typically condylar fractures cause neck pain, occipitocervical tenderness, reduced craniocervical motion, and retropharyngeal soft tissue swelling.[61] The most commonly associated cranial nerve palsy is CN XII, because of the close relationship of the hypoglossal canals to the condyles.[62] This neuropathy, as well as CN IX to XI palsy or CN VI palsy, can be acute or delayed, and temporary or permanent. Other neurologic deficits may include limb weakness, vertigo, and hyperreflexia.

Treatment

Following the classification by Tuli et al,[60] type I fractures do not require any specific treatment, type IIA may require a rigid collar, and type IIB are instable and require surgical instrumentation or halo traction.[63,64]

- Immobilization with a hard collar is often recommended in cases of stable occipital condyle fractures without bone fragment displacement because of the need for pain management and because of the possibility of bone fragment migration due to head movements. It is recommended for a duration of 1 to 3 months.[63]
- The most popular treatment is the use of an external immobilization (cervical collar or halo-vest immobilization). In rare cases, surgery may be indicated to remove bone fragments, especially when causing neurologic deficits. Occipitocervical dislocation or instability requires occipitocervical internal fixation and fusion.

■ Traumatic Carotid-Cavernous Fistula

- Traumatic carotid-cavernous fistula is a rare vascular complication of traumatic brain and facial injury. It represents an anomalous vascular communication between the carotid artery system and the venous channels within the cavernous sinuses of the sphenoid in the skull base.[65]
- It can occur in up to 2.4% of anterior SBFs, 8.3% of middle SBFs (especially with transverse or oblique fractures), and 1.7% of posterior SBFs.[66]
- Direct or indirect craniofacial trauma can lead to weakness in the muscular layer of the ICA or produce the fistula as a result of a laceration. This creates a vascular shunt from a high-flow arterial system to a low-flow venous sinus, potentially leading to a temporal/orbital bruit, proptosis, chemosis, or cranial nerve palsy (predominatly CN VI). Trigeminal nerve involvement, high intraocular pressure, pulsating exophthalmus, ptosis, papilledema, optic nerve atrophy, and ischemia have also been described.[67]

Signs and Symptoms

Signs and symptoms include pulsatile exophthalmos, orbital bruit, chemosis, and visual disturbances.

Types

The fistula can be direct or indirect.

Treatment

Prompt diagnosis and intervention should be emphasized in the management of such patients, and noninvasive endovascular techniques for early detection of traumatic carotid cavernous fistula should be considered in cases of facial or middle fossa fractures (see Chapter 12, page 298).[66]

- Ligation or trapping of the carotid artery is one of the alternatives, but these procedures have a high incidence of vision loss, recurrence, and stroke.[68] Endovascular treatment by means of detachable balloon occlusion is another possible method.[69,70] Embolization may be performed via a transarterial route or a trasvenous approach, through the superior ophthalmic vein.[71] The successful treatment may lead to immediate resolution of the proptosis, chemosis, and bruits, whereas ophthalmoplegia and optic nerve dysfunction may take up to 4 months to resolve.[72,73]
- Rarely the carotid-cavernous fistula can be associated with brainstem and basal ganglia venous congestion when the pericarotid vascular structures are involved (uncal vein with a hypoplastic second segment of the basal vein of Rosenthal, thrombosed or hypoplastic superior petrosal sinus, etc.). This situation requires emergency treatment.[74]
- In the very rare event of bilateral fistulae requiring treatment, a one-step endovascular detachable balloon treatment has been shown to be an effective method.[75]
- Balloon occlusion test may be helpful in assessing the risk of sacrificing one ICA.

■ Gunshot Wounds

The anterior skull base is the most common site for penetrating bullet injuries to the skull base that are most often caused by low-energy guns (82% of the cases).[76]

- Gunshot wounds involving the anterior skull base may be associated with orbital/ocular injury, CSF leak (from the nose, orbit, or wound), hematoma, brain contusion/laceration, and pneumocephalus.[77]
- In some cases, the removal of the bullet is required to prevent secondary complications and infections. Removal of the bullet and surgical repair can be done by means of a coronal subfrontal approach, or a middle or posterior fossa approach, depending on the location of the injury. A case treated by means of an endoscopic endonasal approach has been published as well.[78]

■ Posttraumatic Cerebrospinal Fluid Leak

Twenty-five percent of patients with head injury have fractures of the anterior skull base,[79] of which 12 to 30% may develop a CSF leak.[23,80]

The management algorithm[81] of such patients includes the ABC of life support and trauma protocols (airway, breathing, and circulation), exclusion of other life-threatening injuries, initial neurologic evaluation with GCS and neurologic screening exam, CSF leak diagnostics (Valsalva, glucose test strip, "halo" or "double ring" sign, β_2-transferrin), and head CT (see also Chapter 32).

- In patients with SBF, low-flow CSF leak, and GCS of 14 or 15 without surgical indications of other injuries, a conservative management approach is often sufficient. If there is no significant mass effect or risk of herniation and a low-flow leakage, lumbar drainage may be useful in stopping the persistent leak. Lumbar drainage may also be considered for high-flow leaks or those lasting more than 2 days. If a period of 3 days of lumbar drainage is not enough to stop the leak, CT contrast cisternography, MRI cisternography, or intrathecal fluorescein assay may be an option to use to localize the site of leak prior to surgery. Assuming there is a leak without confirmatory evidence in a stable patient may lead to unsuccessful surgery.

- For patients with a GCS ≤ 13, more intensive care is indicated. The neurologic and clinical status and the risk of meningitis should be assessed frequently. Persistent CSF leaks should be investigated as above, but intervention may need to be delayed until the resolution of cerebral edema in unconscious patients. Those with extensive fractures of the frontal skull base frequently have multiple other injuries (e.g., facial) so management should be planned in conjunction with other specialists, such as plastic surgeons. Those without an indication for emergency surgery can often be managed conservatively until brain edema resolves and the clinical condition improves. Pericranial flaps used for emergency procedures such as an acute subdural hematoma should always be preserved in the event that it is required for CSF leak repair.

■ References

Boldfaced references are of particular importance.

1. Wani AA, Ramzan AU, Raina T, et al. Skull base fractures: an institutional experience with review of the literature. Indian J Neurotrauma 2013;10:120–126
2. de Boussard CN, Bellocco R, af Geijerstam JL, Borg J, Adami J. Delayed intracranial complications after concussion. J Trauma 2006;61:577–581
3. **Samii M, Tatagiba M. Skull base trauma: diagnosis and management. Neurol Res 2002;24:147–156**

4. Perheentupa U, Kinnunen I, Grénman R, Aitasalo K, Mäkitie AA. Management and outcome of pediatric skull base fractures. Int J Pediatr Otorhinolaryngol 2010; 74:1245–1250
5. Somasundaram A, Laxton AW, Perrin RG. The clinical features of periorbital ecchymosis in a series of trauma patients. Injury 2014;45:203–205
6. Remmler D, Denny A, Gosain A, Subichin S. Role of three-dimensional computed tomography in the assessment of nasoorbitoethmoidal fractures. Ann Plast Surg 2000; 44:553–562, discussion 562–563
7. Ali QM, Dietrich B, Becker H. Patterns of skull base fracture: a three-dimensional computed tomographic study. Neuroradiology 1994;36:622–624
8. Fatterpekar GM, Doshi AH, Dugar M, Delman BN, Naidich TP, Som PM. Role of 3D CT in the evaluation of the temporal bone. Radiographics 2006;26(Suppl 1):S117–S132
9. **Ringl H, Schernthaner R, Philipp MO, et al. Three-dimensional fracture visualisation of multidetector CT of the skull base in trauma patients: comparison of three reconstruction algorithms. Eur Radiol 2009;19:2416–2424**
10. **Ringl H, Schernthaner RE, Schueller G, et al. The skull unfolded: a cranial CT visualization algorithm for fast and easy detection of skull fractures. Radiology 2010;255:553–562**
11. Perheentupa U, Mäkitie AA, Karhu JO, Koivunen P, Blanco Sequieros R, Kinnunen I. Frontobasilar fractures: proposal for image reviewing algorithm. J Craniomaxillofac Surg 2014;42:305–312
12. Kubal WS. Updated imaging of traumatic brain injury. Radiol Clin North Am 2012; 50:15–41
13. Donat TL, Endress C, Mathog RH. Facial fracture classification according to skeletal support mechanisms. Arch Otolaryngol Head Neck Surg 1998;124:1306–1314
14. Biffl WL, Moore EE, Offner PJ, et al. Optimizing screening for blunt cerebrovascular injuries. Am J Surg 1999;178:517–522
15. Sakas DE, Beale DJ, Ameen AA, et al. Compound anterior cranial base fractures: classification using computerized tomography scanning as a basis for selection of patients for dural repair. J Neurosurg 1998;88:471–477
16. Madhusudan G, Sharma RK, Khandelwal N, Tewari MK. Nomenclature of frontobasal trauma: a new clinicoradiographic classification. Plast Reconstr Surg 2006;117:2382–2388
17. **Manson PN, Stanwix MG, Yaremchuk MJ, Nam AJ, Hui-Chou H, Rodriguez ED. Frontobasal fractures: anatomical classification and clinical significance. Plast Reconstr Surg 2009;124:2096–2106**
18. **Buitrago-Téllez CH, Schilli W, Bohnert M, Alt K, Kimmig M. A comprehensive classification of craniofacial fractures: postmortem and clinical studies with two- and three-dimensional computed tomography. Injury 2002;33:651–668**
19. **Bächli H, Leiggener C, Gawelin P, et al. Skull base and maxillofacial fractures: two centre study with correlation of clinical findings with a comprehensive craniofacial classification system. J Craniomaxillofac Surg 2009;37:305–311**
20. **Fusetti S, Hammer B, Kellman R, Matula C, Strong EB, Di Ieva A. AO Foundation Surgery Reference: Cranial Vault and Skull Base. https://www2.aofoundation**

.org/wps/portal/surgery?showPage=diagnosis&bone=CMF&segment=Cranium. Accessed September 2014

21. Di Ieva A, Audigé L, Kellman RM, et al. The Comprehensive AOCMF Classification: skull base and cranial vault fractures—level 2 and 3 tutorial. Craniomaxillofac Trauma Reconstr 2014;7(Suppl 1):S103–S113

22. Audigé L, Cornelius PC, Kunz C, Buitrago-Tellez C, Prein J. AO Comprehensive Injury Automatic Classifier. https://www.aofoundation.org/Structure/resource/AO-OTA -Fracture-Dislocation-Classification/comprehensive-injury-automatic-classifier/ Pages/Comprehensive-Injury-Automatic-Classifier.aspx. Accessed August 2014

23. Kral T, Zentner J, Vieweg U, Solymosi L, Schramm J. Diagnosis and treatment of frontobasal skull fractures. Neurosurg Rev 1997;20:19–23

24. Piccirilli M, Anichini G, Cassoni A, Ramieri V, Valentini V, Santoro A. Anterior cranial fossa traumas: clinical value, surgical indications, and results—a retrospective study on a series of 223 patients. J Neurol Surg B Skull Base 2012;73:265–272

25. Rodriguez ED, Stanwix MG, Nam AJ, et al. Twenty-six-year experience treating frontal sinus fractures: a novel algorithm based on anatomical fracture pattern and failure of conventional techniques. Plast Reconstr Surg 2008;122:1850–1866

26. Pollock RA, Hill JL Jr, Davenport DL, Snow DC, Vasconez HC. Cranialization in a cohort of 154 consecutive patients with frontal sinus fractures (1987-2007): review and update of a compelling procedure in the selected patient. Ann Plast Surg 2013;71: 54–59

27. Tedaldi M, Ramieri V, Foresta E, Cascone P, Iannetti G. Experience in the management of frontal sinus fractures. J Craniofac Surg 2010;21:208–210

28. Gerbino G, Roccia F, Benech A, Caldarelli C. Analysis of 158 frontal sinus fractures: current surgical management and complications. J Craniomaxillofac Surg 2000;28: 133–139

29. Lakhani RS, Shibuya TY, Mathog RH, Marks SC, Burgio DL, Yoo GH. Titanium mesh repair of the severely comminuted frontal sinus fracture. Arch Otolaryngol Head Neck Surg 2001;127:665–669

30. Poon A, McCluskey PJ, Hill DA. Eye injuries in patients with major trauma. J Trauma 1999;46:494–499

31. Roth FS, Koshy JC, Goldberg JS, Soparkar CN. Pearls of orbital trauma management. Semin Plast Surg 2010;24:398–410

32. Haug RH, Van Sickels JE, Jenkins WS. Demographics and treatment options for orbital roof fractures. Oral Surg Oral Med Oral Pathol Oral Radiol Endod 2002;93:238–246

33. Cossman JP, Morrison CS, Taylor HO, Salter AB, Klinge PM, Sullivan SR. Traumatic orbital roof fractures: interdisciplinary evaluation and management. Plast Reconstr Surg 2014;133:335e–343e

34. Bell RB, Chen J. Frontobasilar fractures: contemporary management. Atlas Oral Maxillofac Surg Clin North Am 2010;18:181–196

35. Brodie HA, Thompson TC. Management of complications from 820 temporal bone fractures. Am J Otol 1997;18:188–197

36. Yalçıner G, Kutluhan A, Bozdemir K, Cetin H, Tarlak B, Bilgen AS. Temporal bone fractures: evaluation of 77 patients and a management algorithm. Ulus Travma Acil Cerrahi Derg 2012;18:424–428

37. Singh G, Singh B, Singh D. Prospective study of "otological injury secondary to head trauma." Indian J Otolaryngol Head Neck Surg 2013;65(Suppl 3):498–504
38. Saraiya PV, Aygun N. Temporal bone fractures. Emerg Radiol 2009;16:255–265
39. Kwong Y, Yu D, Shah J. Fracture mimics on temporal bone CT: a guide for the radiologist. AJR Am J Roentgenol 2012;199:428–434
40. Desikan RS, Chen JY. Imaging of temporal bone trauma. Operative Techniques in Otolaryngology-Head and Neck Surgery 2014;25:110–117
41. Asha'ari ZA, Ahmad R, Rahman J, Yusof RA, Kamarudin N. Patterns of intracranial hemorrhage in petrous temporal bone fracture. Auris Nasus Larynx 2012;39:151–155
42. Yeakley JW. Temporal bone fractures. Curr Probl Diagn Radiol 1999;28:65–98
43. Rafferty MA, Mc Conn Walsh R, Walsh MA. A comparison of temporal bone fracture classification systems. Clin Otolaryngol 2006;31:287–291
44. Kang HM, Kim MG, Boo SH, et al. Comparison of the clinical relevance of traditional and new classification systems of temporal bone fractures. Eur Arch Otorhinolaryngol 2012;269:1893–1899
45. Dubey KN, Bajaj A, Kumar I. Fracture of the styloid process associated with the mandible fracture. Contemp Clin Dent 2013;4:116–118
46. Blythe JN, Matthews NS, Connor S. Eagle's syndrome after fracture of the elongated styloid process. Br J Oral Maxillofac Surg 2009;47:233–235
47. Arechvo I, Giniunaite AM, Balseris S. Bilateral fracture of the styloid process with parapharyngeal emphysema. Otol Neurotol 2014;35:e155–e156
48. Lin DT, Lin AC. Surgical treatment of traumatic injuries of the cranial base. Otolaryngol Clin North Am 2013;46:749–757
49. Ochalski PG, Spiro RM, Fabio A, Kassam AB, Okonkwo DO. Fractures of the clivus: a contemporary series in the computed tomography era. Neurosurgery 2009;65:1063–1069, discussion 1069
50. Corradino G, Wolf AL, Mirvis S, Joslyn J. Fractures of the clivus: classification and clinical features. Neurosurgery 1990;27:592–596
51. **Menkü A, Koç RK, Tucer B, Durak AC, Akdemir H. Clivus fractures: clinical presentations and courses. Neurosurg Rev 2004;27:194–198**
52. Dashti R, Ulu MO, Albayram S, Aydin S, Ulusoy L, Hanci M. Concomitant fracture of bilateral occipital condyle and inferior clivus: what is the mechanism of injury? Eur Spine J 2007;16(Suppl 3):261–264
53. **Ochalski PG, Adamo MA, Adelson PD, Okonkwo DO, Pollack IF. Fractures of the clivus and traumatic diastasis of the central skull base in the pediatric population. J Neurosurg Pediatr 2011;7:261–267**
54. Bala A, Knuckey N, Wong G, Lee GY. Longitudinal clivus fracture associated with trapped basilar artery: unusual survival with good neurological recovery. J Clin Neurosci 2004;11:660–663
55. Bloom AI, Neeman Z, Slasky BS, et al. Fracture of the occipital condyles and associated craniocervical ligament injury: incidence, CT imaging and implications. Clin Radiol 1997;52:198–202
56. Noble ER, Smoker WR. The forgotten condyle: the appearance, morphology, and classification of occipital condyle fractures. AJNR Am J Neuroradiol 1996;17:507–513

57. Leone A, Cerase A, Colosimo C, Lauro L, Puca A, Marano P. Occipital condylar fractures: a review. Radiology 2000;216:635–644

58. **Debernardi A, D'Aliberti G, Talamonti G, et al. Traumatic injuries to the craniovertebral junction: a review of rare events. Neurosurg Rev 2014;37:203–216, discussion 216**

59. **Anderson PA, Montesano PX. Morphology and treatment of occipital condyle fractures. Spine 1988;13:731–736**

60. **Tuli S, Tator CH, Fehlings MG, Mackay M. Occipital condyle fractures. Neurosurgery 1997;41:368–376, discussion 376–377**

61. Theodore N, Aarabi B, Dhall SS, et al. Occipital condyle fractures. Neurosurgery 2013; 72(Suppl 2):106–113

62. Alcelik I, Manik KS, Sian PS, Khoshneviszadeh SE. Occipital condylar fractures. Review of the literature and case report. J Bone Joint Surg Br 2006;88:665–669

63. Caroli E, Rocchi G, Orlando ER, Delfini R. Occipital condyle fractures: report of five cases and literature review. Eur Spine J 2005;14:487–492

64. Waseem M, Upadhyay R, Al-Husayni H, Agyare S. Occipital condyle fracture in a patient with neck pain. Int J Emerg Med 2014;7:5–1

65. Fabian TS, Woody JD, Ciraulo DL, et al. Posttraumatic carotid cavernous fistula: frequency analysis of signs, symptoms, and disability outcomes after angiographic embolization. J Trauma 1999;47:275–281

66. **Liang W, Xiaofeng Y, Weiguo L, Wusi Q, Gang S, Xuesheng Z. Traumatic carotid cavernous fistula accompanying basilar skull fracture: a study on the incidence of traumatic carotid cavernous fistula in the patients with basilar skull fracture and the prognostic analysis about traumatic carotid cavernous fistula. J Trauma 2007;63:1014–1020, discussion 1020**

67. Palestine AG, Younge BR, Piepgras DG. Visual prognosis in carotid-cavernous fistula. Arch Ophthalmol 1981;99:1600–1603

68. Fattahi TT, Brandt MT, Jenkins WS, Steinberg B. Traumatic carotid-cavernous fistula: pathophysiology and treatment. J Craniofac Surg 2003;14:240–246

69. Jimenez DF, Gibbs SR. Carotid-cavernous sinus fistulae in craniofacial trauma: classification and treatment. J Craniomaxillofac Trauma 1995;1:7–15

70. Polin RS, Shaffrey ME, Jensen ME, et al. Medical management in the endovascular treatment of carotid-cavernous aneurysms. J Neurosurg 1996;84:755–761

71. Zhang Z, Wang C, Yang K, et al. Endovascular embolization of refractory traumatic carotid cavernous fistula with micro-coils: a preliminary experience. Turk Neurosurg 2014;24:190–195

72. Corradino G, Gellad FE, Salcman M. Traumatic carotid-cavernous fistula. South Med J 1988;81:660–663

73. Niamtu J III, Campbell RL. Carotid cavernous fistula. J Oral Maxillofac Surg 1982;40: 52–56

74. Ract I, Drier A, Leclercq D, et al. Extensive basal ganglia edema caused by a traumatic carotid-cavernous fistula: a rare presentation related to a basal vein of Rosenthal anatomical variation. J Neurosurg 2014;121:63–66

75. Chiriac A, Iliescu BF, Dobrin N, Poeata I. One-step endovascular treatment of bilateral traumatic carotid-cavernous fistulae with atypical clinical course. Turk Neurosurg 2014;24:422–426

76. Betz P, Stiefel D, Hausmann R, Eisenmenger W. Fractures at the base of the skull in gunshots to the head. Forensic Sci Int 1997;86:155–161

77. Bhatoe HS. Missile injuries of the anterior skull base. Skull Base 2004;14:1–8, discussion 8

78. Villaret AB, Zenga F, Esposito I, Rasulo F, Fontanella M, Nicolai P. Intracerebral bullet removal through an endoscopic transnasal craniectomy. Surg Neurol Int 2012;3:155–178

79. Rocchi G, Caroli E, Belli E, Salvati M, Cimatti M, Delfini R. Severe craniofacial fractures with frontobasal involvement and cerebrospinal fluid fistula: indications for surgical repair. Surg Neurol 2005;63:559–563, discussion 563–564

80. Wax MK, Ramadan HH, Ortiz O, Wetmore SJ. Contemporary management of cerebrospinal fluid rhinorrhea. Otolaryngol Head Neck Surg 1997;116:442–449

81. Sherif C, Di Ieva A, Gibson D, et al. A management algorithm for cerebrospinal fluid leak associated with anterior skull base fractures: detailed clinical and radiological follow-up. Neurosurg Rev 2012;35:227–237, discussion 237–238

35 Emergencies and Acute Situations in Skull Base Surgery

■ Pituitary Apoplexy

Pituitary apoplexy is acute hemorrhage or infarction of the pituitary gland.

Incidence

The incidence is six in 100,000 people, occurring in 1 to 9% of surgically treated pituitary adenomas. It has a male predilection, and the average age at presentation is 47 years. There is a 10% risk of apoplexy in incidentally discovered macroadenomas.[1]

- Pituitary adenomas often show asymptomatic bleeding, which is detected during surgery, on pathology, or on magnetic resonance imaging (MRI); 14 to 25% of patients with a pituitary adenoma have asymptomatic bleeding.[2–5] Pituitary apoplexy, therefore, is a clinical and not a pathological diagnosis.
- Prolactinomas, which are also the most frequent functional pituitary adenomas, have the highest incidence of apoplexy. Macroadenomas with suprasellar extensions are also prone to apoplexy.[4]
- In pituitary tumors, apoplexy/ischemia may occur because of the rapid growth of the tumor.[3,6]
- The risk of apoplexy is 0.6 to 10% in incidentally discovered macroadenomas.[5–10]
- About 80% of patients who present with apoplexy have no prior pituitary tumor diagnosis.[6]

Pituitary apoplexy can also occur in the nonneoplastic pituitary gland (after postpartum hypotension, for example, in Sheehan's syndrome) and rarely in other sellar lesions, such as tuberculosis, craniopharyngioma, and lymphocytic hypophysitis.[11–13]

Apoplexy Progression

Progression occurs as follows: tumor expansion → hemorrhage or infarct → compression on the surrounding pituitary parenchyma → partial destruction of the normal pituitary gland → acute compression of surrounding structures → potential extravasation of blood in the subarachnoid space.[14]

The increased intrasellar pressure, due to the acute expansion of the hematoma, may be the cause of ischemic necrosis following hypopituitarism.[15]

Risk Factors

Various precipitating factors have been implicated in pituitary apoplexy, such as hypertension,[16,17] dopamine agonists,[18] antithrombotic therapy,[18,19] estrogen therapy, radiation therapy, major surgery, and head trauma.[3,17] Pregnancy has also been related to pituitary apoplexy[20,21] leading to Sheehan's syndrome.

Pituitary stimulation tests with gonadotropin-releasing hormone, thyrotropin-releasing hormone, and corticotropin-releasing hormone may also induce pituitary apoplexy; thus, these patients should be closed monitored for apoplexy if they have been previously diagnosed with a pituitary tumor or if this diagnosis is suspected.[17]

Signs and Symptoms

There is atypical triad of symptoms: acute headache, visual deficits, and panhypopituitarism.

- Acute severe headache, often retro-orbital and sometimes occipital, has an onset and severity similar to that in subarachnoid hemorrhage. Headache is the most common symptom in pituitary apoplexy, occurring in 95% of cases, typically accompanied by nausea and vomiting (43–80% of cases), and less commonly by photophobia, fever, and decreased level of consciousness.[1] It may be mistaken for a subarachnoid hemorrhage or missed in the emergency department by clinicians or radiologists who fail to consider pituitary apoplexy in the differential diagnosis because pituitary apoplexy is less likely to cause meningeal signs.
- Visual field deficits are generally bitemporal superior quadrantanopsia or bitemporal hemianopsia. Decreased visual acuity occurs in 46 to 82% of patients,[5,8,16,22–24] with a range of symptoms from blurry vision to blindness.
- Diplopia occurs in 40 to 69% of patients. It is generally due to cranial nerve (CN) III palsy (unilateral dilated pupil, ptosis, eyeball deviated inferolaterally). Less frequently due to CN IV or VI palsy.[8,16,22,25] Up to 40% of patients can have combined deficits, generally involving CNs III and VI together.[8,16,22]
- Hypopituitarism: The most significant and life-threatening deficiency is secondary hypoadrenalism, although the most frequent is secondary hypo-

gonadism. Diabetes insipidus occurs in fewer than 8% of cases of pituitary apoplexy.[16]

- Other possible signs include Horner's syndrome, facial pain, and sensory loss due to trigeminal involvement (generally in CN V_1 or V_2).
- Rarely, pituitary apoplexy may lead to meningismus, stupor, and coma,[25] or neurologic symptoms related to vasospasm due to subarachnoid bleeding or internal carotid artery (ICA) compression.[5,26]

Imaging

- Computed tomography (CT) scans show blood hyperdensity in the sella in cases of bleeding. Injection of contrast shows increased uptake in the residual pituitary parenchyma. CT scan detects pituitary apoplexy in fewer than 28% of cases.[16,17]
- MRI is the best way to detect pituitary hemorrhage if apoplexy is suspected clinically.[16,17] In the early acute phase, it is characterized by isointense or slightly hypointense signal on T1 and T2 images and compression of the surrounding structures; a hyperintense signal is seen on fluid-attenuated inversion recovery (FLAIR) imaging. The signal becomes hyperintense on T1 and isointense/hyperintense on T2 in the subacute phase. In the chronic phase, the signal is hypointense on T1 and hyperintense on T2. Restricted diffusion is present in the adenoma on diffusion-weighted imaging. Enhancement of the rim after contrast and thickening of the sphenoid mucosa may be signs of apoplexy.[27]
- Pituitary apoplexy is in the differential diagnosis of subarachnoid bleeding due to aneurysm, arteriovenous malformation rupture, meningitis, cavernous sinus thrombosis, septic shock, encephalitis, migraine, and optic neuritis.

Medical Management

Management can entail either conservative measures or surgical treatment (see surgical technique on page 503). Conservative management is a viable option if the patient shows little to no neuro-ophthalmologic deficit.[17]

- If hypopituitarism is suspected, high-dose steroids are recommended.[28]
- Check for diabetes insipidus as well.
- Patients with suspected pituitary apoplexy should undergo visual field testing as soon as possible (ideally within 24 hours).[17]
- Emergency department management: patients with visual loss should be stabilized from an endocrinologic and hemodynamic perspective and then taken to surgery for urgent decompression.[17]
- Otherwise, patients with pituitary apoplexy should initially be assessed hourly for any change in vital signs, neurologic symptoms, or vision. After stability is noted, then the frequency of this assessment can be decreased.

Urine output, urine-specific gravity, serum, and urine electrolytes should be assessed frequently for signs of diabetes insipidus. Serum cortisol should be measured at 8 a.m. If at any point during this monitoring process the patient becomes unstable or the patient's condition worsens, or if there is a deterioration in the level of consciousness, then surgery should be considered.[1,17]

Outcome

Death is very rare in pituitary apoplexy, and in generally is related to intraoperative complications (vascular injury) or acute secondary adrenal insufficiency. Extraocular cranial neuropathy in general resolves over time, regardless of the treatment. Pituitary hormone deficiency can be permanent, but there may be partial or complete restoration of pituitary function in up to 50% of cases.[15,17] Hormone replacement therapy after surgery is necessary in the majority of patients, especially in those who had low serum prolactin levels before surgery.[16,17] There may be a delay in the presentation of thyroid dysfunction following surgery, so test thyroid function 7 to 10 days after surgery and again at 6 to 8 weeks.

- The complications encountered in surgery for pituitary apoplexy are no different from those for all surgery to the sellar and suprasellar region.
- Patients who are blind before surgery are less likely to recover, although partial recovery is still possible, whereas the majority of patients with partial deficits prior to surgery have a drastic improvement after surgery, either immediately after surgery or gradually over the following weeks.[16,17,29,30]
- For follow-up, it is recommended that patients undergo an MRI scan 3 to 6 months after apoplexy,[17] in order to detect any possible tumor regrowth or recurrent bleeding. Further MRI scans should be repeated yearly for the first 5 years following apoplexy and thereafter based on clinical indications.[17]

■ Facial Nerve Palsy

See page 199.

■ Optic Nerve Decompression

See page 482.

■ Oculomotor Nerve Palsies

See Chapters 3 and 10.

■ Traumatic Cerebrospinal Fluid Leak

See Chapter 32 and Chapter 34, page 853.

■ References

Boldfaced references are of particular importance.
1. **Singh TD, Valizadeh N, Meyer FB, Atkinson JL, Erickson D, Rabinstein AA. Management and outcomes of pituitary apoplexy. J Neurosurg 2015 ;122:1450–1457**
2. Wakai S, Fukushima T, Teramoto A, Sano K. [Pituitary apoplexy: its incidence and clinical significance (author's transl.)]. No To Shinkei 1981;33:561–568
3. Cardoso ER, Peterson EW. Pituitary apoplexy: a review. Neurosurgery 1984;14:363–373
4. Fraioli B, Esposito V, Palma L, Cantore G. Hemorrhagic pituitary adenomas: clinico-pathological features and surgical treatment. Neurosurgery 1990;27:741–747, discussion 747–748
5. **Semple PL, De Villiers JC, Bowen RM, Lopes MB, Laws ER Jr. Pituitary apoplexy: do histological features influence the clinical presentation and outcome? J Neurosurg 2006;104:931–937**
6. Jingsenl C, Gao C, Kai Q, et al. Transsphenoidal surgical decompression in pituitary apoplexy: clinical experience with 72 patients. Neurosurg Q 2014;24:139–142
7. Nishizawa S, Ohta S, Yokoyama T, Uemura K. Therapeutic strategy for incidentally found pituitary tumors ("pituitary incidentalomas"). Neurosurgery 1998;43:1344–1348, discussion 1348–1350
8. Sibal L, Ball SG, Connolly V, et al. Pituitary apoplexy: a review of clinical presentation, management and outcome in 45 cases. Pituitary 2004;7:157–163
9. Semple PL, Webb MK, de Villiers JC, Laws ER Jr. Pituitary apoplexy. Neurosurgery 2005;56:65–72, discussion 72–73
10. Arita K, Tominaga A, Sugiyama K, et al. Natural course of incidentally found non-functioning pituitary adenoma, with special reference to pituitary apoplexy during follow-up examination. J Neurosurg 2006;104:884–891
11. Podgórski JK, Rudnicki SZ, Potakiewicz Z, Delimat L, Siwik JW. [A case of intrasellar craniopharyngioma with the symptoms of pituitary apoplexy]. Neurol Neurochir Pol 1991;25:689–693
12. Arunkumar MJ, Rajshekhar V. Intrasellar tuberculoma presenting as pituitary apoplexy. Neurol India 2001;49:407–410
13. Lee MS, Pless M. Apoplectic lymphocytic hypophysitis. Case report. J Neurosurg 2003; 98:183–185
14. **Krisht AF, Vaphiades M, Husain M. Pituitary apoplexy. In: Krisht AF, Tindall GT, eds. Pituitary Disorders: Comprehensive Management. Baltimore: Lippincott Williams & Wilkins; 1999:295–303**
15. Zayour DH, Selman WR, Arafah BM. Extreme elevation of intrasellar pressure in patients with pituitary tumor apoplexy: relation to pituitary function. J Clin Endocrinol Metab 2004;89:5649–5654

16. Randeva HS, Schoebel J, Byrne J, Esiri M, Adams CB, Wass JA. Classical pituitary apoplexy: clinical features, management and outcome. Clin Endocrinol (Oxf) 1999;51: 181–188

17. Rajasekaran S, Vanderpump M, Baldeweg S, et al. UK guidelines for the management of pituitary apoplexy. Clin Endocrinol (Oxf) 2011;74:9–20

18. **Liu ZH, Tu PH, Pai PC, Chen NY, Lee ST, Chuang CC. Predisposing factors of pituitary hemorrhage. Eur J Neurol 2012;19:733–738**

19. Möller-Goede DL, Brändle M, Landau K, Bernays RL, Schmid C. Pituitary apoplexy: re-evaluation of risk factors for bleeding into pituitary adenomas and impact on outcome. Eur J Endocrinol 2011;164:37–43

20. Vaphiades MS, Simmons D, Archer RL, Stringer W. Sheehan syndrome: a splinter of the mind. Surv Ophthalmol 2003;48:230–233

21. de Heide LJ, van Tol KM, Doorenbos B. Pituitary apoplexy presenting during pregnancy. Neth J Med 2004;62:393–396

22. Ayuk J, McGregor EJ, Mitchell RD, Gittoes NJ. Acute management of pituitary apoplexy—surgery or conservative management? Clin Endocrinol (Oxf) 2004;61: 747–752

23. Lubina A, Olchovsky D, Berezin M, Ram Z, Hadani M, Shimon I. Management of pituitary apoplexy: clinical experience with 40 patients. Acta Neurochir (Wien) 2005; 147:151–157, discussion 157

24. Nielsen EH, Lindholm J, Bjerre P, et al. Frequent occurrence of pituitary apoplexy in patients with non-functioning pituitary adenoma. Clin Endocrinol (Oxf) 2006;64: 319–322

25. Reid RL, Quigley ME, Yen SS. Pituitary apoplexy. A review. Arch Neurol 1985;42:712–719

26. Warwar RE, Bhullar SS, Pelstring RJ, Fadell RJ. Sudden death from pituitary apoplexy in a patient presenting with an isolated sixth cranial nerve palsy. J Neuroophthalmol 2006;26:95–97

27. Osborn AG, Salzman KL, Barkovich AJ. Diagnostic Imaging: Brain, 2nd ed. Manitoba, Canada: Amirsys Publishing; 2010

28. Veldhuis JD, Hammond JM. Endocrine function after spontaneous infarction of the human pituitary: report, review, and reappraisal. Endocr Rev 1980;1:100–107

29. **Kerrison JB, Lynn MJ, Baer CA, Newman SA, Biousse V, Newman NJ. Stages of improvement in visual fields after pituitary tumor resection. Am J Ophthalmol 2000;130:813–820**

30. **Gruber A, Clayton J, Kumar S, Robertson I, Howlett TA, Mansell P. Pituitary apoplexy: retrospective review of 30 patients—is surgical intervention always necessary? Br J Neurosurg 2006;20:379–385**

36 Pediatric Skull Base

Skull base development is a dynamic process owing its complexity to the progressively changing relative size and orientation of the anterior, middle, and posterior cranial fossae (see Chapter 4). The temporal differences in the fusion of suture lines and the progressive pneumatization of the paranasal sinus and mastoid provide an additional element of complexity in skull base surgery in the pediatric patient.

■ Tumors in Children

Skull base tumors in children are rare.

- Most commonly, they have a mesenchymal origin and the majority of malignant tumors are sarcomas (**Fig. 36.1**). The anterior and middle cranial fossae are more frequently affected.[1] However, overall, malignant intrinsic tumors, such as medulloblastomas, are the predominant tumor, and they have a male predilection (69%).[2]
- Developmental tumors such as teratomas, choristomas, epidermoids, dermoids, nasal gliomas, and lipomas occur more frequently in children than in adults. In childhood, meningiomas are less common than benign sheath tumors (**Fig. 36.2**). These tumors are amenable to surgical resection and consequently have a good prognosis.[3]

■ Tumors of the Anterior Cranial Fossa

Esthesioneuroblastoma

Review pathology on page 161.

- The estimated incidence of esthesioneuroblastoma is 0.1/100,000 in children up to 15 years of age. It is the most common malignancy of the nasal cavity.[4]

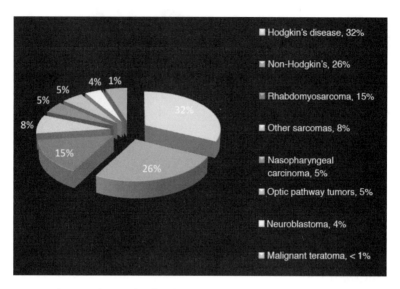

Fig. 36.1 Pediatric malignant head and neck tumors.

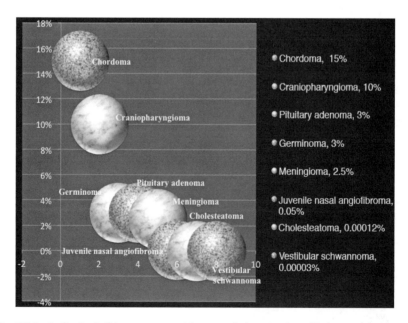

Fig. 36.2 Pediatric skull base tumors with generally benign clinical behavior (chordomas and juvenile nasal angiofibroma are locally aggressive. Chordomas and malignant meningiomas can metastasize).

- Esthesioneuroblastoma has a bimodal age distribution, with one peak in young adult patients and another peak in the 5th to 6th decades. The pediatric age ranges from 11 to 20 years.[5]
- The differential diagnosis includes lymphoma, sarcoma, anaplastic carcinoma, rhabdomyosarcoma, and transitional cell carcinoma.
- Epistaxis (76%), nasal obstruction and difficulty breathing (71%), pain (11%), anosmia, proptosis, and endocrinopathies are the most frequent symptoms.[6]
- Metastases to cervical lymph nodes, lungs, and bone can be observed in 8 to 30% of cases.[7] In patients with metastasis, the 5-year survival is near 0%.[3]
- The Kadish staging system is widely used to predict outcome and prognosis (see page 653).[8]
- Surgical resection of low-grade tumors with tumor-free margins is the treatment of choice.
- Esthesioneuroblastoma is radiosensitive. Either pre- or postoperative radiotherapy can be used.[3]

Juvenile Nasopharyngeal Angiofibroma

Juvenile nasopharyngeal angiofibroma (JNA) is a benign but locally aggressive and highly vascular tumor. Review the pathology on page 155.

- Juvenile nasopharyngeal angiofibroma accounts for 0.05% of head and neck tumors.[9]
- It occurs in prepubescent boys, starting adjacent to the sphenopalatine foramen. It grows toward adjacent structures, and can invade one nasal cavity and push the nasal septum contralaterally. It can also invade the skull base and intracranial structures, such as the cavernous sinus superiorly and posteriorly, and the maxillary sinus, pterygopalatine fossa, and the orbit laterally.
- A hormonal etiology has been proposed because of its prevalence in adolescent boys.
- Symptoms include difficulty breathing through the nose (80–90%), epistaxis (45–60%), headache (25%), facial swelling (10–18%), rhinorrhea, anosmia, rhinolalia, and otalgia.[10] Some patients present with life-threatening epistaxis.
- Since JNA is a highly vascular tumor, marked contrast enhancement is seen on computed tomography (CT) and magnetic resonance imaging (MRI). Prominent flow voids, seen on most MRI sequences, give rise to the characteristic "salt-and-pepper" appearance.[11]
- The differential diagnosis includes rhabdomyosarcoma, nasopharyngeal carcinoma, and nasopharyngeal teratoma. Lymphangioma and encephalocele do not show contrast enhancement.
- The treatment of choice is complete surgical removal. A staging classification has been proposed.[12] In stage 1 and 2, surgery is the treatment of choice.[3]

- Preoperative embolization can help to prevent excessive bleeding,[12,13] but is only an adjuvant to treatment. Recently, a direct intratumoral embolization has been proposed[14]
- Radiotherapy has been used as both a primary treatment and as an adjunct to surgery.[3]
- Because of the rarity of JNA, very few trials of chemotherapy have been reported. The presurgical use of flutamide (a testosterone receptor blocker) for the treatment of JNA has also been reported. In the four cases presented, the average tumor shrinkage was 44% following flutamide use.[3] A good preoperative volume reduction with flutamide in postpubertal patients has been reported, but a minimal response is found in prepubertal patients.[15] Another series treated five patients for recurrent JNA with doxorubicin, vincristine, dactinomycin, and cyclophosphamide, resulting in tumor remission in all cases.[16] Another published report used Adriamycin and dacarbazine in a patient with advanced disease; extensive tumor regression was reported following treatment.[17] Chemotherapy, therefore, potentially can be an alternative to radiation in cases of aggressive, unresectable JNA.

Rhabdomyosarcoma

Rhabdomyosarcoma (RMS) is a rare malignant tumor of striated muscle tissue. It is the most common of the soft tissue sarcomas in children; 35 to 40% of RMSs are located in the head and neck. See pathology on page 166.

- Patients with genetic diseases (e.g., Li-Fraumeni syndrome, neurofibromatosis, fetal alcohol syndrome, and nevoid basal cell carcinoma) have an increased risk of developing RMS. In addition, intrauterine exposure to alkylating agents, parental use of marijuana and cocaine, and exposure to X-rays are considered risk factors for RMS.[18]
- Rhabdomyosarcoma arises from undifferentiated mesenchymal cells, the rhabdomyoblasts. Different histological types are described: embryonal, alveolar, botryoid, and pleomorphic. Embryonal RMS is the most common in the head, neck, and genitourinary tract. In this tumor, the cells are similar to embryo cells of age 6 to 8 weeks. In alveolar RMS, a more aggressive subtype, the cells have a similar appearance to embryo cells of age 10 to 12 weeks. In the botryoid subtype, the cells are similar to embryonal RMS and present as grape lesions. Pleomorphic RMS, most common in adults, is an undifferentiated sarcoma. Alveolar and undifferentiated RMS have a poor prognosis.[19]
- Presenting symptoms depend on the tumor size and location. Usually RMS presents as an expanding mass. Superficial tumors are detected sooner, but deeply located tumors can be large once they are diagnosed. Typical presentation can include nasal obstruction, pain, and upper respiratory symptoms. Rhabdomyosarcoma often recurs and metastasizes. Metastases involve local

lymph nodes in 5% of cases. Lung, liver, bone, and bone marrow are other common sites of RMS metastases.

- Rhabdomyosarcoma is classified into stage I through IV based on the amount of tumor spread and the size of residual tumor after surgery.[20]
- A tumor, node, metastasis (TNM) staging system has been developed and incorporated in the Intergroup Rhabdomyosarcoma Study Group (IRSG)-IV protocol.[21]
- Treatment of RMS includes surgery, chemotherapy, and radiotherapy.
- Whenever possible, surgical removal should be performed with wide (> 1 cm) margins of normal tissue. However, this goal often cannot be achieved in skull base RMS.
- Radiotherapy combined with chemotherapy appears to provide the best local control. Several case series have described a survival rate of 60% in patients treated with chemotherapy and radiotherapy. However, the survival rate was only 19% in cases that utilized other treatment regimens.[22-25] Older patients, histological alveolar type, and tumor size > 6 cm are risk factors associated with a poor prognosis.[22]

Fibrous Dysplasia

Fibrous dysplasia is a benign developmental disease. See pages 164 and 533.

- Fibrous connective tissue replaces normal lamellar bone. The ribs or craniofacial bones, in particular the maxilla and sphenoid, are often involved. Frequently, fibrous dysplasia may occur in one site as a monostotic form. The polyostotic form, as a part of McCune-Albright syndrome, is rare but has endocrine implications. When more than 50% of the skeleton is involved, fractures and deformities are also common.
- Fibrous dysplasia can be asymptomatic or can present with local pain, local swelling or deformity, pathological fracture, cranial nerve involvement with progressive visual or hearing loss, seizures, elevated serum alkaline phosphatase (33%), and spontaneous scalp hemorrhage.[26] Fibrous dysplasia can also be associated with Cushing's syndrome and acromegaly, although this is rare.
- Surgery is indicated in cases of neurologic symptoms or progressive deformity. Some authors have advocated early aggressive surgery,[27] but complete resection may be difficult and may still be associated with recurrence in up to 25% of patients.[28] After adolescence, progression may slow down, so treatment is tailored to specific symptoms.

■ Tumors of the Central and Middle Skull Base

Pituitary Adenoma

In children, pituitary adenoma (PAs) represent less than 3% of all supratentorial tumors.[29] Review pathology on page 143.

- The most frequent functional adenomas in children are prolactin (PRL)-secreting, followed by adrenocorticotropic hormone (ACTH)-secreting and growth hormone (GH)-secreting tumors. Nonfunctional tumors are rare, and are usually diagnosed when suprasellar growth has caused compression of the optic chiasm with bitemporal hemianopia. This may be associated with varying degrees of hypopituitarism.
- In females, prolactinoma causes failure of menarche and galactorrhea; in males, it causes impotence. GH-secreting tumors in children cause gigantism instead of acromegaly, because the epiphyseal plates in the long bones have yet to completely undergo ossification.
- ACTH-secreting adenomas cause Cushing's syndrome, with stunted growth, hypertension, central fat deposition, abdominal purple striae, diabetes or glucose intolerance, and osteoporosis.
- Review radiology (**Table 5.4**, page 118), endocrinology (Chapter 8), and surgical treatment (page 499).
- The transsphenoidal endoscopic endonasal approach is the gold standard for PA resection,[30,31] but it can be limited in young children due to the small sizes of the nostrils. See endonasal approaches in Chapter 16.

Craniopharyngioma

Review pathology (page 148) and radiology (**Table 5.4**, page 119).

- Craniopharyngioma accounts for 1.8 to 10% of intracranial tumors in children.[3,32]
- Clinical symptoms include headache, visual deficits, varying degrees of hypopituitarism, diabetes insipidus, and significant weight gain.[33] In cases of hydrocephalus, intracranial hypertension can be the first symptom; it occurs more frequently in children than in adults.[32]
- Attempts to remove as much of the tumor as possible are preferable for long-term control; however, unfavorable tumor locations (e.g., optic nerve with or without hypothalamic involvement) may be associated with a higher risk of vascular and hypothalamic injury. In these cases, a limited resection followed by radiotherapy may be more prudent. Cyst drainage with insertion of an Ommaya reservoir and judicious use of radiotherapy may lead to long-term control. Intensity-modulated proton therapy in pediatric craniopharyngiomas has been reported to achieve significantly better coverage while minimizing the dosage to normal tissue in comparison to double scattering proton therapy.[34]
- Extended endoscopic endonasal transsphenoidal approaches and craniotomy are performed with or without orbital cranial osteotomy. Endoscopic endonasal surgery has been shown to have gross total resection high rates in the pediatric population.[35] The risks of complications are higher in recurrent cases.

- The overall survival rate is 92%, but relapses and reduced quality of life are also frequent.[36]

■ Tumors of the Posterior Cranial Fossa

Chordoma

Review pathology (page 165) and radiology (page 117).

- Chordoma is a slow-growing, locally aggressive tumor that occurs most frequently in the clivus in children and in the sacral region in adults.
- Chordoma accounts for 15% of intracranial tumors in children.[3]
- Metastases occur to lungs, lymph nodes, liver, bone, and adrenals.
- A more aggressive behavior in children than in adults has been reported for a prevalent atypical type.[37] Malignant transformations into fibrosarcoma or malignant fibrous histiocytoma can also occur, although these transformations are generally quite rare.
- Presenting symptoms are cranial nerve (CN) palsies (usually CN III or VI), pain, and obstruction of the sinonasal structures.[3]
- The best option is radical surgical excision, but gross tumor removal can be difficult to achieve in some cases.
- Adjunctive radiotherapy can be used before[38] and after surgery.[39,40]
- Proton beam therapy may achieve better results in children than in adults.[41,42]
- The treatment of choice can be considered surgery followed by local proton beam therapy.

Meningioma

Review pathology (page 138) and radiology (page 114).

- Meningiomas are rare and account for 1.5 to 1.8% of intracranial tumors in children.[43]
- They are associated with neurofibromatosis types 1 and 2 (NF1 and NF2) (see pages 135 and 137). Multiple meningiomas in children are one of the hallmarks of NF2, and their presence should quite clearly suggest this diagnosis.[44]
- There is a male predilection, with a high incidence of cystic tumors, high-grade meningiomas, and an increased recurrence rate.[45]
- The treatment of choice is total resection.
- When the resection is subtotal, close observation for at least 10 years is recommended.
- Patients with NF2 should be considered a special risk, necessitating lifelong follow-up.[46]

- Papillary meningiomas are malignant subtypes that are more common in pediatric patients.
- Malignant subtypes may metastasize outside the central nervous system (CNS) to lungs, liver, lymph nodes, and heart.
- Adjuvant radiation therapy is indicated in malignant subtypes, recurrences, or in partial resections.

Vestibular Schwannoma

Review pathology (page 135) and radiology (page 117).

- In children, vestibular schwannomas are almost always found in cases of NF2, often with bilateral tumors.
- Frequent symptoms are progressive hearing loss, disequilibrium, headache, facial weakness, obstructive hydrocephalus, nystagmus, and ataxia. Usually, tumors are already large at the time of diagnosis.
- Whenever possible, because of rich vascularization of schwannoma in children, preoperative embolization should be considered.[47,48]
- Surgical is the treatment of choice in order to preserve hearing, especially in bilateral schwannomas. If needed, the translabyrinthine approach can be used, but it is generally reserved for cases of unilateral deafness. With small tumors, radiosurgery in children has been advocated not only to stop the tumor growth but also to avoid deafness after surgery, especially in cases of bilateral schwannomas.[49]

Cholesteatoma or Epidermoid Tumor

- The incidence of congenital cholesteatomas is 0.12 cases per 100,000 people.[50] See pathology (page 153) and radiology (page 126).
- Cholesteatomas are benign tumors with a congenital or acquired origin. Congenital tumors can be located intracranially or within the skull bones, with almost all bone tumors occurring in the temporal bone.
- Intracranial cholesteatomas originate from ectodermal implants trapped in the CNS. In the calvarial location, the ectoderm is trapped in the skull, within the diploe, and expands both the inner and outer tables; secondarily, the calvarial cholesteatoma can involve dural sinuses and intracranial structures.[26]
- Acquired tumors can originate from epithelium migration after otitis media or tympanic membrane perforation.[51]
- Symptoms depend on tumor location. These tumors can cause hearing loss or sometimes recurrent episodes of septic meningitis (when a cyst ruptures its contents).
- Treatment is typically surgical with the goal of preserving hearing. For temporal bone cholesteatomas, two main strategies have been described: the

canal-wall-down mastoidectomy and the canal-wall-up tympanomastoid-ectomy. The canal-wall-down provides better exposure due to the aggressive removal of the posterior ear canal wall; a common cavity is intentionally formed so that it exists as a bowl after the procedure. This is done with the purpose of improved postoperative surveillance of the disease.[52] The canal-wall-up technique is less aggressive in order to preserve hearing, but also carries a high recurrence rate.[3] In these techniques, a second look to check for tumor recurrence is needed. When attempting a second look, an endoscopic approach can be less invasive and is more readily accepted by patients.[53]

- Clinical and radiological long-term follow-up is essential, given the high recurrence rate of 57% after 5 years.[54]

Ewing's Sarcoma

Ewing's sarcoma is a primitive neuroectodermal tumor. See pathology on page 166.

- Ewing's sarcoma is the second most common malignant tumor in children. More often located in the spine, Ewing's sarcoma can involve the skull base in children, sometimes in a massive way.
- The presenting symptoms are local pain and swelling. Spectral karyotyping has shown a 11;22 translocation and a frequent Ewing's sarcoma/FLI1 fusion transcript in cases of Ewing's sarcoma.[55]
- Surgery is indicated to decompress neural structures followed by adjuvant chemotherapy, with good reported results. Radiotherapy is used when there is no response to chemotherapy or for localized tumors as an adjunct to surgery.[55]

■ Malformations

Encephalocele

See Chapter 37.

Craniofacial Dysmorphic Syndromes (Table 36.1)

Craniofacial dysmorphic syndromes are the result of disordered development. Normal development of the face and the skull is interrupted, resulting in a wide group of congenital craniofacial anomalies. Two major categories can be distinguished: those associated with craniosynostoses and those associated with cleft.[56] The most common syndromes associated with craniosynostoses are

Table 36.1   Overview of Major Forms of Syndromic Craniosynostoses

	Apert Syndrome	Crouzon Syndrome	Pfeiffer Syndrome
Skull phenotype	Bilateral coronal synostosis	Bilateral coronal synostosis, pancranio-synostosis, cloverleaf skull	Bilateral coronal synostosis, cloverleaf skull in type 2 Pfeiffer
Facial features	Hypertelorism, down-slanting palpebral fissures, cleft palate, high arched palate, midface hypoplasia	Hypertelorism, beaked nose, proptosis, rarely cleft palate, mandibular prognathism, midface hypoplasia	Hypertelorism, down-slanting palpebral fissures, proptosis, rarely cleft palate, midface hypoplasia
Neurocognitive	Severe intellectual disability and/or developmental delay, conductive hearing loss common	Intellect usually normal; conductive hearing loss common	Intellect normal in type 1 Pfeiffer; in types 2 and 3 Pfeiffer, intellectual disability and developmental delay common, conductive hearing loss common

Source: Adapted from Nneamaka B, Solomon BD, Muenke M. Impact of genetics on the diagnosis and clinical management of syndromic craniosynostoses. Childs Nerv Syst 2012;28:1447–1463. Reprinted with permission.

Crouzon, Apert, Pfeiffer, Muenke, and Saethre-Chotzen syndromes. The most common syndromes associated with clefts are Pierre Robin, Treacher Collins, Nager, Binder, and Stickler syndromes. All cases exhibit autosomal dominant inheritance and require a multidisciplinary approach. Timing of surgery has to be planned in consideration of the growing skull. Surgical intervention should be done in stages: craniotomy aims to decompress the brain and is done in infancy; advancement of the middle third improves nasal airflow and may be done in puberty; finally, orthognathic surgery improves occlusion and dental esthetics and may be done in adolescence.[57]

Crouzon Syndrome (Craniofacial Dysostosis)

- Crouzon syndrome is the most common craniosynostosis syndrome and it accounts for 48% of general craniosynostoses.[58]

Muenke Syndrome	Saethre–Chotzen Syndrome	Craniofrontonasal Syndrome
Unilateral or bilateral coronal synostosis, macrocephaly	Unilateral or bilateral coronal synostosis, metopic synostosis	Unilateral or bilateral coronal synostosis
Hypertelorism, down-slanting palpebral fissures, high arched palate, mild midface hypoplasia	Ptosis, ear anomalies—small ears with prominent crus, low frontal hairline, rarely cleft palate, midface hypoplasia	Hypertelorism, broad nasal bridge, broad or bifid nasal tip; rarely cleft lip and/or palate (females more severely affected)
Intellectual disability and/ or developmental delay common, low-frequency sensorineural hearing loss common	Intellect usually normal, developmental delays common in those with gene deletions, conductive, mixed, and profound sensorineural hearing loss	Normal intellect in > 50%, 10–50% with developmental delay, occasionally learning difficulties (mild), sensorineural hearing loss

- Mutation of the *FGFR2* (fibroblast growth factor receptor) gene has been described.[59] Acanthosis nigricans is associated with the mutation of *FGFR3*.[60]
- Crouzon syndrome is characterized by craniosynostoses of coronal and basal sutures, with brachycephalia, maxillary hypoplasia, shallow orbits, and proptosis. Hearing loss occurs in 30 to 55% of patients, and anomalies of the palatal swelling occur in 50%; cleft palate is not common.[58]
- Childhood surgery is performed in stages with fronto-orbital and midfacial advancement to correct synostosis in the first year of life.[61] Hypertelorism is usually corrected with facial bipartition at age 7.[62] Maxillary advancement is performed after skeletal growth is completed.[58]

Apert Syndrome (Acrocephalosyndactyly Type 1)

- Apert syndrome accounts for 4.5% of craniosynostosis[58] and is associated with syndactyly of the hands and the feet. Other symptoms include closure of the coronal suture with acrocephaly, prominent forehead, pituitary fossa

and basiocciput larger than normal, amblyopia with visual impairment, depression of nasal bridge, dental anomalies, malocclusion, and, often, mental retardation, obstructive sleep apnea, and cleft palate in about 30% of cases.[58]
- Mutations of the *FGFR2* gene have been found.[63]
- If obstructive sleep apnea occurs, an early midfacial distraction can been performed with good results.[64]

Pfeiffer Syndrome

- Three clinical types of Pfeiffer syndrome have been described. Type 1 is associated with craniosynostosis of the coronal suture; midface hypoplasia; broad, medially deviated halluces; and variable soft tissue syndactyly. Mutations in *FGFR1* or *FGFR2* have been described.[63] Type 2 is characterized by, in addition to the above, pansynostosis, in which all calvarial sutures prematurely fuse, frequent elbow ankylosis/synostosis, and additional unusual anomalies. Type 3 is characterized by a very short anterior cranial base, ocular proptosis, elbow ankylosis/synostosis, and additional unusual anomalies.[63]

Muenke Syndrome

- Muenke syndrome is characterized by wide radiological and clinical variability. A single mutation in *FGFR3* is associated with Muenke syndrome.[65] The clinical findings are craniosynostosis, most commonly of the coronal suture, carpal or tarsal bone fusion, and hearing loss.[63]

Craniofrontonasal Syndrome

- Craniofrontonasal syndrome is an X-linked developmental malformation. Due to an unusual inheritance pattern, females are more severely affected than males. Craniofrontonasal syndrome is caused by mutations in the *EFNB1* (*Ephrin B1*) gene, which encodes one of eight known ephrin ligands. Clinical features include coronal suture synostosis, hypertelorism, cleft palate, and a broad or bifid nasal tip. It is more frequently found in females.[63]

■ Pediatric Skull Base Trauma

Cranial base fractures are associated with dural tears and cerebrospinal fluid (CSF) leak, brain and cranial nerve injury, and brain herniation.

- The most common skull base fractures in children are temporal bone fractures (64%), followed by sphenoethmoidal complex (41%) and orbital fractures (35%)[66] (**Fig. 36.3**).

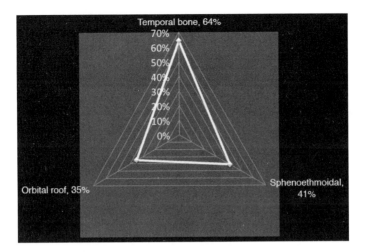

Fig. 36.3 Skull base fractures in children.

- Anterior cranial base and orbito-naso-ethmoidal fractures are frequent in children younger than 5 years of age as a consequence of nonpneumatized nasal sinuses. Among orbital roof fractures, the most common are blowout fractures.
- The most common causes are falls (35%), recreational activities (29%), motor vehicle accidents (24%), and child abuse (12%).[67]
- Anterior cranial fossa fractures often involve the frontal sinus and ethmoid planum with pneumoencephalos and CSF rhinorrhea, whereas middle cranial fossa fractures involve the sphenoid sinus and temporal bone with CSF rhinorrhea and otorrhea. Lastly, posterior skull base fractures involving the clivus are caused by severe head trauma. In clival fractures the mortality and morbidity rate is high due to injuries to blood vessels, the brainstem, and the lower cranial nerves. In adults, the majority of cases occur following frontal or axial impact, whereas all reported pediatric cases occurred secondary to occipital impact.[68]
- Generally, surgical treatment is not needed in linear fractures.
- Treatment of pediatric basilar fractures has to respect the growth of the bone, and for this reason rigid bone fixation is achieved by resorbable bone fixation.[69] Surgical treatment is often challenging and requires a multidisciplinary team approach.
- Surgical treatment consists of reconstruction and stabilization of the fracture, along with sealing off dural tears to avoid CSF leak.

■ Surgical Approaches in the Pediatric Skull Base

Standard surgical approaches to skull base lesions, with dedicated modifications, can be used in children; the developing craniofacial skull has to be considered in the surgical planning. Particular care and attention must be given to the management of blood loss, temperature control, and electrolyte balance. Because of the small size of pediatric patients, minimal blood loss can be significant, requiring transfusion. The immaturity of pediatric sinuses that are not yet well pneumatized should also be considered in endonasal approaches. Unerupted dentition can be compromised by maxillotomy. Several landmarks that differ from adult landmarks have been described in children, and the surgeon must have a working knowledge of these differences.[70]

- Endoscopic endonasal approaches and extended endoscopic endonasal approaches enable the surgeon to reach the midline aspect of sphenoethmoid planum, sphenoid sinus, and upper, middle, and lower clivus lesions.[30,31,71–81] More lateral lesions involving the cavernous sinus and pterygomaxillary fossa can be resected by an endonasal transmaxillary-transpterygoid approach.[82] These approaches can be done via one or two nostrils and can be combined with other transcranial techniques. The main advantage is the direct access to the pathology without brain retraction and without facial deformities. A direct endoscopic view is more favorable to protect basilar neurovascular structures. The absent or partial pneumatization of nasal sinuses in younger children is the main disadvantage, when sinuses are not eroded by tumor. In these cases, neuronavigation is essential to guide the surgeon, and more drilling is required. Furthermore, narrow nasal cavities require smaller endoscopes and meticulous surgical techniques. Transfacial, transoral, and transmaxillary approaches are limited by the budding teeth.[83]
- Transfacial approaches in many studies do not result in disruption of facial growth, as most osteotomies do not pass through growth centers.[2] A shallow anterior fossa in the developing skull makes the frontotemporal-orbitozygomatic (FTOZ) approach easier.[83] In cases of vestibular schwannomas, the approach that is chosen must be one that preserves hearing. The future implications of partial resection of occipital condyle and hemilaminectomy of C1 in a far-lateral transcondylar approach in children are still unclear.[3]
- Even if skull base tumors in children are more aggressive, minimal surgical-related morbidities and good long-term tumor control have been reported.[2,70,83,84]

Outcomes

- In a series of 55 children who underwent skull base approaches, a 11% rate of permanent neurologic morbidity was reported.[70]

Pearl

Because of the benign histology of many skull base tumors in children, the higher rate of complete resection, the good response to adjuvant therapy, and the plasticity of the developing nervous system, complex skull base procedures in children carry better outcomes than in adults.

- In a series of 23 pediatric patients who underwent skull base approaches for resection of tumors with a median follow-up of 60 months, gross total resection was achieved in 52%. The survival rate was 87% and the rate of permanent neurologic morbidity was 9%.[84] In another series of 26 cases of skull base tumors, a 30.7% complication rate of permanent deficits was reported, with a 92% complete resection rate and 81% tumor-free survival rate at 2 years postoperatively.[2] A retrospective series of 67 children operated for skull base pathologies during a 6-year period[85] reported that 80% of children were alive and well after 2½ years, with no severe postoperative complications. The series also reported no perioperative mortality. The publication concluded that the complication and mortality rates are lower than those in adults and that long-term cosmetic effects of subcranial approaches are negligible.[85]

■ References

Boldfaced references are of particular importance.
1. **Hanbali F, Tabrizi P, Lang FF, DeMonte F. Tumors of the skull base in children and adolescents. J Neurosurg 2004;100(2, Suppl Pediatrics):169–178**
2. **Teo C, Dornhoffer J, Hanna E, Bower C. Application of skull base techniques to pediatric neurosurgery. Childs Nerv Syst 1999;15:103–109**
3. Bauer AM, Baskaya MK. Tumors of the Pediatric Skull, Skull base and orbit. In: G Narenthiran ed. Textbook of Paediatric Neurosurgery. Madison: Annals of Neurosurgery; 2008
4. Bisogno G, Soloni P, Conte M, et al. Esthesioneuroblastoma in pediatric and adolescent age. A report from the TREP project in cooperation with the Italian Neuroblastoma and Soft Tissue Sarcoma Committees. BMC Cancer 2012;12:117
5. Becker LE, Hinton D. Primitive neuroectodermal tumors of the central nervous system. Hum Pathol 1983;14:538–550
6. Hlavac PJ, Henson SL, Popp AJ. Esthesioneuroblastoma: advances in diagnosis and treatment. Contemp Neurosurgery 1998;20:1–5
7. Oskouian RJ Jr, Jane JA Sr, Dumont AS, Sheehan JM, Laurent JJ, Levine PA. Esthesioneuroblastoma: clinical presentation, radiological, and pathological features, treatment, review of the literature, and the University of Virginia experience. Neurosurg Focus 2002;12:e4
8. Kadish S, Goodman M, Wang CC. Olfactory neuroblastoma. A clinical analysis of 17 cases. Cancer 1976;37:1571–1576

9. Tewfik TL. Juvenile nasopharyngeal angiofibroma. http://emedicine.medscape.com. 2014. Accessed September 1, 2014

10. Nicolai P, Castelnuovo P. Benign tumors of the sinonasal tract. In: Flint PW, Haughey BH, Lund LJ, et al, eds. Cummings Otolaryngology: Head and Neck Surgery. Philadelphia: Mosby Elsevier; 2010:Chapter 49

11. Seo CS, Han MH, Chang KH, Yeon KM. Angiofibroma confined to the pterygoid muscle region: CT and MR demonstration. AJNR Am J Neuroradiol 1996;17:374–376

12. Radkowski D, McGill T, Healy GB, Ohlms L, Jones DT. Angiofibroma. Changes in staging and treatment. Arch Otolaryngol Head Neck Surg 1996;122:122–129

13. Moulin G, Chagnaud C, Gras R, et al. Juvenile nasopharyngeal angiofibroma: comparison of blood loss during removal in embolized group versus nonembolized group. Cardiovasc Intervent Radiol 1995;18:158–161

14. Jang HU, Kim TH, Park CM, Kim JS. Direct intratumoral embolization of intranasal vascular tumors. Auris Nasus Larynx 2013;40:103–105

15. Thakar A, Gupta G, Bhalla AS, et al. Adjuvant therapy with flutamide for presurgical volume reduction in juvenile nasopharyngeal angiofibroma. Head Neck 2011;33: 1747–1753

16. Goepfert H, Cangir A, Lee YY. Chemotherapy for aggressive juvenile nasopharyngeal angiofibroma. Arch Otolaryngol 1985;111:285–289

17. Schick B, Kahle G, Hässler R, Draf W. [Chemotherapy of juvenile angiofibroma—an alternative?]. HNO 1996;44:148–152

18. Cripe T. Pediatric rhabdomyosarcoma. Medscape July 2011. http://emedicine.medscape .com/article/988803-overview. Accessed August 30, 2014

19. Newton WA Jr, Gehan EA, Webber BL, et al. Classification of rhabdomyosarcomas and related sarcomas. Pathologic aspects and proposal for a new classification—an Intergroup Rhabdomyosarcoma Study. Cancer 1995;76:1073–1085

20. Crist W, Gehan EA, Ragab AH, et al. The Third Intergroup Rhabdomyosarcoma Study. J Clin Oncol 1995;13:610–630

21. Crist WM, Anderson JR, Meza JL, et al. Intergroup Rhabdomyosarcoma study–IV: results for patients with nonmetastatic disease. J Clin Oncol 2001;19:3091–3102

22. Callender TA, Weber RS, Janjan N, et al. Rhabdomyosarcoma of the nose and paranasal sinuses in adults and children. Otolaryngol Head Neck Surg 1995;112:252–257

23. Carrau RL, Myers NE. Neoplasms of the nose and paranasal sinuses. In: Head and Neck Surgery/Otolaryngology. Philadelphia: Lippincott Williams & Wilkins; 2001

24. Gerber ME, Cotton RT. Pediatric malignancies. In: Head and Neck Surgery/Otolaryngology. Philadelphia: Lippincott Williams & Wilkins; 2001

25. Harnsberger HR, Hudgins PA, Wigins RH, Davidson HC. Tête et Cou. Paris: Maloine; 2004

26. Greenberg MS, Ed. Handbook of Neurosurgery. New York: Thieme; 2010

27. Camilleri AE. Craniofacial fibrous dysplasia. J Laryngol Otol 1991;105:662–666

28. Jones NF, Schramm VL, Sekhar LN. Reconstruction of the cranial base following tumour resection. Br J Plast Surg 1987;40:155–162

29. Keil MF, Stratakis CA. Pituitary tumors in childhood: update of diagnosis, treatment and molecular genetics. Expert Rev Neurother 2008;8:563–574

30. Cusimano MD, Di Ieva A, Lee J, Anderson J. Canula-assisted endoscopy in bi-portal transphenoidal cranial base surgery: technical note. Acta Neurochir (Wien) 2013; 155:909–911

31. Cusimano MD, Kan P, Nassiri F, et al. Outcomes of surgically treated giant pituitary tumours. Can J Neurol Sci 2012;39:446–457

32. Lasky JL, ed. Pediatric Craniopharyngioma. http://emedicine.medscape.com. 2014. Accessed August 8, 2014

33. Müller HL. Diagnostics, treatment, and follow-up in craniopharyngioma. Front Endocrinol (Lausanne) 2011;2:70

34. Yeung D, McKenzie C, Indelicato DJ. A dosimetric comparison of intensity-modulated proton therapy optimization techniques for pediatric craniopharyngiomas: a clinical case study. Pediatr Blood Cancer 2014;61:89–94

35. **Koutourousiou M, Gardner PA, Fernandez-Miranda JC, Tyler-Kabara EC, Wang EW, Snyderman CH. Endoscopic endonasal surgery for craniopharyngiomas: surgical outcome in 64 patients. J Neurosurg 2013;119:1194–1207**

36. Müller HL. Childhood craniopharyngioma: treatment strategies and outcomes. Expert Rev Neurother 2014;14:187–197

37. Borba LA, Al-Mefty O, Mrak RE, Suen J. Cranial chordomas in children and adolescents. J Neurosurg 1996;84:584–591

38. Crockard A, Macaulay E, Plowman PN. Stereotactic radiosurgery. VI. Posterior displacement of the brainstem facilitates safer high dose radiosurgery for clival chordoma. Br J Neurosurg 1999;13:65–70

39. al-Mefty O, Borba LA. Skull base chordomas: a management challenge. J Neurosurg 1997;86:182–189

40. Catton C, O'Sullivan B, Bell R, et al. Chordoma: long-term follow-up after radical photon irradiation. Radiother Oncol 1996;41:67–72

41. Austin-Seymour M, Munzenrider J, Goitein M, et al. Fractionated proton radiation therapy of chordoma and low-grade chondrosarcoma of the base of the skull. J Neurosurg 1989;70:13–17

42. Hoch BL, Nielsen GP, Liebsch NJ, Rosenberg AE. Base of skull chordomas in children and adolescents: a clinicopathologic study of 73 cases. Am J Surg Pathol 2006;30:811–818

43. Arivazhagan A, Devi BI, Kolluri SV, Abraham RG, Sampath S, Chandramouli BA. Pediatric intracranial meningiomas—do they differ from their counterparts in adults? Pediatr Neurosurg 2008;44:43–48

44. Fuchs HE, Tomita T. Neurocutaneous syndromes and meningiomas of childhood. In: McLone DG, Marlin AE, Scott RM, et al, eds. Pediatric Neurosurgery. Surgery of the developing Nervous System. Philadelphia: Saunders; 2001:778–779

45. Lakhdar F, Arkha Y, El Ouahabi A, et al. Intracranial meningioma in children: different from adult forms? A series of 21 cases. Neurochirurgie 2010;56:309–314

46. Kotecha RS, Pascoe EM, Rushing EJ, et al. Meningiomas in children and adolescents: a meta-analysis of individual patient data. Lancet Oncol 2011;12:1229–1239

47. **Allcutt DA, Hoffman HJ, Isla A, Becker LE, Humphreys RP. Acoustic schwannomas in children. Neurosurgery 1991;29:14–18**

48. Rushworth RG, Sorby WA, Smith SF. Acoustic neuroma in a child treated with the aid of preoperative arterial embolization. Case report. J Neurosurg 1984;61:396–398

49. Kondziolka D, Lunsford LD, Flickinger JC. Stereotactic radiosurgery in children and adolescents. Pediatr Neurosurg 1990-1991;1991;16:219–221

50. Tos M. A new pathogenesis of mesotympanic (congenital) cholesteatoma. Laryngoscope 2000;110:1890–1897

51. Bluestone C, Klein J. Intratemporal complications and sequelae of otitis media. In: Bluestone C, Stool S, Kenna M, eds. Pediatric Otolaryngology. Philadelphia: WB Saunders; 1996:604–635

52. Forsen J. Chronic disorders of the middle ear and mastoid. In: Wetmore R, Muntz H, McGill T, eds. Pediatric Otolaryngology: Principles and Practice Pathways. New York: Thieme; 2000:293–303

53. Thomassin JM, Braccini F. [Role of imaging and endoscopy in the follow up and management of cholesteatomas operated by closed technique]. Rev Laryngol Otol Rhinol (Bord) 1999;120:75–81

54. Rosenfeld RM, Moura RL, Bluestone CD. Predictors of residual-recurrent cholesteatoma in children. Arch Otolaryngol Head Neck Surg 1992;118:384–391

55. Tsai EC, Santoreneos S, Rutka JT. Tumors of the skull base in children: review of tumor types and management strategies. Neurosurg Focus 2002;12:e1

56. Buchanan EP, Xue AS, Hollier LH Jr. Craniofacial syndromes. Plast Reconstr Surg 2014;134:128e–153e

57. Carneiro GVS, Farias JG, Santos FA, Lamberti PL. Apert syndrome: review and report a case. Braz J Otorhinolaryngol 2008;74:640

58. Tewfik TL. Manifestations of craniofacial syndromes. http://emedicine.medscape.com. 2013. Accessed August 8, 2014

59. Aleck K. Craniosynostosis syndromes in the genomic era. Semin Pediatr Neurol 2004; 11:256–261

60. Meyers GA, Orlow SJ, Munro IR, Przylepa KA, Jabs EW. Fibroblast growth factor receptor 3 (FGFR3) transmembrane mutation in Crouzon syndrome with acanthosis nigricans. Nat Genet 1995;11:462–464

61. Kirmi O, Lo SJ, Johnson D, Anslow P. Craniosynostosis: a radiological and surgical perspective. Semin Ultrasound CT MR 2009;30:492–512

62. Tandon YK, Rubin M, Kahlifa M, Doumit G, Naffaa L; TandonY K. Bilateral squamosal suture synostosis: a rare form of isolated craniosynostosis in Crouzon syndrome. World J Radiol 2014;6:507–510

63. Agochukwu NB, Solomon BD, Muenke M. Impact of genetics on the diagnosis and clinical management of syndromic craniosynostoses. Childs Nerv Syst 2012;28:1447–1463

64. Mitsukawa N, Kaneko T, Saiga A, Akita S, Satoh K. Early midfacial distraction for syndromic craniosynostotic patients with obstructive sleep apnoea. J Plast Reconstr Aesthet Surg 2013;66:1206–1211

65. Singh A, Goyal M, Kumar S, Kress W, Kapoor S. Phenotypic variability in two families of Muenke syndrome with FGFR3 mutation. Indian J Pediatr 2014;81:1230–1232

66. Perheentupa U, Kinnunen I, Grénman R, Aitasalo K, Mäkitie AA. Management and outcome of pediatric skull base fractures. Int J Pediatr Otorhinolaryngol 2010;74: 1245–1250

67. Caviness AC. Skull fractures in children, Uptodate. New York: Wolters Kluwer; 2014

68. Ono H, Uchida M, Tanaka Y, Tanaka K, Hashimoto T. Traumatic longitudinal clival fracture in a child—case report. Neurol Med Chir (Tokyo) 2011;51:707–710

69. Clauser L, Dallera V, Sarti E, Tieghi R. Frontobasilar fractures in children. Childs Nerv Syst 2004;20:168–175

70. Brockmeyer D, Gruber DP, Haller J, Shelton C, Walker ML. Pediatric skull base surgery. 2. Experience and outcomes in 55 patients. Pediatr Neurosurg 2003;38: 9–15

71. Alfieri A, Jho HD. Endoscopic endonasal cavernous sinus surgery: surgical approaches. Neurosurgery 2001;49:354–362

72. Alfieri A, Jho HD, Tschabitscher M. Endoscopic endonasal approach to the ventral cranio-cervical junction: anatomical study. Acta Neurochir (Wien) 2002;144:219–225, discussion 225

73. Alfieri A, Jho HD, Schettino R, Tschabitscher M. Endoscopic endonasal approach to the pterygopalatine fossa: anatomic study. Neurosurgery 2003;52:374–378, discussion 378–380

74. Alfieri A, Moreau JJ. Abord endoscopique endonasal de la base du crâne. Neurochirurgie 2003;49:457–458

75. de Divitiis E, Cappabianca P, Gangemi M, Cavallo LM. The role of the endoscopic trans-sphenoidal approach in pediatric neurosurgery. Childs Nerv Syst 2000;16:692–696

76. de Divitiis E, Cavallo LM, Esposito F, Stella L, Messina A. Extended endoscopic trans-sphenoidal approach for tuberculum sellae meningiomas. Neurosurgery 2008;62(6, Suppl 3):1192–1201

77. Komatsu F, Komatsu M, Di Ieva A, Tschabitscher M. Endoscopic approaches to the trigeminal nerve and clinical consideration for trigeminal schwannomas: a cadaveric study. J Neurosurg 2012;117:690–696

78. Komatsu F, Komatsu M, Di Ieva A, Tschabitscher M. Endoscopic extradural subtemporal approach to lateral and central skull base: a cadaveric study. World Neurosurg 2013;80:591–597

79. Komatsu F, Komatsu M, Di Ieva A, Tschabitscher M. Endoscopic far-lateral approach to the posterolateral craniovertebral junction: an anatomical study. Neurosurg Rev 2013;36:239–247, discussion 247

80. Jho HD, Ha HG. Endoscopic endonasal skull base surgery: Part 1—The midline anterior fossa skull base. Minim Invasive Neurosurg 2004;47:1–8

81. Jho HD, Ha HG. Endoscopic endonasal skull base surgery: Part 3—The clivus and posterior fossa. Minim Invasive Neurosurg 2004;47:16–23

82. Frank G, Pasquini E. Endoscopic endonasal cavernous sinus surgery, with special reference to pituitary adenomas. Front Horm Res 2006;34:64–82

83. Lang DA, Neil-Dwyer G, Evans BT, Honeybul S. Craniofacial access in children. Acta Neurochir (Wien) 1998;140:33–40

84. Hayhurst C, Williams D, Yousaf J, Richardson D, Pizer B, Mallucci C. Skull base surgery for tumors in children: long-term clinical and functional outcome. J Neurosurg Pediatr 2013;11:496–503

85. Gil Z, Constantini S, Spektor S, et al. Skull base approaches in the pediatric population. Head Neck 2005;27:682–689

37 Congenital Encephaloceles

■ General Principles

- Encephaloceles refers to a herniation of brain tissue, which protrudes through a defect in the skull base and maintains a connection to the subarachnoid space.[1]
- They can broadly be classified as either primary or secondary:
  - Primary encephaloceles **(Table 37.1)** are congenital and are present at birth. They are a type of neural tube defect and can occur in isolation or with other syndromes, resulting from the failure of separation from the surface ectoderm and the neuroectoderm.
  - Secondary encephaloceles are more common and can be a result of trauma (accidental or iatrogenic), infection, tumor related, or possibly secondary to elevated intracranial pressures (i.e., spontaneous).[3] Frequently associated with cerebrospinal fluid (CSF) fistula (see Chapter 32).
- By definition, cephalocele refers to the sac-like protrusion of cranial contents through a defect in the skull base/cranium.
  - An encephalocele contains brain tissue alone.
  - A meningoencephalocele contains brain tissue and meninges.
  - A meningocele contains only meninges.

> **Surgical Anatomy Pearl**
>
> Treatment of encephaloceles requires an intimate understanding of both skull base embryology and anatomy (see Chapter 2 and Chapter 4).

■ Epidemiology

- Incidence: 0.8 to 5 per 10,000 live births.[4,5] Males and females are equally affected. Occipital encephaloceles are most frequent in North America and Western Europe,[6] and sincipital and basal encephaloceles are more frequent

Table 37.1   Classification of Primary Encephaloceles Based on Location and Anatomic Defect

Location	Type (Congenital)	Cranial Defect Location
Anterior cranial fossa	Sincipital	At the junction of the frontal and ethmoid bones
	Basal	At the junction of the sphenoid and ethmoid bones
Posterior cranial fossa	Occipital	Between the lambda and the foramen magnum
Middle cranial fossa	Temporal lobe	Can involve defects of the temporal, parietal, and sphenoid bones

Source: Adapted from David DJ, Proudman TW. Cephaloceles: classification, pathology, and management. World J Surg 1989;13:349–357. Reprinted with permission.

in Southeast Asia, Russia, and central Africa (incidence of 1 in 3,500 to 1 in 5,000 live births).[7]
- Isolated encephaloceles are generally not familial.

■ Clinical Features

Occipital Encephaloceles[2,8]

- Present at birth.
- May be diagnosed prenatally by ultrasound.
- Neural tissue is covered with skin.
- Neural tissue can involve nonfunctioning gliotic tissue, cerebral tissue, or cerebellar tissue.
- Can have cranial nerve defects, developmental delay, blindness, seizures.
- Neurologic symptoms often related to degree of cerebral or cerebellar dysplasia.
- May be progressive if hydrocephalus develops after birth.
- May be associated with Chiari malformations or other syndromes (e.g., Meckel-Gruber syndrome).[9]

Sincipital Encephaloceles[10]

- Are typically visible on the face.
- Can range from small occult lesions to large pulsatile masses with significant facial deformity.

- They can be classified according to the exit point on the face[11]: interfrontal, nasofrontal, nasoethmoidal, naso-orbital.
- Unlike dermoids and gliomas, sincipital encephaloceles on the face are pulsatile because of their connection to the subarachnoid space.

Basal Encephaloceles[2,10]

- Because of their location at the base of the skull, basal encephaloceles may not have any external manifestations.
- Some patients may have a concurrent broad nasal bridge or other midfacial anomalies.
- Frequently presents as nasal obstruction, CSF rhinorrhea, or recurrent meningitis. They may not become apparent until later in life.
- Have been classified based on their anatomic location along the skull base[12]: transethmoidal, sphenoethmoidal, spheno-orbital, sphenomaxillary, transsphenoidal.

Temporal Lobe Encephaloceles

- Can be further classified based on location[13] (**Table 37.2**):
  - Congenital temporal encephaloceles are present at birth but may not have significant clinical symptoms until adulthood.[14]
  - Diagnosis is challenging, as symptoms may be nonspecific and can include otorrhea, recurrent ear infections, conductive hearing loss, and recurrent meningitis.[15]
  - Occasionally, the associated CSF leak may present as clear rhinorrhea, as the CSF flows into the nasal cavity via the eustachian tube.
  - Medically refractory temporal lobe epilepsy has been associated with temporal encephaloceles.[16]

Table 37.2   Types of Temporal Lobe Encephaloceles Based on the Location

Location of the Temporal Lobe Encephalocele	Involvement
Temporal	
• Lateral	Pterion/asterion/cranial vault
• Anteroinferior/transalar	Anteroinferior portion of middle fossa
• Posteroinferior	Tegmen tympani
Sphenoidal	
• Spheno-orbital/posterior-orbital	Sphenoid wing
• Anteromedial	Anteromedial portion of the middle fossa

- ○ Temporal lobe encephaloceles involving the sphenoid sinus may not present until adulthood with CSF rhinorrhea or recurrent meningitis.
- ○ Association between bony defects and formation of temporal encephaloceles is unclear. The incidence of middle fossa/tegmen skull base defects found in pathologic specimens with no history of infection/surgery to this region ranges from 21 to 31%, which is much higher than the incidence of congenital temporal encephaloceles.[17]

■ Investigations

Imaging

If an encephalocele is suspected, a comprehensive neuroimaging workup is mandatory. This includes a high-resolution computed tomography (CT) of the skull base and facial bones to assess any bony defects and a magnetic resonance imaging (MRI) to evaluate the contents of the encephalocele as well as any associated cranial abnormalities (e.g., microcephaly, hydrocephalus). If extensive facial deformity exists, three-dimensional reconstruction of the facial bones is useful for planning the reconstructive surgery.

Prenatal Imaging

With the advancements in prenatal imaging, ultrasound can detect approximately 80% of congenital encephaloceles. Findings include a cystic or solid mass contiguous with the brain through a defect in the skull.[18] Prenatal MRI has an even higher sensitivity for detecting encephaloceles and can be used where the diagnosis is uncertain.

Cerebrospinal Fluid Rhinorrhea

For basal encephaloceles, nasal obstruction may not be readily apparent in a newborn. However, unexplained clear rhinorrhea should be tested for β_2-transferrin to confirm the presence or absence of CSF.

■ Treatment

The general goals of treatment of encephaloceles are removal of the herniated brain tissue and closure of the dural and skull base defect to prevent further complications. Because of the varied location of the encephaloceles, the specific surgical options are described below.

Occipital Encephaloceles

Surgical management depends on the neural tissue that occupies the herniated sac. This may be ascertained with preoperative MRI, but often requires intra-operative assessment. Gliotic tissue can be removed safely and the skull base defect is closed. If normal brain is present within the sac, attempts are made to preserve the neural elements.

Surgical options include the following:

- Expansion cranioplasty using titanium mesh.[19]
- Ventricular volume reduction (two-stage procedure)[20]:
  - First stage: The dural sac is closed to increase ventricular pressure and create hydrocephalus.
  - Second stage: As ventriculomegaly develops, a ventriculoperitoneal shunt is placed to reduce the ventricles size.
- The additional intracranial space can now accommodate the herniated brain tissue.
- The tentorium can be divided to create infratentorial space for the herniated brain tissue.[21]

Sincipital Encephaloceles

Because of their involvement with the facial skeleton, sincipital encephaloceles require a multidisciplinary team composed of a neurosurgeon, a craniofacial surgeon, and an otolaryngologist. Sincipital encephaloceles are treated early in infancy because of their association with facial deformity and the deformity's impact on social and skeletal development. Surgical approaches to these kinds of encephaloceles often include a coronal incision, bifrontal craniotomy, and bilateral orbitotomy.[6] These components may be combined with transfacial approaches (e.g., lateral rhinotomy or midfacial degloving), depending on the exit point of the encephalocele. Once the encephalocele is resected or reduced to the bony defect, a watertight duraplasty is performed. Therefore, craniofacial surgeons and otolaryngologists repair any associated facial defects. Orbital trans-location may be required for cases with hypertelorism.

- Temporal lobe encephaloceles[13]: Treatment is recommended for symptomatic temporal encephaloceles. The approach depends on the location of the defect in the middle cranial fossa and may involve either intra- or extracranial routes.
  - Intracranial routes involve frontotemporal or temporal craniotomies to adequately visualize and repair the skull base defect (can be combined with zygomatic osteotomy). The encephalocele is typically amputated at the bony defect. The osseous defect is then repaired and duraplasty is performed.

- ○ Extracranial approaches can include the following:
  - ▪ Transfacial approaches (e.g., lateral rhinotomy or midfacial degloving) for anteromedial and anteroinferior encephaloceles. Transfacial approaches are discussed elsewhere (see Chapter 15).
  - ▪ Transmastoid approaches for posteroinferior encephaloceles (i.e., involving the tegmen).
  - ○ Can be combined with a subtemporal craniotomy
  - ○ Endonasal approaches for middle fossa anteromedial encephaloceles extending into the sphenoid sinus (see transpterygoid approaches on page 428)

Basal Encephaloceles

If associated with a CSF leak, basal encephaloceles require urgent treatment because of the ongoing risks of ascending meningitis. Traditionally, open transfacial approaches to the anterior skull base were used (see Chapter 15), particularly in the pediatric population.[6] They can be combined with a bifrontal craniotomy (i.e., anterior craniofacial approach) to provide excellent exposure to the skull base and paranasal sinuses. Although there have been concerns regarding facial growth disturbances with these approaches, many studies have reported no changes in facial development.[22]

- With the advent of endoscopic approaches, many basal encephaloceles can now be approached and treated successfully via a purely endonasal approach[23] (see Chapter 16). The limiting factor is often the anatomic size of the paranasal sinuses relative to the endoscopic equipment and the degree of sinus pneumatization (particularly the sphenoid sinus).

■ References

Boldfaced references are of particular importance.
1. **Di Ieva A, Bruner E, Haider T, et al. Skull base embryology: a multidisciplinary review. Childs Nerv Syst 2014;30:991–1000**
2. **David DJ, Proudman TW. Cephaloceles: classification, pathology, and management. World J Surg 1989;13:349–357**
3. Woodworth BA, Bolger WE, Schlosser RJ. Nasal cerebrospinal fluid leaks and encephaloceles. Oper Tech Otolaryngol 2006; 17(2):111–116.
4. Stevenson RE, Allen WP, Pai GS, et al. Decline in prevalence of neural tube defects in a high-risk region of the United States. Pediatrics 2000;106:677–683
5. Siffel C, Wong LY, Olney RS, Correa A. Survival of infants diagnosed with encephalocele in Atlanta, 1979-98. Paediatr Perinat Epidemiol 2003;17:40–48
6. **Tsai EC, Santoreneos S, Rutka JT. Tumors of the skull base in children: review of tumor types and management strategies. Neurosurg Focus 2002;12:e1**

7. Suwanwela C. Geographic distribution of fronto-ethmoidal encephalomeningocele. Br J Prev Soc Med 1972;26:193–198
8. Simpson DA, David DJ, White J. Cephaloceles: treatment, outcome, and antenatal diagnosis. Neurosurgery 1984;15:14–21
9. Agrawal A, Lakhkar BB, Lakhkar B, Grover A. Giant occipital encephalocele associated with microcephaly and micrognathia. Pediatr Neurosurg 2008;44:515–516
10. **David DJ. Cephaloceles: classification, pathology, and management—a review. J Craniofac Surg 1993;4:192–202**
11. Suwanwela C, Suwanwela N. A morphological classification of sincipital encephalomeningoceles. J Neurosurg 1972;36:201–211
12. Gerhardt HJ, Mühler G, Szdzuy D, Biedermann F. [Therapy problems in sphenoethmoidal meningoceles]. Zentralbl Neurochir 1979;40:85–94
13. Wind JJ, Caputy AJ, Roberti F. Spontaneous encephaloceles of the temporal lobe. Neurosurg Focus 2008;25:E11
14. Mulcahy MM, McMenomey SO, Talbot JM, Delashaw JB Jr. Congenital encephalocele of the medial skull base. Laryngoscope 1997;107:910–914
15. Kamerer DB, Caparosa RJ. Temporal bone encephalocele—diagnosis and treatment. Laryngoscope 1982;92(8 Pt 1):878–882
16. Mayeno JK, Korol HW, Nutik SL. Spontaneous meningoencephalic herniation of the temporal bone: case series with recommended treatment. Otolaryngol Head Neck Surg 2004;130:486–489
17. Kapur TR, Bangash W. Tegmental and petromastoid defects in the temporal bone. J Laryngol Otol 1986;100:1129–1132
18. Graham D, Johnson TR Jr, Winn K, Sanders RC. The role of sonography in the prenatal diagnosis and management of encephalocele. J Ultrasound Med 1982;1:111–115
19. Gallo AE Jr. Repair of giant occipital encephaloceles with microcephaly secondary to massive brain herniation. Childs Nerv Syst 1992;8:229–230
20. Oi S, Saito M, Tamaki N, Matsumoto S. Ventricular volume reduction technique—a new surgical concept for the intracranial transposition of encephalocele. Neurosurgery 1994;34:443–447, discussion 448
21. Bozinov O, Tirakotai W, Sure U, Bertalanffy H. Surgical closure and reconstruction of a large occipital encephalocele without parenchymal excision. Childs Nerv Syst 2005;21:144–147
22. **Teo C, Dornhoffer J, Hanna E, Bower C. Application of skull base techniques to pediatric neurosurgery. Childs Nerv Syst 1999;15:103–109**
23. Woodworth BA, Schlosser RJ, Faust RA, Bolger WE. Evolutions in the management of congenital intranasal skull base defects. Arch Otolaryngol Head Neck Surg 2004;130:1283–1288

38 Biology and Genetics of Skull Base Tumors

This chapter summarizes our current knowledge of the cell biology and genetics of common skull base tumors, including aspects of stem cell biology, genetics, epigenetics, proteomics, receptor signaling, cell cycle and cell death pathways, predictors of aggressive biological behavior, and associations.

■ Cartilaginous Tumors

Chondroblastoma

Stem Cell Biology

Lactoferrin expression is shared with fetal chondroblasts and osteoblasts.[1]

Genetics

These tumors have no recurrent chromosomal aberrations or *IDH1* mutations.[2]

Proteomics

These tumors demonstrate Sox9 transcription factor expression. Sox9 is involved in signaling differentiation from chondrogenic mesenchymal cells to early chondroblasts.[3]

Receptor Signaling

Growth plate signaling involves Indian hedgehog and parathyroid hormone–related protein (IHH/PThrP) and fibroblast growth factor (FGF) pathways.[4]
Sex-hormone receptor signaling is also present.[5]

- Diffuse expression of SRD5A1, an enzyme that catalyzes the conversion of testosterone to dihydrotestosterone. Diffuse expression of CYP19, converts testosterone to estrogen. Diffuse expression of ESR1 (estrogen receptor alpha). Low/absent expression of CA-RP X (carbonic anhydrase protein X).

Biological Predictors

Malignant transformation to chondrosarcoma can occur after radiotherapy, and therefore radiation should be avoided in this tumor.[6]

Association

This tumor shares similar histological and molecular features with chondromyxoid fibroma.

Enchondroma

Stem Cell Biology

Liver kinase b1 (Lkb1)-dependent inhibition of mammalian target of rapamycin (mTOR) C1 regulates the transition from mitotic chondrocytes to mature post-mitotic chondrocytes. Loss of Lkb1 function results in enchondroma-like masses in mice, and this phenotype can be reversed with the mTOR C1 inhibitor.[7]

Genetics

Seventy-one percent of patients with this tumor harbor the *IDH1* mutation (R132C is the most frequent).[8] The *IHD2* mutation is also observed, but is infrequent (2% in Ollier disease and Maffucci syndrome patients).

In one study, the R150C mutation in the parathyroid hormone receptor 1 *(PTHR1)* gene was found in two of six patients with Ollier disease and was shown to be pathogenic for chondromas in mice by slowing chondrocyte differentiation.[9]

Epigenetics

The epigenetics of this tumor are evident as hypermethylation.[10]

Proteomics

Expression of IDH1 R132H mutant protein shows intraneoplastic mosaicism.[10] Overexpression of the Gli2 transcription factor is sufficient to cause enchondroma-like lesions in mice.[9]

Biological Predictors

Among patients with multiple enchondromas (Maffucci and Ollier disease), there is a 44–50% risk of developing chondrosarcoma when the enchondromas are located in the axial skeleton.[11]

Association

Ollier disease is associated with multiple enchondromas. Maffucci syndrome is associated with multiple enchondromas and subcutaneous spindle cell hemangiomas.

Ollier disease and Maffucci syndrome are also associated with somatic mosaic mutations in *IDH1* and *IDH2*.[12]

Chondrosarcoma

Stem Cell Biology

Chondrosarcoma types recapitulate the cellular phenotypic heterogeneity found during fetal chondrogenesis, suggesting that the most likely origin of the neoplastic cell is multipotent mesenchymal cells.[13] Expression of mutant *IDH2* in murine mesenchymal progenitor cells generates undifferentiated sarcomas in vivo.[14]

Genetics

Forty-six percent to 59% of patients carry the *IDH1/2* mutations, with the *IDH1* R132C mutation occurring most frequently.[15,16] The alpha chain of type II collagen, the major cartilage collagen, is encoded by the *COL2A1* gene. Mutations that affect the coding sequence of *COL2A1* are found in 44% of chondrosarcomas. These mutations are predicted to affect the collagen maturation process and may therefore impair chondrocyte differentiation.[16] COL2A1 gene mutations are more frequent in higher grade chondrosarcoma.[16]

Epigenetics

Tumors with the *IDH* mutation show C–phosphate–G (CpG) island hypermethylation in regions containing genes involved in stem cell differentiation and lineage specification.[14]

Proteomics

Chondrosarcoma expresses Sox9, a transcription factor that regulates the synthesis of type II collagen.[17]

Receptor Signaling

The IHH signaling pathway is affected in 18% of cases.[16]

Cell-Cycle Pathways

Six to nine percent of high-grade chondrosarcomas harbor alterations in the retinoblastoma protein (pRb) tumor suppressor signaling pathway involving decreased CDKN2A expression, increased CDK4 expression, and/or expression of cyclin D1.[18] A subset of high-grade tumors shows inactivation of wild-type p53 by mouse double-minute 2-homologue (MDM2) overexpression.[18]

Cell-Death Pathways

Expression of antiapoptotic proteins (Bcl-2, Bcl-xL, XIAP) confers radio- and chemoresistance.[19,20]

Biological Predictors

Leukemia/lymphoma-related factor (LRF) expression is a survival factor for chondrosarcoma cells and correlates with malignancy and chemoresistance.[21] High expression of hypoxia inducible factor 2α and low expression of Beclin-1 are associated with poor overall survival.[22]

Association

Chondrosarcoma can arise from enchondroma.

■ Noncartilaginous Tumors

Osteosarcoma

Stem Cell Biology

Genes under the transcriptional control of the transcription factor activator protein 1 (AP-1) regulate chondroblast/osteoblast growth. The components of the AP-1 heterodimer are c-Jun and c-Fos which are overexpressed in osteosarcomas and chondrosarcomas.[23] Interaction of runt-related transcription factor 2 (RUNX2) with p27, which is required for osteoblast differentiation, is disrupted in osteosarcoma.

Genetics

Genomic instability is present, possibly due to chromothripsis.[24] A gain of chromosome 6p, 8q, and 17p is seen.[24] Up to 50% of patients harbor a *p53* gene alteration (allelic loss, point mutation, gene rearrangement).[25] *Rb1* gene alterations occur in 70% of cases.

Proteomics

Osteosarcoma expresses vascular endothelial growth factor (VEGF).[26]
   The absence of biglycan expression may contribute to defective mineralization of collagen fibrils.[27]

Receptor Signaling

The hepatocyte growth factor receptor (MET) is overexpressed and is associated with tumor progression.

Cell-Cycle Pathways

Increased CDK4 expression is seen, as are CDKN2A mutations and gene methylation.[28]

Biological Predictors

- High survivin expression correlates with the presence of metastasis and with poor survival.[29] High expression of *CCN3* gene correlates with a worse prognosis.[30]
- Polymorphisms in nucleotide excision repair genes may predict the response to cisplatin therapy.[31]

Association

- Osteosarcoma is associated with previous radiation, Paget's disease, fibrous dysplasia, and chronic osteomyelitis.
- Hereditary retinoblastoma patients have a 1,000-fold higher risk of osteosarcoma as compared with the general population.

Chordoma

Stem Cell Biology

Chordomas are characterized by expression of brachyury (T-gene), a transcription factor expressed in the developing notochord.[32] Chordoma cells lose stem-cell marker expression and can differentiate along an osteogenic lineage when exposed to all-*trans*-retinoic acid.[33] It is thought that chordoma arises from the embryonic notochord cell remnant in the vertebral body or nucleus pulposus. However, a chordoma cell of origin has not been proven, and it is important to note that benign notochordal cell tumors do not transform into chordoma.[34]

Genetics

Most skull base chordomas have normal karyotypes (74%). Abnormal karyotypes are observed in 75% of recurrent tumors, involving chromosome 3 or 13 in most cases.[35] Chromosomal alterations resulting in gain of the T-gene locus are found in at least 50% of sporadic chordomas.[36] T-gene (Chr 6) duplication is associated with familial chordoma.[37] Other familial susceptibility loci have been mapped to 1p36 and 7q33.[38] CDKN2A/2B gene loss is a feature of 70% of sacral chordomas but only 22% of skull base chordomas.[39,40] No *IDH1/2* mutations are present in chordoma.[15]

Epigenetics

Hypermethylation of three known tumor suppressor genes *(RASSF1, KL, HIC1)* has been described in a series of 10 chordomas.[41]

Proteomics

Expression levels of brachyury are the same whether the T-gene encoding brachyury is amplified or not[36]; 94% of chordomas express at least one type of FGF receptor.[42] Fragile histidine triad protein (FHIT) tumor suppressor (Chr3) expression is lost in 98% of sacral and 67% of clival chordomas.[40]

Receptor Signaling

Increases in copy number of the epidermal growth factor receptor (EGFR) gene are observed in 40% of chordomas.[43] Receptor tyrosine kinases located on the cell membrane are triggered by specific ligands involved in paracrine and autocrine growth signaling. Chordoma cells express platelet-derived growth factor receptors (PDGFR) α and β, epidermal growth factor receptor, human epidermal growth factor receptor 2 (HER2), KIT, and c-MET.[44]

Cell-Death Pathways

Chordomas express anti-apoptotic proteins Bcl-xL and MCL1.[45]

Cell-Cycle Pathways

T-gene expression is required for chordoma cell proliferation in vitro.[36] Decreased expression of micro-RNA (miRNA) 1 and associated overexpression of its target genes c-MET and histone deacetylase 4 (HDAC4) is observed in chordoma. Reintroduction of miRNA 1 into chordoma cells reduces cell proliferation.[46]

Biological Predictors

No biological predictors of chordomas have been identified yet.

Association

Chordomas arising in patients with tuberous sclerosis have been reported.[47]

Head and Neck Paraganglioma

Stem Cell Biology

Paraganglioma cells express neural stem cell markers (Nestin and CD33) as well as lineage-specific markers of differentiated cells of neural stem cell origin. Norepinephrine- or dopamine-secreting tumors show high expression of hypoxia-inducible factor 2α (HIF2α). Cells expressing high HIF2α levels show a less mature chromaffin cell developmental phenotype. This fact implicates HIF2α activation as an early event in tumor development, maintaining an undifferentiated phenotype in paragangliomas with loss of function mutations in von Hippel–Landau (VHL) disease or succinate dehydrogenase genes.[48]

Genetics

Hereditary tumors with germline mutation occur in 35% of patients, and sporadic tumors are found in 65%. Among sporadic tumors, 14% cluster with transcriptional profiles similar to those of tumors with germline mutations[49]; 54% of head and neck paragangliomas harbor a germline mutation in one of the succinate dehydrogenase genes (*SDHx*).[50] *IDH* mutations are extremely rare (< 1%).[51] Genes involved in the hypoxia-angiogenesis pathway are overexpressed in paragangliomas associated with von Hippel–Landau *(VHL)* or *SDHx* gene mutations.[48] Head and neck paragangliomas also have *VHL* or *SDH AF2/B/C/D* mutations. Only one patient with multiple head and neck paragangliomas has shown a *TMEM127* mutation. *RET, NF1,* or *MAX* mutations are not seen in head and neck paragangliomas, but are found in paragangliomas at other sites.[52] The risk of malignant paraganglioma varies according to mutation type as follows, in order of decreasing risk: *SDHB* (66–83%), *SDHD* (< 5%), *VHL* (3%), *SDHC* (< 2%), and *TMEM127*.[53] *SDHD*-linked paragangliomas are associated with loss of the maternally imprinted chromosome 11.[49]

Epigenetics

Accumulation of succinate in SDHx mutant tumors inhibits histone demethylases, resulting in increased histone H3 methylation.[54]

Proteomics

SDHx- and VHL-related tumors do not produce epinephrine because they lack PNMT. VHL-related tumors produce norepinephrine, whereas SDHx tumors produce dopamine and its O-methylated metabolite methoxytyramine.[55]

Biological Predictors

Recurrences are associated with the presence of germline mutations.[56]

Association

Paragangliomas are associated with VHL disease arising from *VHL* gene germline mutation. Familial paragangliomas are associated with autosomal dominant germline mutations, as follows:

- PGL-1: *SDHD* gene on chromosome 11q23
- PGL-2: *SDHAF2* gene on chromosome 11q13
- PGL-3: *SDHC* gene on chromosome 1q21
- PGL-4: *SDHB* gene on chromosome 1p36

The Carney triad is a very rare condition with gastrointestinal stromal tumor, pulmonary chondroma, and extra-adrenal paragangliomas.

Esthesioneuroblastoma

Stem Cell Biology

Tumor cells express the human homologue of the Drosophila achaete-scute gene (HASH1) that is a marker of immature olfactory neurons.[57] Expression of neuroendocrine granules, chromogranins, neurofilament proteins, and synaptophysin point to a neural crest cell origin.[58–60]

Genetics

Complex chromosomal aberrations and copy number changes over the entire genome are found in esthesioneuroblastoma. These tumors also exhibit copy number changes shared with carcinomas such as 7q11.2 gain, chr 2 losses, and 6q21-22 loss.[61] Aneuploidy is associated with higher Kadish stage.[61]

Epigenetics

The epigenetics of esthesioneuroblastoma are unknown.

Receptor Signaling

Marked Trk-A and Trk-B neurotrophin receptor expression is frequent (90%).[62] Sonic hedgehog receptor PTCH1 as well as downstream signaling molecules Gli1 and Gli2 are upregulated in esthesioneuroblastoma.[63]

Cell-Cycle Pathways

Maintenance of the cell-cycle in esthesioneuroblastoma cells requires sonic hedgehog signaling.[63]

Cell-Death Pathways

About 70% of tumors show expression of the antiapoptotic factor Bcl-2.[64] Bcl-2 expression increases with histopathological grade.[65]

Biological Predictors

Tumors with lower Hyams grade histopathology have a lower recurrence rate and longer overall and disease-free survival.[66]

Associations

None.

Schwannoma

Stem Cell Biology

Ligand-mediated activation of EGFR and PDGFR results in enhanced expression of stem-cell genes in vestibular schwannoma cells.[67] Loss of Merlin (*NF2* gene) expression results in increased expression of CD44 and Nestin stem cell markers in human Schwann cells.[68]

Genetics

It has been found that 88% of sporadic schwannomas harbor a mutation in the *NF2* gene (located on chromosome 22q12.2).[69] Schwannomas are a feature of three autosomal dominant inherited syndromes: neurofibromatosis type 2, schwannomatosis, and Carney complex type 1 (see Associations, below). Inactivation of the *NF2* tumor suppressor gene follows the Knudson's two-hit hypothesis, whereby germline mutation of the gene locus on one allele combines with somatic loss of heterozygosity or subsequent mutation of the wild-type allele, resulting in loss of function of the tumor suppressor.[70]

Receptor Signaling

The *NF2* gene encodes Merlin, which is a membrane protein that acts as a negative growth regulator. Merlin protein shares sequence similarity with the Ezrin-Radixin-Moesin family proteins that function to link the actin cytoskeleton to extracellular glycoproteins; 86% of sporadic schwannomas show reduced expression of Merlin protein, and lower expression is related to a higher growth index.[71]

Vestibular schwannomas express neuroregulin-1 (NRG1) and its receptors ERBB2 (Her2/neu) and ERBB3, which are involved in signaling proliferation of Schwann cells.[72–74]

Vestibular schwannoma cells also express VEGF receptor 1 and VEGF protein. Recurrent tumors are characterized by high VEGF expression.[75]

Cell-Death Pathways

Expression of antiapoptotic protein Bcl-2 is frequent in vestibular schwannomas (64%).[76] Schwannoma cells also express the antiapoptotic protein Survivin.[77]

Cell-Cycle Pathways

Merlin is a negative regulator of at least three key factors involved in signaling cell proliferation: Rac, Akt, and mTOR. Thus, loss of Merlin serves to release a cellular block on cell division.[78]

Biological Predictors

Some vestibular schwannomas may not respond to standard radiation doses due to the action of multiple radioresistance molecular pathways.[79]

Associations

Schwannoma is associated with neurofibromatosis type 2 (NF2). A germline mutation in *NF2* observed in 33 to 60% of patients with NF2. Mutations that result in a truncated protein produce a more severe clinical phenotype.[70]

- Carney complex type 1 is characterized by psammomatous melanotic schwannomas. These tumors show loss of heterozygosity in the gene encoding type 1A regulatory subunit of protein kinase A (*PRKAR1A*) on chromosome 17. *PRKAR1A* mutation in the remaining allele produces a nonfunctional protein, resulting in activation of protein kinase A, decreased expression of neurofibromin, and enhanced activation of Rac1. Protein kinase A phosphorylates Merlin at residue serine 518, which results in inactivation of Merlin function, a key feature in sporadic and NF2-related schwannomas.[78]

Meningioma

Stem Cell Biology

The inner part of the dura (dural border cells) and the outer part of the arachnoid (arachnoid barrier cells) derive from a common prostaglandin D-synthase (PGDS) expressing progenitor. Inactivation of *NF2* in the PTGDS-expressing common progenitor resulted in meningothelial (arachnoid barrier cell derived) or fibroblastic (dural border cell derived) meningiomas. Meningiomas only formed if *NF2* was inactivated in fetal or neonatal meninges.[80]

Genetics

The majority (> 60%) of meningiomas are monoclonal.[81] Typical meningiomas (World Health Organization [WHO] grade I) show a normal karyotype or loss of one chromosome 22 in all or some of the cells.[82] Loss of heterozygosity for chromosome 22 markers flanking the *NF2* gene is observed in 60% of sporadic meningiomas. The majority of these tumors carry an inactivating mutation in the remaining *NF2* gene.[83] *NF2* loss is most commonly observed in fibroblastic meningiomas.[84] Atypical or anaplastic meningiomas show loss of up to six further chromosomes in addition to chromosome 22 or partial/complete loss of the short arm of chromosome 1.[82]

Deletion of 1p36 (including the alkaline phosphatase gene *ALPL*) is found in 27% of typical meningiomas, 70% of atypical meningiomas, and 100% of anaplastic meningioma.[85] Suppressor of fused (SUFU) homologue is a negative regulator of sonic hedgehog signaling and important for control of stem cell differentiation in adults. Loss of SUFU due to frequent chromosome 10 long arm deletion is thought to contribute to meningioma development. This is supported by the observation that a SUFU loss of function germline mutation segregates with family members affected with meningioma in a family with five siblings affected with meningioma.[86] Mutation of the chromatin-remodeling gene *SMARCB1* has been observed in familial multiple meningioma.[87]

Epigenetics

Atypical and anaplastic meningiomas are associated with aberrant CpG island hypermethylation of multiple genes.[88] Tissue inhibitor of metalloproteinase 3 gene located on 22q12.3 is hypermethylated in meningiomas that have allelic loss of 22q12. Increased frequency of tissue inhibitor of metalloproteinase-3 (TIMP3) hypermethylation is observed in higher grade meningiomas (67% anaplastic, 22% atypical, 17% typical). Hypermethylation results in decreased TIMP3 expression levels. TIMP3 normally acts to inhibit matrix metalloproteinases, thereby blocking invasion and metastasis. TIMP3 also functions to induce apoptosis and suppression of tumor growth and angiogenesis.[88]

Receptor Signaling

Basic FGF, a potent mitogen for mesoderm-derived cells, is abundantly produced in meningiomas.[89] Activation of the WNT/beta-catenin, Notch, sonic hedgehog, phosphoinositide 3-kinase (PI3K)/Akt, and mitogen-activated protein kinase (MAPK) pathways is observed in meningiomas[83,90]; 72% of genes in the sonic hedgehog signaling pathway are differentially expressed in meningioma compared with normal tissue.[91]

Multiple autocrine ligand-receptor signaling pathways involved in growth response are upregulated in meningioma including PDGF BB and its receptor PDGFR-β. Transforming growth factor-α (TGF-α) and epidermal growth factor (EGF) and its receptor EGFR, stromal cell derived factor 1 and its receptor CXCR, as well as bone morphogenic protein and its receptors are also found.[90]

Cell-Cycle Pathways

Loss of cell-cycle regulatory factors encoded by *CDKN2A*, *CDKN2B*, and *ARF* takes place in the majority of anaplastic meningiomas.[83]

Biological Predictors

High expression of insulin-like growth factor II is associated with anaplastic histology and tumor invasiveness.[92] Radiation-induced meningiomas are more often atypical and show aggressive clinical features such as multiplicity, brain invasion, and recurrence.[93]

Associations

Meningiomas are seen in 50% of patients with NF2.[94] Meningiomas have also been reported in other inherited tumor syndromes including Cowden, Werner, Gorlin, Li- Fraumeni, Turcot, Gardener, VHL, and multiple endocrine neoplasia type I.[83]

- The risk of developing meningioma is increased with exposure to low- or high-dose radiation, and the latency period for development of the tumor is dependent on the dose and age at exposure.[93]

Hemangiopericytoma

Stem Cell Biology

Hemangiopericytoma is thought to derive from a mesenchymal progenitor that gives rise to pericytes and expresses prostaglandin D synthase.[95]

Genetics

Harbor translocations and inversions are seen on chromosome 12.[96] Hemangiopericytoma shares the same fusion gene as peripheral solitary fibrous tumors (*NAB2–STAT6* fusion). The presence of this fusion gene can be obtained indirectly by immunohistochemistry for *STAT6*, which will show nuclear localization in tumors with *NAB2-STAT6* fusion.[97]

Proteomics

Hemangiopericytoma expresses vimentin and β and γ actin.[98]

Cell-Cycle Pathways

Loss of p16 expression due to homozygous deletion of the *CDKN2A* gene is observed in 25% of tumors.[99]

Biological Predictors

Ki-67 staining is > 15% in anaplastic hemangiopericytoma.[100]

Pituitary Adenoma

Stem Cell Biology

The adenohypophysis is derived from Rathke's pouch stem cells that follow a coordinated program of differentiation in response to secreted growth factor (SHH, BMP, FGF, Wnt) signaling. Experimental evidence in mice and rats indicates continued slow cell turnover in the adenohypophysis. New secretory cells are formed in response to loss of negative feedback from target organs. These cells arise from nonsecretory progenitors and are not the product of mitosis of differentiated secretory cells. The dynamic cell population changes that occur in the pituitary involving expansion and regression is thought to make this tissue susceptible to acquisition of genetic aberrations and tumor formation.[101] Cells with stem-like features such as sphere formation in growth factor–rich media and expression of stem cell markers have been identified from a somatotroph tumor, although it is not yet clear if these cells meet all the requirements for the definition of a cancer stem cell.[102]

Genetics

The majority of pituitary adenomas demonstrate a normal karyotype.[103]

Genetic alterations and chromosomal imbalances are more often found in functional adenomas (52%) compared with nonfunctional adenomas (43%). The most frequent chromosomal aberration is a gain in chromosome 10 (32% of all adenomas).[104]

Germline mutations in aryl hydrocarbon interacting protein *(AIP)* gene in patients with familial pituitary adenoma predispose to formation of growth hormone–secreting pituitary adenomas and less commonly prolactinomas, adrenocorticotropic hormone (ACTH)-secreting adenomas, and nonfunctional adenomas.[105] In growth hormone (GH)-producing adenomas harboring the *AIP* mutation, the $G\alpha_{1-2}$ and $G\alpha_{1-3}$ proteins are defective and this results in elevated cyclic adenosine monophosphate (cAMP) levels that trigger downstream signaling involved in cell proliferation.[105] Changes in the expression of genes involved in pituitary development are found in nonfunctional pituitary adenomas.[106] Up to 40% of patients with acromegaly harbor activating mutations in the *GNAS* gene.[105]

Epigenetics

Aberrant methylation of CpG sites within gene associated CpG islands is observed in each of the adenoma subtypes.[107] Hypermethylation of *SOCS-1* gene is found in the majority (83%) of nonfunctional pituitary adenomas and some GH- and ACTH-producing adenomas. This methylation pattern is associated with transcriptional silencing of the *SOCS-1* gene, resulting in activation of JAK/STAT signaling, which is known to be tumorigenic.[108] Methylation-dependent gene silencing is a common feature of pituitary adenomas. The following genes have been found to be under epigenetic regulation in pituitary adenoma: *RB1, p16(INK4a), p15 (INK4b), p14 (ARF), p21 (WIPF/Cip1), GADD45G, DAP kinase, PTAG, MEG3A, ZAC.*

Proteomics

Heat shock protein 110 and bradykinin B2 are overexpressed, whereas C-terminal src kinase and annexin II are underexpressed in all pituitary adenomas.[109]

Receptor Signaling

Upregulated signaling through receptor tyrosine kinases regulating mitogenic pathways is frequently observed in pituitary adenomas. The two major pathways that have been identified are the PI3K/Akt/mTOR and Raf/MEK/extracellular signal-regulated kinase (ERK) pathways.[110] Dysregulation of cAMP signaling is a feature of GH-secreting pituitary adenomas. This is found in both sporadic and McCune-Albright syndrome–related cases and is associated with mutation or loss of genetic imprinting of the α-subunit of the stimulatory G-protein gene *(GNAS)*.[111]

Cell-Cycle Pathways

Dysregulation of the cell-cycle by promoter hypermethylation of cyclin-dependent kinase inhibitor genes or enhanced degradation of p27 is frequent in pituitary adenoma. Overexpression of a mitochondrial enzyme that catalyzes conversion of cholesterol to pregnenolone (P450scc) in response to steroid is regulated by the steroid responsive transcription factor SF1 in rat pituitary adenomas. P450scc *(CYP11A1* gene) is expressed at high levels at the messenger RNA (mRNA) and protein level in gonadotroph adenomas and functions in promoting proliferation of tumor cells.[112] BMP4 stimulates lactotroph proliferation by signaling expression of c-Myc, an important driver of the cell cycle. Prolactinomas express high levels of BMP4.[113]

Cell-Death Pathways

PLAGL1 is a tumor suppressor gene that induces apoptosis and G1 cell cycle arrest. Expression of this gene is reduced in pituitary adenomas. Furthermore, knockdown of *AIP* expression leads to a reduction in *PLAGL1* expression indicating a link between *AIP* mutation and dysregulated cell-death pathways.[114]

Biological Predictors

Loss of death-associated protein kinase expression is associated with an invasive phenotype.[115] Expression of pituitary tumor transforming gene *(PTTG)* mRNA is associated with an invasive phenotype in pituitary macroadenomas.[116] Tumors with *AIP* mutations are larger and have a respond less to somatostatin analogues than do sporadic tumors.[105] Somatotroph adenomas that express low levels of E-cadherin and RORC have a blunted insulin-like growth factor I (IGF-I) and tumor size response to somatostatin analogue therapy.[117] Low levels of Raf kinase inhibitory protein (RKIP) correlate with a poor clinical response to somatostatin analogue therapy. RKIP acts to attenuate MAPK signaling and blocks internalization of G-protein–coupled receptors.[118]

Overexpression of Galectin-3 (a β-ganglioside binding lectin) and a Ki-67 index of > 3% are associated with tumor recurrence/progression in prolactin and ACTH-secreting adenomas.[119] Only minor gene expression differences have been found between recurrent and nonrecurrent nonfunctional pituitary adenomas.[120]

Associations

Pituitary adenomas are seen in several germline mutation syndromes: McCune-Albright syndrome *(GNAS)*, multiple endocrine neoplasia type 1 *(MEN1)*, Carney complex *(PRKAR1A)*, multiple endocrine neoplasia type 4 *(CDKN1B)*, and pituitary adenoma predisposition syndrome *(AIP)*.

Craniopharyngioma

Stem Cell Biology

The current hypothesis for the origins of craniopharyngioma is that adamantinomatous craniopharyngioma (aCP) derives from remnants of the craniopharyngeal duct, whereas papillary craniopharyngioma (pCP) arises from metaplasia of adenohypophyseal cells in the pars tuberalis.[121] Expression of mutant β-catenin in periluminal progenitors of the developing Rathke's pouch results in formation of aCP-like tumors in mice. This supports Wnt pathway activation in stem cell precursors that generate the adenohypophysis as the likely origin of aCPs.[122]

Genetics

Chromosomal gains and losses are infrequent in aCP. In tumors that show chromosomal imbalance, gains are more prominent.[123]

aCPs, but not pCPs, harbor β-catenin *(CTNNB1)* missense mutations in exon 3. β-catenin is an important signaling molecule in the Wnt pathway that controls cell proliferation, morphology, and development.[124] Upregulation of β-catenin-mediated genes *Axin 2* and *BMP4* is observed in aCP.[125] pCPs, but not aCPs, harbor a point mutation in the *BRAF* oncogene that results in an amino acid substitution (Val600Glu). This substitution is known to constitutively activate BRAF, resulting in kinase signaling involved in cell division and differentiation.[126]

Proteomics

Cyst formation is associated with overexpression of VEGF.[127] Carbonic anhydrase IX protein expression level correlates with cyst size.[128] aCPs express odontogenic markers (enamelin, amelogenin, enamelysin), which are absent in pCPs.[129]

Receptor Signaling

aCPs demonstrate aberrant localization of β-catenin to the nucleus at the center of epithelial whorls adjacent to mesenchymal fibrosis, or adjacent to ghost cells. β-catenin is localized to the cell membrane in pCPs.[130]

Cell-Cycle Pathways

Cell clusters with nuclear β-catenin expression within aCPs show expression of p21$^{WAF1/Cip1}$, which is a key factor maintaining cells in the G1 phase of the cells cycle, thereby limiting sensitivity to radiation injury. These cell clusters may be responsible for high recurrence of aCPs, given their expression of stem cell and radioresistance biomarkers—p21$^{WAF1/Cip1}$, β-catenin, CD 133, and CD44.[131]

Biological Predictors

The invasive phenotype of aCPs with finger-like extensions into surrounding brain contributes to the difficulty in surgical resection of these tumors and possibly associated hypothalamic-pituitary dysfunction compared with pCPs, which form well-circumscribed masses. This invasive phenotype may also explain the higher recurrence rate associated with aCPs as compared with pCPs.[132]

■ References

1. Ieni A, Barresi V, Grosso M, Rosa MA, Tuccari G. Immunolocalization of lactoferrin in cartilage-forming neoplasms. J Orthop Sci 2009;14:732–737
2. Damato S, Alorjani M, Bonar F, et al. IDH1 mutations are not found in cartilaginous tumours other than central and periosteal chondrosarcomas and enchondromas. Histopathology 2012;60:363–365
3. Konishi E, Nakashima Y, Iwasa Y, Nakao R, Yanagisawa A. Immunohistochemical analysis for Sox9 reveals the cartilaginous character of chondroblastoma and chondromyxoid fibroma of the bone. Hum Pathol 2010;41:208–213
4. Romeo S, Bovée JV, Jadnanansing NA, Taminiau AH, Hogendoorn PC. Expression of cartilage growth plate signalling molecules in chondroblastoma. J Pathol 2004;202: 113–120
5. Romeo S, Szuhai K, Nishimori I, et al. A balanced t(5;17)(p15;q22-23) in chondroblastoma: frequency of the re-arrangement and analysis of the candidate genes. BMC Cancer 2009;9:393
6. Weatherby RP, Dahlin DC, Ivins JC. Postradiation sarcoma of bone: review of 78 Mayo Clinic cases. Mayo Clin Proc 1981;56:294–306
7. Lai LP, Lilley BN, Sanes JR, McMahon AP. Lkb1/Stk11 regulation of mTOR signaling controls the transition of chondrocyte fates and suppresses skeletal tumor formation. Proc Natl Acad Sci U S A 2013;110:19450–19455

8. Amary MF, Bacsi K, Maggiani F, et al. IDH1 and IDH2 mutations are frequent events in central chondrosarcoma and central and periosteal chondromas but not in other mesenchymal tumours. J Pathol 2011;224:334–343

9. Hopyan S, Gokgoz N, Poon R, et al. A mutant PTH/PTHrP type I receptor in enchondromatosis. Nat Genet 2002;30:306–310

10. Pansuriya TC, van Eijk R, d'Adamo P, et al. Somatic mosaic IDH1 and IDH2 mutations are associated with enchondroma and spindle cell hemangioma in Ollier disease and Maffucci syndrome. Nat Genet 2011;43:1256–1261

11. Verdegaal SH, Bovée JV, Pansuriya TC, et al. Incidence, predictive factors, and prognosis of chondrosarcoma in patients with Ollier disease and Maffucci syndrome: an international multicenter study of 161 patients. Oncologist 2011;16:1771–1779

12. Amary MF, Damato S, Halai D, et al. Ollier disease and Maffucci syndrome are caused by somatic mosaic mutations of IDH1 and IDH2. Nat Genet 2011;43:1262–1265

13. Aigner T. Towards a new understanding and classification of chondrogenic neoplasias of the skeleton—biochemistry and cell biology of chondrosarcoma and its variants. Virchows Arch 2002;441:219–230

14. Lu C, Venneti S, Akalin A, et al. Induction of sarcomas by mutant IDH2. Genes Dev 2013;27:1986–1998

15. Arai M, Nobusawa S, Ikota H, Takemura S, Nakazato Y. Frequent IDH1/2 mutations in intracranial chondrosarcoma: a possible diagnostic clue for its differentiation from chordoma. Brain Tumor Pathol 2012;29:201–206

16. Tarpey PS, Behjati S, Cooke SL, et al. Frequent mutation of the major cartilage collagen gene COL2A1 in chondrosarcoma. Nat Genet 2013;45:923–926

17. Wehrli BM, Huang W, De Crombrugghe B, Ayala AG, Czerniak B. Sox9, a master regulator of chondrogenesis, distinguishes mesenchymal chondrosarcoma from other small blue round cell tumors. Hum Pathol 2003;34:263–269

18. Schrage YM, Lam S, Jochemsen AG, et al. Central chondrosarcoma progression is associated with pRb pathway alterations: CDK4 down-regulation and p16 overexpression inhibit cell growth in vitro. J Cell Mol Med 2009;13:2843–2852

19. Kim DW, Seo SW, Cho SK, et al. Targeting of cell survival genes using small interfering RNAs (siRNAs) enhances radiosensitivity of Grade II chondrosarcoma cells. J Orthop Res 2007;25:820–828

20. Kim DW, Kim KO, Shin MJ, et al. siRNA-based targeting of antiapoptotic genes can reverse chemoresistance in P-glycoprotein expressing chondrosarcoma cells. Mol Cancer 2009;8:28

21. Kumari R, Li H, Haudenschild DR, et al. The oncogene LRF is a survival factor in chondrosarcoma and contributes to tumor malignancy and drug resistance. Carcinogenesis 2012;33:2076–2083

22. Chen C, Ma Q, Ma X, Liu Z, Liu X. Association of elevated HIF-2a levels with low Beclin 1 expression and poor prognosis in patients with chondrosarcoma. Ann Surg Oncol 2011;18:2364–2372

23. Papachristou DJ, Pirttiniemi P, Kantomaa T, Papavassiliou AG, Basdra EK. JNK/ERK-AP-1/Runx2 induction "paves the way" to cartilage load-ignited chondroblastic differentiation. Histochem Cell Biol 2005;124:215–223

24. Szuhai K, Cleton-Jansen AM, Hogendoorn PC, Bovée JV. Molecular pathology and its diagnostic use in bone tumors. Cancer Genet 2012;205:193–204

25. Sandberg AA, Bridge JA. Updates on the cytogenetics and molecular genetics of bone and soft tissue tumors: osteosarcoma and related tumors. Cancer Genet Cytogenet 2003;145:1–30

26. Oda Y, Yamamoto H, Tamiya S, et al. CXCR4 and VEGF expression in the primary site and the metastatic site of human osteosarcoma: analysis within a group of patients, all of whom developed lung metastasis. Mod Pathol 2006;19:738–745

27. Benayahu D, Shur I, Marom R, Meller I, Issakov J. Cellular and molecular properties associated with osteosarcoma cells. J Cell Biochem 2001;84:108–114

28. Sandberg AA. Genetics of chondrosarcoma and related tumors. Curr Opin Oncol 2004;16:342–354

29. Osaka E, Suzuki T, Osaka S, et al. Survivin expression levels as independent predictors of survival for osteosarcoma patients. J Orthop Res 2007;25:116–121

30. Perbal B, Zuntini M, Zambelli D, et al. Prognostic value of CCN3 in osteosarcoma. Clin Cancer Res 2008;14:701–709

31. Caronia D, Patiño-García A, Milne RL, et al. Common variations in ERCC2 are associated with response to cisplatin chemotherapy and clinical outcome in osteosarcoma patients. Pharmacogenomics J 2009;9:347–353

32. Vujovic S, Henderson S, Presneau N, et al. Brachyury, a crucial regulator of notochordal development, is a novel biomarker for chordomas. J Pathol 2006;209:157–165

33. Aydemir E, Bayrak OF, Sahin F, et al. Characterization of cancer stem-like cells in chordoma. J Neurosurg 2012;116:810–820

34. Iorgulescu JB, Laufer I, Hameed M, et al. Benign notochordal cell tumors of the spine: natural history of 8 patients with histologically confirmed lesions. Neurosurgery 2013;73:411–416

35. Almefty KK, Pravdenkova S, Sawyer J, Al-Mefty O. Impact of cytogenetic abnormalities on the management of skull base chordomas. J Neurosurg 2009;110:715–724

36. Presneau N, Shalaby A, Ye H, et al. Role of the transcription factor T (brachyury) in the pathogenesis of sporadic chordoma: a genetic and functional-based study. J Pathol 2011;223:327–335

37. Yang XR, Ng D, Alcorta DA, et al. T (brachyury) gene duplication confers major susceptibility to familial chordoma. Nat Genet 2009;41:1176–1178

38. Larizza L, Mortini P, Riva P. Update on the cytogenetics and molecular genetics of chordoma. Hered Cancer Clin Pract 2005;3:29–41

39. Hallor KH, Staaf J, Jönsson G, et al. Frequent deletion of the CDKN2A locus in chordoma: analysis of chromosomal imbalances using array comparative genomic hybridisation. Br J Cancer 2008;98:434–442

40. Diaz RJ, Guduk M, Romagnuolo R, et al. High-resolution whole-genome analysis of skull base chordomas implicates FHIT loss in chordoma pathogenesis. Neoplasia 2012;14:788–798

41. Rinner B, Weinhaeusel A, Lohberger B, et al. Chordoma characterization of significant changes of the DNA methylation pattern. PLoS ONE 2013;8:e56609

42. Shalaby AA, Presneau N, Idowu BD, et al. Analysis of the fibroblastic growth factor receptor-RAS/RAF/MEK/ERK-ETS2/brachyury signalling pathway in chordomas. Mod Pathol 2009;22:996–1005

43. Shalaby A, Presneau N, Ye H, et al. The role of epidermal growth factor receptor in chordoma pathogenesis: a potential therapeutic target. J Pathol 2011;223:336–346

44. Diaz RJ, Cusimano MD. The biological basis for modern treatment of chordoma. J Neurooncol 2011;104:411–422

45. Yang C, Schwab JH, Schoenfeld AJ, et al. A novel target for treatment of chordoma: signal transducers and activators of transcription 3. Mol Cancer Ther 2009;8:2597–2605

46. Duan Z, Choy E, Nielsen GP, et al. Differential expression of microRNA (miRNA) in chordoma reveals a role for miRNA-1 in Met expression. J Orthop Res 2010;28:746–752

47. McMaster ML, Goldstein AM, Parry DM. Clinical features distinguish childhood chordoma associated with tuberous sclerosis complex (TSC) from chordoma in the general paediatric population. J Med Genet 2011;48:444–449

48. Richter S, Qin N, Pacak K, Eisenhofer G. Role of hypoxia and HIF2a in development of the sympathoadrenal cell lineage and chromaffin cell tumors with distinct catecholamine phenotypic features. Adv Pharmacol 2013;68:285–317

49. Burnichon N, Vescovo L, Amar L, et al. Integrative genomic analysis reveals somatic mutations in pheochromocytoma and paraganglioma. Hum Mol Genet 2011;20:3974–3985

50. Burnichon N, Rohmer V, Amar L, et al; PGL.NET network. The succinate dehydrogenase genetic testing in a large prospective series of patients with paragangliomas. J Clin Endocrinol Metab 2009;94:2817–2827

51. Gaal J, Burnichon N, Korpershoek E, et al. Isocitrate dehydrogenase mutations are rare in pheochromocytomas and paragangliomas. J Clin Endocrinol Metab 2010;95:1274–1278

52. Galan SR, Kann PH. Genetics and molecular pathogenesis of pheochromocytoma and paraganglioma. Clin Endocrinol (Oxf) 2013;78:165–175

53. Ricketts CJ, Forman JR, Rattenberry E, et al. Tumor risks and genotype-phenotype-proteotype analysis in 358 patients with germline mutations in SDHB and SDHD. Hum Mutat 2010;31:41–51

54. Xiao M, Yang H, Xu W, et al. Inhibition of a-KG-dependent histone and DNA demethylases by fumarate and succinate that are accumulated in mutations of FH and SDH tumor suppressors. Genes Dev 2012;26:1326–1338

55. Fishbein L, Nathanson KL. Pheochromocytoma and paraganglioma: understanding the complexities of the genetic background. Cancer Genet 2012;205:1–11

56. Crona J, Nordling M, Maharjan R, et al. Integrative genetic characterization and phenotype correlations in pheochromocytoma and paraganglioma tumours. PLoS ONE 2014;9:e86756

57. Carney ME, O'Reilly RC, Sholevar B, et al. Expression of the human Achaete-scute 1 gene in olfactory neuroblastoma (esthesioneuroblastoma). J Neurooncol 1995;26:35–43

58. Mills SE, Frierson HF Jr. Olfactory neuroblastoma. A clinicopathologic study of 21 cases. Am J Surg Pathol 1985;9:317–327

59. Taxy JB, Bharani NK, Mills SE, Frierson HF Jr, Gould VE. The spectrum of olfactory neural tumors. A light-microscopic immunohistochemical and ultrastructural analysis. Am J Surg Pathol 1986;10:687–695

60. Trojanowski JQ, Lee V, Pillsbury N, Lee S. Neuronal origin of human esthesioneuroblastoma demonstrated with anti-neurofilament monoclonal antibodies. N Engl J Med 1982;307:159–161

61. Guled M, Myllykangas S, Frierson HF Jr, Mills SE, Knuutila S, Stelow EB. Array comparative genomic hybridization analysis of olfactory neuroblastoma. Mod Pathol 2008; 21:770–778

62. Weinreb I, Goldstein D, Irish J, Perez-Ordonez B. Expression patterns of Trk-A, Trk-B, GRP78, and p75NRT in olfactory neuroblastoma. Hum Pathol 2009;40:1330–1335

63. Mao L, Xia YP, Zhou YN, et al. Activation of sonic hedgehog signaling pathway in olfactory neuroblastoma. Oncology 2009;77:231–243

64. Kim JW, Kong IG, Lee CH, et al. Expression of Bcl-2 in olfactory neuroblastoma and its association with chemotherapy and survival. Otolaryngol Head Neck Surg 2008;139: 708–712

65. Fukushima S, Sugita Y, Niino D, Mihashi H, Ohshima K. Clincopathological analysis of olfactory neuroblastoma. Brain Tumor Pathol 2012;29:207–215

66. Bell D, Saade R, Roberts D, et al. Prognostic utility of Hyams histological grading and Kadish-Morita staging systems for esthesioneuroblastoma outcomes. Head Neck Pathol 2014

67. Yi D, Kuo SZ, Zheng H, et al. Activation of PDGFR and EGFR promotes the acquisition of a stem cell-like phenotype in schwannomas. Otol Neurotol 2012;33:1640–1647

68. Ahmad Z, Brown CM, Patel AK, Ryan AF, Ongkeko R, Doherty JK. Merlin knockdown in human Schwann cells: clues to vestibular schwannoma tumorigenesis. Otol Neurotol 2010;31:460–466

69. Jacoby LB, MacCollin M, Barone R, Ramesh V, Gusella JF. Frequency and distribution of NF2 mutations in schwannomas. Genes Chromosomes Cancer 1996;17:45–55

70. Sughrue ME, Yeung AH, Rutkowski MJ, Cheung SW, Parsa AT. Molecular biology of familial and sporadic vestibular schwannomas: implications for novel therapeutics. J Neurosurg 2011;114:359–366

71. Bian LG, Tirakotai W, Sun QF, Zhao WG, Shen JK, Luo QZ. Molecular genetics alterations and tumor behavior of sporadic vestibular schwannoma from the People's Republic of China. J Neurooncol 2005;73:253–260

72. Hansen MR, Roehm PC, Chatterjee P, Green SH. Constitutive neuregulin-1/ErbB signaling contributes to human vestibular schwannoma proliferation. Glia 2006;53: 593–600

73. Baek SY, Kim SU. Proliferation of human Schwann cells induced by neu differentiation factor isoforms. Dev Neurosci 1998;20:512–517

74. Maurel P, Salzer JL. Axonal regulation of Schwann cell proliferation and survival and the initial events of myelination requires PI 3-kinase activity. J Neurosci 2000;20: 4635–4645

75. Uesaka T, Shono T, Suzuki SO, et al. Expression of VEGF and its receptor genes in intracranial schwannomas. J Neurooncol 2007;83:259–266

76. Mawrin C, Kirches E, Dietzmann K, Roessner A, Boltze C. Expression pattern of apoptotic markers in vestibular schwannomas. Pathol Res Pract 2002;198:813–819

77. Katoh M, Wilmotte R, Belkouch MC, de Tribolet N, Pizzolato G, Dietrich PY. Survivin in brain tumors: an attractive target for immunotherapy. J Neurooncol 2003;64: 71–76

78. Carroll SL. Molecular mechanisms promoting the pathogenesis of Schwann cell neoplasms. Acta Neuropathol 2012;123:321–348

79. Yeung AH, Sughrue ME, Kane AJ, Tihan T, Cheung SW, Parsa AT. Radiobiology of vestibular schwannomas: mechanisms of radioresistance and potential targets for therapeutic sensitization. Neurosurg Focus 2009;27:E2
80. Kalamarides M, Stemmer-Rachamimov AO, Niwa-Kawakita M, et al. Identification of a progenitor cell of origin capable of generating diverse meningioma histological subtypes. Oncogene 2011;30:2333–2344
81. Zhu J, Frosch MP, Busque L, et al. Analysis of meningiomas by methylation- and transcription-based clonality assays. Cancer Res 1995;55:3865–3872
82. Zang KD. Meningioma: a cytogenetic model of a complex benign human tumor, including data on 394 karyotyped cases. Cytogenet Cell Genet 2001;93:207–220
83. Mawrin C, Perry A. Pathological classification and molecular genetics of meningiomas. J Neurooncol 2010;99:379–391
84. Hartmann C, Sieberns J, Gehlhaar C, Simon M, Paulus W, von Deimling A. NF2 mutations in secretory and other rare variants of meningiomas. Brain Pathol 2006;16:15–19
85. Müller P, Henn W, Niedermayer I, et al. Deletion of chromosome 1p and loss of expression of alkaline phosphatase indicate progression of meningiomas. Clin Cancer Res 1999;5:3569–3577
86. Aavikko M, Li SP, Saarinen S, et al. Loss of SUFU function in familial multiple meningioma. Am J Hum Genet 2012;91:520–526
87. van den Munckhof P, Christiaans I, Kenter SB, Baas F, Hulsebos TJ. Germline SMARCB1 mutation predisposes to multiple meningiomas and schwannomas with preferential location of cranial meningiomas at the falx cerebri. Neurogenetics 2012;13:1–7
88. Barski D, Wolter M, Reifenberger G, Riemenschneider MJ. Hypermethylation and transcriptional downregulation of the TIMP3 gene is associated with allelic loss on 22q12.3 and malignancy in meningiomas. Brain Pathol 2010;20:623–631
89. Takahashi JA, Mori H, Fukumoto M, et al. Gene expression of fibroblast growth factors in human gliomas and meningiomas: demonstration of cellular source of basic fibroblast growth factor mRNA and peptide in tumor tissues. Proc Natl Acad Sci U S A 1990;87:5710–5714
90. Choy W, Kim W, Nagasawa D, et al. The molecular genetics and tumor pathogenesis of meningiomas and the future directions of meningioma treatments. Neurosurg Focus 2011;30:E6
91. Laurendeau I, Ferrer M, Garrido D, et al. Gene expression profiling of the hedgehog signaling pathway in human meningiomas. Mol Med 2010;16:262–270
92. Nordqvist AC, Mathiesen T. Expression of IGF-II, IGFBP-2, -5, and -6 in meningiomas with different brain invasiveness. J Neurooncol 2002;57:19–26
93. Umansky F, Shoshan Y, Rosenthal G, Fraifeld S, Spektor S. Radiation-induced meningioma. Neurosurg Focus 2008;24:E7
94. Evans DG, Huson SM, Donnai D, et al. A genetic study of type 2 neurofibromatosis in the United Kingdom. I. Prevalence, mutation rate, fitness, and confirmation of maternal transmission effect on severity. J Med Genet 1992;29:841–846
95. Kawashima M, Suzuki SO, Yamashima T, Fukui M, Iwaki T. Prostaglandin D synthase (beta-trace) in meningeal hemangiopericytoma. Mod Pathol 2001;14:197–201
96. Henn W, Wullich B, Thönnes M, Steudel WI, Feiden W, Zang KD. Recurrent t(12;19)(q13;q13.3) in intracranial and extracranial hemangiopericytoma. Cancer Genet Cytogenet 1993;71:151–154

97. Schweizer L, Koelsche C, Sahm F, et al. Meningeal hemangiopericytoma and solitary fibrous tumors carry the NAB2-STAT6 fusion and can be diagnosed by nuclear expression of STAT6 protein. Acta Neuropathol 2013;125:651–658

98. Schürch W, Skalli O, Lagacé R, Seemayer TA, Gabbiani G. Intermediate filament proteins and actin isoforms as markers for soft-tissue tumor differentiation and origin. III. Hemangiopericytomas and glomus tumors. Am J Pathol 1990;136:771–786

99. Ono Y, Ueki K, Joseph JT, Louis DN. Homozygous deletions of the CDKN2/p16 gene in dural hemangiopericytomas. Acta Neuropathol 1996;91:221–225

100. Zhou JL, Liu JL, Zhang J, Zhang M. Thirty-nine cases of intracranial hemangiopericytoma and anaplastic hemangiopericytoma: a retrospective review of MRI features and pathological findings. Eur J Radiol 2012;81:3504–3510

101. Vankelecom H. Pituitary stem cells drop their mask. Curr Stem Cell Res Ther 2012; 7:36–71

102. Xu Q, Yuan X, Tunici P, et al. Isolation of tumour stem-like cells from benign tumours. Br J Cancer 2009;101:303–311

103. Larsen JB, Schrøder HD, Sørensen AG, Bjerre P, Heim S. Simple numerical chromosome aberrations characterize pituitary adenomas. Cancer Genet Cytogenet 1999; 114:144–149

104. Trautmann K, Thakker RV, Ellison DW, et al. Chromosomal aberrations in sporadic pituitary tumors. Int J Cancer 2001;91:809–814

105. Tuominen I, Heliovaara E, Raitila A, et al. AIP inactivation leads to pituitary tumorigenesis through defective Galpha-cAMP signaling. Oncogene 2014

106. Moreno CS, Evans CO, Zhan X, Okor M, Desiderio DM, Oyesiku NM. Novel molecular signaling and classification of human clinically nonfunctional pituitary adenomas identified by gene expression profiling and proteomic analyses. Cancer Res 2005; 65:10214–10222

107. Duong CV, Emes RD, Wessely F, Yacqub-Usman K, Clayton RN, Farrell WE. Quantitative, genome-wide analysis of the DNA methylome in sporadic pituitary adenomas. Endocr Relat Cancer 2012;19:805–816

108. Buslei R, Kreutzer J, Hofmann B, et al. Abundant hypermethylation of SOCS-1 in clinically silent pituitary adenomas. Acta Neuropathol 2006;111:264–271

109. Ribeiro-Oliveira A Jr, Franchi G, Kola B, et al. Protein western array analysis in human pituitary tumours: insights and limitations. Endocr Relat Cancer 2008;15:1099–1114

110. Dworakowska D, Wlodek E, Leontiou CA, et al. Activation of RAF/MEK/ERK and PI3K/AKT/mTOR pathways in pituitary adenomas and their effects on downstream effectors. Endocr Relat Cancer 2009;16:1329–1338

111. Mantovani G, Lania AG, Spada A. GNAS imprinting and pituitary tumors. Mol Cell Endocrinol 2010;326:15–18

112. Lee M, Marinoni I, Irmler M, et al. Transcriptome analysis of MENX-associated rat pituitary adenomas identifies novel molecular mechanisms involved in the pathogenesis of human pituitary gonadotroph adenomas. Acta Neuropathol 2013;126:137–150

113. Paez-Pereda M, Giacomini D, Refojo D, et al. Involvement of bone morphogenetic protein 4 (BMP-4) in pituitary prolactinoma pathogenesis through a Smad/estrogen receptor crosstalk. Proc Natl Acad Sci U S A 2003;100:1034–1039

114. Theodoropoulou M, Stalla GK, Spengler D. ZAC1 target genes and pituitary tumorigenesis. Mol Cell Endocrinol 2010;326:60–65
115. Simpson DJ, Clayton RN, Farrell WE. Preferential loss of death associated protein kinase expression in invasive pituitary tumours is associated with either CpG island methylation or homozygous deletion. Oncogene 2002;21:1217–1224
116. Jia W, Lu R, Jia G, Ni M, Xu Z. Expression of pituitary tumor transforming gene (PTTG) in human pituitary macroadenomas. Tumour Biol 2013;34:1559–1567
117. Lekva T, Berg JP, Heck A, et al. Attenuated RORC expression in the presence of EMT progression in somatotroph adenomas following treatment with somatostatin analogs is associated with poor clinical recovery. PLoS ONE 2013;8:e66927
118. Fougner SL, Borota OC, Berg JP, Hald JK, Ramm-Pettersen J, Bollerslev J. The clinical response to somatostatin analogues in acromegaly correlates to the somatostatin receptor subtype 2a protein expression of the adenoma. Clin Endocrinol (Oxf) 2008; 68:458–465
119. Righi A, Morandi L, Leonardi E, et al. Galectin-3 expression in pituitary adenomas as a marker of aggressive behavior. Hum Pathol 2013;44:2400–2409
120. Marko NF, Coughlan C, Weil RJ. Towards an integrated molecular and clinical strategy to predict early recurrence in surgically resected non-functional pituitary adenomas. J Clin Neurosci 2012;19:1535–1540
121. Garrè ML, Cama A. Craniopharyngioma: modern concepts in pathogenesis and treatment. Curr Opin Pediatr 2007;19:471–479
122. Gaston-Massuet C, Andoniadou CL, Signore M, et al. Increased Wingless (Wnt) signaling in pituitary progenitor/stem cells gives rise to pituitary tumors in mice and humans. Proc Natl Acad Sci U S A 2011;108:11482–11487
123. Yoshimoto M, de Toledo SR, da Silva NS, et al. Comparative genomic hybridization analysis of pediatric adamantinomatous craniopharyngiomas and a review of the literature. J Neurosurg 2004;101(1, Suppl):85–90
124. Buslei R, Nolde M, Hofmann B, et al. Common mutations of beta-catenin in adamantinomatous craniopharyngiomas but not in other tumours originating from the sellar region. Acta Neuropathol 2005;109:589–597
125. Hölsken A, Kreutzer J, Hofmann BM, et al. Target gene activation of the Wnt signaling pathway in nuclear beta-catenin accumulating cells of adamantinomatous craniopharyngiomas. Brain Pathol 2009;19:357–364
126. Brastianos PK, Taylor-Weiner A, Manley PE, et al. Exome sequencing identifies BRAF mutations in papillary craniopharyngiomas. Nat Genet 2014;46:161–165
127. Vaquero J, Zurita M, de Oya S, Coca S, Morales C, Salas C. Expression of vascular permeability factor in craniopharyngioma. J Neurosurg 1999;91:831–834
128. Proescholdt M, Merrill M, Stoerr EM, Lohmeier A, Dietmaier W, Brawanski A. Expression of carbonic anhydrase IX in craniopharyngiomas. J Neurosurg 2011;115:796–801
129. Sekine S, Takata T, Shibata T, et al. Expression of enamel proteins and LEF1 in adamantinomatous craniopharyngioma: evidence for its odontogenic epithelial differentiation. Histopathology 2004;45:573–579
130. Cao J, Lin JP, Yang LX, Chen K, Huang ZS. Expression of aberrant beta-catenin and impaired p63 in craniopharyngiomas. Br J Neurosurg 2010;24:249–256

131. Holsken A, Stache C, Schlaffer SM, et al. Adamantinomatous craniopharyngiomas express tumor stem cell markers in cells with activated Wnt signaling: further evidence for the existence of a tumor stem cell niche? Pituitary 2014;17:546–556
132. Stache C, Holsken A, Schlaffer SM, et al. Insights into the infiltrative behavior of adamantinomatous craniopharyngioma in a new xenotransplant mouse model. Brain Pathol 2015;25:1–10

39 Quality of Life in Skull Base Surgery

■ Definition of Quality of Life

The World Health Organization defines quality of life (QOL) as an individual's perception of their position in life in the context of the culture and value systems in which they live and in relation to their goals, standards, and concerns. It is a broad-ranging concept affected in a complex way by the person's physical health, psychosocial state, level of independence, social relationships, and their relationships to the salient features of their environment.[1-3]

■ Evaluation of QOL in Patients with Skull Base Tumors

For several decades, skull base surgeons have struggled to improve survival rates. Recently, increasing attention has been paid to improving and evaluating QOL. However, the surgeon's perception of the patient's QOL is not sufficiently accurate to correctly estimate the patient's QOL status.[4] Therefore, a patient-reported measurement is important. A detailed understanding of the different aspects of QOL may help surgeons improve the assessment and management of patients before and after treatment, and provide a patient-centered guide to the choices of medical interventions.[5] QOL questionnaires may help to compare the results of surgery.[3]

■ QOL Assessment

Site-Specific Questionnaires (Table 39.1)

1. Anterior Skull Base Questionnaires (ASBQ)[6-8]
2. Sino-Nasal Outcome Test (SNOT-22)[8,9]

3. ASK Nasal Inventory-9 and ASK Nasal Inventory-12 (Anterior Skull Base Nasal Inventory-9 and -12)[10-12]
4. Functional Assessment of Cancer Therapy–Meningioma (FACT-MNG)[13,14]
5. Glasgow Benefit Inventory (GBI)[15,16]
6. Skull Base Inventory (SBI)[17]

Global QOL Measures (Table 39.2)

1. Karnofsky Performance Status (KPS)[10,18]
2. The 36-Item Short Form Health Survey (SF-36)[14]
3. Functional Assessment of Cancer Therapy-General (FACT-G)[3,19,20]
4. Sickness Impact Profile (SIP) to assess quality of life[3,14]

QOL Indexes Used for Various Skull Base Surgery Approaches (Tables 39.3 and 39.4)

1. Patients with anterior skull base tumors undergoing open skull base surgery: ASBQ[6,7,10,21,22] **(Table 39.3)**
2. QOL after transnasal endoscopic surgery: ASBQ[5,23–25], SNOT-22[8,24,26] **(Table 39.3)**
3. Comparison of QOL after transnasal endoscopic versus open skull base resection:
   a. Comparisons are complicated by the heterogeneity of the two populations, the inherently different indications for each approach, the varying proportions of malignant tumors included in studies, differences in the rates of radiotherapy, as well as the varying extents of surgical resection achieved by the two approaches.[10]
   b. However, some authors have reported the following:
      • Improvements in QOL seem to appear earlier in the endoscopic group.[10,27]
      • Patients better tolerated the endoscopic procedure than the microscopic procedure.[28]
      • Patients who underwent endoscopic surgery had significantly better ASBQ scores in physical function and impact on emotions compared with patients who underwent open surgery.[23]
      • Malignant histological type and adjuvant radiation therapy had a poor impact on QOL in patients undergoing open surgery, whereas such differences were absent in the endoscopic group.[23]
4. QOL of patients with skull base meningioma[29] **(Table 39.4)**
5. QOL of patients with vestibular schwannoma **(Table 39.4)**
6. QOL of patients with chordoma[14] **(Table 39.4)**

Table 39.1 Summary of Site-Specific Questionnaires

Questionnaire	Description	Scoring	Multi-dimensional	Disadvantage
ASBQ	A cancer-specific QOL instrument designed to measure QOL of patients with anterior base pathology.	A 35-item survey divided into six QOL domains: performance, physical function, vitality, pain, influence on emotions, and specific symptoms. Responses are recorded on a five-item Likert scale, ranging from 1 (worst QOL) to 5 (best QOL) for each item. Total scores range from 35 to 175, and overall scores are reported as mean item scores ranging from 1.0 to 5.0, with a higher score indicating better QOL.	Yes	Only for patients with anterior skull base tumor
SNOT-22	A disease-specific instrument designed for the assessment of QOL related to benign sinonasal disease.	Twenty-two items that can be divided into domains. Responses are recorded on a six-item Likert scale, ranging from 0 (no problem) to 5 (worst) for each item. Total scores range from 0 to 110, with a higher score indicating worse QOL.	Yes	Not tailored for patients undergoing skull base surgery
ASK Nasal Inventory-9	A self-reported QOL survey for assessing nasal outcomes following endonasal pituitary and skull base surgery.	A nine-question patient survey focusing on the most common postoperative complaints, including crusting, sinusitis, pain, and ease of breathing. Questions determine how often patients experience specific symptoms, with scores ranging from 1 (never) to 5 (all of the time).	No	Unidimensional
ASK Nasal Inventory-12	ASK Nasal Inventory-12 was developed from the ASK Nasal Inventory-9.	Same as the ASK Nasal Inventory-9.	No	Unidimensional

FACT-MNG	A tumor site-specific web-based outcome instrument for meningioma patients, as an amalgamation of the Functional Assessment of Cancer Therapy-Brain (FACT-BR) and SF-36, and newly formulated questions addressing tumor site-specific signs and symptoms.	Six QOL domains: physical well-being, emotional well-being, social/family well-being, functional well-being, additional concerns and tumor site-specific questions for 11 intracranial meningioma sites.	Yes	Not yet validated
GBI	Designed to provide an assessment of the patient's perceived benefit from otolaryngological interventions.	Eighteen questions addressing changes in health status resulting from management. Response to each question is based on a five-point Likert scale. Total score ranges from −100 to +100, with negative scores representing deterioration in status, zero as no change, and positive scores as a benefit.	Yes	
SBI	A disease-specific instrument for anterior and central skull base pathology.	Forty-one items; total score ranges from 0 to 100.	Yes	Further validation is needed; lack of duplicate coding

Abbreviations: ASBQ, Anterior Skull Base Questionnaire; SNOT-22, Sinonasal Outcome Test-22; ASK Nasal Inventory, Anterior Skull Base Nasal Inventory; FACT-MNG, Functional Assessment of Cancer Therapy-Meningioma; GBI, Glasgow Benefit Inventory; QOL, quality of life; SBI, Skull Base Inventory; SF-36, 36-Item Short Form Health Survey.

Table 39.2 Summary of Global Quality of Life (QOL) Measures

Instrument	Description	Scoring	Multidimensional	Disadvantage
KPS	A rating scale of functional status (not truly a QOL instrument; it is more like a performance score)	0 to 100, with higher score indicating better functional status	No	Scores are determined by health care providers, not patients
SF-36	A widely validated patient-oriented outcome instrument of 36 questions across eight health domains: physical functioning, role limitations due to physical health problems, bodily pain, social functioning, general mental health, role limitations due to emotional problems, vitality, and general health perception	0 to 100, with 100 representing the best possible health state	Yes	May not be optimal for evaluating cranial nerve deficit
FACT-G	Psychometric and functional assessment of QOL in cancer patients; 27 items in four primary domains: physical well-being, social/family well-being, emotional well-being, functional well-being	0 (not at all) to 4 (very much)	Yes	
SIP	136 yes/no items and 12 subscales	Higher score indicates a poor QOL	No	May be of limited use in a clinical setting

Abbreviations: KPS, Karnofsky Performance Scale; SF-36, 36-Item Short Form Health Survey; FACT-G, Functional Assessment of Cancer Therapy-General; SIP, sickness Impact Profile to assess quality of life.

Table 39.3 Summary of QOL Questionnaires for Use in Skull Base Surgery Patients

Treatment	Questionnaire	Main findings
Open skull base surgery	ASBQ	Overall QOL: 74% reported a significant improvement or no change within 6 months after open skull base surgery.[7]
		Significantly improved at 12 months postoperatively.[6,7,10,21,22]
		Worst impact: financial and emotional domains[22]
		Negative prognostic factors: old age, malignancy, comorbidity, wide resection, and radiotherapy[6,7]
Transnasal endoscopic surgery	ASBQ	No significant association with reduced QOL
		Age, comorbidity, adjuvant radiation therapy, prior surgery, histological type (benign vs malignant),[5,23] type of surgery (pituitary tumors vs nonpituitary tumors), anatomic region involved (cribriform, planum, sella, or clivus),[23] functioning tumors were not associated with postoperative ASBQ score.[24]
	SNOT-22	Scores worsened at 3 weeks postoperatively and returned to baseline thereafter; at 12 months postoperatively.[8]
		Scores worsened at 3 weeks postoperatively and significant improved at the 12 months.[8]
		Sinonasal morbidity is increased temporarily; the vast majority of patients have good QOL by 4 to 6 months after surgery.[26]
		An expanded endonasal approach with vascularized septal flap induces more nasal symptoms (olfactory loss and posterior nasal discharge) compared with routine pituitary surgery.[24]

Table 39.4 Summary of QOL Questionnaires for Use in Specific Skull Base Pathologies

Tumor	Treatment	Questionnaire	Main findings
Skull base meningioma[29]			14 to 35% of patients do not regain their premorbid working ability after surgery.
			The age of patients significantly influenced cognitive performance: young patients tended to experience a longer period for recovery despite successful surgery, and were also less confident about their cognitive performance status compared to older patients.
Vestibular schwannoma (VS)	Before treatment	SF-36	Significantly decreased when compared with healthy controls.[30]
			Vertigo was the symptom causing the most pronounced negative effect.[30-32]
			Unilateral hearing loss and tinnitus had a less impact on QOL.[30]
			Some evidence suggests that patients with a larger tumor (> 3 cm) may experience lower QOL when compared with patients with smaller tumors, although this has not been confirmed in all studies.[33]
	Conservative management	SF-36	QOL was similar to that of the normal population when QOL was measured using SF-36.[30,32]
		GBI	Conservative management of VS did not lead to changes in QOL.[30,32]
	Surgery		Many authors have reported that surgery for VS resulted in a significant reduction in QOL for patients, but mostly for physical dimensions of QOL, at 1 to 3 months postoperatively.[30,34,35]
			At 3 to 12 months postoperatively, patients who had experienced these declines reported recovery to at least baseline levels of QOL.[30]
			The major effect is psychological, with increased rates of emotional distress and impaired social functioning even in comparison with patients with major illness.[30]

	SF-36	Patients with large VS (grade III or IV) undergoing surgery had lower scores in all SF-36 categories except pain, when compared with data from other studies.[30,36] Tinnitus and vertigo may have significant underestimated impacts on postoperative course and QOL.[35,37]
Gamma Knife radiosurgery	SF-36	No significant decline in SF-36 results were noticed after Gamma Knife radiosurgery.[38] QOL did not differ significantly between conservative management and Gamma Knife radiosurgery.[31]
Chordoma[17]	SF-36	Patients with skull base chordomas report a lower QOL compared with the general population. The most significant determinants of QOL in the posttreatment phase in this patient population were neurologic deficits (sensory deficit and bowel/bladder dysfunction), pain medication use, corticosteroid use, and levels of depression.

Abbreviations: GBI, Glasgow Benefit Inventory; SF-36, 36-Item Short Form Health Survey.

■ References

Boldfaced references are of particular importance.

1. Rehabilitation after cardiovascular diseases, with special emphasis on developing countries. Report of a WHO Expert Committee. World Health Organ Tech Rep Ser 1993;831:1–122

2. **de Almeida JR, Witterick IJ, Gullane PJ, et al. Quality of life instruments for skull base pathology: systematic review and methodologic appraisal. Head Neck 2013; 35:1221–1231**

3. **Cusimano MD. Quality-of-life assessment in patients with lesions of the cranial base. Skull Base Surg 1999;9:259–264**

4. Gil Z, Abergel A, Spektor S, Khafif A, Fliss DM. Patient, caregiver, and surgeon perceptions of quality of life following anterior skull base surgery. Arch Otolaryngol Head Neck Surg 2004;130:1276–1281

5. Cavel O, Abergel A, Margalit N, Fliss DM, Gil Z. Quality of life following endoscopic resection of skull base tumors. J Neurol Surg B Skull Base 2012;73:112–116

6. **Gil Z, Abergel A, Spektor S, Shabtai E, Khafif A, Fliss DM. Development of a cancer-specific anterior skull base quality-of-life questionnaire. J Neurosurg 2004;100: 813–819**

7. Gil Z, Abergel A, Spektor S, et al. Quality of life following surgery for anterior skull base tumors. Arch Otolaryngol Head Neck Surg 2003;129:1303–1309

8. **McCoul ED, Anand VK, Schwartz TH. Improvements in site-specific quality of life 6 months after endoscopic anterior skull base surgery: a prospective study. J Neurosurg 2012;117:498–506**

9. Piccirillo JF, Merritt MG Jr, Richards ML. Psychometric and clinimetric validity of the 20-item Sino-Nasal Outcome Test (SNOT-20). Otolaryngol Head Neck Surg 2002;126: 41–47

10. Kirkman MA, Borg A, Al-Mousa A, Haliasos N, Choi D. Quality-of-life after anterior skull base surgery: a systematic review. J Neurol Surg B Skull Base 2014;75:73–89

11. Little AS, Kelly D, Milligan J, et al. Prospective validation of a patient-reported nasal quality-of-life tool for endonasal skull base surgery: the Anterior Skull Base Nasal Inventory-12. J Neurosurg 2013;119:1068–1074

12. Little AS, Jahnke H, Nakaji P, Milligan J, Chapple K, White WL. The anterior skull base nasal inventory (ASK nasal inventory): a clinical tool for evaluating rhinological outcomes after endonasal surgery for pituitary and cranial base lesions. Pituitary 2012; 15:513–517

13. Zlotnick D, Kalkanis SN, Quinones-Hinojosa A, et al. FACT-MNG: tumor site specific web-based outcome instrument for meningioma patients. J Neurooncol 2010;99: 423–431

14. **Diaz RJ, Maggacis N, Zhang S, Cusimano MD. Determinants of quality of life in patients with skull base chordoma. J Neurosurg 2014;120:528–537**

15. Swan IR, Guy FH, Akeroyd MA. Health-related quality of life before and after management in adults referred to otolaryngology: a prospective national study. Clin Otolaryngol 2012;37:35–43

16. Robinson K, Gatehouse S, Browning GG. Measuring patient benefit from otorhinolaryngological surgery and therapy. Ann Otol Rhinol Laryngol 1996;105:415–422

17. de Almeida JR, Vescan AD, Gullane PJ, et al. Development of a disease-specific quality-of-life questionnaire for anterior and central skull base pathology—the skull base inventory. Laryngoscope 2012;122:1933–1942

18. Karnofsky DA, Burchenal JH. Present status of clinical cancer chemotherapy. Am J Med 1950;8:767–788

19. Palme CE, Irish JC, Gullane PJ, Katz MR, Devins GM, Bachar G. Quality of life analysis in patients with anterior skull base neoplasms. Head Neck 2009;31:1326–1334

20. Weitzner MA, Meyers CA, Gelke CK, Byrne KS, Cella DF, Levin VA. The Functional Assessment of Cancer Therapy (FACT) scale. Development of a brain subscale and revalidation of the general version (FACT-G) in patients with primary brain tumors. Cancer 1995;75:1151–1161

21. Abergel A, Fliss DM, Margalit N, Gil Z. A prospective evaluation of short-term health-related quality of life in patients undergoing anterior skull base surgery. Skull Base 2010;20:27–33

22. **Gil Z, Fliss DM. Quality of life in patients with skull base tumors: current status and future challenges. Skull Base 2010;20:11–18**

23. Abergel A, Cavel O, Margalit N, Fliss DM, Gil Z. Comparison of quality of life after transnasal endoscopic vs open skull base tumor resection. Arch Otolaryngol Head Neck Surg 2012;138:142–147

24. **Alobid I, Enseñat J, Mariño-Sánchez F, et al. Expanded endonasal approach using vascularized septal flap reconstruction for skull base tumors has a negative impact on sinonasal symptoms and quality of life. Am J Rhinol Allergy 2013;27:426–431**

25. **Castelnuovo P, Lepera D, Turri-Zanoni M, et al. Quality of life following endoscopic endonasal resection of anterior skull base cancers. J Neurosurg 2013;119:1401–1409**

26. Pant H, Bhatki AM, Snyderman CH, et al. Quality of life following endonasal skull base surgery. Skull Base 2010;20:35–40

27. Karabatsou K, O'Kelly C, Ganna A, Dehdashti AR, Gentili F. Outcomes and quality of life assessment in patients undergoing endoscopic surgery for pituitary adenomas. Br J Neurosurg 2008;22:630–635

28. Lwu S, Edem I, Banton B, et al. Quality of life after transsphenoidal pituitary surgery: a qualitative study. Acta Neurochir (Wien) 2012;154:1917–1922

29. Chen CM, Huang AP, Kuo LT, Tu YK. Contemporary surgical outcome for skull base meningiomas. Neurosurg Rev 2011;34:281–296, discussion 296

30. Breivik CN, Nilsen RM, Myrseth E, et al. Conservative management or gamma knife radiosurgery for vestibular schwannoma: tumor growth, symptoms, and quality of life. Neurosurgery 2013;73:48–56, discussion 56–57

31. Breivik CN, Varughese JK, Wentzel-Larsen T, Vassbotn F, Lund-Johansen M. Conservative management of vestibular schwannoma—a prospective cohort study: treatment, symptoms, and quality of life. Neurosurgery 2012;70:1072–1080, discussion 1080

32. Gouveris HT, Mann WJ. Quality of life in sporadic vestibular schwannoma: a review. ORL J Otorhinolaryngol Relat Spec 2010;72:69–74

33. Gauden A, Weir P, Hawthorne G, Kaye A. Systematic review of quality of life in the management of vestibular schwannoma. J Clin Neurosci 2011;18:1573–1584

34. Cheng S, Naidoo Y, da Cruz M, Dexter M. Quality of life in postoperative vestibular schwannoma patients. Laryngoscope 2009;119:2252–2257

35. Scheich M, Ginzkey C, Reuter E, Harnisch W, Ehrmann D, Hagen R. Quality of life after microsurgery for vestibular schwannoma via the middle cranial fossa approach. Eur Arch Otorhinolaryngol 2014;271:1909–1916
36. Rameh C, Magnan J. Quality of life of patients following stages III-IV vestibular schwannoma surgery using the retrosigmoid and translabyrinthine approaches. Auris Nasus Larynx 2010;37:546–552
37. Grauvogel J, Kaminsky J, Rosahl SK. The impact of tinnitus and vertigo on patient-perceived quality of life after cerebellopontine angle surgery. Neurosurgery 2010;67:601–609, discussion 609–610
38. Park SS, Grills IS, Bojrab D, et al. Longitudinal assessment of quality of life and audiometric test outcomes in vestibular schwannoma patients treated with gamma knife surgery. Otol Neurotol 2011;32:676–679

40 Training in Skull Base Surgery

Skull base surgery is one of the most complex kinds of surgery because it requires a deep understanding of surgical anatomy, technical skills, and interdisciplinary collaboration among different specialists (e.g., neurosurgeons, otorhinolaryngologists, and craniomaxillofacial/plastic surgeons).

A natural progression for learning surgery is as follows: (1) studying surgical anatomy and procedures; (2) observing live surgery; (3) performing anatomic dissections and surgical simulations in anatomy labs and/or with surgery simulators; (4) assisting in surgical procedures; and (5) performing live surgery, initially supervised and later alone, in collaboration with other specialists. The importance of developing clinical decision-making skills to understand when to operate and the optimal surgical approach cannot be understated.

- The role of residency and fellowships is of paramount importance. Imitation of senior surgeons is the most powerful method by which surgeons learn to operate.[1] A stepwise educational progression undertaken by surgical residents provides better surgical outcomes with lower morbidity.[2, 3]
- Skull base surgery has a particularly steep learning curve, and the skull base surgeon has to master both endoscopic and microscopic techniques.

■ Anatomy Lab

- Cadaver dissection in the anatomy lab enables trainees to acquire a practical knowledge of surgical anatomy, giving them the chance to improve their dissecting and surgical techniques.[4,5]
- Laboratory training is imperative to acquire expertise in microsurgical techniques (as emphasized by Yasargil)[6] and endoscopic techniques.[4]
- A cadaver lab is the place where beginners can learn and train, experts can test their skills, and good surgeons can become better surgeons.[4]
- The training checklist in the anatomy lab is as follows[4]:
  1. Manual training
  2. Anatomy orientation

3. Simulation surgery
4. Confirmation of the technical feasibility of an approach
5. Comparison of microscopic and endoscopic approaches, and use of both in endoscope-assisted microsurgical approaches
6. Analysis of tools and instruments

- Developing the ability to handle different instruments, such as endoscopes and microscopes, including those provided with angled endoscopes, and learning three-dimensional (3D) anatomy orientation are important goals of trainees in the lab. Angled endoscopes increase the ability to view structures "around the corner," but they also increase the risk of disorientation.[7] The combined use of endoscopes and microscopes provides different points of view of the same object at the gross, mesoscopic, and surgical microscopic levels.[8]
- The cadaver lab can be used for simulating the surgical approach and testing its feasibility. Novel approaches should seek to be minimally traumatic rather than minimally invasive.[4]
- In the cadaver lab, it is possible to analyze the ergonomics of the setting and the instrumentation[9] by testing drills, aspirators, ultrasonic aspirators, and aneurysms clips, and by studying the position of the monitors and tools to ensure an optimal setup in the operating room.[4]
- Surgical techniques and approaches for removing mass lesions may be tested using skull base tumor models. By using resin polymer injections (the resin can be injected via the endonasal route in different locations), it is possible to simulate a skull base tumor and its surgical resection.[10]
- Anaglyphic 3D stereoscopic printing is a relatively easy technique for 3D prints of anatomic structures.[11,12]
- In mastoidectomy training, the drilling of the bone can be performed after injection of indocyanine green in the arteries of the cadaver, which enables fluorescence-guided bone drilling. Techniques such as skeletonization of the facial nerve and semicircular canals can then be practiced.[13] The indocyanine diffuses into the more vascularized regions, such as the mucosa covering the mastoid air cells, so that the fluorescent zone can be safely drilled, while the nonfluorescent regions indicate solid bone, such as the one covering the facial and the semicircular canals.
- Inexpensive and ultraportable systems for laboratory training in skull base endoscopic dissections have been developed. These systems cost a fraction of a standard high-definition endoscopy system.[14]
- For institutions with more resources, the lab can be equipped with radiological imaging tools (neuronavigation, C-arm fluoroscopy, computed tomography [CT]), surgical robots, 3D endoscopes, exoscopes, and others.
- Recording of anatomy dissections (photographs and videos) is useful for didactic purposes and training. Trainees may review their performance and implement changes to enhance their technical skills.

- A modular/incremental approach to endonasal skull base surgery is useful in endoscopy training.
- Mastering one level of difficulty of each procedure before proceeding to the next level is a natural way of progressing trainees' learning.
- These levels of difficulty that can be mastered using cadavers are based on related surgical procedures of increasing complexity[7,15–17]:
  1. Ligation of the sphenopalatine artery, endoscopic sphenoethmoidectomy, exposure of the nasofrontal recess.
  2. Frontal sinusotomy and management of intrasellar region, as well as medial orbital decompression. In surgery, this level is often used for the resection of pituitary tumors, cerebrospinal fluid (CSF) leak repair, and surgical decompression of the optic nerve in Graves' disease.
  3. Extrasellar region; extended approaches to the clivus, odontoid, and petrous apex.
  4. Extended approach to the planum, exposure of the internal carotid artery, intradural approach to the odontoid process, approaches to the parapharyngeal space, and craniofacial resection.
  5. Approach to the circle of Willis and cranial nerves.
- Fresh/frozen specimens rather than skulls or formaldehyde-fixed specimens are the most realistic specimens for anatomic dissection and surgical training, although they are not readily available in many institutions. They may also carry risks of infections, and their use is limited to a short timeframe.

> **Pearl**
>
> Dried skulls are not recommended for endonasal transsphenoidal simulations.

- Dried skulls can be used for simulation of craniotomies/craniectomies, petrosectomy, etc.
- Fixation enables preserving specimens for long periods of time. Formaldehyde-based embalming is the most commonly used technique for specimen preservation. Fixation in formaldehyde, however, does render the tissue quite tough and rigid. The use of fabric softener (methyl bis[tallow amido ethyl] 2-hydroxyethyl ammonium methyl sulfate) has been proposed for softening the tissue following formaldehyde fixation and obtaining ideal tissue texture.[18] Otherwise, a customized formula made of ethanol (62.4%), glycerol (17%), phenol (10.2%), formaldehyde (2.3%), and water (8.1%) has been shown to prevent decay of the specimen, giving the brain a consistency very similar to that of tissues obtained in cryopreserved specimens.[19]
- Blood vessels of specimens can be injected with colored silicone rubber (e.g., red for the arteries and blue for the veins), latex, and other solutions.[20,21] The injection of blood vessels can be performed via the cannulation of the carotid and vertebral arteries at the neck, as well as the jugular veins, whenever required. Arterial injections are generally considered to be enough for most

approaches, but this depends on the anatomic target; dissection of the orbits, pineal gland, and cavernous sinus, for example, also requires venous injection. Latex injections result in deeper penetration of the solution into small cerebral vessels than silicone,[21] although the latter makes the vessels softer for surgical manipulation.

- Pressurized dynamic filling of the cerebral vasculature and subarachnoid cisterns makes the anatomic dissection an experience very similar to actual surgery on patients.[22, 23]
- Lack of perfusion and in vivo elasticity may be compensated for by introducing animal training, as in in-vivo swine models[24] or anesthetized rats. The latter can be used especially for bypass surgery training.
- Plastination techniques give persistently dry, odorless and durable specimens, which can also be used for skull base anatomy training.[25,26] The rigidity of the specimens typically only allows for training on rigid structures, such as the petrous bone, rather than on soft parenchyma, such as the brain. Despite these limitations, plastination remains a fascinating technique for preserving organs and learning anatomy (especially plastinated slices of anatomic regions, such as brain slices in all axes).[27,28]

> **Pearl**
>
> A surgical dissection laboratory without an instructor available is of limited benefit.[29]

■ Artificial Models

To address a potential lack of cadavers and animal models, 3D plastic models have been developed for microsurgery and endoscopy training, including suturing, performing duraplasty and cranioplasty, and other procedures.[30-36] Such models contain colored blood vessels and dural sinuses, cranial nerves, brain, silicon structures that can also be used for bypasses, bone-like structures that can be drilled, and synthetic dura mater that can be sutured. CT/magnetic resonance imaging (MRI)–based 3D models produced using laser-sintered powdered polymers and 3D printers are also used for anatomy training and surgery simulation,[37-42] allowing for biomodeling of skull base and associated tumors and other lesions.

■ Imaging-Guided and Virtual Surgical Planning

- In some institutions that lack anatomy labs, image-guided dedicated workstations are used for virtual surgery planning as part of surgery education.[43]

- Spatially complex surgical skills can be improved by means of surgical simulations.[44]
- Endoscopic endonasal surgery requires meticulous manipulation of the instruments. As in laparoscopic surgery, training is mandatory for residents and trainees.[45]
- Preoperative segmentation of the anatomic structures and surgical targets is highly recommended. This can be done on neuronavigation systems and on virtual surgical planning platforms for endoscopic and microsurgical skull base surgery that function by rendering and fusing CT and MRI (multimodal imaging, e.g., MRI with computed tomography angiography [CTA] and positron emission tomography [PET], using shareware software, e.g., OsiriX®).[46–51]
- Virtual simulations of surgery on 3D image–based models can be performed on dedicated workstations equipped with stereovision systems, such as the Dextroscope or Dextrobeam® (Volume Interactions Pte, Ltd., Singapore), NeuroTouch® (National Research Council Canada, Boucherville, Quebec, Canada), and others.[52–60]
- For acquiring psychomotor skills for endoscopic endonasal surgery, a portable personal trainer using a virtual reality simulator equipped with a webcam has been developed.[61]

■ References

Boldfaced references are of particular importance.

1. Di Ieva A. Memetics in neurosurgery and neuroscience. NeuroQuantology 2008;6: 182–193
2. Ebner FH, Dimostheni A, Tatagiba MS, Roser F. Step-by-step education of the retrosigmoid approach leads to low approach-related morbidity through young residents. Acta Neurochir (Wien) 2010;152:985–988, discussion 988
3. Roser F, Pfister G, Tatagiba M, Ebner FH. Live surgery in neurosurgical training courses: essential infrastructure and technical set-up. Acta Neurochir (Wien) 2013;155:541–545
4. Tschabitscher M, Di Ieva A. Practical guidelines for setting up an endoscopic/skull base cadaver laboratory. World Neurosurg 2013;79(2, Suppl):16.e1–16.e7
5. Salma A, Chow A, Ammirati M. Setting up a microneurosurgical skull base lab: technical and operational considerations. Neurosurg Rev 2011;34:317–326, discussion 326
6. Yaşargil MG. A legacy of microneurosurgery: memoirs, lessons, and axioms. Neurosurgery 1999;45:1025–1092
7. Kassam A, Snyderman CH, Mintz A, Gardner P, Carrau RL. Expanded endonasal approach: the rostrocaudal axis. Part I. Crista galli to the sella turcica. Neurosurg Focus 2005;19:E3
8. Cappabianca P, Magro F. The lesson of anatomy. Surg Neurol 2009;71:597–598, discussion 598–599

9. Resch KD. Postmortem inspection for neurosurgery: a training model for endoscopic dissection technique. Neurosurg Rev 2002;25:79–88

10. **Gragnaniello C, Nader R, van Doormaal T, et al. Skull base tumor model. J Neurosurg 2010;113:1106–1111**

11. Ribas GC, Bento RF, Rodrigues AJ Jr. Anaglyphic three-dimensional stereoscopic printing: revival of an old method for anatomical and surgical teaching and reporting. J Neurosurg 2001;95:1057–1066

12. Isolan GR, Rowe R, Al-Mefty O. Microanatomy and surgical approaches to the infratemporal fossa: an anaglyphic three-dimensional stereoscopic printing study. Skull Base 2007;17:285–302

13. Gragnaniello C, Kamel M, Al-Mefty O. Utilization of fluorescein for identification and preservation of the facial nerve and semicircular canals for safe mastoidectomy: a proof of concept laboratory cadaveric study. Neurosurgery 2010;66:204–207

14. Dias LA, Gebhard H, Mtui E, Anand VK, Schwartz TH. The use of an ultraportable universal serial bus endoscope for education and training in neuroendoscopy. World Neurosurg 2013;79:337–340

15. Kassam A, Snyderman CH, Mintz A, Gardner P, Carrau RL. Expanded endonasal approach: the rostrocaudal axis. Part II. Posterior clinoids to the foramen magnum. Neurosurg Focus 2005;19:E4

16. Kassam AB, Gardner P, Snyderman C, Mintz A, Carrau R. Expanded endonasal approach: fully endoscopic, completely transnasal approach to the middle third of the clivus, petrous bone, middle cranial fossa, and infratemporal fossa. Neurosurg Focus 2005;19:E6

17. **Snyderman C, Kassam A, Carrau R, Mintz A, Gardner P, Prevedello DM. Acquisition of surgical skills for endonasal skull base surgery: a training program. Laryngoscope 2007;117:699–705**

18. Krishnamurthy S, Powers SK. The use of fabric softener in neurosurgical prosections. Neurosurgery 1995;36:420–423, discussion 423–424

19. Benet A, Rincon-Torroella J, Lawton MT, González Sánchez JJ. Novel embalming solution for neurosurgical simulation in cadavers. J Neurosurg 2014;120:1229–1237

20. Sanan A, Abdel Aziz KM, Janjua RM, van Loveren HR, Keller JT. Colored silicone injection for use in neurosurgical dissections: anatomic technical note. Neurosurgery 1999;45:1267–1271, discussion 1271–1274

21. Alvernia JE, Pradilla G, Mertens P, Lanzino G, Tamargo RJ. Latex injection of cadaver heads: technical note. Neurosurgery 2010;67(2, Suppl Operative):362–367

22. **Aboud E, Al-Mefty O, Yaşargil MG. New laboratory model for neurosurgical training that simulates live surgery. J Neurosurg 2002;97:1367–1372**

23. Olabe J, Olabe J, Sancho V. Human cadaver brain infusion model for neurosurgical training. Surg Neurol 2009;72:700–702

24. Regelsberger J, Heese O, Horn P, et al. Training microneurosurgery—four years experiences with an in vivo model. Cent Eur Neurosurg 2011;72:192–195

25. Maeta M, Uno K, Saito R. The potential of a plastination specimen for temporal bone surgery. Auris Nasus Larynx 2003;30:413–416

26. Qiu MG, Zhang SX, Liu ZJ, et al. Plastination and computerized 3D reconstruction of the temporal bone. Clin Anat 2003;16:300–303

27. Weiglein AH. Plastination in the neurosciences. Keynote lecture. Acta Anat (Basel) 1997;158:6–9

28. Riederer BM. Plastination and its importance in teaching anatomy. Critical points for long-term preservation of human tissue. J Anat 2014;224:309–315

29. Cusimano MD. Virtual reality surgery: neurosurgery and the contemporary landscape a three-dimensional interactive virtual dissection model to simulate transpetrous surgical avenues. Neurosurgery 2003;53:1010–1011, author reply 1011–1012

30. Chen G, Ling F. A new plastic model of endoscopic technique training for endonasal transsphenoidal pituitary surgery. Chin Med J (Engl) 2010;123:2576–2579

31. Mori K, Yamamoto T, Nakao Y, Esaki T. Development of artificial cranial base model with soft tissues for practical education: technical note. Neurosurgery 2010;66(6, Suppl Operative):339–341, n. 341

32. Matula C, Kjærsgaard L, Di Ieva A. Watertight dural closure in brain surgery: a simple model for training. J Neurol Surg A Cent Eur Neurosurg 2014;75:241–245

33. Zymberg S, Vaz-Guimarães Filho F, Lyra M. Neuroendoscopic training: presentation of a new real simulator. Minim Invasive Neurosurg 2010;53:44–46

34. Mori K. Dissectable modified three-dimensional temporal bone and whole skull base models for training in skull base approaches. Skull Base 2009;19:333–343

35. Mori K, Yamamoto T, Oyama K, Ueno H, Nakao Y, Honma K. Modified three-dimensional skull base model with artificial dura mater, cranial nerves, and venous sinuses for training in skull base surgery: technical note. Neurol Med Chir (Tokyo) 2008;48:582–587, discussion 587–588

36. Almeida DB, Hunhevicz S, Bordignon K, et al. A model for foramen ovale puncture training: technical note. Acta Neurochir (Wien) 2006;148:881–883, discussion 883

37. Wanibuchi M, Ohtaki M, Fukushima T, Friedman AH, Houkin K. Skull base training and education using an artificial skull model created by selective laser sintering. Acta Neurochir (Wien) 2010;152:1055–1059, discussion 1059–1060

38. Grunert R, Strauss G, Moeckel H, et al. ElePhant—an anatomical electronic phantom as simulation-system for otologic surgery. Conf Proc IEEE Eng Med Biol Soc 2006;1:4408–4411

39. D'Urso PS, Anderson RL, Weidmann MJ, et al. Biomodelling of skull base tumours. J Clin Neurosci 1999;6:31–35

40. Waran V, Narayanan V, Karuppiah R, Owen SL, Aziz T. Utility of multimaterial 3D printers in creating models with pathological entities to enhance the training experience of neurosurgeons. J Neurosurg 2014;120:489–492

41. Mashiko T, Otani K, Kawano R, et al. Development of three-dimensional hollow elastic model for cerebral aneurysm clipping simulation enabling rapid and low cost prototyping. World Neurosurg 2013;83:351–361

42. Waran V, Menon R, Pancharatnam D, et al. The creation and verification of cranial models using three-dimensional rapid prototyping technology in field of transnasal sphenoid endoscopy. Am J Rhinol Allergy 2012;26:e132–e136

43. Anastakis DJ, Regehr G, Reznick RK, et al. Assessment of technical skills transfer from the bench training model to the human model. Am J Surg 1999;177:167–170

44. Wanzel KR, Hamstra SJ, Anastakis DJ, Matsumoto ED, Cusimano MD. Effect of visual-spatial ability on learning of spatially-complex surgical skills. Lancet 2002;359:230–231

45. Bahrami P, Graham SJ, Grantcharov TP, et al. Neuroanatomical correlates of laparoscopic surgery training. Surg Endosc 2014;28:2189–2198

46. Caversaccio M, Langlotz F, Nolte LP, Häusler R. Impact of a self-developed planning and self-constructed navigation system on skull base surgery: 10 years experience. Acta Otolaryngol 2007;127:403–407
47. Krüeger A, Kubisch C, Straub G, Preim B. Sinus endoscopy—application of advanced GPU volume rendering for virtual endoscopy. IEEE Trans Vis Comput Graph 2008; 14:1491–1498
48. Haerle SK, Daly MJ, Chan HH, Vescan A, Kucharczyk W, Irish JC. Virtual surgical planning in endoscopic skull base surgery. Laryngoscope 2013;123:2935–2939
49. **de Notaris M, Topczewski T, de Angelis M, et al. Anatomic skull base education using advanced neuroimaging techniques. World Neurosurg 2013;79(2, Suppl): 16.e9–16.e13**
50. Yao WC, Regone RM, Huyhn N, Butler EB, Takashima M. Three-dimensional sinus imaging as an adjunct to two-dimensional imaging to accelerate education and improve spatial orientation. Laryngoscope 2014;124:596–601
51. **Harput MV, Gonzalez-Lopez P, Türe U. Three-dimensional reconstruction of the topographical cerebral surface anatomy for presurgical planning with free OsiriX Software. Neurosurgery 2014;10(Suppl 3):426–435, discussion 435**
52. Hilbert M, Müller W. Virtual reality in endonasal surgery. Stud Health Technol Inform 1997;39:237–245
53. **Spicer MA, Apuzzo ML. Virtual reality surgery: neurosurgery and the contemporary landscape. Neurosurgery 2003;52:489–497, discussion 496–497**
54. **Bernardo A, Preul MC, Zabramski JM, Spetzler RF. A three-dimensional interactive virtual dissection model to simulate transpetrous surgical avenues. Neurosurgery 2003;52:499–505, discussion 504–505**
55. Wolfsberger S, Forster MT, Donat M, et al. Virtual endoscopy is a useful device for training and preoperative planning of transsphenoidal endoscopic pituitary surgery. Minim Invasive Neurosurg 2004;47:214–220
56. Spicer MA, van Velsen M, Caffrey JP, Apuzzo ML. Virtual reality neurosurgery: a simulator blueprint. Neurosurgery 2004;54:783–797, discussion 797–798
57. Neubauer A, Wolfsberger S, Forster MT, Mroz L, Wegenkittl R, Bühler K. Advanced virtual endoscopic pituitary surgery. IEEE Trans Vis Comput Graph 2005;11:497–507
58. Kockro RA, Hwang PY. Virtual temporal bone: an interactive 3-dimensional learning aid for cranial base surgery. Neurosurgery 2009;64(5, Suppl 2):216–229, discussion 229–230
59. Delorme S, Laroche D, DiRaddo R, Del Maestro RF. NeuroTouch: a physics-based virtual simulator for cranial microneurosurgery training. Neurosurgery 2012;71(1, Suppl Operative):32–42
60. Rosseau G, Bailes J, del Maestro R, et al. The development of a virtual simulator for training neurosurgeons to perform and perfect endoscopic endonasal transsphenoidal surgery. Neurosurgery 2013;73(Suppl 1):85–93
61. Hirayama R, Fujimoto Y, Umegaki M, et al. Training to acquire psychomotor skills for endoscopic endonasal surgery using a personal webcam trainer. J Neurosurg 2013; 118:1120–1126

41 Nursing in Skull Base Surgery

- A team-based approach is essential for managing skull base patients. It requires expertise from several medical disciplines, such as neurosurgery, otolaryngology, craniomaxillofacial and plastic surgery, vascular surgery, pathology, neuroradiology and interventional neuroradiology, nuclear medicine and radiotherapy, as well as multiple nursing disciplines, such as operating room nurses, clinical nurses with competence in skull base pathologies, and home care staff. Further interprofessional collaboration is often required: speech pathologists, social workers, dietitians, physiotherapists, occupational therapists, radiation therapist, cancer care navigators, social workers, and psychologists among others.
- All skull base nurses should be involved in teaching and research activity to improve the care and experiences of the patient and family.

■ Longitudinal Care of Patients and Families by Nurses

- The multidisciplinary management of patients affected by skull base pathologies should also include nurses and a nurse manager, for the best care of patients and family in the pre- and postoperative management of the disease (instrumental tests, follow-up, quality of life assessment, data collection, etc.).
- Lack of information is the main reason for patients' and families' inability to cope with skull base pathologies, management of complications, and related issues.[1]
- Ideally, the nurse should also be part of the skull base team and should meet the patient during the first encounter with the surgical team. The nurse can aid in the discussion about treatment options and in the informed consent process.[1] The medical staff should also discuss potential facial deformities related to skull base tumors and radical surgery with the patients and their family.[2]

- In the preoperative assessment, nurses are involved in identifying comorbidities, social and other risk factors, and neuropsychological issues, which may affect the surgical and treatment outcome. Nurses are also involved in informing patients about medical issues relevant to the patient's disease and care plan, and possible complications and their management. Nurses also assist patients in coping with anxiety and fear.[3–5]
- Nurse managers or practitioners can also provide a continuity of care along with support for patients and families during prolonged surgeries and postoperative follow-up treatment and surveillance.
- Nurses who provide care in the preoperative and postoperative community phase of care can also be pivotal in helping to tailor patient-specific care by inpatient ward nurses and intensive care unit (ICU) nurses in the immediate postoperative period.

■ Ward and Intensive Care Unit Nurses

- Nurses are directly involved in the management of the following:
  - Patients' pain and side effects of analgesics
  - Nutrition, based on the dietitian's plan
  - Postoperative complications (e.g., facial palsy, for which the patient's eyes have to be kept moistened; skin flaps, for which perfusion of the skin has to be monitored; fluid imbalances, such as diabetes insipidus in pituitary surgery)
  - Psychological status, with or without the help of a psychologist
- Handover with colleagues at the change of shift is fundamental in all areas: from the ward to ICU and the operating room.

■ Operating Room Nurses

- A perfect synergy and communication between the circulating nurse and the scrubbing nurse is fundamental for avoiding errors and delays.
- Preoperative briefing with the surgeon and anesthesia team is essential to determine which surgical instruments will be needed during surgery, in order to avoid delays (e.g., fibrin glue, angulated endoscopes, etc.), as well to discuss the patient positioning, surgical draping, and any relevant issues. Complementary maneuvers should be discussed as well: intraoperative angiography, pre- or postoperative lumbar drainage, ventricular drainage, tarsorrhaphy, skin flaps/fascia/fat grafts, intraoperative monitoring, and surgical draping.
- Operating room nurses need expertise in handling the specific tools and technologies used in skull base surgery, such as head frames, microscopes,

endoscopes, irrigating bipolars, hemostatic material, ultrasonic aspirators, lasers, ultrasound, image guidance, as well as new technologies.

- Operating room nurses are involved in the positioning and padding of the patient to ensure the avoidance of pressure ulcers and neurovascular injuries.
- Operating room nurses manage compression stockings, catheters, vascular accesses, and lumbar drains.
- Operating room nurses are responsible for the appropriate administration of medication intraoperatively, such as bacitracin for bone flaps, topical adrenaline for nasal decongestion, and fibrin glue for reconstruction.
- As in any surgery, keeping count of the pre- and postoperative instruments and gauze/cottonoids is imperative.
- The circulating nurse has the responsibility of recording, collecting, and labeling the surgical specimens for the pathology examinations. The communication among the surgeon, scrub nurse, and circulating nurse is fundamental for avoiding mistakes (for example, in correctly labeling all the surgical margins).
- Operating room nurses and nurses involved in the postoperative phase have the task of evaluating the clinical and neurologic status of the patient, performing examinations and recording scores (e.g., Glasgow Coma Scale score, intracranial pressure, amount of drained cerebrospinal fluid, etc.).
- Operating room nurses should have standardized procedures of patient handover to the next set of nurses involved in care to avoid costly errors that could have impact on the well-being of the patient or on the resources being used for patient care.

■ References

1. Sievers AEF, Borcyckowski D. Nursing care of skull base surgery patients. In: Donald PJ, ed. Surgery of the Skull Base. Philadelphia: Lippincott-Raven; 1998:119–139
2. Borozny M, Gray E, Ratel M. Nursing concerns associated with radical skull base surgery: a case study. J Neurosci Nurs 1993;25:45–51
3. Burkhart LE. The nurse's role as clinical coordinator for the Center for Cranial Base Surgery. J Neurosci Nurs 1991;23:61–63
4. Durity MB, Wyness A, Durity F, Ratel M. Education and information needs identified by patients and key family members prior to surgery for a skull base neoplasm: implications for practice. Axone 2000;22:32–45
5. Wyness MA, Durity MB, Durity F. Narratives of patients with skull base tumors and their family members: lessons for nursing practice. Axone 2002;24:18–35

Index

Note: The use of *f*, *t*, or *b* following a page number indicates a figure, table, or box.